KV-699-400

Greer's Ocular Pathology

To my wife Kay

Greer's Ocular Pathology

DAVID R. LUCAS
MD (London), FRCPath
Senior Lecturer in Ophthalmic Pathology
University of Manchester
Honorary Consultant Ophthalmic Pathologist
Manchester Royal Eye Hospital

FOURTH EDITION

BLACKWELL SCIENTIFIC PUBLICATIONS

OXFORD LONDON EDINBURGH

BOSTON MELBOURNE

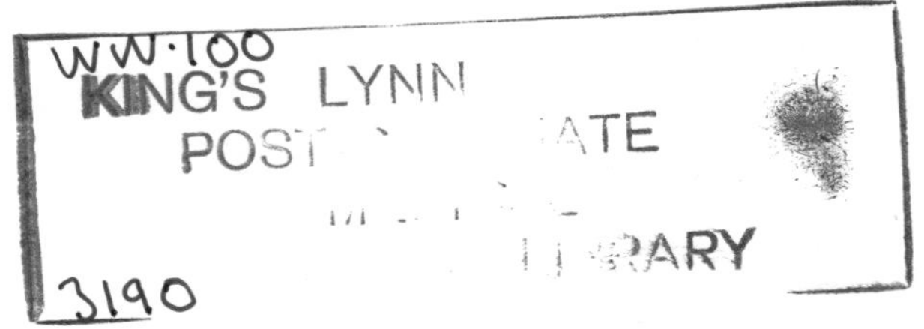
WW.100
KING'S LYNN
POST ATE
RARY
3190

© 1963, 1972, 1979, 1989 by
Blackwell Scientific Publications

Editorial offices:
Osney Mead, Oxford OX2 0EL
(*Orders*: Tel. 0865–240201)
8 John Street, London WC1N 2ES
23 Ainslie Place, Edinburgh EH3 6AJ
3 Cambridge Center, Suite 208
Cambridge, Massachusetts 02142, USA
107 Barry Street, Carlton
Victoria 3053, Australia

All rights reserved. No part of this publication may be reproduced, stored in a retrieval system, or transmitted, in any form or by any means, electronic, mechanical, photocopying, recording or otherwise without the prior permission of the copyright owner

First published 1963
(under the title *Ocular Pathology* by C.H. Greer)
Second edition 1972
Third edition 1979
Fourth edition 1989

Set by Setrite Typesetters Ltd, Hong Kong;
printed and bound in Great Britain by
William Clowes Ltd, Beccles and London

DISTRIBUTORS

USA
Year Book Medical Publishers
200 North LaSalle Street
Chicago, Illinois 60601
(*Orders*: Tel. 312–726–9733)

Canada
The C.V. Mosby Company
5240 Finch Avenue East
Scarborough, Ontario
(*Orders*: Tel. 416–298–1588)

Australia
Blackwell Scientific Publications
(Australia) Pty Ltd
107 Barry Street
Carlton, Victoria 3053
(*Orders*: Tel. 03–347–0300)

British Library
Cataloguing in Publication Data

Greer, Courtenay Hugh
Greer's ocular pathology. — 4th ed.
1. Man. Eyes. Pathology
I. Title II. Lucas, D.R.
617.7′1

ISBN 0–632–01513–6

Contents

Colour plates

Preface to fourth edition

Preparing the fourth edition of a well liked and trusted text by a distinguished and now sadly deceased author is not an easy task and has involved some difficult decisions.

Though extensive revisions had been made, the original format and size of the book had remained almost unchanged through the three editions published between 1963 and 1979. The time thus seemed ripe for a considerably more radical review of the scope and format. The present edition does, therefore, differ markedly from its predecessors. The text has been increased by four new chapters and the content of some of the original chapters extensively revised and redistributed. Many illustrations have been replaced and many more added. The additional text and illustrations have inevitably added considerably to the size of the book, but have not, I hope, made it unbearably long.

The primary aim of the fourth edition remains the same as that of the previous editions, namely to provide ophthalmologists and those training in the specialty with an elementary survey of the pathological aspects of their specialty. It has been my experience that pathologists in training also found the previous editions useful and I hope the alterations and additions I have made will increase its value to them as well.

The bibliographies at the end of each chapter have been greatly expanded and brought up to date, though no claim is made that they are comprehensive. Those who are stimulated by the necessarily rather superficial coverage will, therefore, be able to gain an entry into the literature to read more deeply. Since it is an elementary text, authors' names have generally not been cited in the text except in relation to rare conditions or controversial areas. I have also listed a number of recent texts on ophthalmic pathology in a general bibliography at the end. These should be consulted for topics not covered and for a more detailed treatment and possibly different view of the topics that are covered in the present text.

Four appendices have also been added. The first outlines a systematic guide to tackling eye sections. The second lists the various types of collagen and other connective tissue components. The third provides a guide to the various complex carbohydrates, many of which are of great importance in the eye, and the fourth lists and explains some of the common staining reactions used. It is hoped they will prove useful for reference purposes.

D.R. LUCAS

Departments of Ophthalmology and Pathology
University of Manchester

Preface to first edition

This book is for ophthalmologists and those training as ophthalmologists. It is based on the author's course of instruction in ocular pathology for the Diploma of Ophthalmology of Melbourne University and for the Fellowship in Ophthalmology of the Royal Australasian College of Surgeons.

The book makes no claim to be an exhaustive account of its subject but is an attempt to present, in brief but not synoptic form, most of what the postgraduate student should know about ocular pathology in order to face his examiners with confidence. Its more general but no less important aim is to emphasise the pathological basis of the signs and symptoms of ophthalmic diseases.

In selecting topics for inclusion, preference has been given to those which students find difficult to grasp and to material which, by reason of its dispersal in books and journals, is not always readily available.

C.H. GREER

Acknowledgements

I must first express my thanks to the ophthalmologists in the north-west of England and elsewhere who have supported me with their interest and entrusted me with their material.

Numerous colleagues, mainly in the Departments of Ophthalmology and Pathology in the University of Manchester and in the Royal Eye Hospital, have been generous with their time in reading sections of the text and making helpful comments and criticisms. Of these I particularly mention Mr S.K. Bhargava, Miss J. Duvall, Dr A.G. Freemont, Dr I.J.M. Jeffrey, Mr A.E.A. Ridgway, Dr R.W. Stoddart (who prepared Appendix III), Mr A.B. Tullo, Dr H. Whitwell and Professor P.O. Yates. I am also indebted to various more junior members of the staff of the Royal Eye Hospital who kindly sampled parts of the text and made useful suggestions.

I owe a great deal to my now retired colleague, Dr J.L.S. Smith, formerly Consultant Ophthalmic Pathologist to St Paul's Eye Hospital, Liverpool, with whom I have spent many happy hours discussing cases and from whose perceptive eye I have learned much.

Much of the material from which the photomicrographs were taken was prepared by Miss Kathleen Hughes who worked in the laboratory in the Royal Eye Hospital for 37 years and I freely acknowledge my gratitude to her. Since her retirement, the ophthalmic material has been processed in the Surgical Histology Laboratory in the Manchester Royal Infirmary and I am indebted to its technical staff for the skill and willingness which they have shown in tackling the technical problems of handing eyes. I have also depended heavily on the skill of Mrs L. Thomas who prepared the material for both scanning and transmission electron microscopy.

Various colleagues have kindly allowed me to use their material to supplement my own. The source of such material is acknowledged after the caption. I am most grateful to Mrs Jane Crosby and Miss Margaret Banton, photographers in the University Department of Pathology, for their patience and skill in photographing specimens and printing my numerous negatives. I also have to thank various authors for kindly providing illustrations from original articles and to the editors of the journals for allowing them to be reproduced. The source of such material is acknowledged after the caption.

Finally, it is a pleasure to acknowledge the help I have received from staff at Blackwell Scientific Publications. I am particularly grateful to Mr Peter Saugman for his encouragement during the writing and to Mrs Vicky Murray for her patient, meticulous editing.

D.R. LUCAS

Chapter 1 Inflammation, immunity and the eye

ACUTE INFLAMMATION

Acute inflammation may be defined as the immediate vascular, exudative and cellular reaction of living tissue to injury. The injury may be inflicted by living or non-living agents.

Injury by living organisms: the injurious agent is self-reproducing and continuously produces toxins which damage the tissues. The inflammatory response continues as long as the organisms survive and proliferate in the tissues and may therefore be of short or long duration. This is reflected in the terms acute, subacute and chronic which are used to characterise the inflammatory response.

Injury by physical agents: injury by physical agents such as mechanical trauma, heat, chemicals, etc., is usually incurred in a single incident of limited duration. The resulting inflammation is excited by the products of tissue destruction and, when these have been removed, the inflammation subsides.

The sequelae of acute inflammation may be:

1 Resolution. If the exciting cause is eliminated rapidly and tissue destruction is minimal, return to normality ensues.

2 Suppuration. When the local accumulation of exudate, products of tissue breakdown, dead leucocytes and micro-organisms is sufficiently great an abscess containing pus is formed.

3 Organisation and repair. When there is suppuration or when an excess of exudate and necrotic debris persists, ingrowth of capillaries and fibroblasts occurs and the area becomes walled off. The pus or other material is gradually absorbed and a fibrous scar formed.

4 If the causal agent is not eliminated, the process may become chronic. However, chronic inflammation often arises without a preceding acute phase.

Acute inflammation is a rapidly developing reaction to swiftly acting noxious agents such as pyogenic cocci and is non-specific in that it is invoked chiefly by the products of tissue destruction rather than by the injurious agents themselves. Acute inflammation often subsides relatively quickly.

The well known features of acute inflammation are:

1 Vasodilatation which causes local redness.

2 Exudation of fluid into the tissues which causes local swelling.

3 Migration of leucocytes into the tissues.

These processes and the factors by which they are mediated will now be considered briefly.

Vasodilatation

Arterioles: after a brief transitory contraction, the arterioles relax, blood flow through them is increased and the hydrostatic pressure at the capillaries is raised.

Capillaries and venules: dilatation of capillaries occurs as a result of relaxation of the precapillary sphincters. At the same time, opening of the gaps between the endothelial cells under the influence of chemical mediators (see below) permits the rapid exudation of fluid into the tissues.

Exudation

Normal capillaries do not allow the passage of solutes exceeding a molecular weight of about 10 000. Opening of the gaps allows plasma proteins to pass into the tissues. In mild inflammation, only small amounts pass through and the exudate is watery. In severe inflammation, gamma globulins and fibrinogen escape. The latter is deposited in the tissues.

The functions of the exudate are:

1 Dilution of bacterial toxins.

2 Limitation of bacterial spread by entrapping the organisms in a fibrin net.

3 The γ-globulins may include antibodies which neutralise toxins and opsonins which promote the phagocytosis of bacteria.

Drainage of the exudate takes place through lymphatic channels to the regional lymph nodes where the first step in the immune response is set in motion (p.7).

Migration of leucocytes

Circulating leucocytes in peripheral blood migrate into the exudate. In acute bacterial inflammation, these are predominantly neutrophil polymorphonuclear leucocytes (neutrophils) followed somewhat later by monocytes.

With the loss of plasma into the tissues, flow through the capillaries becomes sluggish and circulating neutrophils, which have a natural tendency to adhere to endothelial surfaces, stick to the capillary walls. In histological sections this is described as 'margination'. The cells pass through intercellular junctions between endothelial cells of the capillary wall.

Chemotaxis

Within the tissue, movement of leucocytes is governed by chemotactic factors liberated in the inflammatory process. These comprise:

1 Bacterial products.

2 Factors derived from injured tissues.

3 Factors derived from neutrophils and mast cells (leukotrienes).

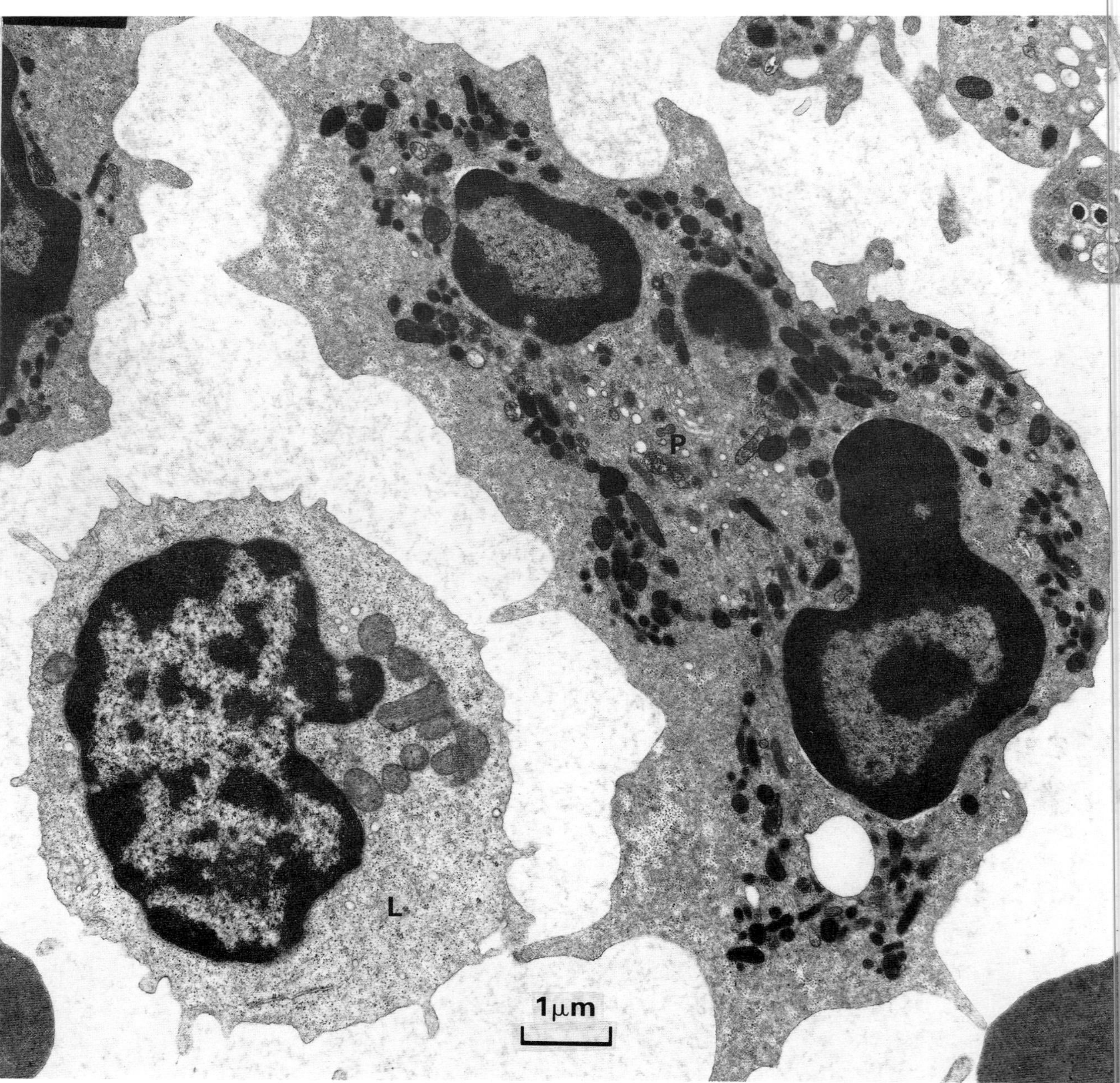

Fig. 1.1. Electron micrograph showing a normal lymphocyte (L) and a normal neutrophil polymorph (P). Note the large number of organelles, mainly mitochondria and lysosomes, in the cytoplasm of the polymorph in comparison with that of the lymphocyte whose cytoplasm contains, in addition to a few mitochondria, only a tiny fragment of rough endoplasmic reticulum and some small dense particles. (×13 700). (Micrograph by courtesy of Dr Carolyn Jones.)

4 Factors derived from blood plasma, particularly the complement system.

Chemotaxis is essential to attract the leucocytes to the site of injury in the tissues.

Leucocytes participating in the acute inflammatory process

Neutrophil leucocytes

Neutrophil leucocytes (Fig. 1.1) are derived from specific precursors in the bone marrow. They have a short life-span of only 3 to 4 days. In their cytoplasm are two types of granule:

1 *Azurophilic lysosomal granules* which contain enzymes including phosphatases, myeloperoxidase, nucleases, nucleotidase, lysozyme, cathepsin, β-glycuronidase, collagenase, elastase, kallikrein and plasminogen (precursor of plasmin or fibrinolysin).

2 *Specific granules* which are more numerous and contain the microbicidal factors lysozyme and lactoferrin.

The main functions of neutrophils are:

1 Ingestion and killing of invading bacteria. They are the first cells to try to repel an acute bacterial infection.

2 Digestion of dead tissue cells and fibrin which is accomplished by release of the enzymes listed above from their granules when they die.

Eosinophil leucocytes

In acute inflammation provoked by helminths or in hypersensitivity reactions, eosinophils are often numerous. The cytoplasm of these cells is packed with large granules which stain brilliantly with eosin and contain enzymes capable of degrading certain chemical mediators of acute inflammation such as histamine.

Basophil leucocytes and mast cells

Basophil leucocytes are present in peripheral blood in smaller numbers than eosinophils and mast cells are widely distributed in connective tissue throughout the body mainly in the adventitia of blood vessels. The cytoplasm of mast cells is normally crammed with large prominent granules which stain by the PAS (periodic-acid-Schiff) method and by toluidine blue (see Appendix IV). The granules themselves contain histamine, heparin and, in rodents, serotonin (5-hydroxy tryptamine). The cell surface is characterised by striking filopodia (Fig. 1.2).

Macrophages

Macrophages are derived from blood monocytes. They have a longer life-span than neutrophils and are able to divide at the inflammatory site. They appear in large numbers in the later stages of the acute inflammatory process when the bacterial invasion has been contained by the neutrophils. Though they are capable of ingesting and killing bacteria, their principal role in the inflammatory process is the phagocytosis and disposal of tissue and cell debris which they are able to do more comprehensively than neutrophils.

Macrophages play a crucial role in immune reactions because they process antigens before presentation to immunocompetent lymphocytes.

Phagocytosis

The mechanism involves engulfing the micro-organism in the cell membrane of the leucocyte. The infolded cell membrane with the entrapped micro-organism is a phagosome.

Pathogenic bacteria resist phagocytosis by two principal methods:

1 Provision of antiphagocytic properties in the cell wall which may take several forms:

(i) Polysaccharide capsule, e.g. pneumococci. The effect of this may be overcome by the production of opsonins which are specific antibodies and facilitate phagocytosis by coating the wall.

(ii) Antiphagocytic protein components in the cell wall such as M protein in streptococci. Staphylococci produce A protein in their cell wall which neutralises binding sites for opsonins on the surface of neutrophils.

(iii) High lipid content in cell wall as in mycobacteria. This interferes with fusion between phagosome and lysosome so that the organism can remain alive within the macrophage.

2 Production of exotoxins which kill leucocytes, e.g. streptolysins by streptococci and α-toxin by staphylococci.

Phagocytic killing mechanisms

In the neutrophil, fusion of the phagosome with a lysosome exposes the micro-organism to the action of the lysosomal agents which are capable of killing and digesting many organisms. The most important killing mechanism is the hydrogen peroxide–halide–myeloperoxidase system in which halogenation of the bacterial cell wall occurs. The oxygen required for this mechanism is trapped by NADPH. A superoxide anion is then formed by the enzyme NADPH oxidase and subsequently converted to hydrogen peroxide by superoxide dismutase. Myeloperoxidase and hydrogen peroxide also damage the cell wall by converting amino acids into aldehydes and by reacting with unsaturated lipids. Both

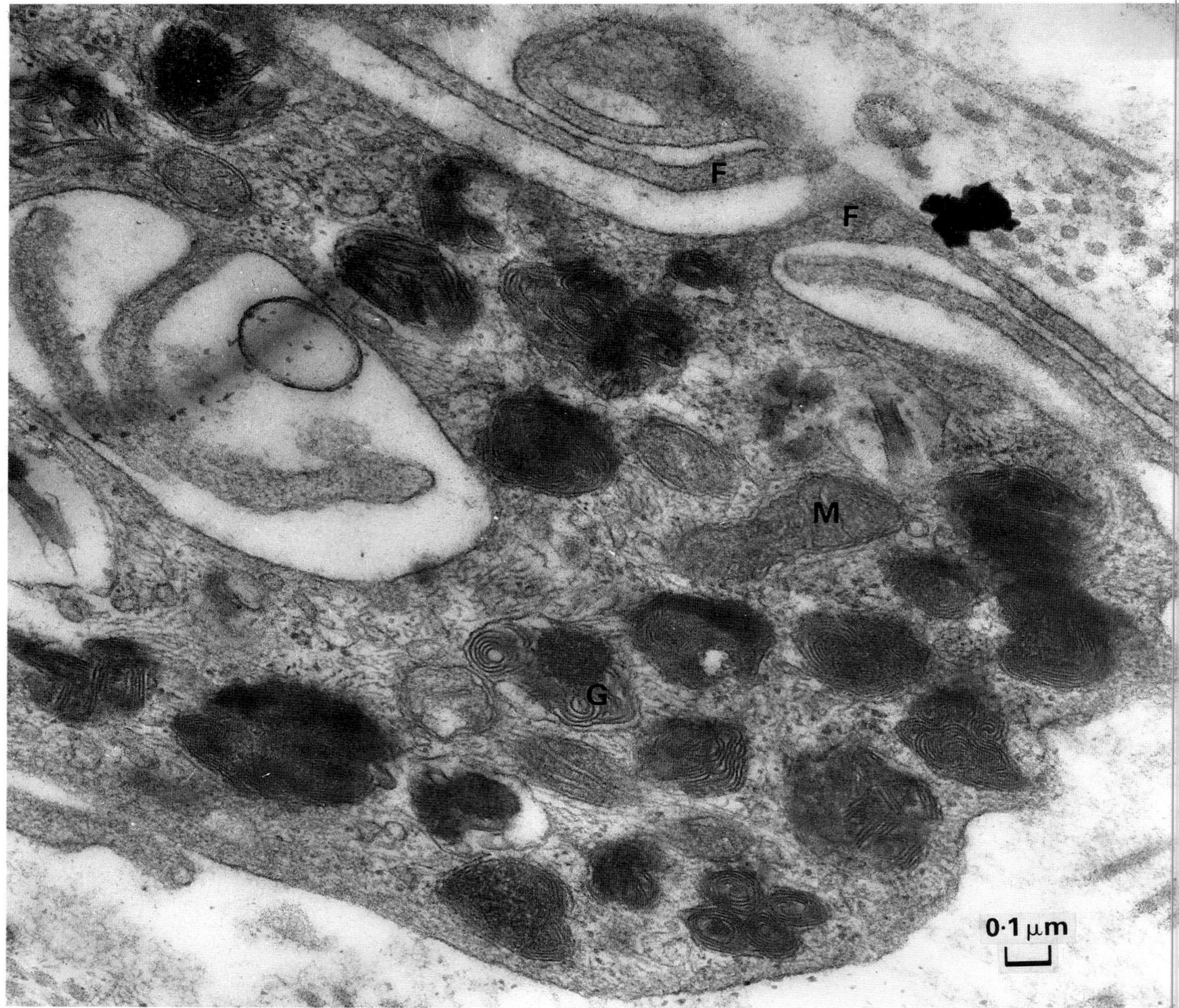

Fig. 1.2. Part of a mast cell showing filopodia (F), typical wholed granules (G) and mitochondria (M). (×59 400).

the hydrogen peroxide and intermediate products are highly toxic. The operation of this process is reflected in the burst of oxygen uptake and activation of the hexose monophosphate shunt which follows active phagocytosis of bacteria by neutrophils. Some micro-organisms produce catalase which breaks down the hydrogen peroxide and thus renders this mode of killing ineffective.

The other lysosomal agents are independent of oxygen and, while some such as lysozyme and elastase are capable of damaging the cell wall, they are probably more important in the digestion of dead organisms.

Macrophages lack myeloperoxidase, but probably operate a hydrogen peroxide killing mechanism by the use of catalase. As in neutrophils, a burst in oxygen consumption and activation of the hexose monophosphate shunt also occurs following phagocytosis. The anti-microbial activity of macrophages is greatly enhanced by the presence of soluble factors produced by lymphocytes known as lymphokines (p.9).

Chemical mediators of inflammation

Control of the inflammatory process depends on the liberation or activation at the inflammatory site of a large number of interrelated chemical factors.

Histamine

Histamine is important in the early stages of acute inflammation. It is found, as already noted, in blood basophils and mast cells and also in platelets. Pharmacologically it causes:

1 Vascular dilatation and an increase in capillary permeability by the formation of gaps between the endothelial cells.

2 Contraction of extravascular smooth muscle.

Histamine plays an important role in immediate-type hypersensitivity reactions (p. 14) such as hay fever and asthma. Its effects may be counteracted by 'antihistamine' drugs. In the tissues it is inactivated by histaminase or acetylation.

Bradykinin

Bradykinin is the most important of a group of polypeptides known as kinins. It is a nonapeptide generated from kininogen (an α-globulin), which is a precursor present in plasma, by the action of kallikrein, an enzyme also present in plasma. It is so named because the contractile response of smooth muscle to it is slower than it is to histamine (in Greek *bradys* = slow). Apart from its action on smooth muscle it causes vasodilatation and increased vascular permeability.

The Hageman factor

The Hageman factor is a serum β-globulin which is present in inactive form in plasma. It is activated by tissue damage and its primary effects are:

1 Activation of prekallikreins in plasma to form kallikrein (see above).

2 Activation of the intrinsic clotting mechanism and the fibrinolytic system.

A secondary effect is activation of the complement cascade.

Complement

Complement is one of four important and interrelated enzymic cascades (Figs 1.3 and 1.4). The other three are:

1 The blood clotting mechanism.

2 Fibrinolysis.

3 Kinin formation (see above).

The complement system consists of an enzymatic chain reaction in which nine components participate. The components are referred to as C1 to C9, but the first four steps are not in numerical order; the order is C1–C4–C2–C3. During the reaction, smaller fragments become split off from some of the components, notably 3 and 5 (C3a, C5a, etc.). The reaction may be triggered in two ways:

1 *The classical pathway* is triggered by an antibody–antigen reaction which in traditional terminology is said to 'fix' complement.

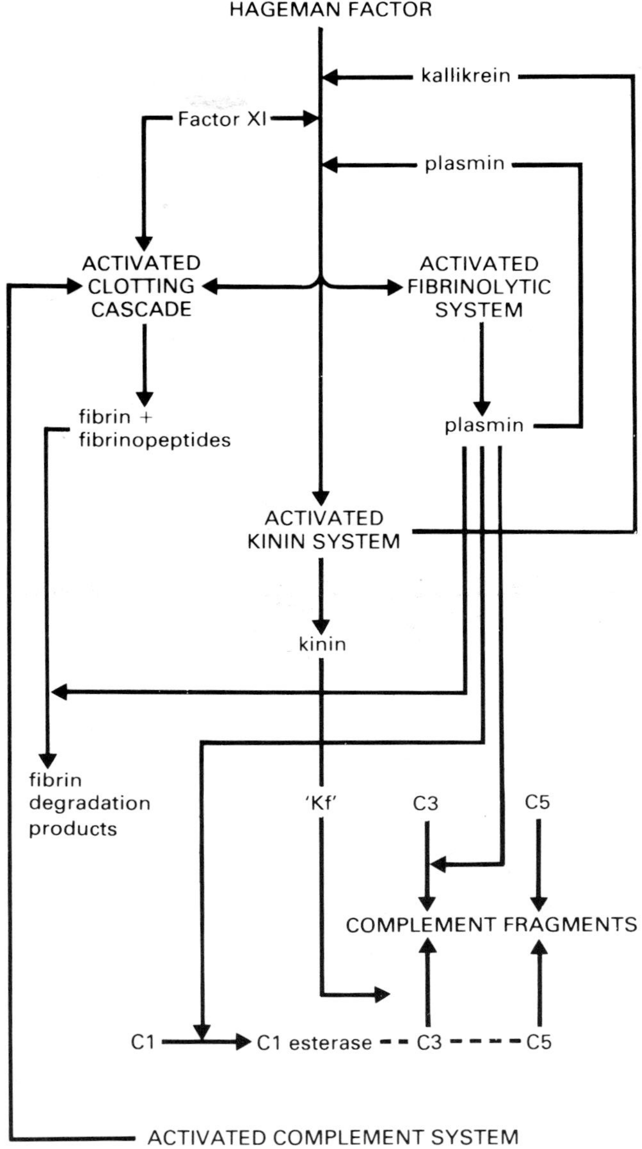

Fig. 1.3. Schema of the relationships between the kinin, clotting, fibrinolytic and complement systems. (Redrawn with permission from Ryan & Majno, 1977.)

2 *The alternative pathway* in which the first three steps are by-passed and activation of C3 occurs as a result of contact with non-antibodies such as the bacterial endotoxin or polysaccharide and properdin (an activator present in plasma).

Both pathways can be activated by plasmin and thrombin as well as by lysosomal enzymes released from dead leucocytes.

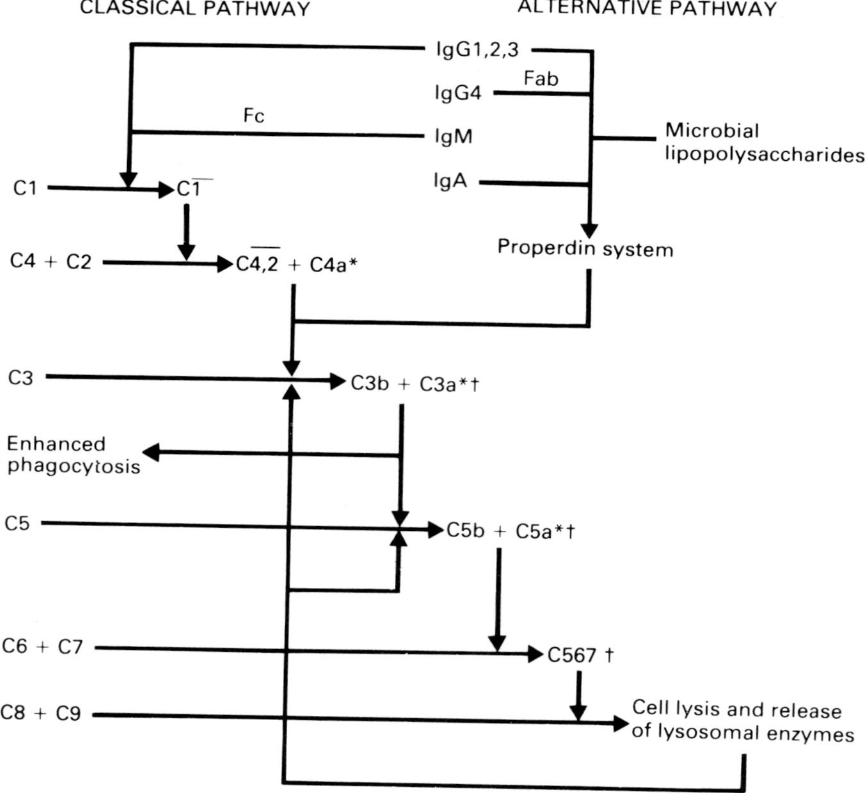

Fig. 1.4. The inflammatory sequelae of complement activation. The asterisks show increased vascular permeability and smooth muscle contraction, and the daggers indicate leukocyte chemotaxis. (Redrawn with permission from Ryan & Majno, 1977.)

Active components of the complement system

1 C3a and C5a are known as anaphylatoxins which release histamine from mast cells and are strongly chemotactic for neutrophils. Local injection into the skin also causes inflammatory oedema.
2 C3b, the larger residual part of C3, is important in facilitating the action of opsonic antibodies by binding to receptors which are present both on the antibody and on the surface of the phagocyte.
3 C5, C6 and C7 form an activated complex (C567) which is chemotactic for neutrophils.
4 C8 and C9 are the end product lyse cells or bacterial membranes.

The destructive potential of complement is limited by the short life of the components and the presence in plasma of natural inhibitors.

The complement system is, in effect, the first line of defence against microbial invasion in that it is ubiquitous. Contact with invading microbes triggers the generation of chemotactic factors which attract neutrophils to the site.

Plasmin (fibrinolysin)

Plasmin is generated from an inactive precursor plasminogen which is present in plasma by activated Hageman factor. Its principal action is fibrinolysis, but it has two secondary actions:
1 Cleavage of C3 and C5 to produce the active fragments C3a and C5a referred to above.
2 Reaction with activated Hageman factor to generate the sub-units which trigger the prekallikrein system and result in kinin formation.

Prostaglandins and leukotrienes

Prostaglandins are 20-carbon polyunsaturated fatty acid derivatives of arachidonic acid containing a 5-carbon ring. They are extremely widespread in tissues. The most important are PGE1 and PGE2 (the figure refers to the number of double bonds outside the ring) which cause vasodilatation and increased permeability when injected into skin. However, these agents have also been found to inhibit the release of granules from mast cells and lysosomal enzymes from polymorphs. It appears that they can act both as mediators and regulators of inflammation according to concentration.

Leukotrienes are also polyunsaturated fatty acids derived from arachidonic acid, but differ from prostaglandins in not having a 5-carbon ring. They were first described in leucocytes and are known to be produced by leucocytes and mast cells. The most important are LTB4 which is chemotactic for neutrophils and also causes them to stick to capillary endothelium. LTC4 and LTD4 are able to cause a weal and flare reaction when injected into skin.

Slow reacting substance A is a mixture of three leukotrienes including LTC4 and LTD4. It is so called because it causes a slower, but more sustained contraction of smooth muscle than histamine. It is released when mast cells are degranulated.

Prostaglandins and leukotrienes are thought to be important in sustaining the inflammatory reaction after the initial acute phase. The anti-inflammatory effects of aspirin and indomethacin result from blockage of the synthesis of prostaglandins and leukotrienes from arachidonic acid, but anti-inflammatory steroids inhibit the formation of arachidonic acid itself.

Extraneous factors

Certain micro-organisms produce active factors which affect the course of the inflammatory response they initiate. The most important are:

1 *Hyaluronidase* is produced by streptococci, *Clostridium welchii* and some staphylococci. This enzyme liquefies ground substance and, therefore, tends to promote a cellulitis.

2 *Coagulase* is produced by pathogenic staphylococci. Since it activates the blood coagulation mechanism, spread of the organisms through the tissues is hampered and the inflammatory reaction is localised.

C-reactive protein

C-reactive protein, which is so called because it reacts with the C polysaccharide of pneumococci, is the best known of a number of α-2 globulins which are synthesised by the liver and appear in excess in the plasma following injury or inflammation. C-reactive protein binds to other polysaccharides present in bacterial and fungal cell walls and also phospholipids. The resulting complex is efficient at triggering the complement chain through the classical pathway.

The role of C-reactive protein in the inflammatory process is uncertain, but measurement of plasma levels may be of value in the diagnosis of infections and in the assessment of inflammatory diseases such as rheumatoid arthritis, etc.

Pus formation

Suppuration is the natural result of the invasion of the tissues by pyogenic organisms. The inflammatory reaction brings a large force of neutrophils to the infected area to combat the invading bacteria. In the ensuing struggle, bacteria are ingested and killed while tissue cells and polymorphs die from the effects of bacterial toxins. Enzymes liberated from dead cells, particularly the neutrophils, digest the dead cells, collagen fibres, serum proteins, etc. to form pus which thus contains products of protein breakdown, nucleoproteins, lipids and fluid exudate together with both living and dead polymorphs and bacteria. Suppuration can also be induced in the absence of bacteria by the injection of bacterial proteins, turpentine, silver nitrate and other substances which cause an accumulation of neutrophils and tissue necrosis.

In the eye, pus is commonly found as a dense yellowish blob suspended in the vitreous (vitreous abscess) or as a yellowish-grey sediment in the inferior part of the anterior chamber (hypopyon). In H & E (haematoxylin and eosin) sections, pus is recognisable as a dense purplish mass composed mainly of polymorphs in various stages of disintegration.

CHRONIC INFLAMMATION

Chronic inflammation may follow an acute inflammatory reaction when the causal agent is not completely eliminated. More often, it is the response to slowly acting, persistent injurious agents and may be a seriously destructive process. It evolves slowly along one of several paths and the inflammatory changes are commonly accompanied by those of synchronous repair.

Exudation of fluid occurs, but is usually less marked than in acute inflammation. The cells which enter the inflamed area are chiefly monocytes, lymphocytes and sometimes eosinophils.

Chronic inflammation is traditionally classified as granulomatous or non-granulomatous. As will be seen when the immune system is reviewed, the distinction, although not absolute, has some practical and conceptual value. In non-granulomatous inflammation the cells seen are predominantly lymphocytes, plasma cells derived from B-lymphocytes and macrophages. In granulomatous inflammation the picture is dominated by macrophages and their epithelioid and giant cell derivatives which usually show a characteristic follicular arrangement.

The cells observed in chronic inflammation are responsible for the immune response discussed below.

THE IMMUNE RESPONSE

Participating cells

Lymphocytes

Lymphocytes vary in size from small, which are about the size of a red blood cell, to large which are perhaps 50% larger in diameter. By light microscopy they have a densely staining nucleus surrounded by a thin pale rim of cytoplasm. Even under the electron microscope few organelles are seen in the cytoplasm other than occasional mitochondria and small amounts of endoplasmic reticulum (see Fig. 1.1).

Lymphocytes are an indispensable component of the body's immune system, because of their capacity to recognise and respond to antigens.

Most lymphocytes continually recirculate between the lymphoid tissues and the bloodstream. They enter the lymph nodes and gut-associated lymphoid tissue through venules lined by high endothelium and are returned to the general circulation via the lymphatics and thoracic duct.

In a somewhat oversimplified view, there are two functionally distinct populations which are, however, both derived from stem cells in the bone marrow.

B-lymphocytes migrate from the bone marrow to the lymphoid follicles in lymph nodes and gut- associated lymphoid tissue. The latter is thought in man to correspond to a lymphoid organ in birds called the *bursa of Fabricius* from which the prefix B- is derived. The surface of the cell carries immunoglobulins which function as specific antigen-recognition units and antigen receptors and also as receptors for the Fc portion of antibodies and the C3b component of complement. After antigen combines with the antigen receptors, B-lymphocytes undergo transformation into blast cells and can then differentiate into plasma cells which are able to secrete specific antibodies to the antigen. This process requires T-lymphocyte co-operation.

Plasma cells: these distinctive cells which, paradoxically, are not normally present in circulating blood, are easily

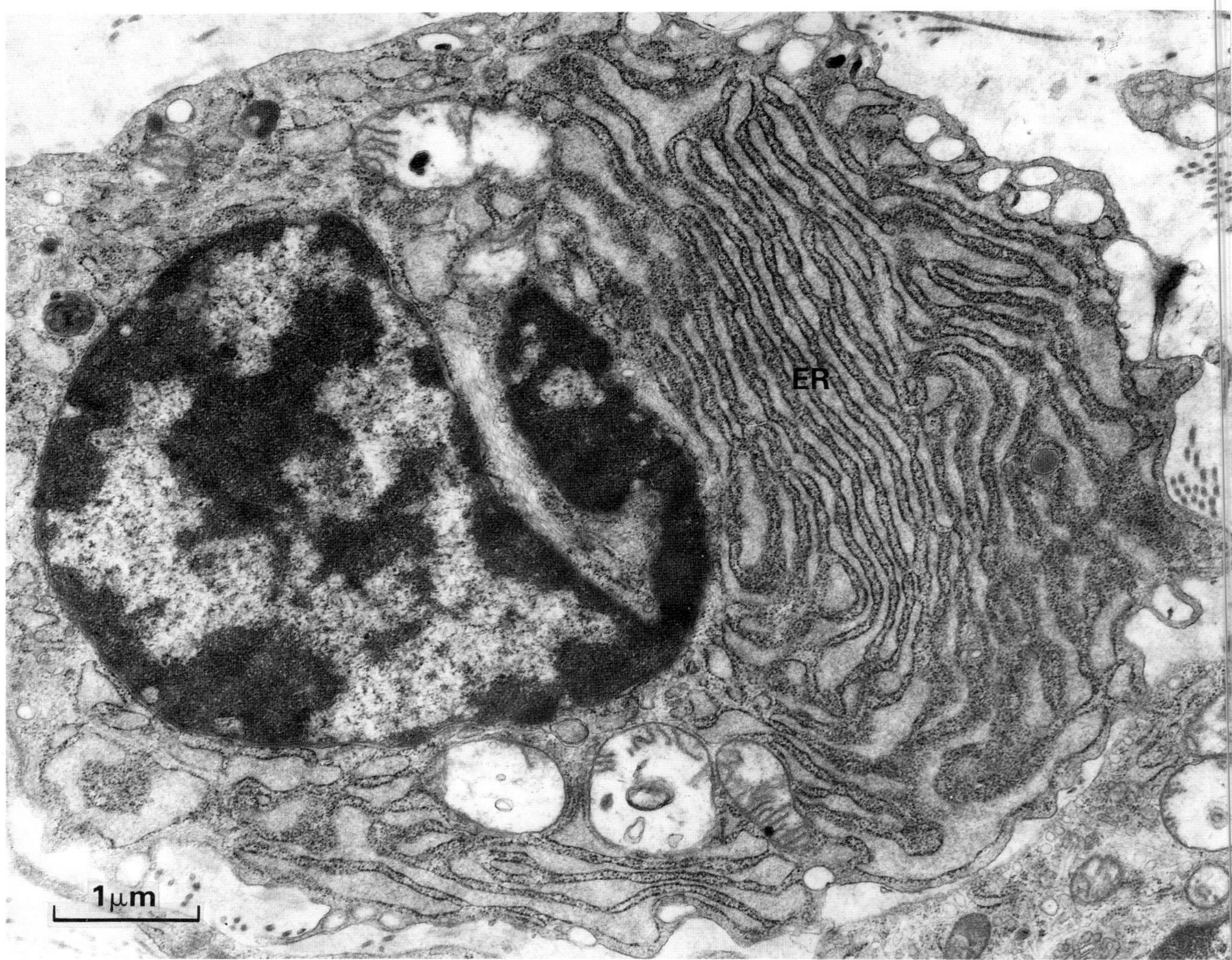

Fig. 1.5. A plasma cell. Note the large content of rough endoplasmic reticulum (ER) in the cytoplasm. (×20 900).

recognisable in H & E stained tissue sections by their purple cytoplasm rich in RNA and round eccentric nuclei wherein the coarse chromatin is sometimes arranged like the spokes of a wheel or the figures of a clock face.

By electron microscopy (Fig. 1.5) the cytoplasm is seen to contain abundant rough endoplasmic reticulum and a Golgi apparatus. These organelles reflect the high rate of protein synthesis necessary for antibody production. Occasionally, the antibody appears not to be released and accumulates in the cell. This gives rise to a large rounded hyaline eosinophilic body long known as a Russell body to light microscopists.

T-lymphocytes are thought to be derived from stem cells which migrate to the thymus from the bone marrow in foetal life. This differentiation proceeds under the influence of thymic epithelial cells and is independent of any immunological stimulus. At about the time of birth, T-lymphocytes are seeded to the paracortical areas of lymph nodes, the periarteriolar lymphoid sheaths in the spleen and the interfollicular regions of the gut-associated lymphoid tissue. T-lymphocytes constitute the bulk of the population of recirculating lymphocytes mentioned above.

T-lymphocytes carry somewhat immunoglobulin-like proteins on their surface membranes which act as antigen receptors. Macrophages play an important role in processing antigen before passing it to the T-cell receptors. T-cells do not possess C3b or Fc receptors.

Following contact with antigen, T-cells undergo transformation into blast cells which proliferate and produce a force of antigen-sensitised effector cells with various functions:

1 Elaboration of lymphokines, of which the most important are:

(i) Migration inhibition factor which prevents macrophages and leucocytes from leaving sites of T-cell–antigen interaction.

(ii) Macrophage activating factor which increases cell membrane activity and stickiness.

(iii) Chemotactic factor which attracts macrophages and other leucocytes.

(iv) Cytotoxic factor which is directed against cells expressing relevant antigens.

(v) Mitogenic factor which enhances the proliferation of sensitised T-cells and possibly recruits uncommitted leucocytes to undergo blast cell transformation.

(vi) Transfer factor. This is capable of transferring reactivity to a given antigen from a sensitised to a non-sensitised individual.

2 Regulation of antibody production by B-cells. This is accomplished by two sub-populations of T-cells:

(i) Helper T-cells which cooperate with B-cells in the production of specific antibodies.

(ii) Suppressor T-cells which inhibit the ability of B-cells to produce antibody.

3 Production of killer cells which attack sensitised target cells.

4 Provision of long-term memory cells which have a life-span of 5 to 10 years.

Null cells lack the characteristics of either T- or B-cells. They constitute some 5% of the lymphocyte population. This sub-population may include at least some of the so-called natural killer (NK) cells that are capable of non-specific cytotoxicity *in vitro*.

Epithelioid cells

Epithelioid cells are derived from macrophages by a process of maturation, the stimulus for which is unknown. They are so called because the nucleus has a prominent nucleolus which gives them a superficial resemblance to epithelial cells. By electron microscopy the cell membrane is seen to be highly convoluted and the cytoplasm contains abundant endoplasmic reticulum and lysosomes. They have a life of 1 to 3 weeks. During maturation they lose some of their phagocytic activity, but can take up subcellular particles and their function is thought to be the removal of small irritant matter. Large aggregations are seen in tuberculomata, sarcoid granulomata and, in the eye, in granulomatous endophthalmitis such as sympathetic ophthalmitis.

Giant cells

Giant cells arise by the fusion of macrophages. The stimulus to their formation apears to be the presence of foreign material which is too large to be phagocytosed by ordinary macrophages. The nuclei may be distributed randomly through the cytoplasm or arranged in the form of a ring around the periphery of the cytoplasm (Fig. 1.6). Both types of distribution may be seen in foreign body granulomata such as those arising in response to sutures. Langhans type cells, which have a markedly peripheral arrangement of the nuclei, predominate in tuberculous and lepromatous granulomata. Touton giant cells, which are characteristically seen in xanthogranulomatous lesions, are generally smaller than Langhans cells and the nuclei are arranged in a ring in the centre of the cell. In an ocular context, giant cells are most commonly seen in granulomata arising in the eyelid in response to spillage of sebaceous secretion from the Meibomian glands.

Langerhans cells

Langerhans cells are dendritic cells derived from bone

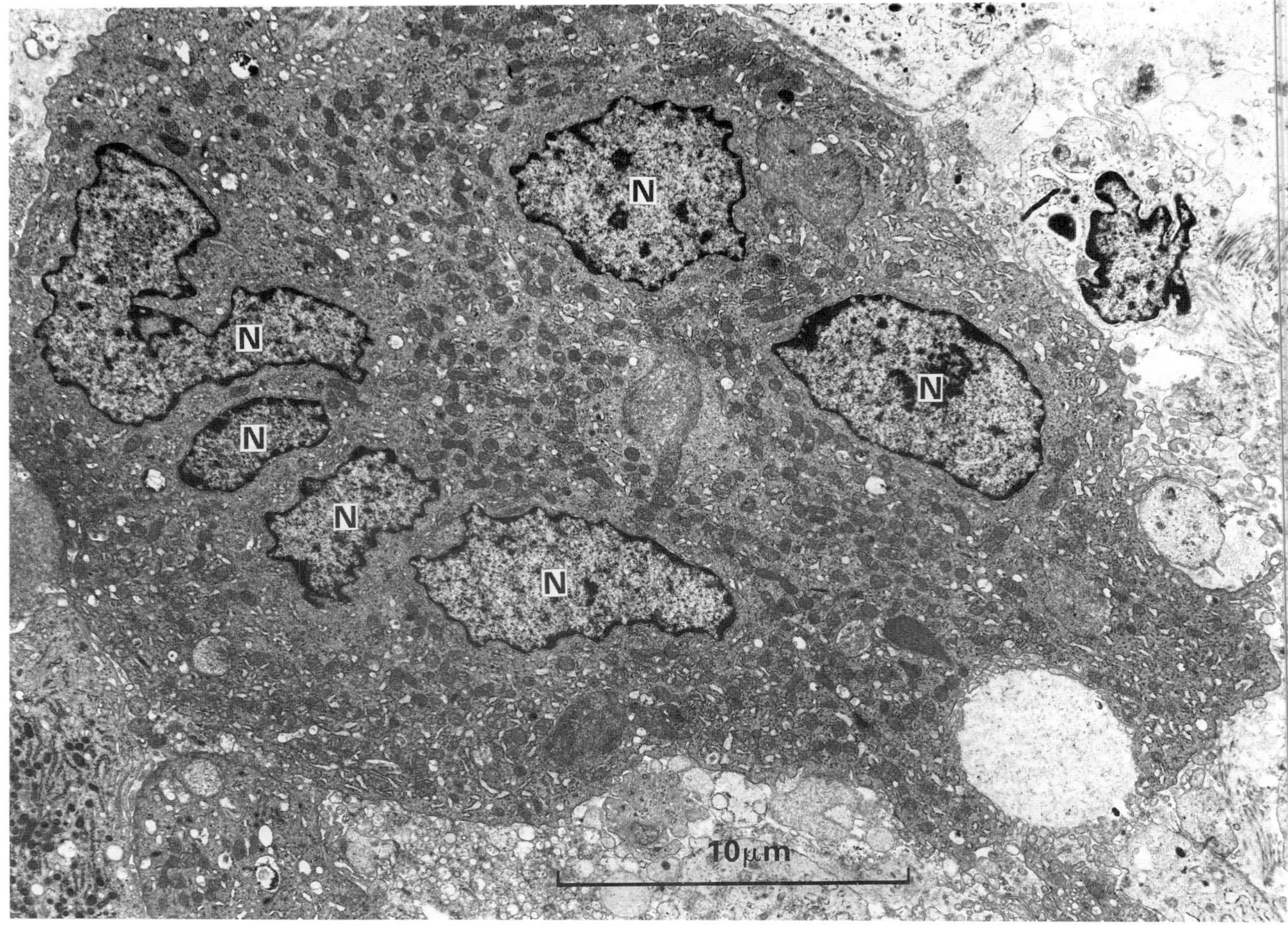

Fig. 1.6. A multinucleate giant cell. Note the ring of nuclei (N). (×4800).

marrow mesenchyme which are found in dermis, mucous membranes, cornea and lymphatic tissue. They are characterised by the presence of a unique racquet-shaped organelle known as the Birkbeck granule. Their function is similar to that of macrophages in that they scavenge foreign small molecular material and process it for presentation to immunocompetent lymphocytes. They thus play an essential role in the sensitisation of skin and mucous membranes and are probably involved in corneal graft reactions.

Antigens

An antigen may be defined as a foreign substance capable of stimulating the production of antibodies. Proteins are the most antigenic substances. Molecular weight is important. It is rare for proteins of a molecular weight less than 5000 to be antigenic. Insulin is an important exception to this generalisation.

Antigenic determinants: binding between antigen and antibody occurs at small areas on the surface of the antigen molecule. These binding sites are known as antigenic determinants or epitopes. The number of sites determines the strength of the binding. A complex antigen has a variety of binding sites. When complex antigens have common determinants, cross-reactions can occur.

Haptens: low molecular weight substances, which are not themselves antigenic, but competitively inhibit the binding of antigen to antibody. They may become attached to a larger protein molecule where they act as an antigenic determinant and stimulate the production of specific antibody. This will react not only with the complex, but also with the unattached small molecules. Such substances are of great importance because they include not only low molecular weight proteins, but drugs and polysaccharide components of microbial cells.

Histocompatibility antigens

Histocompatibilty antigens play a leading role in graft rejection. They are collectively known as the HLA (histocompatibility locus antigen) system because they were originally described on human leucocytes. There are four major groups of antigens known as -A, -B, -C and -D/DR which are coded by four or five genetic loci known as the major histocompatibility complex. This complex is located on the short arm of chromosome 6 in man. An individual derives one gene for each antigen from each parent. The products of HLA-A, -B and -C (class I) resemble immunoglubulins structurally and are found on all nucleated cells. Those of the -D/DR locus (class II), however, bear no such resemblance and are present on the surface of specialised immunocompetent cells. They appear to regulate interaction between cell populations involved in the immune response.

There are at least 20 subtypes of -A and -B. Because of the polymorphism of the system, the likelihood of two individuals other than identical twins sharing identical major HLA antibodies is remote.

Apart from their relationship to graft-rejection, these antigens are of considerable interest because of the striking correlation between certain diseases and HLA antigen type. Possible reasons for this are:

1 Linkage disequilibrium: immunoregulatory genes are present within the major histocompatibility complex and are closely associated with the antigens that it defines, especially within the D/DR region. Expression of particular HLA types may, therefore, be linked with abnormalities in immune function which would normally not be apparent. However, an appropriate disturbance of the immune system in such individuals, or its deterioration with ageing, might lead to manifest disease.

2 Direct participation of the antigen: two mechanisms by which the HLA antigen might participate directly in the disease process have been suggested:

(i) The antigen might share determinants with microorganisms so that the latter are tolerated by the immune system.

(ii) The antigen, being situated on the cell surface, might act as a receptor for viruses, toxins or hormones.

Antibodies

Antibodies constitute the globulin fraction of the plasma glycoproteins and are given the generic term immunoglobulin (Ig). There are five main classes known as IgG, IgM, IgA, IgE and IgD. The basic structure of the antibody molecules is illustrated in Fig. 1.7a. It consists of four polypeptide chains — two heavy and two light arranged in the form of a Y. The stem of the Y, however, consists of heavy chains only. It may be separated by

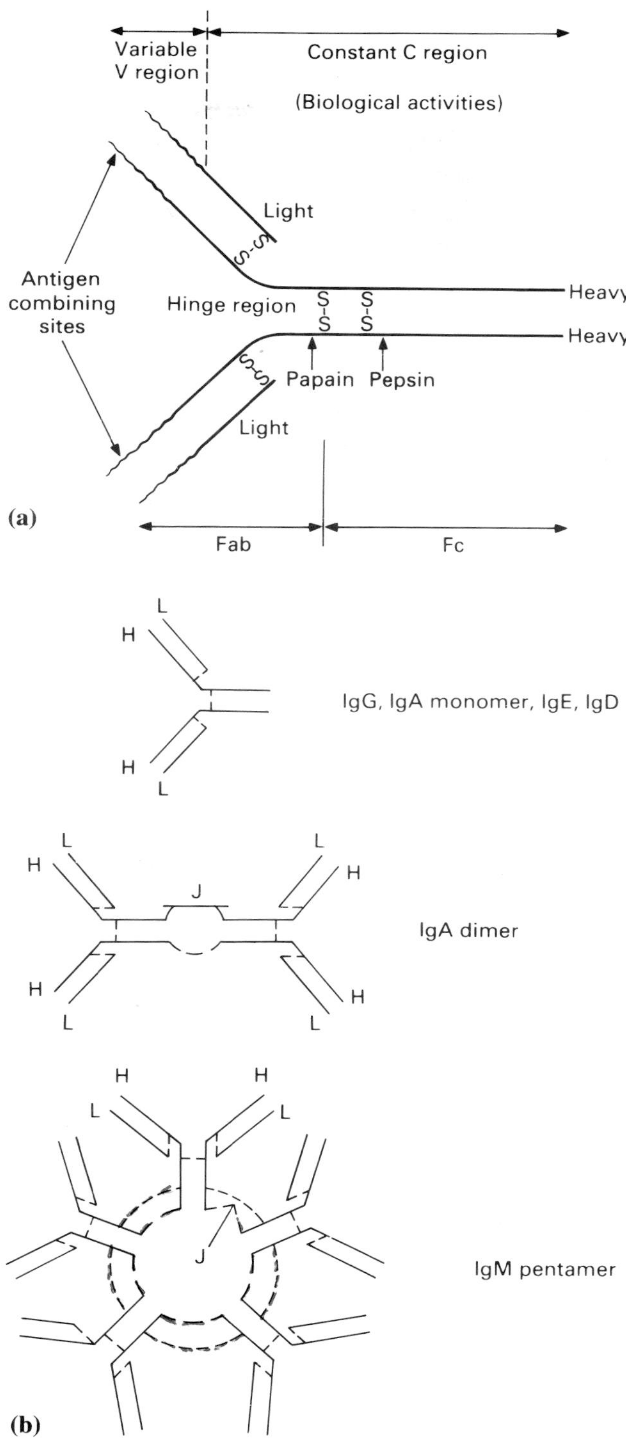

Fig. 1.7. (a) Basic structure of the antibody molecule (the molecule shown is IgG_1). (b) Diagrammatic structures of the antibody molecules of different classes. H = heavy chain; L = light chain; J = joining chain; solid line = polypeptide chain; broken line = disulphide bridge (positions of disulphide bridges are variable and depend on the class). (Redrawn with permission from Taussig, 1984.)

digestion with pepsin and is known as the the Fc fragment since it can be crystallised. It has a binding site which is specific for appropriate surface receptors on cells. The remainder of the molecule is known as the Fab fragment, which contains the variable region and is matched to antigenic determinants. The light chains are of two classes — κ and λ. The pairs within a molecule are always of the same class.

Properties of the different classes

IgG: constitutes about 75% of the plasma immunoglobulin. It consists of the basic molecular unit and has a molecular weight of about 150 000. Functionally, IgG antibodies can neutralise bacterial anti-toxin and circulating viruses. Because of the presence of receptors on the surface of neutrophils for the Fc region of complexed IgG it is an effective opsonin. IgG is also able to fix complement and thus augment opsonisation by a second mechanism. IgG is the only class of antibody able to cross the placental barrier.

IgM: comprises only 7% of the plasma immunoglobulins. Structurally, it consists of five basic molecular units linked by J-chains to form a pentamer (Fig. 1.7b). It has a molecular weight of about 900 000. The structural configuration of the molecule means that there are 10 antigen-binding sites on the surface of a single molecule so that it binds strongly to bacterial, viral or cell surfaces with multiple identical determinants. IgM is produced in large amounts in the early stages of an immune response. The large molecular size and the multiple binding sites of IgM make it the most efficient class of antibody at agglutinating bacteria or red cells. IgM acts as an opsonin only in the presence of complement because neutrophils do not possess a a receptor for its Fc fragment.

IgA: constitutes 20% of plasma immunoglobulin. Structurally it is, like IgG, composed of a single molecular unit and has a molecular weight of about 150 000. It is the antibody found in secretions from mucous membranes, tears, saliva, colostrum and milk. In these situations, it exists as a dimer of two basic molecular units bound by a J-chain (Fig. 1.7b). During passage through the epithelium it has a secretory T-piece added which protects it from digestion. It has been described as an 'immunological paint' which neutralises viruses and toxins and prevents bacteria adhering to mucous membranes. It can also attach to Gram-negative bacteria and, with the aid of complement, render them susceptible to the action of lysozyme.

IgD: forms a very small fraction of the plasma immunoglobulins and has a molecular weight of about 185 000. Though over 50% of B-lymphocytes carry IgD on their surface membrane, its precise function remains uncertain.

IgE (reagin): consists structurally of a single basic molecular unit and has a molecular weight of about 200 000. Circulating levels in blood are very low, but may be raised in allergic subjects. It is responsible for immediate hypersensitivity reactions such as hay fever, asthma, etc. This is related to the unique capacity of its Fc fragment to attach to the surface of mast cells and basophils. IgE also plays a somewhat obscure role in the body's defence mechanism against certain parasites, notably helminths. Blood levels are raised in helminthic infestations.

Monoclonal antibodies

Monoclonal antibodies are playing a rapidly increasing role in medical science in both research and diagnosis and may well have a role in therapy. Conventional antisera produced by injecting antigens into animals consist of a mixture of different classes of antibodies with varying specificity and binding power because they are the product of numerous clones of cells.

Myeloma cells produce monoclonal immunoglobulins in quantity, but to no known antigen. However, it is possible to fuse antibody-producing B-cells obtained from an immunised animal with myeloma cells to produce a so-called hybridoma. The cells of the hybridoma continue to produce antibody, but the specificity of the antibody produced by the hybridoma cell is now determined by that of the B-cell with which it was fused. Large scale cultivation of selected clones enables highly specific antibodies to be produced in quantity.

IMMUNOPATHOLOGICAL MECHANISMS

Tolerance

Natural

During development cells of the immune system acquire the ability to recognise 'self' antigens so that under normal conditions the immune system does not react against the individual's own tissues.

Acquired

Tolerance can be induced artificially. This is accomplished more easily in the foetus and newborn before the immune system is mature. The ease with which tolerance can be induced in the foetus was demonstrated by the classical experiments of Medawar *et al.* They showed that foetal mice which had been injected with cells from an unrelated inbred strain would later tolerate skin grafts from the same strain.

Adult mice may be rendered tolerant to certain antigens by the repeated injection of very large or very small doses of antigen — so-called high and low zone tolerance. Such tolerance is promoted by the simultaneous administration of drugs such as cyclophosphamide which deplete the lymphocyte pool.

Mechanisms involved in tolerance

Natural tolerance may depend on the elimination of 'self' antigen sensitive clones, but suppressor T-cells probably also play an important part. Tolerance due to suppressor T-cells can be transferred to another animal with the cells.

In high zone tolerance both T- and B-lymphocytes become unresponsive, while in low zone tolerance only T-helper cells are unresponsive. This is of importance because low zone tolerance can be broken by the use of a cross-reacting antigen which gives rise to T-cells able to recognise determinants on the tolerated antigen and stimulate antibody production by the B-cells which have remained responsive. The antibody produced cross-reacts with the tolerated antigen so that the unresponsive T-cells are effectively by-passed.

An entirely different mechanism thought to be important in allowing some tumours to resist immunological attack is the production of enhancing antibody. This attaches to antigenic determinants on the cell surface so that they are not recognised by T-cells.

Autoimmune reactions

Autoimmune reactions: breakdown of natural tolerance to the body's own tissues may theoretically occur either because the immune system has become disordered and treats certain normal tissue components as foreign or because the tissue components have become antigenic.

It must be emphasised that antibodies to cell or tissue components (autoantibodies) may be present in certain diseases without there being any evidence that they play any role in pathogenesis. Their detection may, however, be useful for diagnostic purposes.

Autoimmune diseases fall broadly into two categories:

1 Those in which the antibodies are directed against specific target organs such as skin, stomach, adrenal, thyroid, etc.

2 Those in which they are non-organ-specific and directed against widely distributed antigens such as IgG itself or DNA. Diseases in which they are implicated, such as rheumatoid arthritis and systemic lupus erythematosus, tend to be generalised.

The reasons why the immune system becomes unable to recognise 'self' are largely unknown. It has been postulated that normal 'self' antigens may become the target of abnormal immunocytes emanating from a forbidden clone. Another possibility is that production of autoantibodies by B-cells is inhibited by a special subpopulation of suppressor T-cells which for some reason become deficient.

The precise mechanisms by which tissue components become antigenic are also unknown, although there are several hypothetical possibilities:

1 By the unmasking of hidden antigenic determinants to which no natural tolerance has been established. This might possibly be brought about by bacterial enzymes or physical or chemical agents acting on proteins to expose potentially antigenic chemical groupings which are not normally accessible.

2 By immunisation with a foreign antigen which shares antigenic determinants with some host tissue component, e.g. Group A streptococci possess antigens in common with normal heart muscle and glomerular basement membrane.

3 By combination of host proteins with foreign compounds such as drugs or bacterial antigens which by acting as haptens render the complex autoantigenic.

4 By the release of antigenic substances which by virtue of their anatomical location have always been segregated from contact with the immune system, e.g. lens protein.

5 By aberrant expression of class II histocompatibility antigens. T-helper lymphocytes are able to recognise antigen only if it is presented to them by a cell expressing the same class II histocompatibility as themselves. Since the target cells in most organ-specific autoimmune diseases do not normally express class II antigens, any cell-specific surface antigen may effectively never have been presented. Immune tolerance to them would not, therefore, exist. In certain autoimmune diseases such as Hashimoto's thyroiditis and Type 1 diabetes, the target cells (thyroid epithelial cells and β-cells respectively) have been shown to express HLA-DR antigens aberrantly.

Allergic or hypersensitivity reactions

Allergic or hypersensitivity reactions are the terms used to describe a wide range of inflammatory conditions in which damage to body tissues appears to result as an unwanted side-effect of the operation of immune mechanisms. The terms imply that the immune response is altered or exaggerated and it is important to remember that the manner in which the immune system responds to antigenic factors shows a wide individual variation which is governed by genetic factors. Thus the classical allergic and hypersensitivity reactions such as hay fever, asthma, drug sensitivity and serum sickness depend on inherited idiosyncratic factors.

The immune reactions may involve antigens which are foreign to the body, such as bacterial proteins or pollens, or they may be constituents of the body's own tissues which, for various reasons, the immune system will no longer tolerate. In this case, mechanisms intended to repel and destroy invading micro-organisms are turned against the body's own tissues. These are the so-called autoimmune diseases, many of which affect the eye.

Reactions to foreign matter: damage to body tissues occurs as a side-effect of the measures necessary to eliminate the invading micro-organism and neutralise any toxins it may produce. It may be noted in passing that the immune system is apparently incapable of assessing the level of the threat to survival posed by foreign material or organisms. Thus harmless pollen grains may be treated by certain individuals as though they were parasites and egg albumen or serum protein of a different species will excite an immune response comparable with that induced by bacterial toxins.

Although the following reactions are described as separate and distinct responses, it should be appreciated that they rarely occur in isolation.

Type 1 (immediate hypersensitivity) reactions

This type of response is mediated by IgE which is attached to receptors on the surface of mast cells and basophils. Contact between IgE and the appropriate antigen triggers the release from these cells of pharmacologically active substances including histamine, slow reacting substance and eosinophil chemotactic factor. The usual outcome of this reaction is increased capillary permeability in the skin and mucous membranes, contraction of smooth muscle and eosinophilia. This response is responsible for the manifestations of the common allergies to pollen, house dust, fish, etc. About 5–10% of people react in this way to antigens which are apparently harmless to the majority (atopy).

Type 1 hypersensitivity is also responsible for rare and sometimes fatal generalised anaphylactic reactions which are mediated by the same pharmacologically active agents and are characterised by flushing of the skin, bronchospasm and acute hypotension.

Type 2 (cytotoxic hypersensitivity) reactions

IgG and IgM are involved in this type of reaction. By binding to antigenic determinants on cell membranes they activate complement which damages the membrane and results in cell death. Examples of reactions of this type are the haemolytic reaction which occurs in Rhesus incompatibility. Platelets may be involved in drug sensitivity reactions if a drug becomes attached to their surface membrane and acts as a hapten.

Type 3 (immune complex) reactions

Complexes of IgG or IgM form in the circulation or on vascular basement membranes. These complexes bind and activate complement. Release of the activated fragments results in neutrophils being attracted and release of their proteolytic enzymes results in local tissue damage. The immune complexes may also activate the coagulation system resulting in local thrombosis.

In serum sickness, the prototype of Type 3 reactions in which the foreign antigen is horse serum globulin, circulating antibody–antigen complexes localise preferentially in the renal glomeruli and vessels of the heart and joint capsules. Type 3 reactions are thought to participate in a wide variety of other diseases including glomerulonephritis, systemic lupus erythematosus, serum B hepatitis and malarial nephrosis.

When circulating antibody combines with an antigen injected extravascularly, toxic complexes are deposited in the walls of local blood vessels resulting in an inflammatory reaction characterised by haemorrhage, thrombosis, infarction and tissue necrosis (Arthus type reaction). If the supply of antigen is maintained, a more chronic type of reaction may supervene with granuloma formation in some instances.

Type 4 (delayed hypersensitivity) reactions

Unlike the reactions previously described, Type 4 reactions are not mediated by antibodies, but are the result of T-cell activity. The term delayed hypersensitivity reflects the fact that the reaction takes time to become clinically manifest.

After contact with antigen which they have previously encountered, T-cells are transformed into blast cells that proliferate in lymph nodes and other lymphoid aggregates to provide a force of activated cells, some of which find their way back to the source of the antigenic stimulus. There they set in motion cell-mediated reactions by combining with antigens and by the release of lymphokines which in turn initiate an inflammatory response and activate the macrophage system.

The antigens involved may be intrinsic cell components as in graft rejection, chemical agents bound to cell surfaces especially in the skin, or micro-organisms including viruses, protozoa, fungi, chlamydia and mycobacteria. The response to these organisms is clearly directed to killing and eliminating them. Tissue damage results when the release of tissue damaging enzymes from accumulated macrophages is excessive. Macrophages may die and release hydrolytic enzymes as a result of injury sustained by noxious agents produced by the micro-organisms to which they are reacting or because massive accumulation of macrophages causes local ischaemia. The latter will itself also result in tissue damage. Another factor may be some direct killing by cytoxic T-cells of macrophages which have engulfed micro-organisms. The caseous necrosis seen in tuberculosis is partially accounted for by such mechanisms combined with the effect of surfactant lipopolysaccharides liberated from the bacilli.

Type 5 (stimulatory) reactions

In this type of reaction, increased target cell activity results from the stimulatory effect of specific antibody. Although the cells are not damaged, the effect of this excessive activity may be harmful to the host. A good example of this is the action of the anti-thyroid antibody LATS (long acting thyroid stimulator) which mimics the activity of thyroid stimulating hormone.

LOCAL ANATOMICAL FACTORS

Before proceeding to discuss specific intraocular inflammatory diseases, brief mention must be made of certain unique anatomical factors which affect the course of inflammatory and immune reactions in the eye.

Blood–aqueous barrier

The blood–aqueous barrier (Chapter 10) normally restricts the passage of macromolecules such as antibodies into the aqueous, but breakdown occurs as a result of injury or active inflammation.

Conjunctiva

Small numbers of lymphocytes enter the conjunctiva soon after birth and persist throughout life together with a much smaller number of plasma cells which tend to be associated with lacrimal acini of the glands of Krause. The lymphocytes are predominantly T-cells and both suppressor and helper cells are present. Secretory T-piece is added to IgA synthesised by plasma cells in the *substantia propria* and in lacrimal acini on passage through the conjunctival or glandular epithelium. Tear film and lacrimal secretion are rich in IgA. Langerhans and mast cells are normally found in the conjunctiva.

Cornea

All three cellular components of the cornea can express class I HLA antigens in tissue culture, but expression is at a low level in the axial region in normal cornea. Class II antigens have been identified only in the limbal region.

The cornea is traditionally described as a privileged site because of the ease with which grafts between non-identical individuals take. Since it lacks both blood and lymphatic vessels, antigenic material in the cornea reaches the reactive areas of the immune system only slowly through the limbal vessels and aqueous. This situation probably tends to promote tolerance.

Antibody penetrates the cornea freely and can react with antigen in the cornea to form annular precipitates known as Wessely's rings.

Lens

The potentially antigenic proteins of the lens normally have no contact with any reactive cells of the immune system. An autoimmune response may follow capsular rupture, but is by no means inevitable. In hypermature cataracts, slow seepage of liquefied lens matter through the capsule into the aqueous may apparently result in auto-sensitisation (Chapter 4).

Uvea

Lymphocytes are not normally seen in the uvea, but, under certain conditions, lymphoid proliferation and antibody production can be induced as will be discussed later.

Blood–retina barrier

The non-fenestrated capillaries of the retina and the tight junctions between the cells of the pigmented epithelium (Chapter 10) tend to prevent neutrophils from invading the retina in acute inflammation. Cuffing of retinal venules is, however, a common concomitant of inflammatory processes within the eye.

GENERAL EFFECTS OF INFLAMMATION ON THE EYE

Physical signs

Intraocular inflammation is no different from inflammation elsewhere except for the unique circumstance that fluid exudate and migrating cells accumulate in the ocular cavities where they can be seen. This fact has given rise to a special nomenclature for the visible signs of intraocular inflammation, e.g. aqueous flare, keratic precipitates, hypopyon, etc.

Aqueous flare

An aqueous flare is a sign of excess protein in the aqueous fluid and is evidence that the blood–aqueous barrier has been rendered permeable and is allowing the passage of plasma proteins. If fibrinogen escapes, the aqueous may clot in the anterior chamber or after withdrawal. Aqueous flare in phacolytic glaucoma (Chapter 12) is an exception to this rule since it is due to the presence of soluble lens protein.

Keratic precipitates (KPs)

Keratic precipitates are deposits of inflammatory cells on the corneal endothelium.

Monocytes and macrophages in the aqueous show a strong tendency to adhere to one another and to the corneal endothelium, thus forming large deposits (waxy, lardaceous or mutton-fat KPs). These deposits may be so numerous that they coalesce into a continuous layer (conglomerate KPs) which may even become organised into fibrous tissue. Adhesive aggregates of macrophages are also seen at the iris margin (Koeppe nodules), on the iris surface (Busacca nodules) and on the surface of the retina (retinal precipitates). Large deposits of this type are characteristic of granulomatous inflammation. The macrophage clumping may be due to the macrophage activating factor released by antigen-sensitised T-cells.

Neutrophils on the other hand show little tendency to agglutinate. They adhere to the cornea singly or in small groups causing a frosted appearance.

Lymphocytes also form small KPs, but rarely occur alone and are often overshadowed by accompanying macrophages.

Hypopyon

Hypopyon is a sediment composed chiefly of neutrophils (pus cells) and fibrin which forms in the lower part of the anterior chamber. Hypopyon is often evidence of pyogenic organisms within the eye, but the inflammatory reaction to an infected corneal ulcer may release chemotactic agents which attract neutrophils into the anterior chamber from the vessels of the iris and ciliary body. In lens-induced endophthalmitis cataractous lens material in the anterior chamber may attract abundant phagocytes and simulate a hypopyon.

The appearance of hypopyon may also be simulated by diffuse retinoblastoma and occasionally by the discharge of leukaemic cells into the anterior chamber in leukaemia (pseudohypopyon).

Definitions

Panophthalmitis

Panophthalmitis is inflammation of all the ocular tissues including the corneoscleral envelope, Tenon's capsule and often the orbital tissues as well.

Endophthalmitis

Endophthalmitis indicates inflammation involving the ocular cavities and their immediate adjacent structures without extension beyond the sclera. It may be diffuse within the globe or may be confined to either the anterior or posterior segment.

Uveitis

Uveitis means inflammation mainly confined to the uveal tract. It has long been recognised as an unsatisfactory term because in any predominantly uveal inflammation there is likely to be some involvement of the retina, optic nerve, corneoscleral envelope and trabecular meshwork. Conversely, it may be noted that primary inflammation of the cornea, sclera, retina, optic nerve or vitreous may extend into the adjacent uvea.

Classification of intraocular inflammatory disease

The classification of intraocular inflammatory disease has always been problematical. Aetiological classification is desirable, but, after segregating those conditions due to recognisable specific agents, there is a large, heterogeneous, residual group in which causation is obscure. It was traditional to classify this group on the basis of the whether the inflammatory reaction was predominantly 'granulomatous' or 'non-granulomatous'. This was unsatisfactory because the distinction is far from absolute. Indeed, it was often not clear whether the description referred to the clinical or pathological features.

For these reasons a compromise between a purely descriptive and a fully aetiological classification has been adopted:

1 Intraocular inflammation due to specific agents (Chapter 2).

2 Idiopathic intraocular inflammation, which is not uncommonly associated with systemic disease of uncertain pathogenesis (Chapter 3). This is inevitably a mixture of causally unrelated conditions some of which may, however, share pathogenetic mechanisms.

3 Sympathetic ophthalmitis and related conditions (Chapter 4). Although the pathogenesis of these conditions is, like those dealt with in Chapter 3, far from clear, they do form a well-defined group.

BIBLIOGRAPHY

Anderson, J. R., ed. (1985) *Muir's Textbook of Pathology*, 12th Edn. Arnold, Baltimore.

Bhan, A. K., Fujikawa, L. S. & Foster, C. S. (1982) T-cell subsets and Langerhans cells in normal and diseased conjunctiva. *American Journal of Ophthalmology* **94**, 205–212.

Editorial (1982) The Langerhans cell. *Lancet* **ii**, 672–673.

Foulis, A. K. (1986) Class II major histocompatibility complex and organ specific autoimmunity in man. *Journal of Pathology* **150**, 5–11.

Fujikawa, L. S., Colvin, R. B., Bhan, A. K., Fuller, T. C. & Foster, C. S. (1982) Expression of HLA-A/B/C and -DR locus antigens on epithelial, stromal and endothelial cells of the human cornea. *Cornea* **1**, 213–222.

Guttmann, R. D., ed. in chief (1981) *Immunology*. A Scope Publication, Upjohn Co., Kalamazoo.

Jackson, W. B. & Gilmore, N. J. (1981) Ocular immunology: a review. *Canadian Journal of Ophthalmology* **16**, 3–9, 59–65.

Jakobiec, F. A., Lefkowitch, J. & Knowles II, D. M. (1984) B- and T-lymphocytes in ocular disease. *Ophthalmology* **91**, 635–654.

Jakobiec, F. A. (1983) Ocular inflammatory disease: the lymphocyte redivivus. *American Journal of Ophthalmology* **96**, 384–391.

Kunkel, S. L. & Sugar, A. (1983) Inflammatory mechanisms in the eye. In *Immunology of Inflammation*, ed. P. A. Ward. pp 245–278. Elsevier, Amsterdam.

Rahi, A. H. S. & Garner, A. (1976) *Immunopathology of the Eye*. Blackwell Scientific Publications, Oxford.

Roitt, I. M. (1984) *Essential Immunology*, 5th Edn. Blackwell Scientific Publications, Oxford.

Roitt, I., Brostoff, J. & Male, D. (1985) *Immunology*. Churchill Livingstone, London & Gower Medical Publishing, London.

Ryan, G. B. & Majno, G. (1977) *Inflammation*. A Scope Publication, Upjohn Co., Kalamazoo.

Sacks, E., Rutgers, J., Jakobiec, F. A., Bonetti, F. & Knowles, D. M. (1986) A comparison of conjunctival and nonocular dendritic cells utilizing new monoclonal antibodies. *Ophthalmology* **93**, 1089–1097.

Spector, W. G. (1980) *An Introduction to General Pathology*. Churchill Livingstone, Edinburgh.

Taussig, M. J. (1984) *Processes in Pathology and Microbiology*, 2nd Edn. Blackwell Scientific Publications, Oxford.

Woolf, N. (1977) *Cell, Tissue and Disease. The Basis of Pathology*, 2nd Edn. Baillière Tindall, London.

Chapter 2 Intraocular inflammation due to specific agents

PYOGENIC INFECTIONS

Although many different organisms have been incriminated as possible causes of intraocular suppuration, it is usually due to the common pyogenic cocci such as staphylococci, streptococci and pneumococci and occurs in the following circumstances:

1 Following traumatic perforations of the corneoscleral envelope.

2 Following metastatic spread via the bloodstream from an extraocular focus of infection.

3 As a complication of keratitis (hypopyon ulcer).

Disintegrating necrotic intraocular neoplasms may set up an acute inflammatory reaction and simulate intraocular suppuration.

Perforations of the corneoscleral envelope

Perforations of the corneoscleral envelope are the commonest cause of intraocular suppuration. Pyogenic cocci enter the wound through accidental or surgical wounds or perforating corneal ulcers or are carried into the eye by foreign bodies.

1 Post-operative infection is most commonly seen after cataract extractions and occurs soon after operation, but late infections may complicate drainage operations for glaucoma or develop when wound healing is delayed by faulty apposition of the wound margins or incarceration in the wound of uveal tissue or lens capsule. In such instances, organisms enter the wound from the conjunctival sac.

2 Relatively few corneal ulcers progress to perforation. Those due to pneumococcal infection are the most likely to perforate. Ulceration due to *Pseudomonas aeruginosa* infection is acute, destructive and so rapidly progressive that, in the absence of effective treatment, perforation may occur within 2 to 3 days of onset.

3 Introduction of organisms such as *Ps. aeruginosa* and *Bacillus cereus* into the vitreous by foreign bodies may cause a fulminating infection rapidly leading to panophthalmitis and orbital cellulitis. Early treatment must often be empirical since the infecting organisms are inaccessible and may not be identified until pus leaks through the wound or the eye has to be excised.

Metastatic infection

Bacterial infection of the eye leading to suppuration is an uncommon complication of such septic conditions as peritonitis, pneumonia, meningitis, otitis media, osteomyelitis, puerperal sepsis, acute endocarditis, breast abscess and furunculosis.

The blood-borne organisms probably enter the eye along both the central retinal artery and the ciliary arteries but, in the majority of cases, first establish suppurative foci in the retina from where they spread into the vitreous and to the uvea secondarily. Concurrent metastatic infection of the ciliary body and its processes may augment the retinitis. Occasionally the primary suppurative foci are in the iris and ciliary body, but only rarely in the choroid. By contrast, tubercle bacilli and carcinoma cells lodge in the choroid rather than the retina, ciliary body or iris.

In infants and young children with bacterial meningitis, infection of the eye may initiate a silent process which is overlooked until a vitreous abscess or a retinal detachment due to organisation of vitreous exudate forms a 'pseudoglioma'. This possibility must always be considered in the differential diagnosis of retinoblastoma. Bilateral meningococcal endophthalmitis has been reported in meningococcal septicaemia in the absence of signs of meningitis.

Pathology of intraocular suppuration

Intraocular suppuration from any cause is a serious matter. The severity and progress of the inflammation and its eventual outcome depend on the dose and virulence of the infecting organism, the resistance of the host and the availability and efficacy of antibacterial treatment. The balance of these forces determines whether the infection progresses to suppurative panophthalmitis or remains confined to a particular part of the globe. Infection following surgery or accidental trauma does not always provoke an acute suppurative response. If the infecting organisms are of low virulence or are effectively checked by treatment, suppuration may be minimal and the histological picture is dominated by mononuclear cells. Even so, the end result may be disastrous to visual function.

Panophthalmitis

In severe infections the organisms spread to involve all the ocular structures including the lens (if its capsule has been ruptured), the corneoscleral envelope, Tenon's capsule and the orbital tissues (Fig. 2.1). In such cases, there is a danger of meningitis and cavernous sinus thrombosis through spread of the infection from the orbit. Eventually the purulent contents of the globe may be discharged either through the necrotic cornea or through the sclera (usually in the ciliary region) and shrinkage of the eye occurs.

Suppuration in the posterior segment

A *vitreous abscess* results from suppuration localised to the posterior segment This is commonly due to infected foreign bodies penetrating the vitreous cavity, but may be a sequel to metastatic infection. Large masses of pus in the vitreous rarely, if ever, disperse, but are organised and thus result in a traction detachment of the retina. An intact Bruch's membrane forms a barrier to the passage of organisms, although not of toxins, so that, even in the presence of a vitreous abscess, the choroid may show only oedema and lymphocytic infiltration.

Suppuration in the anterior segment

Pus derived from neutrophils entering the the anterior chamber in response to chemotactic products generated in an infected corneal ulcer (hypopyon ulcer) (Fig. 2.2) often disperses without serious consequences as the ulcer heals. On the other hand, suppuration resulting from anterior perforating injuries, retained foreign bodies, perforating corneal ulcers or surgical wounds is much more serious and often progresses to scarring and adhesions.

Microscopic appearances of intraocular suppuration

Acute stage

The acute stage is dominated by neutrophils, exudate and necrosis.

Neutrophils are found as diffuse and perivascular infiltrations throughout the ocular tissues and as large aggregations in the anterior chamber and vitreous cavity. Intense concentrations are seen around perforating vessels in the sclera. The lens capsule resists the passage of bacteria, but, if it has been ruptured, organisms and cells invade the lens substance and a lental abscess is formed.

Proteinous exudate presents as granular or structureless eosinophilic matter best seen in sections in the anterior and posterior chambers. Escaping fibrinogen is converted to fibrin networks recognisable by the fact that small refractile nodes are visible where the fibrin strands intersect. A fibrino-purulent clot may form in the anterior chamber and over the pars plana.

Necrosis: dead cells swell and lose their cellular outlines and their nuclei shrink (pyknosis) or fragment

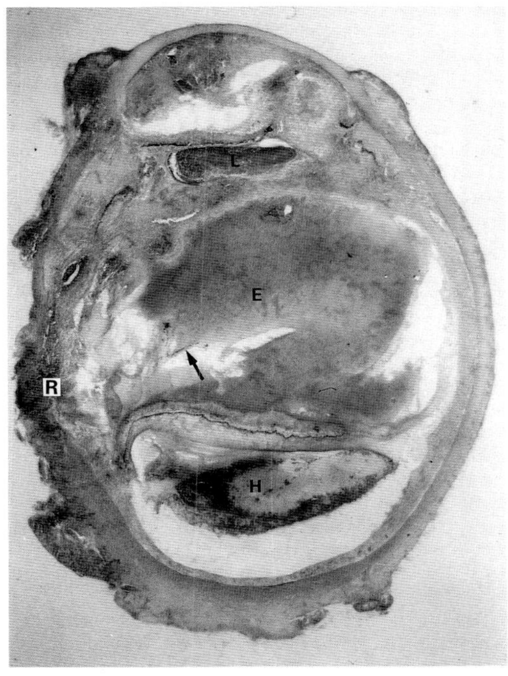

(a)

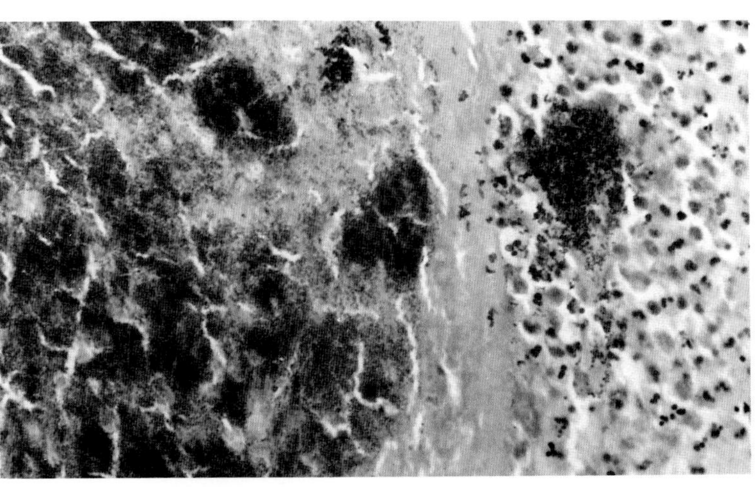

(b)

Fig. 2.1 Catastrophic metastatic suppurative endophthalmitis in a young male student in otherwise good health. (a) Low power view of the eye which is totally disorganised. There is a scleral rupture (R). The capsule of the lens (L) has burst and there is a subretinal haemorrhage (H). Although colonies of bacteria (arrow) could be seen in purulent exudate (E) in the vitreous space, no organisms were recovered in cultures. H & E section. (b) High power of the bacterial colonies in the exudate. H & E (×350).

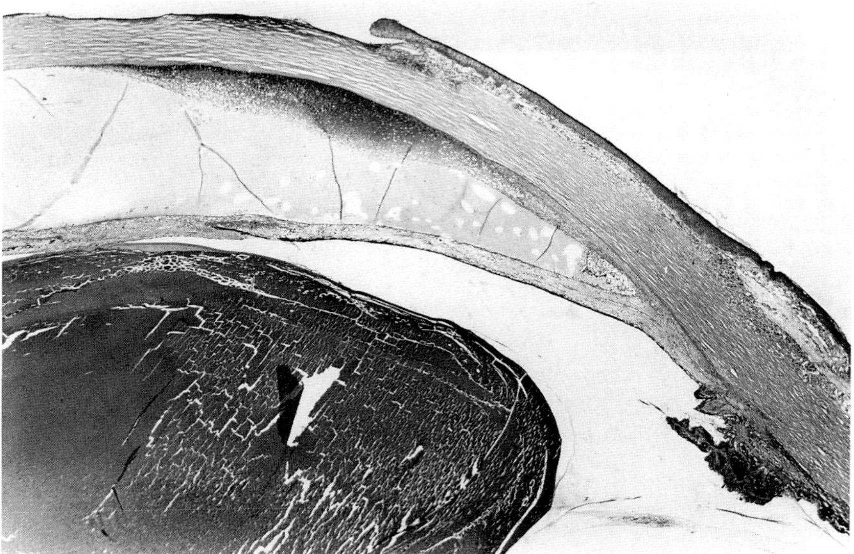

Fig. 2.2 Hypopyon ulcer in a case of end-stage neovascular glaucoma. Note the dense accumulation of pus cells in the anterior chamber posterior to the ulcer.

(karyorrhexis) and eventually disappear. Dead tissue thus appears swollen and eosinophilic. Pigment granules resist destruction, but become scattered and are taken up by macrophages. Toxins diffusing through the cornea may cause an area of central necrosis which is invaded by neutrophils to form a ring abscess which eventually perforates.

Healing stage

As the acute suppurative inflammation subsides, neutrophils are gradually replaced by mononuclear cells, i.e. monocytes, lymphocytes and plasma cells, and the inflammatory exudate in the ocular tissues and chambers commences to absorb or is organised by granulation tissue which is later converted to fibrous scar tissue. Such scarring may be augmented by organising blood clot and by granulation tissue entering the anterior segment from a healing corneal wound. If the inflammation has been confined to one segment of the globe, the less involved segment may return to some semblance of histological normality.

TUBERCULOSIS AND LEPROSY

Tuberculosis

In the older literature, tuberculosis figured as a common cause of intraocular inflammation and hypersensitivity to the tubercle bacillus was thought to play a key role. Nowadays, at least in the northern hemisphere, the incidence of tuberculosis has declined and few cases of endopthalmitis are attributed to it. Pathologically, it may take the form of a destructive granulomatous iritis, retinochoroiditis or miliary choroiditis.

Leprosy

Estimates of eye involvement in cases of leprosy vary greatly (from 20 to 90%). In the eye, the iris and ciliary body are affected by the lepromatous form of the disease which is characterised by massive granuloma formation. In this form, T-cells do not interact effectively with macrophages which have phagoctyosed bacteria so that microscopically giant cells laden with bacteria are seen.

SYPHILIS

Acquired syphilis: chronic or recurrent iridocyclitis or focal choroiditis may occur in secondary syphilis.

Congenital syphilis: may cause acute iridocyclitis, sometimes with associated interstitial keratitis.

Chorioretinal lesions attributable to congenital syphilis are often seen for the first time after the acute phase has passed. They take various forms from the 'pepper and salt' appearance of the fundus to large heavily pigmented or white atrophic areas.

FUNGAL ENDOPHTHALMITIS

The various modes of mycotic infection of the eye are as follows:

1 Exogenous:
   (i) From mycotic corneal ulcers (p. 48).
   (ii) Accidental or surgical trauma.
2 Endogenous:
   (i) Metastatic infections via the bloodstream.
   (ii) Infection spreading from neighbouring structures.

Metastatic infection

Endogenous oculmycosis is most commonly the result of infection by *Candida albicans* and most of the reported cases have been patients who have had recent abdominal surgery, intensive antibiotic treatment and prolonged intravenous catheterisation. *C. albicans* has been cultured from the tips of catheters and from the bloodstream of these patients. In other cases, the source of the fungus has been a primary asymptomatic focus of infection or a clinical infection in the genitourinary or respiratory tracts or in the skin.

Immunosuppressive regimes, diabetes, leukaemia, intravenous drug abuse and chronic debilitating diseases are other factors predisposing to candidial infection. The organisms most commonly lodge in the choroid or retina where they excite a mixed granulomatous and suppurative local inflammatory reaction which tends to spread inwards and give rise to small snowball abscesses in the vitreous. Early diagnosis, which offers a chance of recovery, depends on a high index of suspicion leading to the discovery of an extraocular focus of infection and isolation of the organism from blood cultures and aqeous aspirate.

Metastatic infection is less commonly due to other fungi, but is a recognised complication of aspergillosis (Fig. 2.3), blastomycosis, cryptococcosis and coccidiosis. In the Ohio and Mississipi river basins, choroiditis is sometimes attributed to infection with *Histoplasma capsulatum*, but the diagnosis is only presumptive, being based on the high incidence of pulmonary calcification and positive histoplasmin skin tests among affected individuals. Proven ocular involvement with *Histoplasma capsulatum* may take three forms: (1) disseminated histoplasmosis with retinal and/or uveal involvement; (2) solitary chorioretinal granuloma; and (3) the ocular histoplasmosis syndrome.

Accidental or surgical trauma

Mycotic vitreous abscesses are occasional late complications of accidental or surgical wounds (Chapter 18). Typically there is a latent period after injury varying from days to months before the onset of localised abscesses in the anterior vitreous or on the surface of the ciliary body; *Candida*, *Aspergillus* and *Cephalosporium* are among the many fungi that have been identified. The eye often retains good light projection for a long time. Antibiotic and steroid therapy induce rapid improvement, but this is followed within 2–3 weeks by progressive, painful endophthalmitis often necessitating enucleation.

Infection from neighbouring tissues

Orbitocerebral phycomycosis (mucormycosis) is a destructive inflammatory disease caused by *Mucor* or *Rhizopus* of the class Phycomycetes. These are saprophytic fungi found in soil, decaying food and necrotic tissue. Airborne spores invade and proliferate in the tissues of the nose and paranasal sinuses. Diabetic ketosis is the main predisposing cause, but infection may occur in other debilitating illnesses. From the initial focus, the organisms spread by venous channels to the brain and orbit. Invasion of the eye is thought to be directly through the sclera or via the internal carotid, ophthalmic or posterior ciliary arteries. The fungus, which forms thick, branching, non-septate hyphae measuring 3–12 μm in diameter, shows a tendency to invade the walls of blood vessels causing thrombosis and infarction and induces an acute necrotising panophthalmitis.

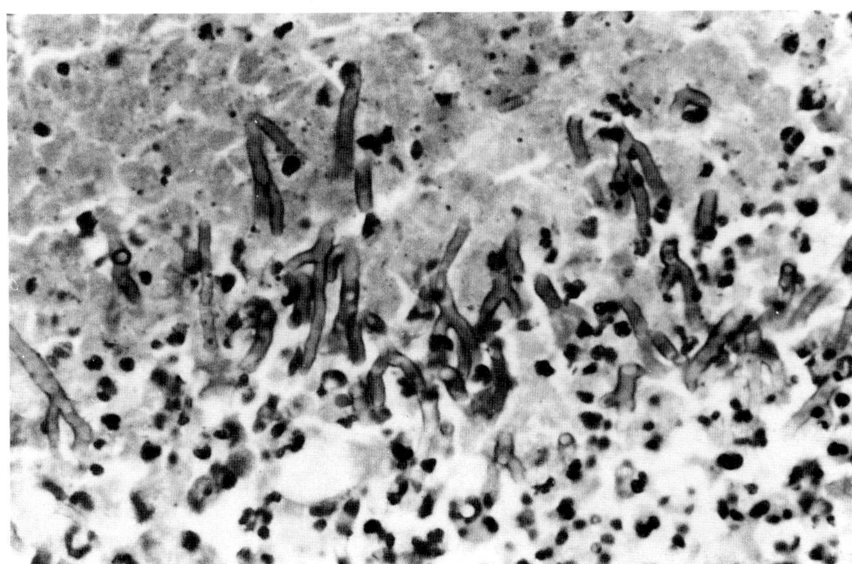

Fig. 2.3 Fungal filaments presumed to be *Aspergillus* in a vitreous abscess in a patient on prolonged treatment with steroids and antibiotics. H & E (×620).

CHAPTER 2

TOXOPLASMOSIS

Toxoplasmosis is due to infection with *Toxoplasma gondii*, a sporozoan belonging to the subclass Coccidia and thus closely related to the malarial parasite. *T. gondii* passes through sexual and asexual phases during its life cycle.

Life cycle

Sexual phase

The sexual phase takes place in the intestinal tract of domestic cats and certain wild felines such as leopards and ocelots, but not in other animals or birds. In this phase oocysts, which may remain infective for many months, are shed in the faeces. After ingestion by an intermediate host, the sporozoites break out of the oocysts, penetrate the gut wall and enter the host's cells wherein they develop into trophozoites and initiate the asexual phase.

Asexual phase

The asexual phase can occur in many species including birds, sheep, cattle, pigs, rodents, foxes, cats and humans. In man *T. gondii* is encountered in two principal forms:

1 *Trophozoites:* these are crescentic organisms approximately half the size of a red blood cell with a rounded posterior end containing the nucelus and a sharper anterior end occupied by an argyrophilic cone. Trophozoites are capable of parasitising any type of nucleated cell within which they multiply until they have filled the cytoplasm and pushed the nucleus aside to form a pseudocyst. This ruptures to release proliferative forms which disseminate via blood, lymph and CSF.

Free trophozoites are eliminated by macrophages. Macrophages can destroy the parasites only after they have been activated by T-lymphocytes. Surviving trophozoites become encysted. This is apparently related to antibody formation as it can be induced in tissue culture by the addition of antibody and complement. Cysts excite little if any tissue reaction and are resistant to pyremethamine and sulphonamide.

2 *Tissue cysts:* as immunity develops, extracellular parasites are destroyed by host defence mechanisms, but the intracellular parasites enclose themselves in a tough PAS-positive membrane (Fig. 2.4) within which they continue to multiply before becoming dormant. Tissue cysts are most abundant in brain, retina and muscles. They vary in size from 8 to 100 μm and contain anything from 4 to 60 000 proliferative-type parasites known as cystizoites.

Modes of infection

Toxoplasmosis is worldwide and the results of dye tests on normal populations indicate that infection without clinical disease is extremely common. It has been variously estimated to be responsible for from 25 to 70% of all cases of posterior uveitis.

Acquired infection

Infection is usually acquired by eating meat containing

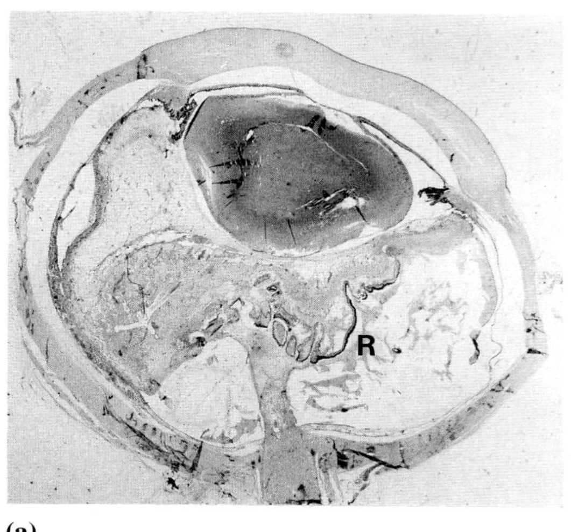

(a)

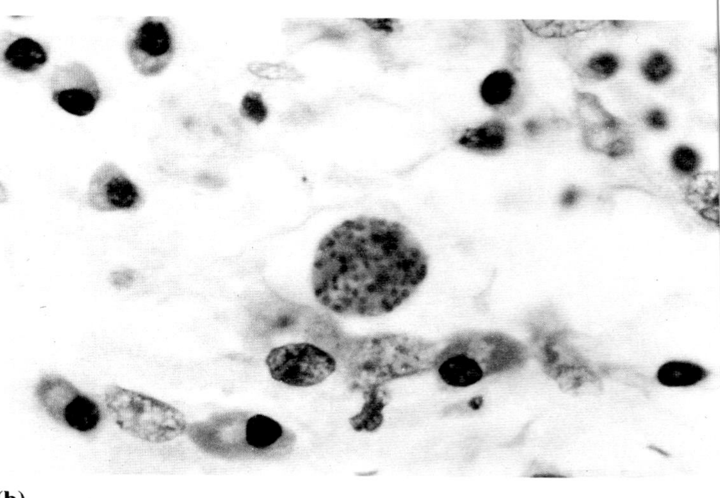

(b)

Fig. 2.4 Congenital toxoplasmosis in an infant of 22 days. (a) Low power showing retinal detachment with much of the retina (R) destroyed and replaced by inflammatory granulation tissue. (b) A small *Toxoplasma* cyst measuring approximately 15 μm in diameter lying in the inflammatory granulation tissue in a light infiltrate of plasma cells and lymphocytes. Nuclei of the parasites are seen as basophilic dots within the cyst, the thin wall of which is inconspicuous in this H & E preparation. (×900).

tissue cysts of *T. gondii*. The cysts are easily destroyed by cooking, smoking or salting. Infection may also result from accidental ingestion of oocysts.

Prenatal infection (congenital toxoplasmosis)

In most prenatal infections, the mother probably suffers her primary infection during pregnancy, although the infection is usually sub-clinical and escapes detection. The unborn child is infected from minute foci in the placenta which discharge toxoplasms into its circulation.

Toxoplasmosis acquired during pregnancy is transmitted to the foetus in approximately 40% of cases. Though the probability of transmission is greatest when the infection is acquired during the last trimester, foetal damage is less severe than when the infection is acquired earlier in pregnancy.

Systemic effects of toxoplasmosis

Prenatal infection (congenital toxoplasmosis)

1 Foetal death and abortion may occur, though toxoplasmosis is not a common cause of abortion.

2 A broad spectrum of disease can result including necrotising encephalitis and retinochoroiditis, lymphadenitis, myocarditis, pneumonitis and hepatitis.

Brain and retina are involved preferentially. Brain damage occurs in the subependymal region of the lateral ventricles and may result in hydrocephalus from blockage of the aqueduct. Glial scarring in the affected area is followed by calcification which is visible in X-rays as characteristic curvilinear streaks. The infant often dies in its first year from encephalitis, but may survive with variable residual cerebral and ocular damage.

3 In less severe infections, bilateral retinochoroiditis may be present at birth or develop during the first 6 months of life.

Postnatal infection

1 The brain and eyes are rarely affected in either children or adults.

2 Primary postnatal infection usually passes unnoticed.

3 Its commonest overt manifestation is a lymphadenopathy which may be febrile and simulate infectious mononucleosis. Sometimes the lymphadenopathy persists for months and malignant lymphoma may be suspected. Occasionally it may be complicated by meningo-encephalitis

4 Very occasionally, the disease presents a typhus-like picture.

5 The ocular manifestations which have occasionally been reported in association with systemic infections include retinochoroiditis, exudative retinitis, papillitis and optic atrophy.

Chronic toxoplasmosis

Chronic toxoplasmosis is predominantly an ocular disease affecting young people in the second and third decades.

Encysted parasites persist in the retina and possibly in brain, muscles and lymph nodes. Antibody is at a low stable level and hypersensitivity to intradermally injected toxoplasmin established.

The initial infection may have occurred many years previously, probably *in utero*, in most cases. There is a suspicion that reactivation of the infection can follow administration of steroids. Chronic toxoplasmosis exhibits two distinct ocular manifestations:

1 *Intermittent attacks:* multiple recurring self-limiting attacks of retinochoroiditis are probably due to the periodic release of trophozoites from dormant cysts. Hypersensitivity to toxoplasmic antigen may be a factor in inflammatory reaction seen in these attacks.

2 *Progressive disease:* in a minority of patients, chronic ocular toxoplasmosis is a progressive disease lasting many months with only minor remissions. In eyes enucleated because of intractable glaucoma, proliferative forms of the parasites have been found.

Toxoplasmosis in immunocompromised patients

Toxoplasmosis has long been recognised as an opportunistic infection of the central nervous system in immunosuppressed patients and fulminant retinochoroiditis has also been reported.

Histological changes in ocular toxoplasmosis

The histological changes depend on the immune state of the patient and the stage and severity of the infection. Characteristically the lesion is an acute circumscribed retinochoroidal ulceration located primarily in the macular area.

Toxoplasms entering the retina from the blood induce a necrotising inflammatory reaction resulting in the disintegration of neural and glial cells with dispersion of their nuclear fragments. The affected area is infiltrated by lymphocytes, macrophages, plasma cells and sometimes neutrophils. Though the local pigmented epithelium is partly destroyed, irregular proliferation occurs at the base of the ulcer. Inflammatory exudation into the vitreous occurs. Bruch's membrane is often breached and an intense granulomatous cellular infiltration of the choroid may develop in which giant cells and epithelioid cells can be seen, sometimes aggregated into pale nests.

The localised retinochoroidal inflammation may

spread into the sclera, episclera and iris thereby eventually resulting in secondary retinal detachment, cataract and secondary glaucoma. Subsequent secondary shrinkage may result in a small eye.

Parasites may be found in the necrotic retina, but not in the choroid. Because there is usually pyknotic nuclear debris present, free proliferative forms are difficult to recognise unless they chance to form a rosette due to incomplete separation of daughter cells after division. Pseudocysts and tissue cysts are seen as round or oval bodies of variable size, packed with small organisms whose nuclei appear as basophilic dots.

Pathogenesis

Though it is likely that release of free parasites from intraretinal cysts is the immediate cause of the inflammatory reaction, other factors may be involved because, in an animal model (Lee *et al.*, 1983), there is little evidence that the cysts provide the focus for the inflammatory reaction. The cysts are found predominantly in the inner retinal layers, particularly in Müller cells, while the cellular reaction is chiefly in the subretinal space, the uvea and around retinal vasculature (Dutton *et al.*, 1986, McMenamin *et al.*, 1986). There is also evidence of an immune reaction against the retina and this may be aggravated by non-specific tissue damage resulting from lysis of inflammatory cells (Dutton *et al.*, 1986).

Laboratory investigations

Isolation of parasites

1 *Acute infection:* the organism may be recovered from cerebrospinal fluid, aqueous or subretinal fluid, bone marrow, blood, saliva or minced biopsy material from lymph nodes, muscle liver or spleen by injection into mice into mouse brain or peritoneal cavity.
2 *Non-acute infection:* the chances of isolation from body fluids or tissue are less, but organism have been recovered from the blood and from enucleated eyes.

Immunological tests

1 *Dye test:* this measures the level of cytoplasm-modifying antibody in the patient's serum. The test system consists of:
(i) Mouse peritoneal exudate containing live toxoplasms.
(ii) Patient's serum.
(iii) Fresh normal human serum to provide accessory complement factor.
(iv) Methylene blue.

In the presence of cytoplasm-modifying antibody and accessory complement factor, the parasite's cytoplasm is modified so that it does not stain with methylene blue. The test is quantified by observing the highest dilution of serum in which 50% of the toxoplasms remain unstained. Although highly specific, the test is cumbersome and not without risk since live organisms are used.

Dye test antibody titres rise to a maximum during the 2 to 6 months after the primary infection. A titre of >1:16 is regarded as diagnostic. Lower titres do not exclude toxoplasmosis, though a negative result does. A rising titre in successive estimations is seen in systemic toxoplasmosis, but rarely during acute exacerbations of retinochoroiditis.
2 *Indirect fluorescent antibody test (IFAT):* smears of killed toxoplasms are exposed to the patient's serum, stained with a fluorescein-conjugated anti-human globulin and examined by fluorescence microscopy. The test can be quantified. The minimum significant titre is 1:8, values below this being regarded as negative. The IFAT correlates well with the dye test and has the advantage of being safer and simpler.

The IFAT has been modified to demonstrate IgM. In the absence of leakage, maternal IgM does not pass the placental barrier, so that the demonstration in the newborn of IgM antibody to toxplasma, especially in rising titre, provides useful evidence for the early diagnosis of congenital toxoplasmosis.
3 *Haemagglutination test:* soluble toxoplasmic antigen is coated onto red blood cells which are then exposed to the patient's serum. Agglutination occurs with positive sera. The responsible antibody appears later than those measured by the dye test and the IFAT and rises slowly to a maximum in the period of 6 to 14 months after infection.

Despite the availability of these serological tests, the diagnosis of ocular toxoplasmosis is often difficult. In the present state of knowledge, a positive serological test of any titre accompanying ocular disease compatible with toxoplasmosis points to a presumptive diagnosis in the absence of any other demonstrable pathology.

VIRUSES

Acquired immune deficiency syndrome

In the developed countries, infection by the human T-cell lymphotropic virus type 3 (HTLV III) has until recently been largely confined to haemophiliacs treated with contaminated Factor VIII, homosexuals and intravenous drug abusers. However, it now appears to be spreading to wider sections of the population. It infects T-helper cells and, to a lesser extent, macrophages and B-cells. The cellular immune response is thus severely compromised and the subject becomes susceptible to a range of opportunistic infective agents such as *Candida*, *Pneumocystis carinii*, *Cryptococcus*, *Mycobacterium avium* and cytomegalovirus.

Cotton wool spots are a common ocular manifestation and often the forerunner of cytomegalovirus infection. Kaposi's sarcoma involving the conjunctiva and eyelids is another important ocular manifestation.

Cytomegalovirus infection

In infants

Intrauterine infection by cytomegalovirus (CMV), a member of the herpes virus group, may result in choroidoretinitis associated with microcephaly or hydrocephalus and periventricular cerebral calcification. At birth, which is often premature, or shortly afterwards, these infants present with jaundice, purpura, anaemia, hepatosplenomegaly, pneumonitis and evidence of neural damage. Many survive and continue to excrete virus in the throat and urine for 2 to 3 years. Retinochoroiditis as the sole manifestation of CMV infection has been reported in neonates, but is rare.

In children up to the age of 5 years, a localised symptomless infection associated with virus inclusions in the salivary glands is quite frequent. In older children, cytomegalovirus infection may result in hepatosplenomegaly with abnormal liver function.

In adults

CMV retinochoroiditis in adults presents as white granular retinal patches with haemorrhages. It affects those who are immunocompromised by diseases such as leukaemia, malignant lymphoma, acquired immune deficiency syndrome or who are undergoing immunosuppressive therapy, particularly renal transplant patients.

The retina shows necrosis which is variable in extent, but involves all layers and is associated with haemorrhage, but little cellular reaction. The infected cell measures up to 40 μm in diameter and its enlarged nucleus contains a single dense basophilic ovoid aggregate of virus particle separated from the nuclear membrane by a clear halo (Fig. 2.5). The cytoplasm may contain basophilic particles.

The choroid may show diffuse granulomatous infiltration.

Laboratory diagnosis

1 *Isolation of virus:* the most reliable method of diagnosis is isolation of virus from blood. The virus has also been isolated from aqueous.

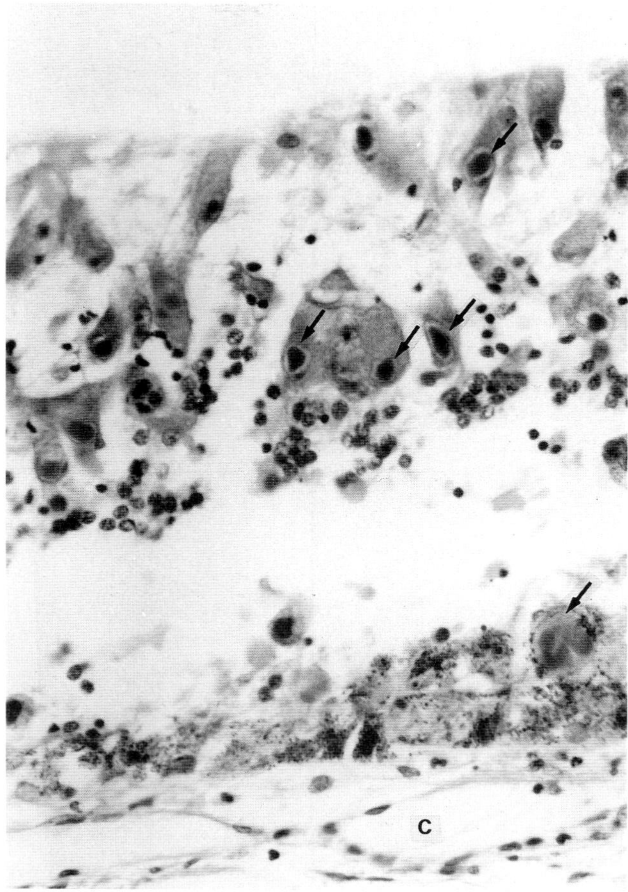

Fig. 2.5 Cytomegalovirus retinitis in a case that had been immunosuppressed following renal transplantation. Necrotic retina containing large cells with nuclei showing perinuclear haloes (arrows). The choroid (C) is not affected. H & E (×440). (Specimen by courtesy of Dr M. Filipic.)

2 *Virus inclusions:* characteristic virus inclusions may be found in the epithelial cells of urinary sediments. They are present in only 50% of neonatal cases and only rarely in older patients.

3 *Complement-fixation test:* the antibody status of an infant is of little help since many newborn babies posses maternal antibodies which are indicative only of maternal infection at some time in the past. A high titre of complement-fixing antibody in the mother or the isolation of virus from her is, however, strong evidence for congenital infection of her infant. In children aged from 6 months to 7 years, the demonstration of complement-fixing antibody almost invariably means active infection. Since 50% of people over the age of 25 years have complement-fixing antibody to CMV, only a rising titre during the course of an illness such as Paul–Bunnell-negative mononucleosis is indicative of infection.

4 *Retinal biopsy*: may provide confirmatory evidence.

Herpes simplex

Iridocyclitis is not uncommon in association with recurrent herpes simplex keratitis. This is manifected clinically by the appearance of 'mutton fat' precipitates on the cornea and Koeppe nodules on the iris. The inflammation may be due to viral infection of the iris and ciliary body. Virus has been recovered from cases with a massive exudative reaction. It is also likely that hypersensitivity plays a role. Atrophy of the iris stroma often follows recurrent attacks.

Herpes simplex virus has been demonstrated in the retina in a case of the acute retinal necrosis syndrome (Culbertson *et al.*, 1982) and antibodies to virus type 1 were found in intraocular fluids in three cases (Sarkies *et al.*, 1986). In this syndrome, an acute necrotising vitreoretinitis and vasculitis, which may be unilateral or bilateral, affects otherwise healthy patients (see Fisher *et al.*, 1982).

Herpes zoster

Iridocyclitis occurs in herpes zoster when the nasociliary division of the fifth cranial nerve is involved. It may be associated with corneal lesions. The occlusive vasculitis characteristic of the disease is seen not only in the iris, but also more remotely in vessels in the retina and sclera. It is not certain whether the vascular changes are a direct effect of the virus. Though possible virus particles have been seen (Witmer & Iwamoto, 1968), it is more likely that they represent a type 3 hypersensitivity reaction.

TOXOCARIASIS

Infestation by *Toxocara* is a comparatively uncommon cause of chronic endophthalmitis with retinal detachment or solitary retinal granulomata. The majority of cases occur between 3 and 13 years of age and over 90% between the ages of 3 and 9 years. The infestation is unilateral and boys and girls are equally affected. A history of contact with puppies is sometimes obtained. *Toxocara canis* is thought to be the principal cause of visceral larva migrans or larval granulomatosis in man.

Clinically, the ocular lesions may simulate Coats' disease, cyclitis, choroiditis, macular degeneration, organising retinal haemorrhage or retinoblastoma. Whenever such diagnoses are entertained, *Toxocara* infestation must be considered.

Life cycle

The nematode *Toxocara* of the family Ascaridae (to which *Ascaris lumbricoides* also belongs) is one of the commonest intestinal parasites of dogs (*T. canis*) and cats (*T. cati*) and is particularly prevalent in puppies during their first 6 months of life. Its distribution is worldwide.

Adult toxocaral worms are 7.5–12.5 cm in length. They live in the intestines of dogs, especially puppies, or cats and shed ova containing first stage larvae in the faeces which when ingested liberate second stage larvae. These larvae, which measure about 400 μm in length and are 20 μm in diameter, penetrate the intestinal wall and spread via liver and lungs.

1 In *adult dogs*, infection may be derived from three possible sources:

(i) Eggs.

(ii) Infected meat from rats, mice, rabbits, etc., containing second stage larvae.

(iii) First and second stage larvae passed in puppy faeces.

Maturation does not proceed beyond the larval stage in adult dogs. The larvae become dormant or encysted and, when the bitch becomes pregnant, they are activated and cross the placenta to cause a prenatal infection of the puppies.

2 In *puppies*, after birth, the larvae migrate to the lungs and are coughed up and swallowed. In the puppy's intestine they mature within 3 weeks, thus completing the life cycle. Ova are then shed in vast numbers in the faeces. One adult worm may shed 200 000 per day.

3 In the *cat*, prenatal infection does not occur. Infection is commonly due to ingestion of eggs or larvae contained in tissues and the complete life cycle takes place in the adult cat.

4 In *intermediate hosts* such as man and a wide variety of other animals including rats, rabbits, mice and monkeys, maturation does not proceed beyond the larval stage. The larvae are disseminated via the liver and lungs to reach the tissues where they can remain infective for considerable periods.

Infestation in man

Infection is by ingestion of ova. Obviously poor hygiene and close contact with infested puppies is likely to increase the risk greatly. However, nearly 25% of soil samples taken from public parks over a wide area in Great Britain showed contamination with viable ova. The ova remain viable in the soil for years.

Heavy infection may give rise to a transitory febrile illness — visceral larval granulomatosis — a disease of childhood characterised by eosinophilia, hypergammaglobulinaemia, pulmonary infiltrations, hepatomegaly and encephalopathy. However, infection is usually asymptomatic.

The larvae may enter the eye directly or may encyst in the tissues to become reactivated later. Entry to the eye may be via the choroidal, ciliary or central retinal arteries.

Ocular lesions

The clinical and pathological manifestations are due to the inflammatory reaction to the larva when it becomes lodged in the eye and dies. There are three common sites where this occurs:

1 *In the anterior vitreous* where organisation of the inflammatory tissue may lead to the formation of a retinal fold, traction on the macula and retinal detachment. The larva or its remains may be found in this inflammatory tissue surrounded by eosinophils, epithelioid cells, foreign body giant cells and scar tissue (Fig. 2.6).

2 *Intraretinally at the ora serrata* with variable extension of the inflammatory exudate into the adjacent vitreous. In such cases, the first intimation of infection may be the sudden appearance of a hypopyon. The histological picture is similar that described above except that the lesion is more circumscribed.

3 *Intraretinally at the posterior pole*. These fundal granulomas are typically raised white circumscribed solitary masses at the posterior pole on the temporal side. Sometimes they exhibit claw-like extensions over the surrounding retina. Papillitis due to a granuloma in the nerve head has also occurred. The following signs may assist the clinical diagnosis:

(i) An ophthalmoscopically visible darker crescentic area in the granuloma indicating the position of the

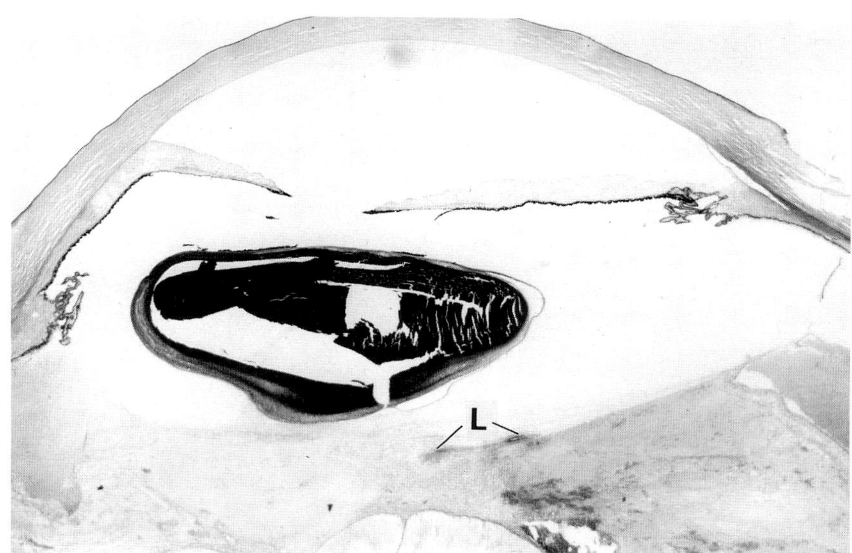

Fig. 2.6 *Toxocara* larva in vitreous of boy aged 6. (a) Low power view showing fibrosis in the vitreous around the larval track (L) which has caused a retinal detachment.

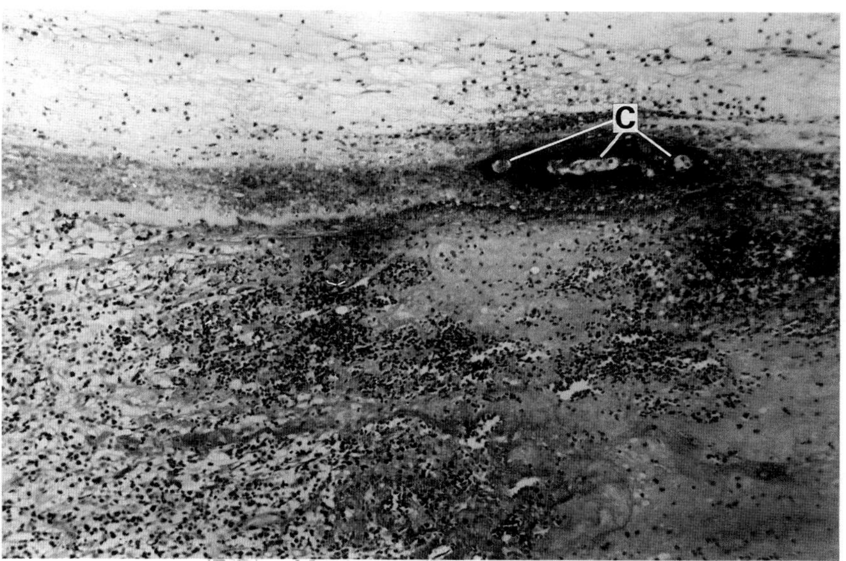

Fig. 2.6 (b) Higher power of the larval track showing chitinous remnants (C). The inflammatory cells round the track are mostly eosinophils. H & E (×95).

larva. When scar formation is minimal, the larval outline may be clearly visible.

(ii) The absence of visible cholesterol deposits in the granuloma in contrast to Coats' disease in which they are a characteristic feature.

(iii) Radiologically detectable calcification in the globe is uncommon, though not unknown, in toxocariasis in contrast to retinoblastomas in which it is a frequent finding (75% of cases).

Microscopically these retinal granulomata consist mainly of scar tissue in which the dead larva is embedded. A variable infiltrate of eosinophils, lymphocytes, plasma cells and foreign body giant cells is present. The mass causes puckering of the adjacent retina and may protrude into the vitreous. It is often firmly adherent to Bruch's membrane. Sometimes it lies almost entirely behind the retina. The subjacent choroid exhibits a localised chronic inflammatory infiltration and eosinophilia. The remainder of the eye appears largely unaffected histologically.

Laboratory diagnosis

Microscopical identification of larva

The diagnosis can be established firmly, if rather late, by demonstrating the second stage larva in sections of the eye after enucleation. This may be a laborious process involving cutting and examining hundreds of serial sections. The larva is recognised in H & E sections by its pale glassy cuticle and small densely stained nuclei which are much smaller than the nuclei of human cells. In cross-section at the level of the mid-gut, the larva shows sharp lateral infoldings of the cuticle, the lateral alae, and an intestine without lumen compressed by two large, non-nucleated granular posterior excretory columns.

Eosinophilia

An increase of eosinophils in peripheral blood in excess of the normal 400 per μl.

Immunological tests

A major problem with these tests has been cross-reactivity to other ascarids, especially *Ascaris lumbricoides*.

1 *The skin test* consists of the intradermal injection of 0.1 ml of saline extract of whole *T. canis*. In sensitised patients, this produces an immediate allergic reaction mediated by IgE and resulting in histamine release and weal formation. The false positive rate is about 2%.

2 *Indirect fluorescent antibody test*: in this test, partially digested *T. canis* larvae are exposed to the test serum and binding of antibody to the cuticle demonstrated by fluorescein-conjugated anti-human globulin. The test can be made more specific by absorbing the test serum with *A. lumbricoides* antigen. While a positive skin test is usually associated with a positive IFAT, the converse is not always true. Thus one in five patients with negative skin tests may be expected to give a positive IFAT.

3 *The enzyme-linked immunoabsorbent assay (ELISA) test*: second stage larval secretory antigen obtained from *in vitro* culture is used in this test. The test is reliable, highly specific and economical in antigen. Unfortunately, the technique does not lend itself to small-scale routine diagnostic use.

BIBLIOGRAPHY

General

Kraus-Mackiw, E. & O'Connor, G. R. , eds (1983) *Uveitis. Patho-Physiology and Therapy*. Thieme Stratton, New York & George Thieme, Stuttgart.

Mycotic infections

Cogan, D. G. (1959) Endogenous intraocular fungous infection. Report of a case. *Archives of Ophthalmology* **42**, 666–682.

Cushman, A. R., Friedman, G. & Capsavage, J. (1976) Systemic candidiasis and endophthalmitis in neurosurgical patients. Report of three cases. *Journal of Neurosurgery* **45**, 95–97.

Doft, B. H., Clarkson, J. G., Rebell, G. & Forster, R. K. (1980) Endogenous Aspergillus endophthalmitis in drug abusers. *Archives of Ophthalmology* **98**, 859–862.

Elliot, J. H., O'Day, D. M., Gutow, G. S., Podgorski, S. F. & Akrabawi, P. (1979) Mycotic endophthalmitis in drug abusers. *American Journal of Ophthalmology* **88**, 66–72.

Feman, S. S., Podgorski, S. F. & Penn, M. K. (1982) Blindness from presumed ocular histoplasmosis in Tennessee. *Ophthalmology* **89**, 1295–1298.

Litricin, O. (1979) Endogenous fungal endophthalmitis (probably Aspergillus). *Ophthalmologica* **179**, 42–47.

Naidoff, M. A. & Green, W. R. (1975) Endogenous Aspergillus endophthalmitis occurring after kidney transplant. *American Journal of Ophthalmology* **79**, 502–509.

Paradis, A. J. & Roberts, L. (1963) Endogenous ocular Aspergillosis. *Archives of Ophthalmology* **69**, 765–769. (Report of a case in an infant with cytomegalic inclusion disease.)

Rippon, J. W. (1982) Mycotic infections of the eye and ear. In *Medical Mycology*, by J. W. Rippon, pp 682–698. W. B. Saunders & Co., Philadelphia.

Scholz, R., Green, W. R., Kutys, R., Sutherland, J. & Richards, R. D. (1984) Histoplasma capsulatum in the eye. *Ophthalmology* **91**, 100–1104.

Servant, J. B., Dutton, G. N., Ong-Tone, L., Barrie, T. & Davey, C. (1985) Candidal endophthalmitis in Glaswegian heroin addicts: report of an epidemic. *Transactions of the Ophthalmological Societies of the UK* **104**, 297–308.

Toxoplasmosis

Akstein, R. B., Wilson, L. A. & Teutsch, S. M. (1982) Acquired toxoplasmosis. *Ophthalmology* **89**, 1299–1302.

Dutton, G. N. (1986) The causes of tissue damage in toxoplasmic retinochoroiditis. *Transactions of the Ophthalmological Society of the UK* **105**, 404–412.

Dutton, G. N., McMenamin, P. G., Hay, J. & Cameron, S. (1986) The ultrastructural pathology of congenital murine toxoplasmic retinochoroiditis. Part II: the morphology of the inflammatory changes. *Experimental Eye Research* **43**, 545–560.

Karim, K. A. & Ludlow, G. B. (1975) The relationship and significance of antibody titres as determined by various serological methods in glandular and ocular toxoplasmosis. *Journal of Clinical Pathology* **28**, 42–49.

Lee, W. R., Hay, J., Hutchison, W. M., Dutton, G. N. & Sim, J. C. (1983) A murine model of congenital toxoplasmosis. *Acta Ophthalmologica* **61**, 818–830.

McMenamin, P. G., Dutton, G. N., Hay, J. & Cameron, S. (1986) The ultrastructural pathology of congenital murine toxoplasmosis. Part I: the localization of *Toxoplasma* cysts in the retina. *Experimental Eye Research* **43**, 529–543.

Perkins, E. S. (1973) Ocular toxoplasmosis. *British Journal of Ophthalmology* **57**, 1–17.

Rothova, A., Van Knapen, F., Baarsma, G. S., Kruit, P. J., Loewer-Sieger, D. H. & Kijlstra, A. (1986) Serology in ocular toxoplasmosis. *British Journal of Ophthalmology* **70**, 615–622.

Scott, E. H. (1974) Toxoplasmosis. *Survey of Ophthalmology* **18**, 255–274.

Shimada, K., O'Connor, G. R. & Yoneda, C. (1974) Cyst formation by *Toxoplasma gondii* (RH strain) *in vitro*. *Archives of Ophthalmology* **92**, 496–500.

Yeo, J. H., Jakobiec, F. A., Iwamoto, T., Richard, G. & Kreissig, I. (1983) Toxoplasmic retinochoroiditis following chemotherapy for systemic lymphoma. *Ophthalmology* **90**, 885–898.

Virus infections

Aaberg, T. M., Cesarz, T. J. & Rytel, M. W. (1972) Correlation of virology and clinical course of cytomegalovirus retinitis. *American Journal of Ophthalmology* **74**, 407–415.

Culbertson, W. W., Blumenkranz, M. S., Haines, H., Gass, J. D. M., Mitchell, K. B. & Norton, E. W. D. (1982) The acute retinal necrosis syndrome. Part 2. *Ophthalmology* **89**, 1317–1325.

de Venecia, G., Zu Rhein, G. M., Pratt, M. V. & Kisken, W. (1971) Cytomegalic inclusion disease in an adult. *Archives of Ophthalmology* **86**, 44–57.

Fisher, J. P., Lewis, M. L., Blumenkrantz, M., Culbertson, W., Flynn, H. W., Clarkson, J. G., Gass, J. D. M. & Norton, E. W. D. (1982) The acute retinal necrosis syndrome. Part 1: clinical manifestations. *Ophthalmology* **89**, 1309–1316.

Friedman, A. H. (1984) The retinal lesions of the acquired immune deficiency syndrome. *Transactions of the American Ophthalmological Society* **82**, 447–488.

Holland, G. N., Pepose, J. S., Pettit, T. H., Gottlieb, M. S., Yee, R. D. & Foos, R. Y. (1983) Acquired immune deficiency syndrome, ocular manifestations. *Ophthalmology* **90**, 859–873.

Humphry, R. C., Parkin, J. M. & Marsh, R. J. (1986) The ophthalmological features of AIDS and AIDS related disorders. *Transactions of the Ophthalmological Society of the UK* **105**, 505–509.

Palestine, A. G., Rodrigues, M. M., Macher, A. M., Chan, C-C., Lane, C., Fauci, A. S., Masur, H., Longo, D., Reichert, C. M., Steis, R., Rook, A. H. & Nussenblatt, R. B. (1984) Ophthalmic involvement in acquired immune deficiency syndrome. *Ophthalmology* **91**, 1092–1099.

Rodrigues, M. M. (1983) Multicentric Kaposi's sarcoma of the conjunctiva in a male homosexual with the acquired immunodeficiency syndrome. *Ophthalmology* **90**, 879–884.

Rosenberg, P. R., Uliss, A. E., Friedland, G. H., Harris, C. A., Small, C. B. & Klein, R. S. (1983) Acquired immunodeficiency syndrome. Ophthalmic manifestations in ambulatory patients. *Ophthalmology* **90**, 874–878.

Sarkies, N., Gregor, Z., Forsey, T. & Darougar, S. (1986) Antibodies to herpes simplex virus type I in intraocular fluids of patients with acute retinal necrosis. *British Journal of Ophthalmology* **70**, 81–84.

Smith, M. E., Zimmerman, L. E. & Harley, R. D. (1966) Ocular involvement in congenital cytomegalic inclusion disease. *Archives of Ophthalmology* **76**, 696–699.

Tsukahara, I., Veno, I. & Kawaniski, H. (1966) Retinal changes in human cytomegalovirus infection. An electron microscopic study. *American Journal of Ophthalmology* **62**, 1153–1160.

Witmer, R. & Iwamoto, T. (1968) Electronmicroscopic observation of herpes-like particles in the iris. *Archives of Ophthalmology* **79**, 331–337.

Toxocariasis

Borg, O. A. & Woodruff, A. W. (1973) Prevalence of infective ova of the toxocara species in public places. *British Medical Journal* **ii**, 470–472.

de Savigny, D. H., Voller, A. & Woodruff, A. W. (1979) Toxocariasis: serological diagnosis by enzyme immunoassay. *Journal of Clinical Pathology* **32**, 284–288.

Molk, R. (1983) Ocular toxocariasis: a review of the literature. *Annals of Ophthalmology* 216–231.

Woodruff, W. A. (1970) Toxocariasis. *British Medical Journal* **ii**, 663–669.

Chapter 3 Idiopathic intraocular inflammation

INTRODUCTION

The inflammatory diseases of the eye to be described in this chapter are a somewhat heterogeneous mixture in which, however, the uvea is the principal seat of an inflammatory process. No cause is usually demonstrable and not infrequently the process is a local manifestation of systemic disease. The inflammation is non-suppurative and usually non-granulomatous, though sarcoid uveitis is a notable exception to this generalisation. In the majority of cases not linked to systemic disease, no cause for the inflammation is demonstrable.

For this group of eye diseases, the term 'uveitis' has been in use for many years and will, no doubt, continue to be used for many more. However, the inflammation is seldom confined to the uveal tract and, in some ways, the term endophthalmitis would be preferable. The term panophthalmitis would be reserved for the rare cases wherein the inflammatory process extends beyond the sclera to involve Tenon's capsule and the orbital tissues.

According to its localisation, uveitis may sub-divided into:

1 Anterior uveitis (iritis, iridocyclitis)
2 Intermediate uveitis (pars planitis, cyclitis)
3 Posterior uveitis (choroiditis)
4 Pan-uveitis

HISTOPATHOLOGICAL CHANGES

The histopathological changes are, in general, of a non-specific character and the resulting picture depends on the severity and duration of the inflammatory process and its principal location within the eye. Tissue destruction is usually less severe than in suppurative inflammation and the inflammatory cells are predominantly lymphocytes, plasma cells and monocytes. Macrophages are less numerous than in typically granulomatous inflammatory exudates while epithelioid and giant cells are seldom seen. The histological features may be resolved into the following components.

Plasmoid exudate

Vaso-dilatation with exudation of protein-rich exudate into the uveal stroma, the ocular chambers and the vitreous is characteristic. The intra-cameral fluids appear eosinophilic in tissue sections and are described as 'plasmoid'. The fluid often contains fibrinogen which clots to form visible fibrin networks.

Cellular infiltrate

This is seen more or less widely distributed throughout the ocular tissues:

In the uvea the infiltrate is predominantly of lymphocytes with a variable admixture of plasma cells (Fig. 3.1a). It is usually light and diffuse with local aggregations in places. Russell bodies are often numerous. Sometimes the infiltrate extends into the scleral vascular channels.

In the retina cuffs of lymphocytes form round the venules and clumps become attached to the internal limiting membrane.

In the vitreous cells may be sprinkled diffusely as well as accumulating over the surface of the ciliary body.

In the anterior chamber lymphocytes form small keratic precipitates and are also found in the trabecular meshwork. Even when the principal location of the inflammation is posterior, inflammatory cells in the anterior chamber are a common feature.

Granulation tissue

Mild inflammation often leaves only focal scars at the site of primary tissue damage. In more severe and protracted inflammation, however, and especially after frequent recurrences, healing by granulation tissue occurs and results in the formation of synechiae, pupillary and cyclitic membranes and chorioretinal adhesions as described below.

In the anterior and posterior chambers exudate is organised by fibroblasts and new vessels from the iris stroma (Fig. 3.1b). This results in adhesions forming between the periphery of the iris and the cornea (anterior peripheral synechiae) and between the pupillary border of the iris and the lens (posterior synechiae) (Fig. 3.2). Organisation along the iris surface forms a fibrovascular membrane which may extend across the pupil and completely seal it. Occasionally the corneal endothelium migrates over the membrane and lays down a new hyaline layer continuous with Desçemet's membrane. Destruction of iris pigmented epithelium releases melanin granules which are carried by macrophages into the iris stroma and to the trabecular meshwork and Schlemm's canal. In severe cases, the resulting fibrosis may obliterate the anterior chamber and the iris and lens become incarcerated in a massive scar. Such a result is, however, more likely to follow a suppurative process.

In the anterior vitreous exudate and haemorrhage are organised by fibroblasts and vessels from the ciliary body, especially the pars plana. A transocular fibrovascular retrolental diaphragm (cyclitic membrane) is thus formed in the anterior vitreous face. This membrane ultimately becomes fibrous and drags the ciliary body and its processes inwards. The ciliary body becomes detached from the sclera except at the scleral spur and traction on the peripheral retina detaches and draws the whole retina forwards.

The ciliary epithelium and and the retinal pigmented epithelium often proliferate into a cyclitic membrane to form elongated pigment strands and tubules. The ciliary processes become shrunken and fibrotic and their vessels obliterated. Aqueous secretion is thus reduced.

In the posterior vitreous exudate and haemorrhage are organised from the nerve head and adjacent retina. Vessels from the latter contribute conspicuous new capillaries (retinitis proliferans).

Large subretinal inflammatory exudates are probably organised mainly by fibroblasts and vessels growing in from the choroid through breaks in Bruch's membrane. The retinal glia plays little if any part, although it may proliferate within the retinal boundaries to take the place

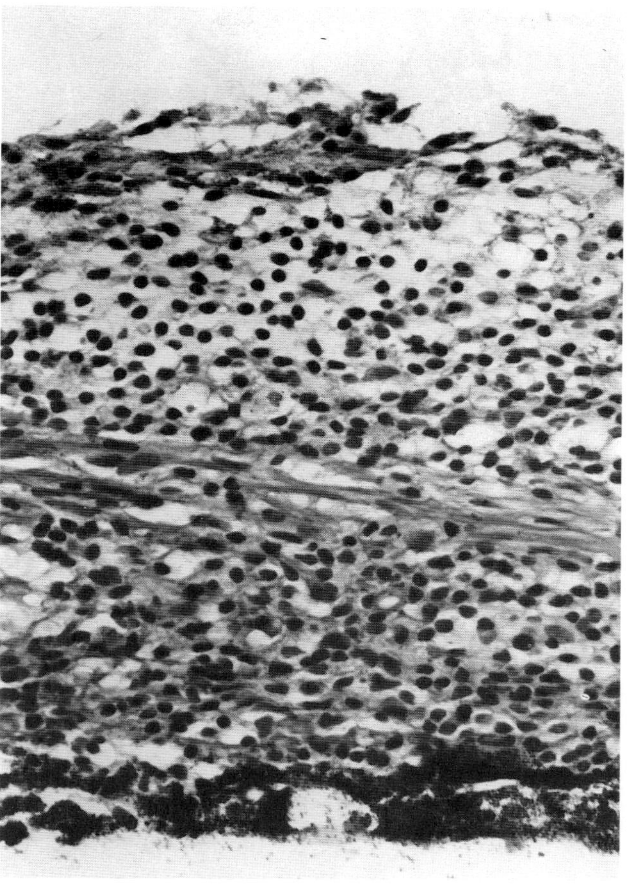

Fig. 3.1 Anterior uveitis. (a) Dense infiltrate of lymphocytes together with some plasma cells in iris stroma. H & E (×440).

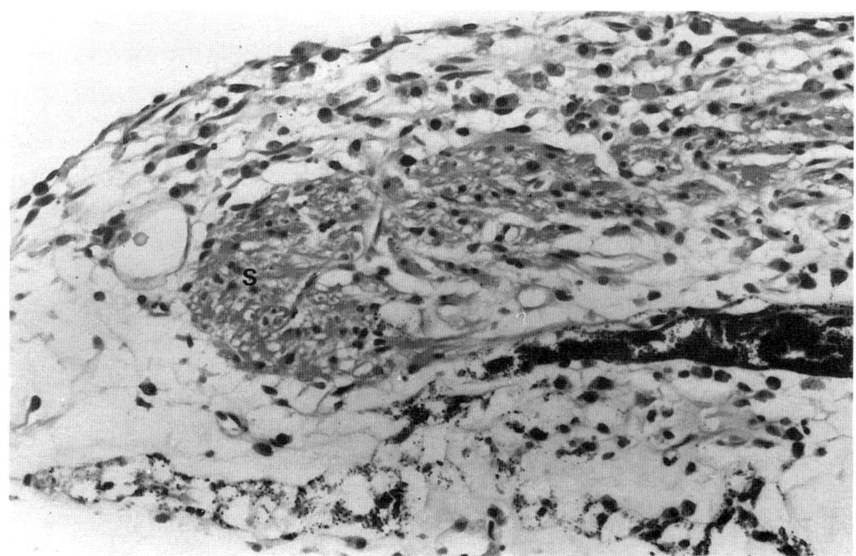

Fig. 3.1 (b) Granulation tissue forming around sphincter pupillae (S). H & E (×410).

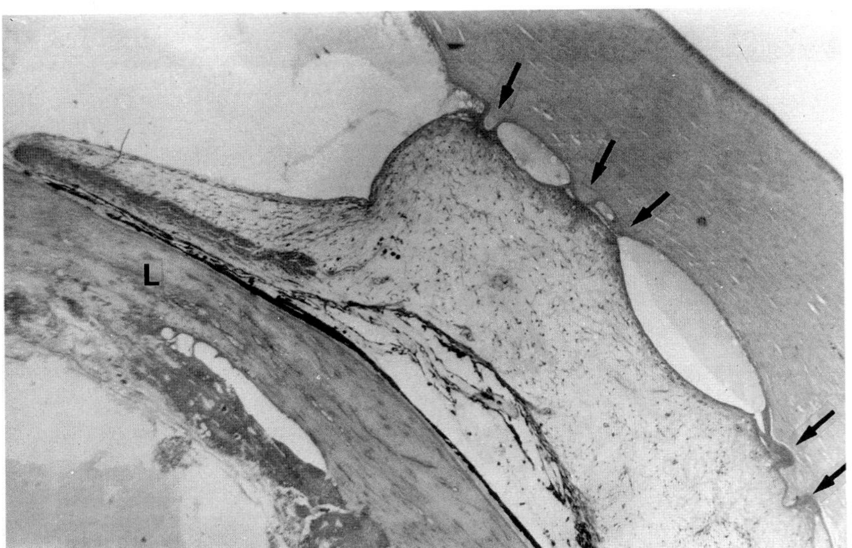

Fig. 3.2 Old case of anterior uveitis due to Behçet's disease showing numerous anterior synechiae (arrows). The pupillary border is also firmly bound down to the lens (L) over a wide area. Masson's trichrome.

of dead neural cells (diffuse retinal gliosis). The retinal pigment epithelium does, however, participate by proliferating and laying down basement membrane material. In this way, nodules and plaques of alternating lamellae of hyalinised fibrous tissue and cells of the pigmented epithelium are formed.

In time, the scarred choroid and subretinal tissue may become indistinguishably fused. After many years, ossification occurs in this composite layer and may extend forwards into the cyclitic membrane. The bone so formed may contain fat or even haemopoietic marrow in its interstices.

Localised areas of chorioretinitis result in focal necrosis of visual cells, pigmented epithelium and choroidal stroma, together with limited local subretinal exudate. The resulting fibroglial scars, which seal the retina to Bruch's membrane and the choroid, are often rimmed by proliferating cells from the pigmented epithelium. Sometimes pigment rodlets released from necrotic pigmented epithelial cells are taken up by macrophages which subsequently migrate along blood vessels where they are seen as black spidery figures.

SEQUELAE

Glaucoma and hypotony

If, as a result of adhesions in the filtration angle or in the pupil, the flow and drainage of aqueous are impeded, secondary glaucoma may ensue. On the other hand, hypotony may result from diminution of aqueous secretion as a result of disorganisation of the ciliary body. Contraction of the intraocular fibrous tissue in such soft eyes eventually results in shrinkage of the globe.

Miscellaneous changes

Among the many interesting but not very important late degenerative changes seen in sections of atrophic post-inflammatory eyes are:

1 Band degeneration of the cornea (Chapter 5).

2 Spherical or placoid, granular or hyaline excrescences formed on Bruch's membrane by the retinal pigmented epithelium (drüsen).

3 Large masses of coarse glia at the ora serrata.

4 Siderocalcific impregnation of the retinal capillaries renders them unnaturally conspicuous and they have, indeed, been mistaken for fungal hyphae.

ANTERIOR UVEITIS

Anterior uveitis may occur:

1 As a secondary reaction to inflammation or injury to the cornea.

2 In the absence of any obvious predisposing factors.

3 In association with a number of systemic diseases.

The disease may take acute, subacute chronic or recurrent forms and involve the iris or iris and ciliary body. Even in the acute form the inflammatory infiltrate is of the type described above. Most cases fall into the second category in which the cause of the inflammatory process eludes discovery. The systemic diseases in which uveitis is a regular occurrence are also mainly conditions wherein the precise pathogenesis remains uncertain.

There is a striking correlation between anterior uveitis and associated syndromes and certain HLA antigens as is shown in Table 3.1. It must, however, be stressed that while, for example, an individual positive for B27 is 100 times more likely to get ankylosing spondylitis than a

Table 3.1 HLA associations of anterior uveitis and related syndromes (from Rahi, 1979).

Disease	Antigen	Frequency percentage: Patients	Frequency percentage: Controls	Relative risk
Acute anterior uveitis	HLA B27	43	7	10
Behçet's disease	HLA B5	60	28	4
Ankylosing spondylitis	HLA B27	90	8	103
Reiter's disease	HLA B27	80	9	40
Rheumatoid arthritis	HLA DRw4	56	15	7
	HLA Dw4	60	12	11

$$\text{Relative risk} = \frac{\%\text{HLA +ve patients}}{\%\text{HLA +ve controls}} \times \frac{\%\text{HLA −ve controls}}{\%\text{HLA −ve patients}}$$

Antigens whose separate identity remains debatable are called w (workshop).

negative individual, the great majority of positive individuals will not get the disease.

Exhaustive immunological studies have been carried out on this group of diseases. These relate mainly to:

1 Levels of immune complexes, immunoglobulins and specific antibodies in aqueous fluid and serum.

2 Lymphocyte sub-populations in such fluids.

3 Isolation of organisms such as *Chlamydia*, *Klebsiella*, *Salmonella* and *Yersinia* which may be implicated in certain types.

Unfortunately, no firm conclusions can yet be drawn. Indeed, the comment by Rahi *et al.* (1976) that 'there appears to be an apparent analogy between uveitis and the legendary Hydra who is reputed to grow four heads when one head is cut off' is still pertinent today.

Ankylosing spondylitis

This is mainly a disease of males aged between 15 and 40 in whom arthritis of rheumatoid type spreads upwards from the sacro-iliac joints to involve those of the spine.

Uveitis occurs in 13–25% of cases and may be the presenting manifestation. It takes the form of an acute recurrent iridocyclitis, the severity of which is unrelated to the severity of the disease in the back.

Cross-reactivity between some strains of *Klebsiella pneumoniae* and the B-27 receptor on lymphocytes of patients with ankylosing spondylitis has been established (see O'Connor, 1983a & b). The disease may thus be an example of molecular mimicry (Chapter 1). However, the role of *Klebsiella* in the pathogenesis remains uncertain (see Beckingsale *et al.*, 1984; Kijlstra *et al.*, 1986).

Reiter's syndrome

This term is used to describe a complex consisting of:

1 Genital infection: acute, often purulent non-gonococcal urethritis is an integral part of the disease and usually precedes the other manifestations. It is often followed by chronic prostatovesiculitis which is invariably present in chronic relapsing cases.

2 Non-suppurative chronic or subacute arthritis principally in the joints of the lower limbs. Concomitant ankylosing spondylitis is uncommon, but sacro-iliac arthritis occurs in approximately 25% of cases and such cases are prone to develop iritis, plantar fasciitis and periostitis of the os calcis.

3 Conjunctivitis and uveitis: the conjunctivitis may be purulent, but papillary or follicular conjunctivitis and superficial punctate keratitis with superficial stromal infiltrates also occur. Iridocyclitis closely resembling that seen in association with ankylosing spondylitis develops in a minority of cases.

The eye manifestations tend to follow a chlamydial urethritis or dysentery caused by *Salmonella* or *Yersinia*. *Chlamydia* may be isolated from the conjunctiva and stools, and *Salmonella* and *Yersinia* from the stools. Antibodies to *Chlamydia* may also be demonstrated by microimmunofluorescence. These micro-organisms presumably act only as a trigger mechanism because the disease progresses long after they have been eliminated. However, evidence of their presence at some stage may be diagnostically useful (see O'Connor, 1983a). There is also a possibility that immune complexes play a role in the disease (see Char *et al.*, 1979), but the antigenic part of the complex has not been categorised.

Psoriasis

Cases of psoriasis often also suffer from ankylosing spondylitis and, in such cases, iridocyclitis resembling that seen in ankylosing spondylitis frequently occurs. In addition to the iridocyclitis, there may be elevated peripheral corneal infiltrates. Immune complex deposition is also likely to be a mechanism in the pathogenesis of the iridocyclitis and arthritis complicating this disease.

Ulcerative colitis

About 10% of patients with ulcerative colitis may develop anterior uveitis or episcleritis. Cases in which there is sacro-iliitis are especially likely to develop uveitis. By contrast with ankylosing spondylitis, however, it is older women who are predominantly affected.

Juvenile rheumatoid arthritis

While uveitis rarely occurs in adult rheumatoid arthritis unless the sclera or cornea are affected, iridocyclitis may complicate the juvenile form. Two types of iridocyclitis have been recognised:

1 Chronic iridocyclitis affecting mainly young girls with pauciarticular disease.

2 Acute iridocyclitis affecting mainly boys with multiple involvement of the joints.

In the majority of the few chronic cases that have been examined, there was a dense infiltrate of plasma cells in the iris and ciliary body in which giant cells were present. Concomitant secondary changes affected other parts of the globe (see Merriam *et al.*, 1983).

Behçet's disease

Behçet's disease affects males more commonly than females. Onset is usually in the third decade. The principal systemic features are recurrent ulceration of the mouth and external genitalia. The gut and central nervous system may also be involved. The disease is rare in Europe, but common in countries bordering the eastern Mediterranean and in the Far East. This is probably related to the distribution of HLA B5.

Ocular involvement in the form of a recurrent iridocyclitis usually occurs later than the systemic manifestations. One or both eyes may be affected. Onset is often acute, sometimes with a hypopyon which resolves within hours. Later the disease may be complicated by retinal vasculitis, vitreous haemorrhage and optic atrophy.

Current thought is that Behçet's disease is another example of an immune complex mediated disease. Circulating immune complexes can be demonstrated in about 70% of cases (see O'Connor, 1983a). The transient hypopyon is presumably a chemotactic response to immune complexes deposited in the anterior uvea.

FUCH'S HETEROCHROMIC IRIDOCYCLITIS

Fuch's heterochromic iridocyclitis is a disease of insidious onset usually between the ages of 20 and 35 which affects males slightly more often than females. By contrast with the diseases in the preceding section, no associated HLA antigens have been demonstrated. The heterochromia is often minimal and easily missed. The affected eye appears lighter as a result of stromal atrophy and loss of stromal pigment. When the atrophy is severe, however, the eye may appear darker because the pigment epithelium is partially exposed. The lens becomes opaque. The cataract is usually posterior polar and eventually progresses through maturity to become hypermature. In a small number of cases focal choroiditis suggestive of toxoplasmosis has been observed.

The main pathological findings based on the small number of globes that have been examined include:

1 Atrophy of iris stroma and pigmented epithelium (Fig. 3.3) and hyalinisation of its blood vessels (iris vessels often appear hyalinised). The ciliary body also shows atrophy.

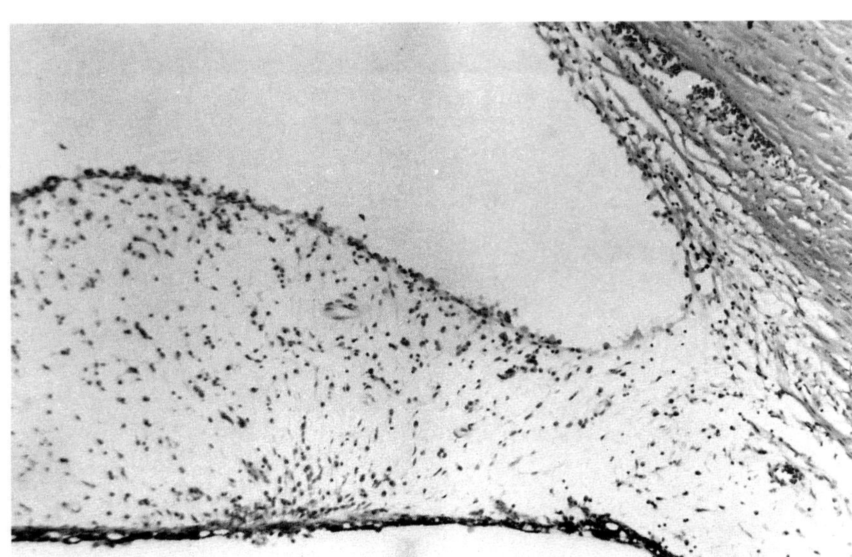

Fig. 3.3 Fuch's heterochromic iridocyclitis. The drainage angle is open. There is a sprinkling of chronic inflammatory cells in the iris stroma and trabecular meshwork and atrophy of the pigmented epithelium. Masson's trichrome (×260).

2 Sparse infiltration of the iris with lymphocytes and plasma cells. Scanty cells are also present in the anterior chamber and trabecular meshwork (Fig. 3.3).

3 Delicate new vessels in the iris stroma and on its surface and occasionally in the chamber angle. These vessels are permeable to fluorescein and also bleed readily if intraocular pressure is reduced (Amsler's sign). A puzzling feature is that they rarely progress to form synechiae sufficient to account for the secondary glaucoma which complicates the disease.

The pathogenesis of heterochromic iridocyclitis has not been established.

SERUM SICKNESS

Signs and symptoms appear 3 days to 3 weeks after an injection of heterologous serum. The disease is characterised by malaise, fever, joint pains, swollen lymph nodes and acute iridocyclitis. Serum sickness is a model for diseases produced by circulating immune complexes which can be demonstrated in the serum. The complexes become deposited under the basement membrane of certain blood vessels, notably those of the uvea and renal glomerulus.

INTERMEDIATE UVEITIS (PARS PLANITIS, CHRONIC POSTERIOR CYCLITIS)

Intermediate uveitis, for which the grammatically dubious term *pars planitis* is persistently used, is a well recognised clinical entity of obscure aetiology. The disease affects both sexes and appears between the ages of 20 and 35. The disease is characterised by fine particulate opacities in the anterior vitreous which eventually form the so-called snowball opacities on the pars plana and peripheral retina, usually in the inferior part of the globe.

Pathological examination of longstanding cases has shown that the vitreous opacities are the result of organisation of the vitreous base by loose fibrovascular tissue containing scattered mononuclear cells. Adjacent hyperplasia of the non-pigmented ciliary epithelium is also present. Probable fibrous astrocytes have been identified by electron microscopy in the organised mass. There was little evidence of uveal inflammation, but lymphocytic cuffing of retinal venules was consistently seen and some cases showed cystoid macular oedema. The condition may well, therefore, be primarily a vitreo-retinitis (see Pederson *et al.*, 1978).

About 50% of cases of pars planitis get serious complications such as cataract, glaucoma and retinal detachment and may end up with phthisis bulbi.

CILIOCHOROIDAL EFFUSION

Exudation into the suprachoroidal space may occur:

1 As a complication of intraocular surgery (Chapter 18).

2 As a complication of scleritis and periocular inflammatory disease.

3 Spontaneously.

The third category occurs for no obvious reason and, if the effusion extends around the globe in annular form, the globe may be enucleated for a suspected ring melanoma of the ciliary body.

Microscopically, an exudate which, in H & E sections, stains with eosin to a variable extent according to its protein content is seen in the external layers of the anterior choroid. The effusion extends forwards in the deep layers of the ciliary body as far as the scleral spur and for a variable distance towards the posterior pole. Lymphocytes and plasma cells in variable numbers are usually seen scattered through the effusion and in the ciliary body.

UVEAL EFFUSION SYNDROME

Sometimes a serous retinal detachment is associated with a spontaneous ciliochoroidal effusion.

POSTERIOR UVEITIS

Inflammation of the choroid not attributable to specific infections such as syphilis, toxoplasmosis, etc. is rare.

PAN-UVEITIS

As already indicated, many of the conditions described in this and the preceding chapter, as well as some to be described later, involve the uveal tract extensively enough to justify the term pan-uveitis. The term is useful, therefore, only to describe the extent of an inflammatory process within the eye rather than to denote a specific entity or group of related diseases.

SARCOID UVEITIS

Sarcoidosis is a systemic disease characterised by non-caseating granulomatous inflammation most commonly affecting the mediastinal and peripheral lymph nodes, lungs, liver, spleen, skin, eyes, phalangeal bones and parotid glands.

Young adults are predominantly affected. The disease is commoner in Negroes than in Caucasians in the United States, but is also common in Sweden and Ireland. Some figures have indicated an association with HLA B8 (see O'Connor, 1983a).

Ocular involvement occurs in about 30% of cases of

systemic sarcoidosis. The most frequent manifestation is anterior uveitis which is bilateral in half the cases. Occasionally the major salivary glands are also affected (uveoparotid fever or Heerfordt's syndrome — see Chapter 15). Many patients with sarcoidosis complain at some time of sore, dry, red eyes. Corneal staining with 1% Bengal Rose solution is positive and Schirmer tests indicate deficient tear secretion, though there is rarely demonstrable disease of the lacrimal glands in such cases. Other less frequent lesions include interstitial keratitis and granulomata in the conjunctiva and orbit. Involvement of the retina and optic nerve is rare, but serious since it is frequently associated with sarcoid lesions of the brain. The retinal lesions include periphlebitis manifest by venous sheathing and haemorrhages, perivenous exudates resembling candle wax drippings and retinochoroidal granulomata.

Microscopic appearances

The histology of the sarcoid lesions is remarkably constant; they consist of small discrete non-caseating nodules of macrophages and giant cells of the Langhans or foreign body type. Many of the macrophages are of the epithelioid type. There is usually a surrounding cuff of lymphocytes and the nodules are encircled, but not penetrated by reticulin fibres. Though the absence of necrosis is important in the histological differential diagnosis of sarcoid granulomata, treatment by steroids may result in necrosis in the nodules. Asteroid bodies, which are proteinaceous in nature, and Schaumann bodies, which are calcific, may be seen in the giant cells, but are of no diagnostic significance.

The lesions closely resemble those induced by deposits of zirconium and beryllium salts, silicious material and sulphonamide crystals. However, the turnover of macrophages is much slower in such granulomata.

Laboratory diagnosis

There are no specific tests other than the Kveim test which depends on the injection of a saline extract of sarcoid granulomata. The antigen tends to be in short supply and carries an inherent risk of hepatitis (O'Connor, 1983a). In favourable cases, with good antigen the result is diagnostic. Often, however, the interpretation of the reaction can be difficult. A possible alternative is the KMIF (Kveim macrophage inhibitor factor) test (Williams *et al.*, 1972) which does not yet, however, appear to be widely used. Both tests may be influenced by steroid therapy.

The following procedures are non-specific, but may, however, provide useful support for a diagnosis based on clinical and radiological findings.

1 Skin hypersensitivity tests with the usual skin-test antigens such as tuberculin, *Candida* and *Trichophyton* are negative.

2 Biopsy of a conjunctival or skin nodule or of a lymph node. While histological diagnosis may not be absolutely conclusive, biopsy is well worthwhile if only to exclude other possibilities.

3 The blood eosinophil count may be raised in the early stages of the disease.

4 Serum globulin, particularly α-2 globulin, is raised when there is pulmonary involvement.

5 Serum lysozyme is elevated even in cases where the disease appears to be confined to the uvea.

6 Serum angiotensin converting enzyme may be elevated. Other conditions in which the level may be raised include, however, primary biliary cirrhosis, hyperthyroidism, diabetes mellitus and leprosy. The level of angiotensin converting enzyme in aqeous may be raised in sarcoid uveitis even when the serum levels are normal.

7 Serum calcium is raised in 12% of cases.

Pathogenesis

The pathogenesis of sarcoidosis remains obscure. The cutaneous anergy is believed to result from a depression in T-cell function and unregulated B-cell proliferation accounts for the raised plasma globulin levels.

BIBLIOGRAPHY

General

Audain, V. P., Quigley, J. H., Vethamanay, S. & Ghose, T. (1977) Immunological studies of human uveitis. *Canadian Journal of Ophthalmology* **12**, 12–15.

Campinchi, R., Faure, J. P., Bloch-Michel, E. & Haut, J. (1973) *Uveitis — Immunologic and Allergic Phenomena* (translated and revised by B. Golden & M. M. Givoiset). Charles C. Thomas, Springfield, Illinois.

Kraus-Mackiw, E. & O'Connor, G. R., eds (1983) *Uveitis — Pathophysiology and Therapy*. Thieme Stratton, New York & George Thieme, Stuttgart.

Maumenee, A. E. (1970) Clinical entities in 'uveitis': an approach to the study of intraocular inflammation. *American Journal of Ophthalmology* **69**, 1–27.

Maumenee, A. E. (1980) Uveitis — then and now. *Transactions of the Ophthalmological Society of the UK* **100**, 9–16.

O'Connor, G. R. (1983a) Endogenous uveitis. In *Uveitis — Pathophysiology and Therapy*, eds E. Kraus-Mackiw & G. R. O'Connor, pp 45–116. Thieme Stratton, New York & George Thieme, Stuttgart.

O'Connor, G. R. (1983b) Factors related to the initiation and recurrence of uveitis. *American Journal of Ophthalmology* **96**, 573–599.

Rahi, A. H. S., Holbrow, E. J., Perkins, E. S. & Dinning, W. J. (1979) What is endogenous uveitis? In *Immunology and Immunopathology of the Eye*, eds A. M. Silverstein & G. R. O'Connor, pp 23–28. Masson, New York.

Schlaegel Jr., T. F. (1969) *Essentials of Uveitis*. J. & A. Churchill, London.

Silverstein, A. M. & O'Connor, G. R., eds (1979) *Immunology and Immunopathology of the Eye*, Masson, New York.

Woods, A. C. (1956) *Endogenous Uveitis*. William Wilkins Co., Baltimore.

HLA associations

DeWolf, W. C., Dupont, B. & Yunis, E. J. (1980) HLA and disease. Current concepts. *Human Pathology* **11**, 332–336.

Rahi, A. H. S. (1979) HLA and eye disease. *British Journal of Ophthalmology* **63**, 283–292.

Immunological aspects

Char, D. H., Stein, P., Masi, R. & Christensen, M. (1979) Immune complexes in uveitis. *American Journal of Ophthalmology* **87**, 678–681.

Deschenes, J., Freeman, W. R., Char, D. H. & Garovov, M. R. (1986) Lymphocyte subpopulations in uveitis. *Archives of Ophthalmology* **104**, 233–236.

Kaplan, H. J., Waldrep, J. C., Nicholson, J. K. A. & Gordon, D. (1984) Immunological analysis of intraocular mononuclear infiltrates in uveitis. *Archives of Ophthalmology* **102**, 572–575.

Kijlstra, A., Luyendijk, L., Van der Gaag, R., Van Kregten, E., Linssen, A. & Willers, J. M. N. (1986) IgG and IgA immune responses against *Klebsiella* in HLA-B27-associated anterior uveitis. *British Journal of Ophthalmology* **70**, 85–88.

McCoy, R., White, L., Tait, B. & Ebringer, R. (1984) Serum immunoglobulins in acute anterior uveitis. *British Journal of Ophthalmology* **68**, 807–810.

Martenet, A. C., Kalin, A. & Grob, P. J. (1980) Newer immunological studies of the aqueous humor in uveitis. *Ophthalmic Research* **12**, 111–117.

Maumenee, A. E. & Silverstein, A. M., eds (1964) *Immunopathology of Uveitis*. William Wilkins Co., Baltimore.

Norn, M. S. (1976) Immunoglobulins in endogenous uveitis. *British Journal of Ophthalmology* **60**, 299–301.

Nussenblatt, R. B., Salinas-Carmona, M., Leake, W. & Scher, I. (1983) T lymphocyte subsets in uveitis. *American Journal of Ophthalmology* **95**, 614–621.

Ozyazgan, Y., Rahi, A., Dinning, W. & Carvalho, G. (1982) Differential lymphocyte count in eye disease. A U-turn in laboratory investigation. *Transactions of the Ophthalmological Society of the UK* **102**, 171–173.

Rahi, A. H. S., Holbrow, E. J., Perkins, E. S., Gungen, Y. Y. & Dinning, W. J. (1976) Immunological investigations in uveitis. *Transactions of the Ophthalmological Society of the UK* **96**, 113–122.

Anterior uveitis

Beckingsale, A. B., Williams, D., Gibson, J. M. & Rosenthal, A. R. (1984) *Klebsiella* and acute anterior uveitis. *British Journal of Ophthalmology* **68**, 866–868.

Brewerton, D. A. (1985) The genetics of acute uveitis. *Transactions of the Ophthalmological Society of the UK* **104**, 248–249.

Merriam, J. C., Chylack, L. T. & Albert, D. M. (1983) Early-onset pauciarticular juvenile rheumatoid arthritis. A histopathologic study. *Archives of Ophthalmology* **101**, 1085–1092.

Pars planitis

Pederson, J. E., Kenyon, K. R., Green, W. R. & Maumenee, A. E. (1979) Pathology of pars planitis. *American Journal of Ophthalmology* **86**, 762–774.

Behçet's disease

Colvard, D. M., Robertson, D. M. & O'Duffy, J. D. (1977) The ocular manifestations of Behçet's disease. *Archives of Ophthalmology* **95**, 1813–1817.

Michelson, J. B. & Chisari, F. V. (1982) Behçet's disease. *Survey of Ophthalmology* **26**, 190–203.

Fuchs' heterochromic iridocyclitis

O'Connor, G. R. (1985) Heterochromic iridocyclitis. *Transactions of the Ophthalmological Society of the UK* **104**, 219–231.

Perry, H. D., Yanoff, M. & Scheie, H. G. (1975) Rubeosis in Fuchs' heterochromic iridocyclitis. *Archives of Ophthalmology* **93**, 337–339.

Sarcoid uveitis

Weinreb, R. N., O'Donnell, J. J., Sandman, R., Char, D. H. & Kimura, S. J. (1979) Angiotensin-converting enzyme in sarcoid uveitis. *Investigative Ophthalmology and Visual Science* **18**, 1285–1287.

Weinreb, R. N., Sandman, R., Ryder, M. I. & Friberg, T. R. (1985) Angiotensin-converting activity in human aqueous humor. *Archives of Ophthalmology* **103**, 34–36.

Williams, W. J., Pioli, E., Jones, D. J. & Dighero, M. (1972) The Kmif (Kveim macrophage induced migration inhibition factor) test in sarcoidosis. *Journal of Clinical Pathology* **25**, 951–954.

Chapter 4 Sympathetic ophthalmitis and related conditions

SYMPATHETIC OPHTHALMITIS

Sympathetic ophthalmitis is a progressive, bilateral uveitis which is extremely uncommon. The incidence has been estimated at between 0.2% and 1.0% of all non-surgical penetrating wounds and less than one case per 10 000 penetrating surgical wounds (Marak, 1979). A recent analysis of nearly 3000 enucleation specimens provided only 17 examples (Mueller-Hermelink, 1983).

Following a perforation of one globe, inflammation develops in both eyes. The perforated eye is called the exciting eye and the other eye the sympathising eye. Uveal prolapse is almost always present in the exciting eye. The relative frequency following perforations of different types is given below:

1 65% of cases follow accidental injuries.

2 25% of cases follow surgical procedures.

3 10% of cases follow perforating corneal ulcers or scleral rupture.

Sympathetic ophthalmitis has occasionally been reported in association with malignant uveal melanomata, but such eyes have probably always suffered a previous perforation of the corneo-scleral coat.

Inflammation begins in the exciting eye at variable intervals after injury — very rarely before 2 weeks and most commonly between 4 and 6 weeks — and synchronously or slightly later in the sympathising eye. Intervals of many years up to half a life-time have been recorded in some cases.

Enucleation of the injured eye within 14 days of injury almost invariably protects the uninjured eye. Enucleation after the other eye is affected does not halt the progress of the disease, though it may possibly ameliorate it. Twenty per cent of cases run a relatively mild, short course without serious ocular damage, but, without treatment, 70% of the remaining cases become permanently blind as a result of protracted relapsing endophthalmitis. Corticosteroids usually control the inflammation which, however, tends to relapse when treatment is withdrawn.

Microscopic appearances

Most histopathological descriptions have been based on surgically enucleated injured eyes. However, a sufficient number of sympathising eyes has been examined to indicate that there is no fundamental difference between the inflammatory changes in the exciting and the sympathising eye.

The cellular infiltrate is characteristically granulomatous, being composed predominantly of masses of lymphocytes in which there are foci of epithelioid macrophages and giant cells. Many of these contain fine pigment granules. Plasma cells are present in variable numbers in the majority of cases. Eosinophils are also found in cases enucleated shortly after the onset of symptoms. Some of these features are illustrated in a typical case (Fig. 4.1)

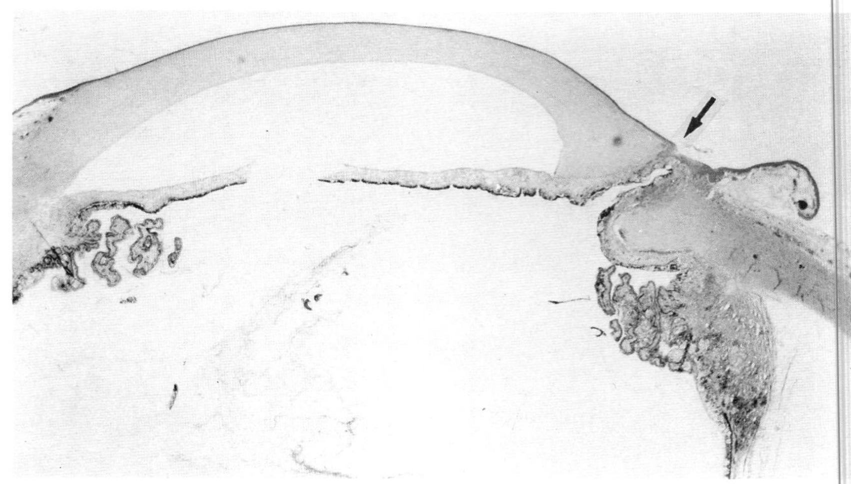

Fig. 4.1 Typical case of sympathetic ophthalmitis in male aged 17 years. Blunt trauma resulted in a traumatic cataract and vitreous haemorrhage. The lens was extracted and 14 days later the other eye became irritable. (a) Anterior segment showing cataract section with prolapse of iris (arrow). Note absence of infiltrate in iris and ciliary body.

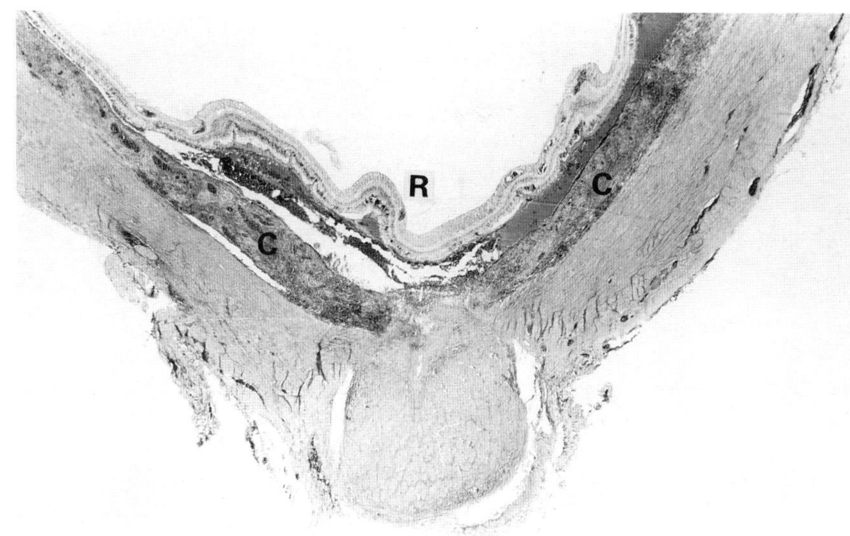

Fig. 4.1 (b) Posterior segment showing massive thickening of the choroid (C). There is a shallow detachment of the retina (R) and there has been avulsion of the retina from the nerve head.

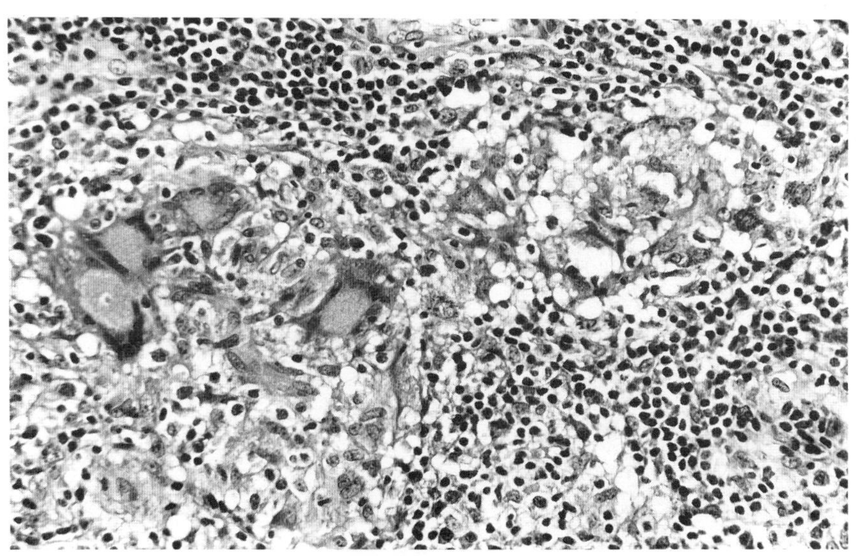

Fig. 4.1 (c) Typical granulomatous infiltrate in the choroid showing groups of giant cells and epithelioid cells surrounded by lymphocytes. H & E (×260).

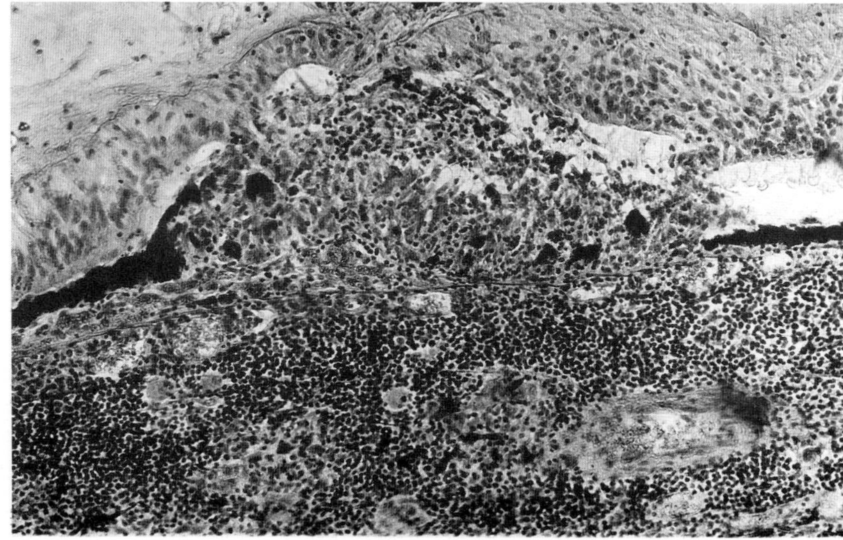

Fig. 4.1 (d) Dalen–Fuchs nodule near ora serrata. In the underlying choroid, pale islands of epithelioid cells are seen in dense lymphocytic infiltration.

Choroid

The posterior choroid is most heavily involved, especially the outer layers. The infiltrate is usually confluent except towards the periphery, but the choriocapillaris is spared and forms a thin cell-free zone immediately beneath Bruch's membrane. The latter usually remains intact. The infiltrate tends to spread along scleral emissary channels and may reach the episclera and orbital tissues.

Ciliary body

The infiltrate first appears in the vascular layers of the ciliary body between the ciliary epithelium and the muscle.

The inflammatory cells erode through the ciliary prolongations of Bruch's membrane and form flat nodules composed of what were thought to be a mixture of proliferating epithelial and epithelioid cells. However, recent work with monoclonal antibodies (Chan *et al.*, 1985) has shown that most of the cells, like those in the choroid, originate from bone marrow derived monocytes. These Dalen–Fuchs nodules may occur in other types of granulomatous uveitis, but are more commonly found and more numerous in sympathetic ophthalmitis.

Migration of cells occurs:

1 Posteriorly through the vitreous. Clumps of macrophages (retinal precipitates) are deposited on the internal limiting membrane of the retina.

2 Anteriorly through the pupil into the anterior chamber where cells are deposited on the surface of the iris and corneal endothelium.

Iris

In the iris, the cellular infiltrate appears as nodular aggregates in the posterior layers. Eventually, the pigmented epithelium is disrupted and the granulomatous infiltrate breaks out onto the lens capsule and into the anterior and posterior chambers.

Retina

The infiltrate rarely spreads into the retina, though the retinal venules may show cuffing by lymphocytes. Pigment migration into the retina and macular oedema are commonly seen. Chorioretinal scarring is a frequent late complication.

Optic nerve

Optic atrophy and or evidence of inflammation is present in about 50% of cases. The latter takes the form of perivascular cuffing or more diffuse lymphocytic infiltration.

Diagnosis

The diagnosis of sympathetic ophthalmitis is based on the following criteria none of which is individually pathognomonic of the disease:

1 The history of peforation of the globe, usually with uveal prolapse.

2 The involvement of the uninjured eye.

3 The presence in the excised eye of a granulomatous infiltrate in the posterior iris, inner layers of the ciliary body and outer layers of the choroid. Although clinically, sympathetic ophthalmitis usually appears to start in the anterior uvea, histologically the whole uvea is involved to some degree even in very early cases. In mild cases, the infiltration may be patchy, leaving normal uveal tissue between inflammatory foci.

4 The presence in the cytoplasm of the epithelioid macrophages and giant cells of pigment granules. This is easily seen in H & E sections, but can be dramatically demonstrated by silver stains such as Masson–Fontana (Appendix IV). Phagocytosis of pigment is unusual in other types of granulomatous uveitis unless there is extensive necrosis of the pigmented epithelium.

5 The absence of caseation or suppuration.

6 The presence of Dalen–Fuchs nodules.

Pathogenesis

Sympathetic ophthalmitis was one of the earliest diseases for which an autoimmune basis was postulated. As long ago as 1910 Elschnig showed that uveal emulsions were autoantigenic. Positive cutaneous hypersensitivity reactions with extracts of uveal tissue were later elicited in cases. However, the results of attempts to demonstrate circulating antibodies to uveal tissue were variable and convincing replicas of the disease in the experimental animal were not achieved with uveal extracts.

The delayed onset and granulomatous nature of the inflammatory reaction clearly indicate a Type 4 (cell-mediated) response. The problem is to identify the antigen(s) involved. In recent years, interest has switched from the uvea, which is after all basically a vascular bed containing pigment, to the retina. Pigment is only weakly antigenic. However, the outer segments of the photoreceptors contain a strong specific antigen — retinal S-antigen. In certain species, a chorioretinitis can be evoked by the use of this antigen. Whether any of the animal models represents a wholly satisfactory model of sympathetic ophthalmitis, however, remains debatable. In small numbers of cases extracts of retina, pigmented epithelium and uveo-retinal tissue as well as uveal pigment have all been reported to stimulate lymphocyte transformation.

The extreme rarity with which sympathetic ophthalmitis follows severe ocular trauma uncomplicated by uveal prolapse provides a clue to a possible pathogenetic mechanism. The intraocular compartment lacks lymphatic drainage and entry of antigens into the bloodstream and thus directly to the spleen tends to promote tolerance. However, a uveal prolapse would allow antigens access to the conjunctival lymphatics and thus to the regional lymph nodes. Subconjunctival injection of retinal S-antigen has been shown to set up a bilateral granulomatous uveitis in the rabbit, whereas intraocular injection did not (Rao *et al.*, 1983).

A possible alternative explanation based on the reported failure to demonstrate auto-antibodies to uvea in sympathetic ophthalmitis is that such antibodies might normally exert a protective effect by coating the tissue component against which the cell-mediated reaction develops.

VOGT–KOYANAGI–HARADA (VKH) SYNDROME

This rare syndrome is commoner in the yellow-skinned races and its onset is usually in middle age. The features comprise a bilateral granulomatous uveitis associated with one or more signs or symptoms such as patchy baldness, greying of the hair, vitiligo and transient deafness. Since the original case reports by Vogt, Koyanagi and Harada, it has become apparent that these signs represent variations in a single disease entity.

In the early stages of the disease there may be evidence of meningeal involvement such as headache and vomiting, with raised cerebrospinal fluid pressure and lymphocytosis up to 300 cells per mm^3.

The first ocular manifestations are diffuse oedema of the posterior retina, vitreous opacitis and gradual retinal detachment due to the accumulation of a subretinal inflammatory effusion. In some case the process is spontaneously arrested at this stage and the retina becomes re-attached with restoration of normal vision (Harada's disease). In other cases, the uveal inflammation spreads to the anterior segment with the formation of lardaceous keratic precipitates and dense posterior adhesions. Only 30% of such patients recover normal vision and many become permanently blind (Vogt–Koyanagi syndrome).

Sometime during the course of the disease, both types of case may develop premature greying or whitening and patchy loss of the scalp and axillary hair, eyebrows and lashes. Patchy depigmentation of the skin and tinnitus with deafness occur less frequently. Depigmentation of the iris is observed in some cases.

Microscopically, the uveal infiltration is strikingly similar to that seen in sympathetic ophthalmitis with foci of epithelioid cells, phagocytosis of pigment and Dalen–Fuchs nodules. The principal described differences are oedema and detachment of the retina and necrosis, exfoliation and depigmentation of the pigmented epithelium. In evaluating the differences between this condition and sympathetic ophthalmitis, it has to be remembered that eyes affected by the former are commonly enucleated at an earlier stage of the disease. It may also be noted that some cases of sympathetic ophthalmitis show poliosis of the lashes and vitiligo.

At present it seems likely that the VKH syndrome is an autoimmune disease closely comparable with sympathetic ophthalmitis, though it is not clear whether the same antigen is involved or how it is 'exposed'. Different reports have incriminated both pigment and human myelin protein. It is difficult to believe that pigment, which is only weakly antigenic, is the antigen primarily responsible, but it may possibly be caught up in the process rather in the same way that the lens may apparently become a secondary target in an immune reaction late in the course of a uveitis. The reaction to myelin may well also be a secondary phenomenon.

LENS-INDUCED ENDOPHTHALMITIS

When disorganised lens matter is released into the ocular cavities it is usually absorbed with little or no disturbance, though the macrophages involved may be numerous enough to cause blockage of the trabecular meshwork (Chapter 12). Sometimes, however, a severe inflammatory reaction results. Such a reaction most commonly follows operations or injuries involving the lens, but occasionally arises spontaneously as a complication of hypermature cataracts.

The inflammation may commence within 48 hours of the release of the lens matter or may be delayed for 10 to 14 days. The reaction may be severe with oedema of the lids, large keratic precipitates and a sterile hypopyon. In rare instances, the fellow eye may be affected and sympathetic ophthalmitis thus simulated. However, the onset of the inflammation in the second eye is later and not synchronous as in sympathetic ophthalmitis.

Microscopical changes

The inflammatory reaction is confined to the anterior segment of the globe and particularly centres in and around the lens or whatever remains of it. The posterior segment is relatively uninvolved, although lymphocytic cuffing of the retinal venules and a sprinkling of lymphocytes in the choroid may be seen.

The cellular infiltrate characteristically contains a large number of neutrophils apparently invading the lens substance. Numerous eosinophils are also often present. The initial cellular infiltrate soon assumes a more granulomatous character with the appearance of macrophages, epithelioid and giant cells (Fig. 4.2). The macrophages form large keratic precipitates while the epithelioid cells tend to pallisade about exposed lens fibres.

A point often overlooked is that while the reaction centred on the lens is granulomatous in character the inflammatory infiltration in the uvea consists almost entirely of lymphocytes and plasma cells. The inflammatory tissue readily organises to form fibrous bands in the anterior chamber, a pupillary membrane, adhesions between the iris and lens and a cyclitic membrane. Post-inflammatory glaucoma may develop.

Pathogenesis

That lenses of many species shared organ-specific antigens has been known for many years and lens proteins have long been regarded as occupying an immunologically privileged situation. As long ago as 1922, Verhoeff and Lemoine put forward the idea that the inflammatory reaction was the result of autoimmunity developing to lens protein which had escaped from its seclusion, and coined the name endophthalmitis anaphylactica (or phacoallergica). Since there is no evidence that lens proteins, even from cataractous lenses, have toxic properties, the term phacotoxic uveitis or endophthalmitis should be abandoned.

Although anti-lens antibodies are readily induced under experimental conditions by extracts of heterologous lens proteins, homologous extracts are much less strongly antigenic (see Misra *et al.*, 1977; Rahi *et al.*, 1977). Under special conditions, it is possible to demonstrate a response to autologous lens protein (Rahi *et al.*, 1977). It has also become clear that lens proteins possess a great variety of antigenic determinants, some of which are shared with other tissues. Clinically, anti-lens antibodies have been found in patients with longstanding uveitis as well as following injury or cataract surgery and even in the absence of demonstrable disease.

The deposition of immune complexes from a reaction between complement-fixing anti-lens antibodies and lens protein would be expected to attract the large number of neutrophils seen in the exudate. Such a mechanism can be demonstrated in the experimental animal (Marak *et al.*, 1976; 1977; 1978). However, since lens proteins are now regarded as only semi-sequestered, the anti-lens antibodies are thought to arise as a result of reversal of low-zone tolerance at the T-cell level (see Chapter 1). This could occur as a result of massive release of antigen; the presence of a contaminant acting as an adjuvant; or if suppressor T-cell activity were, for any reason, depressed (Marak *et al.*, 1978). The hypothesis requires a preponderance of lens protein binding B-cells over T-cells which has, in fact, been demonstrated in the rat (Marak & Rao, 1983).

SYMPATHETIC OPHTHALMITIS ASSOCIATED WITH LENS-INDUCED ENDOPHTHALMITIS

Older reviews showed that 20–25% of cases of sympathetic ophthalmia also showed evidence of lens-induced endophthalmitis. More recent surveys, however, have indicated an association in only 5% of cases. The reason for this change is most likely to be improvement in management (see Marak, 1979).

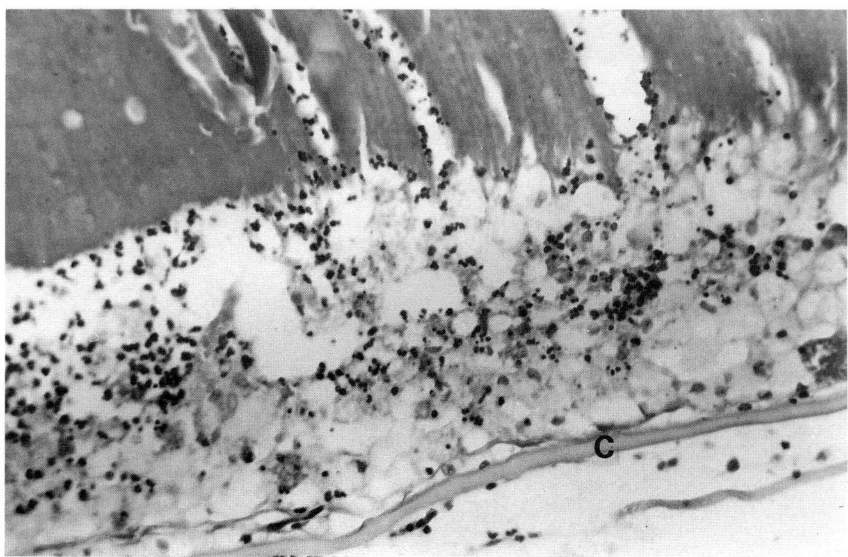

Fig. 4.2 Lens-induced endophthalmitis. Infiltrate of polymorphs and macrophages deep to capsule (C) and spreading between disintegrating fibres. Masson trichrome (×260).

BIBLIOGRAPHY

General

Chan, C.-C., Ben Ezra, D., Hsu, S.-M., Palestine, A. G. & Nussenblatt, R. B. (1985) Granulomas in sympathetic ophthalmia and sarcoidosis. *Archives of Ophthalmology* **103**, 198–202.

Easom, H. A. & Zimmerman, L. E. (1964) Sympathetic ophthalmia and bilateral phacoanaphylaxis. *Archives of Ophthalmology* **72**, 9–15.

Elschnig, A. (1910) Studien zur sympathischen ophthalmie. *Albrecht von Graefes Archiv für Ophthalmologie* **75**, 459–473.

Fuchs, E. (1923) Irido-cyclitic syndrome. In *Text Book of Ophthalmology*, 12th German Edn, translated by A. Duane, pp 254–261. J. B. Lippincott Co., Philadelphia.

Kraus-Mackiw, E. (1983) Exogenous uveitis; sympathetic uveitis. In *Uveitis: Pathophysiology and Therapy*, eds E. Kraus-Mackiw & G. R. O'Connor, pp 117–151. Thieme-Stratton, New York.

Lubin, J. R. & Albert, D. M. (1979) Sympathetic ophthalmia. Ample room for controversy. *Survey of Ophthalmology* **24**, 137–140.

Lubin, J. R., Albert, D. M. & Weinstein, M. (1980) Sixty-five years of sympathetic ophthalmia. A clinicopathologic review of 105 cases (1913–1978). *Ophthalmology* **87**, 109–121.

Marak Jr., G. E. (1979) Recent advances in sympathetic ophthalmia. *Survey of Ophthalmology* **24**, 141–156.

Müeller-Hermelink, H. K. (1983) Recent topics in the pathology of uveitis. In *Uveitis: Pathophysiology and Therapy*, eds E. Kraus-Mackiw & G. R. O'Connor, pp 152–197. Thieme-Stratton, New York.

Rao, N. A., Robin, J., Hartmann, D., Sweeney, J. A. & Marak Jr., G. E. (1983) The role of the penetrating wound in the development of sympathetic ophthalmia. Experimental observations. *Archives of Ophthalmology* **101**, 102–104.

Shammas, H. F., Zubyk, N. A. & Stanfield, T. F. (1977) Sympathetic uveitis following glaucoma surgery. *Archives of Ophthalmology* **95**, 638–641.

Verhoeff, F. H. & Lemoine, A. N. (1922) Endophthamitis phacoanaphylactica. *American Journal of Ophthalmology* **5**, 737–745.

Immunological aspects

Aronson, S. B., Yamamoto, E., Goodner, E. K. & O'Connor, G. R. (1964) The occurrence of an autoanti-uveal antibody in human uveitis. *Archives of Ophthalmology* **72**, 621–625.

Gery, I., Nussenblatt, R. & Ben Ezra, D. (1981) Dissociation between humoral and cellular immune responses to lens antigens. *Investigative Ophthalmology and Visual Science* **20**, 32–39.

Hackett, E. & Thompson, A. (1964) Anti-lens antibody in human sera. *Lancet* **2**, 663–666.

Halbert, S. P., Locatcher-Khorazo, D., Swick, L., Witmer, R., Seegal, B. & Fizgerald, P. (1957) Homologous immunological studies of ocular lens. I. In vitro observations. *Journal of Experimental Medicine* **105**, 439–452.

Hammer, H. (1971) Lymphocyte transformation in sympathetic ophthalmia and Vogt–Koyanagi–Harada syndrome. *British Journal of Ophthalmology* **55**, 850–852.

Hammer, H. (1974) Cellular hypersensitivity to uveal pigment confirmed by leucocyte migration tests in sympathetic ophthalmitis and Vogt–Koyanagi–Harada syndrome. *British Journal of Ophthalmology* **58**, 773–776.

Kraus-Mackiw, E., Georgs, L., Immich, H. & Müller-Ruchholtz, W. (1975) Neuere Angabe zur Häufigkeit und immunologischen Reaktivitat bei Sympathischer Ophthalmie. *Klinische Monatsblätte für Augenheilkunde* **167**, 844–846.

Luntz, M. H. (1964) Auto-immune response to lens and uveal protein. *South African Medical Journal* **38**, 130–133.

Luntz, M. H. (1968) Anti-uveal and anti-lens antibodies in uveitis and their significance.

Manor, R. S., Livni, E. & Cohen, S. (1979) Cell-mediated immunity to human myelin basic protein in Vogt–Koyanagi–Harada syndrome. *Investigative Ophthalmology and Visual Science* **18**, 204–206.

Manski, W. (1973) Immunological studies on normal and pathological lenses. In *The Human Lens in Relation to Cataract* (Ciba Foundation symposium), pp 227–242. Elsevier, Amsterdam.

Marak Jr., G. E., Aye, Mg S. & Alepa, F. P. (1973) Cellular hypersensitivity in penetrating eye injuries. *Investigative Ophthalmology* **12**, 380–382.

Marak Jr., G. E., Font, R. L. & Alepa, F. P. (1976) Experimental lens-induced granulomatous endophthamitis: passive transfer with serum. *Ophthalmic Research* **8**, 117–120.

Marak Jr., G. E., Font, R. L. & Alepa, F. P. (1978) Immunopathogenicity of lens crystallins in the production of experimental lens-induced granulomatous endophthalmitis. *Ophthalmic Research* **10**, 30–35.

Marak Jr., G. E., Font, R. L., Johnson, M. C. & Alepa, F. P. (1972) Lymphocyte-stimulating activity of ocular tissues in sympathetic ophthalmia. *Investigative Ophthalmology* **10**, 770–774.

Marak Jr., G. E., Font, R. L. & Ward, P. A. (1977) Fluorescent antibody studies in experimental lens-induced granulomatous endophthalmitis. *Ophthalmic Research* **9**, 317–320.

Marak Jr., G. E. & Rao, N. A. (1983) Lens protein binding lymphocytes. *Ophthalmic Research* **15**, 6–10.

Marak Jr., G. E., Shichi, H., Rao, N. A. & Wacker, W. B. (1980) Patterns of experimental allergic uveitis induced by rhodopsin and retinal rod outer segments. *Ophthalmic Research* **12**, 165–176.

Mills, P. V. & Shedden, W. I. H. (1965) Serological studies in sympathetic ophthalmitis. *British Journal of Ophthalmology* **49**, 29–33.

Misra, A. N., Rahi, A. H. S. & Morgan, G. (1977) Immunopathology of the lens. II. Humoral and cellular immune responses to homologous lens antigens and their roles in ocular inflammation. *British Journal of Ophthalmology* **61**, 285–296.

Momoeda, S. (1977) Lymphocyte transformation test in Vogt–Koyanagi–Harada syndrome. *Japanese Journal of Ophthalmology* **21**, 488–495.

Rahi, A. H. S., Misra, R. N. & Morgan, G. (1977) Immunopathology of the lens. I. Humoral and cellular immune responses to heterologous lens antigens and their roles in ocular inflammation. *British Journal of Ophthalmology* **61**, 164–176, 371–379.

Rao, N. A., Robin, J., Hartmann, D., Sweeney, J. A. & Marak Jr., G. E. (1983) The role of the penetrating wound in the development of sympathetic ophthalmia. Experimental observations. *Archives of Ophthalmology* **101**, 102–104.

Rao, N. A., Wacker, W. B. & Marak Jr., G. E. (1979) Experimental allergic uveitis, clinicopathologic features associated with varying doses of S-antigen. *Archives of Ophthalmology* **97**, 1954–1958.

Shammas, H. F., Zubyk, N. A. & Stanfield, T. F. (1977) Sympathetic uveitis following glaucoma surgery. *Archives of Ophthalmology* **95**, 638–641

Rahi, A. H. S., Morgan, G., Levy, I. & Dinning, W. (1978) Immunological investigations in post-traumatic granulomatous and non-granulomatous uveitis. *British Journal of Ophthalmology* **62**, 722–728.

Wacker, W. B. (1973) Experimental allergic uveitis. *Internal Archives of Allergy* **45**, 639–656.

Wirostko, E. & Spalter, H. F. (1967) Lens-induced uveitis. *Archives of Ophthalmology* **78**, 1–7.

Wong, V. G., Anderson, R. & O'Brien, P. J. (1971) Sympathetic ophthalmia and lymphocyte transformation.

Woods, A. C. (1925) Sympathetic ophthalmia: the use of uveal pigment in diagnosis and treatment. *Transactions of the Ophthalmological Society of the UK* **45**, 208–249.

Chapter 5 The conjunctiva, cornea and sclera

NORMAL STRUCTURE AND FUNCTION

Cornea

The cornea consists of four layers:

1 The *epithelium* comprises four to five rows of cells of which the basal are columnar and the superficial flat.

2 The *stroma* is composed of collagen fibres 240–340 nm in diameter arranged in orderly lamellae. Transparency depends on regular spacing of the fibrils (Maurice, 1957). This is apparently achieved through there being regularly spaced specific binding sites on the collagen fibrils for the two important proteoglycans in the interfibrillar gel. The proteoglycans (see Appendix III) comprise one or two glycosaminoglycan chains (respectively keratan sulphate and dermatan sulphate) and a protein core (see Scott & Haigh, 1987).

Within the stroma is a sparse population of keratocytes. Deep to the epithelium is Bowman's membrane which is a layer of acellular collagen laid down during foetal life. If it is damaged it is not replaced and an epithelial 'facet' or scar results.

3 *Desçemet's membrane* is the basement membrane of the endothelium. It consists of an anterior collagenous layer laid down during foetal life and a posterior non-collagenous layer of glycoprotein which increases in thickness throughout life. Local dome-shaped excrescences composed of basement membrane material appear at the periphery from age 20 onwards.

4 The *endothelium* is a simple layer of flat hexagonal cells. The endothelium maintains the fluid balance. Its cells probably do not replicate and loss through trauma or disease is made good by expansion of surviving cells. Functional failure results in oedema and loss of stromal clarity.

The corneal endothelium and, indeed the keratocytes, appear to be derived from cells which migrate from the neural crest. The term endothelium is a misnomer as the cells have little in common with vascular endothelium (see Bahn *et al.*, 1984). They do not contain Weibel–Palade bodies and react negatively for Factor VIII, which is a marker for vascular endothelium. On the other hand they react positively for S-100 protein and neuron specific enolase which are found in normal tissues of neural origin.

Conjunctiva

The epithelium of the conjunctiva is a stratified layer of flattened cells three to five rows thick in which mucus-secreting goblet cells are present. These cells are numerous in the caruncle and sparse at the limbus. Deep to the epithelium is a layer of connective tissue, the substantia propria. The latter is adherent to the tarsus, but mobile over the globe except at the limbus where it merges with Tenon's capsule. Lymphocytes and plasma cells populate the substantia propria of the tarsal conjunctiva and antibody therefrom becomes attached to the 'secretory piece' contributed by the conjunctival epithelium. Pilosebaceous units are present in the caruncle.

Surface film

The surface of the cornea and conjunctiva is covered by a film derived from lacrimal and mucous secretions. Apart from immunoglobulins, this contains natural protective agents:

1 *Lysozyme* is a highly basic protein secreted by the lacrimal glands which has lytic, bactericidal and bacteriostatic properties and can also stimulate phagocytosis. Gram-negative bacteria are protected by a lipopolysaccharide coating, but can be rendered susceptible in the presence of antibody and complement.

2 *Lactoferrin* is an iron binding protein which can deprive bacteria of iron which is nutritionally essential to organsims such as coliforms and staphylococci.

Sclera

The scleral stroma is made up of obliquely interwoven bundles of collagen fibres. The fibrils forming these bundles are not uniform in diameter like those of the cornea. A network of elastic fibres is present between the collagen bundles. Flattened melanocytes which are insinuated between the collagen lamellae adjacent to the internal scleral surface form the lamina fusca. The episclera is a thin layer of loose vascular connective tissue on the external surface of the sclera.

CHAPTER 5

CORNEAL OEDEMA

As mentioned above, extensive loss of cells from the corneal endothelium results in failure of the endothelial pump and accumulation of fluid in the cornea.

Causes of endothelial damage

1 *Glaucoma:* the endothelium may be damaged by raised intraocular pressure, which also increases the rate of flow of fluid into the cornea.

2 *Trauma:* the endothelium is particularly susceptible to mechanical damage. This may occur during anterior segment surgery as a result of contact with vitreous or lens. Anterior chamber implants present a particular hazard.

3 Endothelial failure may occur after corneal grafting either because of poorly preserved donor material or because of rejection.

4 *Endothelial dystrophies:* certain dystrophies, especially Fuchs' combined dystrophy, may result in corneal oedema.

Pathological changes

Some epithelial cells may become hydropic, and bullae form between the epithelium and Bowman's membrane (bullous keratopathy) (Fig. 5.1). The bullae contain fluid which is, of course, lost during processing, but serous debris and occasional red cells are usually seen. In chronic cases, fibrovascular pannus grows in from the limbus and downgrowths of epithelium often appear to become cut off and buried in the pannus (Fig. 5.2).

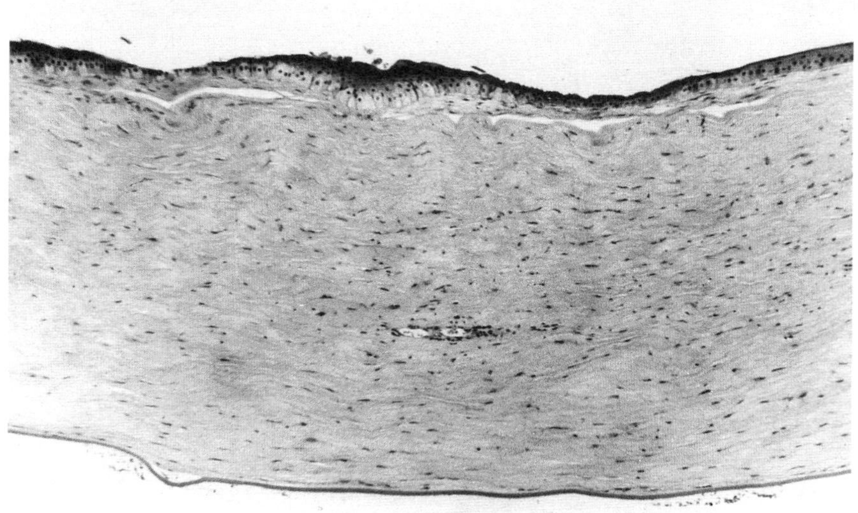

Fig. 5.1 Decompensated cornea resulting from the presence of an anterior chamber lens implant. The epithelium is irregular in thickness, contains hydropic cells and is elevated from Bowman's membrane over a wide area. The stroma is thickened and a vessel is present. No endothelium could be identified. PAS/tartrazine.

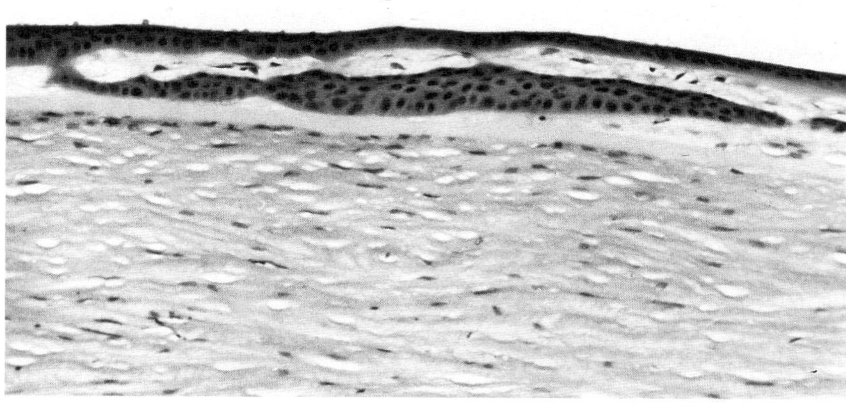

Fig. 5.2 Longstanding degenerative pannus superficial to Bowman's membrane causing layering of the epithelium. H & E (×160).

Stromal oedema is manifested by increased spacing between the stromal lamellae. Oedema sufficient to cause opacification may be difficult to detect in histological sections, but an increase in stromal thickness is demonstrable. In severe cases, Desçemet's membrane becomes undulating in profile. An oedematous cornea is vulnerable to microbial infection and ulceration.

INFLAMMATIONS

Bacterial infections

Coagulase-negative staphylococci and diphtheroid bacilli are normally present in the conjunctival sac and the pathogens mentioned below may also be isolated from apparently healthy eyes.

Acute bacterial conjunctivitis

The pyogenic cocci, especially *Staphylococcus aureus*, pneumococci and *Haemophilus aegyptius* (Koch–Weeks bacillus) are the organisms most commonly isolated from cases of acute bacterial conjunctivitis. *Moraxella lacunata* (diplobacillus of Morax–Axenfeld) is now rather less commonly isolated.

Neisseria gonorrhoeae is equipped with pili which enable it to adhere to undamaged epithelial cells. Infants and young children appear to be especially vulnerable and gonorrhoeal infection may be acquired during birth from an infected mother or occasionally from an infected article such as a towel. Infection by the morphologically indistinguishable *Neisseria meningitidis* occurs sporadically and is a primary infection probably derived in most instances from the nasopharynx of a close contact.

Acute bacterial conjunctivitis is characterised by hyperaemia, oedema and infiltration by neutrophils and mononuclear cells. Secretion and exudation into the conjunctival sac may be mucous, fibrinous or purulent, or a combination of these.

Usually the exudate remains fluid and is discharged as it is formed, but in acute necrotising inflammations dead surface epithelium becomes trapped in coagulated fibrinous or fibrinopurulent exudate to form a pseudomembrane. This occurs particularly in diphtheritic and streptococcal conjunctivitis.

Chronic bacterial conjunctivitis

Chronic infection is manifested by reddening and thickening of the conjunctiva. *Staphylococcus* is again the commonest cause and, in this case, there is usually an associated infection of the lid margin. Various coliforms, epecially *Proteus*, are also able to cause chronic conjunctival infection.

Bacterial ulceration of the cornea

Corneal ulceration due to bacterial infection is commonly central or slightly sub-central. Infection may follow a relatively trivial injury and is especially likely to occur in a cornea affected by chronic oedema. Many bacteria have been incriminated, but the most important are *Staphylococcus aureus*, *Streptococcus pneumoniae* and opportunistic bacteria such as *Proteus mirabilis*. Another organism, *Pseudomonas aeruginosa*, which is found on healthy skin and in the intestinal tract, is of particular importance because it is a common contaminant of eye drops and contact lens solutions and can destroy the cornea with remarkable speed.

The progressive phase of ulcer formation is characterised by oedema, necrosis and invasion by neutrophils. An abscess may form deep to the actual ulcer and, if the two lesions merge to expose Desçemet's membrane, the latter may bulge forward to form a desçemetocele and eventually perforate. Neutrophils are meanwhile attracted from the blood vessels of the iris and ciliary body into the anterior chamber where they form a sediment (hypopyon) (Chapter 2). Dilatation of the capillaries of the substantia propria of the limbal conjunctiva and concomitant infiltration with a mixture of inflammatory cells forms an inflammatory pannus.

As the infection subsides, the necrotic tissues slough away and the crater is epithelialised and gradually filled with fibroblasts derived from neighbouring keratocytes and migrant histiocytes and by capillaries growing in from the limbus. This granulation tissue later matures to a permanent scar. If the loss of tissue is slight and the patient is an infant or child, the scar tends in time to approximate in structure to normal corneal stroma and becomes imperceptible. Past corneal ulceration is indicated by a placoid thickening of the epithelium filling a defect in Bowman's membrane which does not regenerate.

Actinomycetic infections

Actinomyces israeli is a Gram-positive micro-aerophilic branching filamentous organism normally found in the mouth. It may cause an intractable unilateral conjunctivitis as a result of infection of the lacrimal sac or canaliculi. Masses of felted filaments are formed in one or other canaliculus or less commonly in the lacrimal sac. These masses gradually become hard concretions which block the flow of tears and may encourage the growth of pyogenic organisms so that pus can be expelled from the punctum. The surrounding tissues are rarely invaded by the organism. Manual expression through the punctum or surgical removal of the concretion relieves the condition and provides material for smears and cultures.

Mycotic infections

Fungi of various species abound in the environment and various parts of the body including the conjunctival sac, but rarely cause infection in the absence of predisposing factors such as trauma, pre-existing local lesions and prolonged therapy with steroids and antibiotics.

Mycotic conjunctivitis

Mycotic infections of the conjunctiva are uncommon and, like actinomycetic conjunctivitis, are frequently associated with infection of the lacrimal passages. *Candida albicans* and *Aspergillus* may cause chronic conjunctivitis in this way.

Rhinosporidiosis

Infection of the conjunctiva with *Rhinosporidium seeberi* produces polyps in which multiple subepithelial sporangia are visible as greyish-white spots. Infections of the lacrimal sac with this organism results in partial obstruction of the duct by a soft painless mass. Surgical removal of the mass may result in profuse haemorrhage and is often followed by a recurrence of the infection from spores shed into the wound.

Mycotic corneal ulcers

Many fungal species have been isolated from mycotic corneal ulcers, but the most commonly incriminated are *Aspergillus* and *C. albicans*. Among the most destructive is *Fusarium solani*. The infected area of cornea is at first grey and dry and may be outlined by a yellow ring of pus or exhibit grey lines radiating outwards. Satellite lesions, probably representing microabcesses, often appear. Hypopyon is common and may be massive. Sometimes white endothelial plaques are formed, perhaps due to a granulomatous reaction at the level of Desçemet's membrane. Vascularisation is conspicuously absent. The course of infection is characteristically torpid, but eventually a central slough may be discharged to leave a deep ulcer.

Perforation of the cornea is rare, but even without perforation some fungi are capable of invading both anterior and posterior chambers. Sometimes, fungal growth in the posterior chamber results in adhesions between vitreous, lens and iris. Forward displacement of the vitreous–lens–iris complex by aqueous pressure may then cause angle closure and secondary glaucoma.

Laboratory investigation: fungi can be identified in scrapings from the sides and base of the ulcer in wet preparations in 10% potassium hydroxide or in smears stained by Giemsa, Ziehl–Nielsen, PAS and Grocott–Gomori methods (see Appendix IV). Fluorescent antibody staining and affinity to various lectins is of value in identifying the species. Fungi may also be isolated in culture by the use of Sabouraud's agar or broth.

Chlamydial infections

Morphology and life cycle: Chlamydia are small intracellular bacteria which contain both RNA and DNA and have walls resembling those of bacteria. They contain ribosomes of bacterial type and protein synthesis on these is inhibited by broad spectrum antibiotics. The organisms exist in two distinct forms: (1) a highly infectious elementary body measuring 300 nm in diameter which can survive extracellularly and thus act as a transport unit; and (2) a larger and strictly intracellular initial body measuring 500–1200 nm which replicates by binary fission in host cells to produce fresh elementary bodies (Fig. 5.3a). In sub-group A (*v.i.*) these form a perinuclear micro-colony embedded in a glycogen matrix in epithelial cells which stains purple with Giemsa (Fig. 5.3b) and brown with iodine.

Sub-groups: the genus contains two sub-groups.

1 Sub-group A (*C. trachomatis*). This sub-group includes all TRIC (trachoma inclusion conjunctivitis) agents and most isolates from lymphogranuloma venereum (LGV). The organisms are sensitive to sulphadiazine and produce intracytoplasmic inclusions as described. They can be separated into 14 individual serotypes of which A, B and C are responsible for hyperendemic trachoma; D, E, F, G, H, I, J, and K are commonly isolated from eyes and genital tract in areas where trachoma is not hyperendemic; and L1, L2 and L3 give rise to LGV.

2 Sub-group B. This group embraces agents of animal and avian origin such as those causing psittacosis, ornithosis and feline pneumonitis. They form diffuse glycogen-free intracytoplasmic inclusions and are not sensitive to sulphadiazine.

TRIC agent infections: in developed countries chlamydial urethritis, cervicitis, and proctitis are caused mainly by TRIC agents of serotypes D to I. In the UK, they are a common cause of non-specific (non-gonococcal) urethritis in men. Fresh ocular infections are usually due to transfer from the genital tract.

In the rural areas of developing countries where overcrowding, poor hygiene and repeated eye infections are the rule, trachoma and related infections continue to constitute the largest single cause of preventable blindness. In such areas, where trachoma is hyperendemic, eye to eye transmission by eye-seeking flies is very common and infection is mainly by serotypes A, B, and C. Bacteria such as *Haemophilus* which cause seasonal epidemics of acute conjunctivitis are thought to contribute

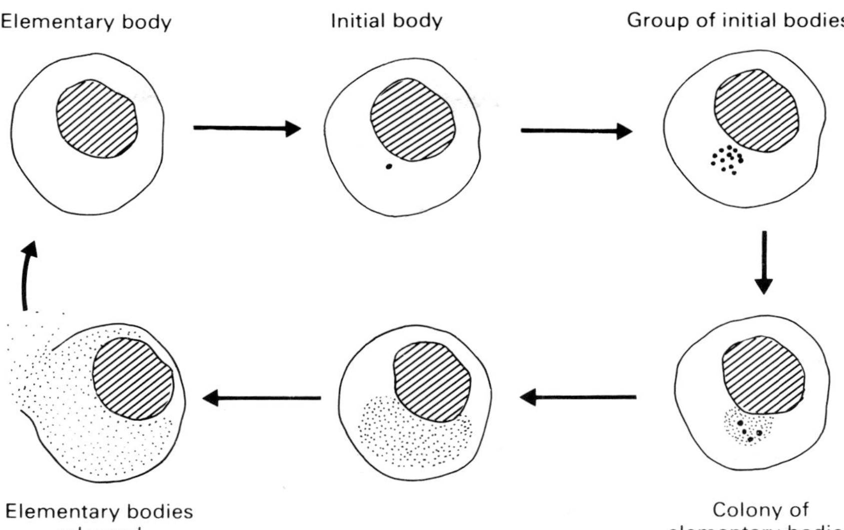

Fig. 5.3 (a) Intracellular cycle of TRIC agent.

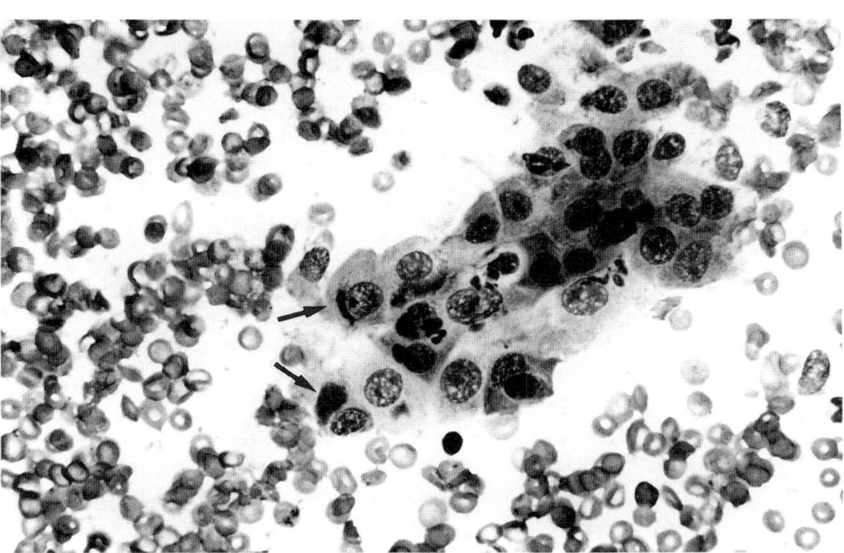

Fig. 5.3 (b) TRIC agent in conjunctival scraping. The epithelial cell (centre) contains a perinuclear inclusion. Giemsa (×410). (Specimen by courtesy of Dr J. L. S. Smith.)

to the severity of hyperendemic trachoma and the prevalence of ensuing blindness, possibly by direct damage to the cornea and enhancement of TRIC agent growth.

There are thus two principal ocular syndromes due to infection with TRIC agents: (1) trachoma; and (2) inclusion conjunctivitis.

Trachoma

Trachoma is almost always bilateral and is characterised clinically by follicle formation mainly in the conjunctiva of the upper tarsus, fornix and limbus, together with epithelial keratitis and scarring. The progress of the disease can be divided into four stages:

Stage I: Incipient. There are minute immature follicles composed of lymphocytes in the upper tarsal conjunctiva. Cytoplasmic inclusions are present in the hyperplastic conjunctival epithelium and the stroma is hyperaemic and oedematous and infiltrated by lymphocytes and neutrophils.

Stage IIa: Follicular hypertrophy. Large soft expressible follicles are present in the conjunctiva of the upper tarsus and fornix and limbal follicles may also be present. Multiple minute punctate erosions appear in the corneal epithelium due to infection of the epithelial cells.

The mature follicles contain germinal centres and necrosis of these centres is characteristic of trachoma. Discharge of their contents to the surface contributes cell debris and macrophages to the cell population of conjunctival scrapings. The stromal infiltration is dominated by plasma cells and macrophages.

Stage IIb: Papillary hypertrophy. This stage represents either trachoma of intense activity or chronic trachoma with superimposed bacterial infection. Follicles are present but are obscured by intense stromal cellular infiltration which causes marked papillary hypertrophy.

Stage III: Cicatrising trachoma. Scarring is proportional to the degree of preceding tissue damage. The surface epithelium becomes stratified squamous in character and the goblet cells disappear while the stromal inflammatory infiltration is gradually replaced, firstly by granulation tissue and then by denser collagenous tissue. As a result, the openings of the lacrimal glands become obstructed and trichiasis, entropion and symblepharon may ensue. A pannus of capillary loops and fibrous tissue descends into the cornea from the upper limbus.

Stage IV: Healed. Inflammation has subsided in the conjunctiva and cornea and both follicles and papillae have been replaced by scar tissue. Scarring of limbal follicles leaves small surface dimples. When these are filled with transparent epithelium they appear as Herbert's pits which are pathognomic of trachoma.

Inclusion conjunctivitis (paratrachoma)

In infants the TRIC agent causes an acute purulent conjunctivitis, which is now the commonest form of ophthalmia neonatorum. The infection is contracted in the birth canal and becomes manifest 5 to 10 days after birth (inclusion blenorrhoea). Occasionally pannus forms and there is conjunctival scarring.

In adults the agent causes a subacute conjunctivitis which is follicular in character and mainly confined to the lower tarsal conjunctiva and lower fornices. Typically, there are no limbal follicles, keratitis is uncommon and the inflammation subsides with appropriate treatment without pannus-formation or scarring. Occasionally, however, the infection may be complicated by persistent punctate keratitis, subepithelial opacities, micropannus and rarely iritis and otitis media.

Laboratory diagnosis of TRIC agent infections

1 *Giemsa-stained smears.* Scrapings from upper tarsal conjunctiva are characteristically pleomorphic showing neutrophils, lymphocytes, macrophages, plasma cells and lymphoblasts. Typical cytoplasmic inclusions are to be found in most cases of inclusion blenorrhoea, but the percentage falls sharply to 40–50% of cases in acute trachoma in adults.
2 *Fluorescent antibody staining.* In adults with ocular or genital infections, a much higher proportion of positive results is obtained by this method than by the examination of Giemsa-stained smears.
3 *Culture.* Chlamydial organisms grow well in cultures of cells such as irradiated McCoy cells or dextran-treated HeLa cells.
4 *Micro-immunofluorescence test.* This test enables the sub-group and serotype to be established. In addition, anti-chlamydial antibodies in serum and tears can be measured. Titres of serum antibody of 1:8 or greater are considered significant.

Amoebic keratitis

Acanthamoeba is a rare cause of intractable corneal ulceration and keratitis which may progress to hypopyon and uveitis. The organism is a free-living amoeba which has been isolated from brackish water and sea water. Infection should be suspected when minor corneal trauma is followed by recalcitrant stromal infiltration. The organism can be cultured by special methods and identified in corneal scrapings examined by immunofluorescent techniques.

Histologically the organisms can be seen in keratoplasty specimens. They are oval in shape, contain a single nucleus and measure up to 20 μm in size. There is accompanying inflammatory infiltration of variable intensity and stromal erosion. Two species, *A. castellani* and *A. polyphaga* have been identified in cases of amoebic keratitis.

Viral infections

Adenovirus infections

The adenoviruses which commonly cause upper respiratory tract, gastrointestinal and ocular infections comprise a group in which more than 35 different serotypes have been identified. The typical features of eye infection are an acute, self-limiting, non-purulent follicular conjunctivitis with regional lymphadenitis. A papillary response is often present in the upper tarsal conjunctiva. The cornea may be involved with variable frequency and degree.

The follicles are aggregates of lymphocytes together with some macrophages. Conjunctival scrapings stained by Giemsa show epithelial cells, lymphocytes and monocytes, but intranuclear inclusions are not readily seen in the epithelial cells.

Adenovirus may be isolated from conjunctival swabs though the cytopathic effect of the virus in culture may take from 5 to 20 days to appear. In the acute stage, immune electron microscopy of tear samples may be helpful in diagnosis. During this stage, a four-fold rise in the serum titre of complement-fixing antibody in samples separated by an interval of 14 days is diagnostic.

The clinical and epidemiological features of ocular adenovirus infection may combine in a number of characteristic ways:

1 *Acute follicular conjunctivitis:* adenovirus infection is the commonest identifiable cause of follicular conjuncti-

vitis. It may occur as isolated cases, or as small community outbreaks. Children and young adults are principally affected and spread may occur via the swimming pool. In a minority of cases, transient corneal opacities are seen. When the ocular signs are associated with upper respiratory tract involvement and pyrexia, it is known as pharyngoconjunctival fever. The serotypes commonly identified are 1, 3, 4 and 7.

2 *Epidemic keratoconjunctivitis:* certain serotypes, notably Type 8, have the capacity to produce explosive outbreaks of eye infection. These occur in industrial situations where ocular trauma is common. They have also affected eye units where lack of hand-washing and use of contaminated towels are responsible for nosocomial infection. The conjunctivitis is severe and may be pseudomembranous. The majority of patients have a keratitis which begins as an epitheliopathy and may progress to characteristic discrete round subepithelial opacities. These lesions, which consist of aggregates of lymphocytes and fibroblastic cells, gradually resolve, though they may persist for years.

Herpes simplex

Modes of infection: herpes simplex virus (HSV) may be transmitted directly between persons or indirectly by contaminated articles such as towels. The source of infection is either a person with an obvious lesion or one who is shedding virus in secretions from the mouth or genitalia. Replication occurs at the site of entry before the virus passes to the regional lymph nodes and possibly the bloodstream.

Primary infection: primary infection with Type 1 virus, which is the usual subtype to involve the nasopharynx and eyes, commonly occurs between 1 and 5 years of age. The infection may not be recognised clinically. Sometimes, however, it results in gingivostomatitis or vesicular eruptions on the lips or face. Primary infection of the eye results in a conjunctivitis which is sometimes accompanied by transient corneal epithelial involvement. Less commonly, primary infection results in meningo-encephalitis or eczema herpeticum or the acute and often fatal disseminated herpes of infancy which involves the skin, mucous membranes, eyes, central nervous system and viscera. Infection of the eyes contracted in the birth canal with Type 2 HSV (genital) herpes virus may result in keratoconjunctivitis or choroidoretinitis. There is also evidence that prenatal infection sometimes results in cataract and peripheral choroidoretinitis.

Recurrent infection: recurrent infections occur despite the presence of serum antibody. After primary infection, the virus remains dormant in sensory nerve ganglia. Type 1 resides in the trigeminal ganglia. A variety of non-specific factors such as fever, trauma, sunburn or menstrual stress may result in a recurrent lesion in the area supplied by the sensory ganglion.

The routes of infection taken by the virus are shown diagrammatically in Fig. 5.4.

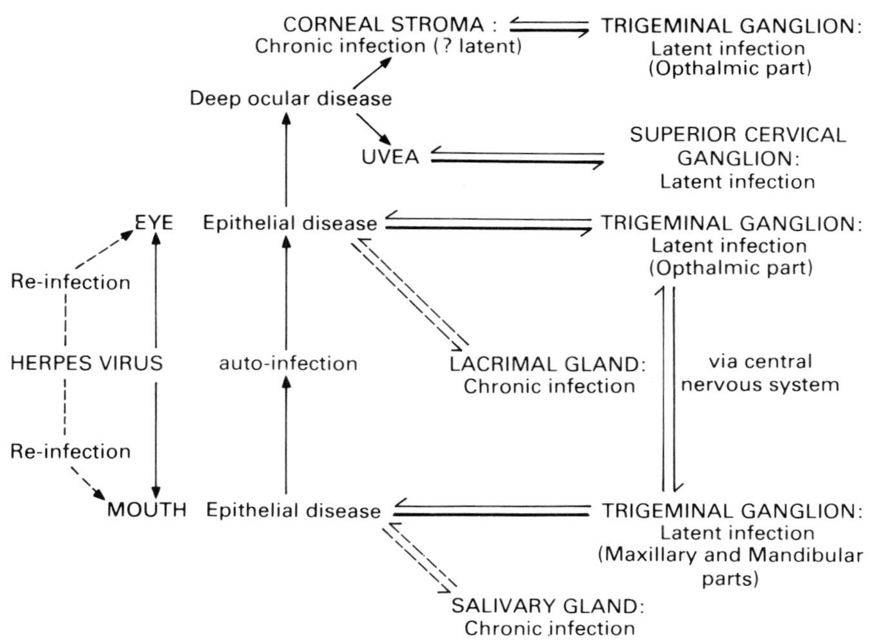

Fig. 5.4 Diagram showing the relationship between re-infection, local manifestations of the disease in the eye and latent infection of the cervical and trigeminal ganglia (arrows). (Reproduced with permission from Easty, 1985.)

Ocular manifestations of herpes simplex

Primary keratoconjunctivitis normally affects only the ocular surface and healing without scarring is the rule. Recurrent infections are, however, more common and may affect the eye in a number of ways:

1 *Epithelial disease*. This commonly takes the form of dendritic ulceration of the cornea. The branches of the ulcer may widen so that it assumes a geographic configuration. After resolution of the infection, a trophic metaherpetic ulcer may occasionally occur as a result of damage to the basement membrane.

2 *Stromal keratitis*. Involvement of the stroma may be diffuse and sometimes a ring similar to a Wessely ring is seen which may well be evidence of an immune hypersensitivity reaction. The commonly observed disciform keratitis is a more localised circumscribed area of stromal oedema. Thinning and vascularisation, usually with underlying keratic precipitates, may eventually occur, especially if involvement is diffuse.

3 *Anterior uveitis*. Herpetic iridocyclitis sometimes complicates keratitis, or may appear in the absence of previous corneal disease. The uveitis usually parallels the keratitis in severity, but is occasionally disproportionately severe or persists after the keratitis has healed. HSV has occasionally been isolated from the aqueous humour of patients with anterior uveitis in the absence of preceding or concurrent keratitis. Secondary cataract and glaucoma are frequent complications.

Microscopic changes in herpes simplex keratitis

1 *Disciform keratitis*. Appearances vary according to the stage. Epithelial oedema with granular degeneration of Bowman's membrane is accompanied by a focal cellular infiltration (Fig. 5.5a & b) which usually includes lymphocytes and polymorphs. Replication of virus within the epithelial cells results in characteristic inclusions within the nuclei (Lipschutz bodies or Type A inclusions). Such inclusions are seldom easy to find in tissue sections. They

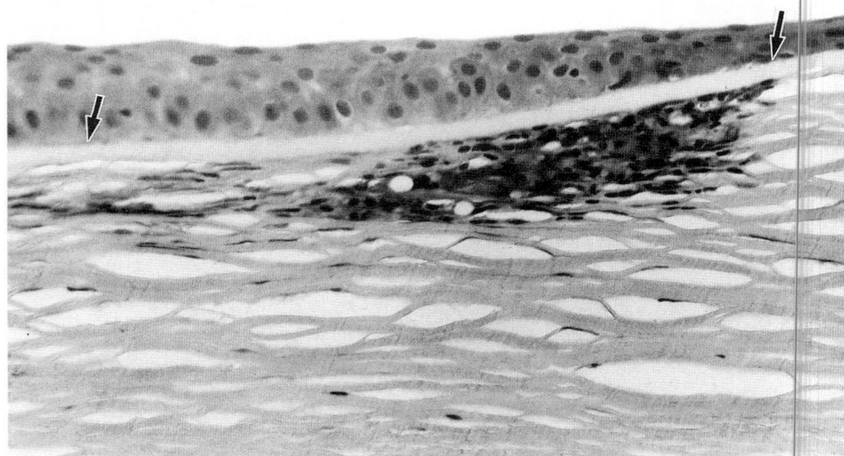

Fig. 5.5 Microscopical changes in herpes simplex keratitis. (a) Dense focal inflammatory infiltrate deep to Bowman's membrane (arrows) which remains intact. H & E (×320).

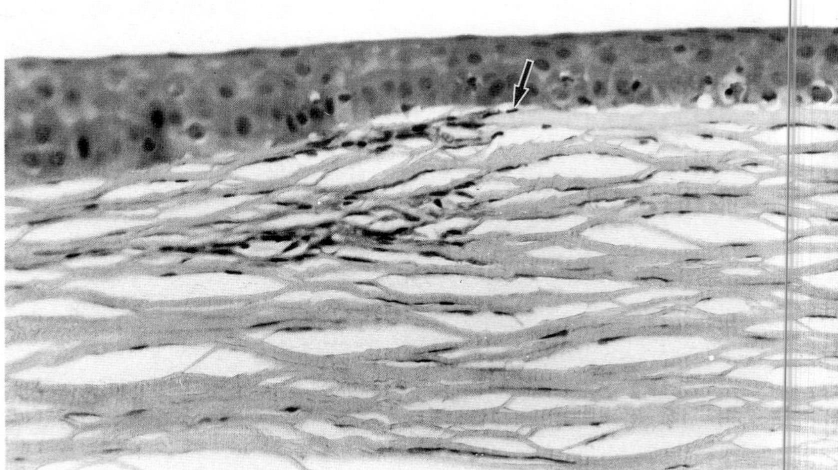

Fig. 5.5 (b) Another focus in the same cornea. The infiltrate is less dense, presumably due to dispersion of the cells, but there is a local break in Bowman's membrane (arrow). H & E (×320).

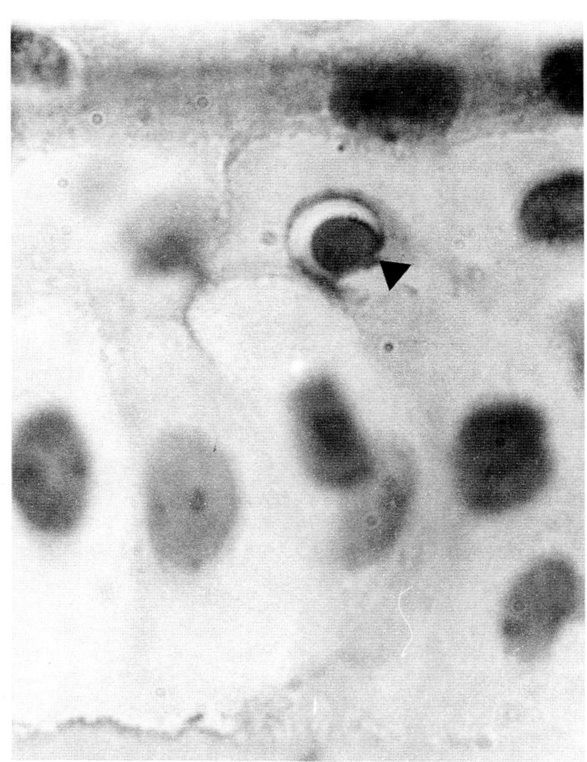

Fig. 5.5 (c) Intranuclear inclusion (arrowhead). Masson's trichrome (×1580).

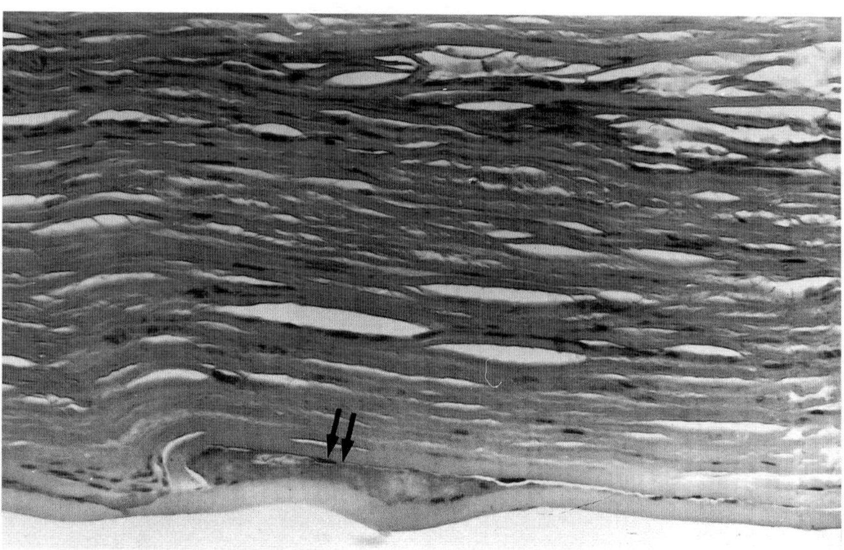

Fig. 5.5 (d) Giant cell closely applied to Desçemet's membrane (double arrow). H & E (×320).

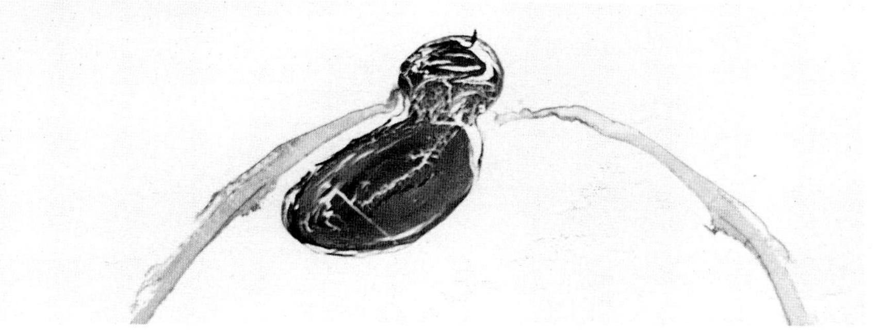

Fig. 5.5 (e) Corneal perforation with prolapse of lens following steroid therapy. H & E.

are usually seen in cells remote from the actively affected area as circular bodies larger than a nucleolus with a clear halo and rim of peripheral cytoplasm. They stain brilliantly with PAS and by the red counterstain of Masson's trichrome (Fig. 5.5c). In H & E sections, they are stained by eosin. The stromal lamellae in the disciform area swell up and there is lymphocytic infiltration of variable intensity. Nuclear fragmentation with the formation of pyknotic debris may be a prominent feature. Later the disciform area may be invaded by blood vessels from the limbus. Deep to the disciform area a granulomatous reaction to Desçemet's membrane is commonly seen (Fig. 5.5d). Desçemet's membrane may be swollen and often fragmented and becomes the target of large foreign body giant cells which are seen closely applied to the surface and capping its broken ends.

2 *Healed disciform keratitis*. Repeated attacks of disciform keratitis may result in stromal scarring. Sections then show an epithelial facet over the scar where Bowman's membrane and the subjacent lamellae have been destroyed. Lymphocytic infiltration may persist in the scar for months or even years after the condition has become clinically quiescent.

3 *Stromal ulceration*. This most commonly follows recurrent epithelial disease which has been treated with steroids and may progress to perforation (Fig. 5.5e). A crater, which may extend down to Desçemet's membrane, is formed. This is bordered by necrotic stromal lamellae infiltrated by lymphocytes and polymorphs. If secondary infection has occurred, micro-organisms may be demonstrable in the necrotic tissue adjacent to the ulcer.

Electron microscopy has occasionally demonstrated HSV in the stromal cells of corneal discs removed from patients undergoing keratoplasty. It has also proved possible to isolate virus from such specimens by prolonged culture.

4 *Kerato-uveitis and uveitis*. Herpetic iridocyclitis is non-granulomatous. HSV-like particles have been observed under the electron microscope in the pigment epithelium, stromal cells, muscle cells and pericytes of iris tissue from a patient with clinically typical herpetic kerato-uveitis. Destruction of iris tissue may leave perforations.

Laboratory diagnosis of herpes simplex keratitis

1 *Cytology*. Scrapings from dendritic ulcers show giant epithelial cells with light blue cytoplasm and multiple nuclei after Giemsa staining, but these are not specific since they also occur in herpes zoster and varicella. Viral antigen can be demonstrated by staining with specific fluorescent antiserum.

2 *Culture*. HSV can be isolated from scrapings from dendritic ulcers in various types of tissue culture.

3 *Serology*. Antibody can be demonstrated by virus neutralisation and complement-fixation tests, but is not diagnostically helpful in recurrent disease since it is present in the serum of most adults and older children.

Herpes zoster

Serological evidence indicates that zoster virus and varicella virus are identical (V-Z virus). Zoster is thought to to be the result of reactivation of virus which has lain dormant in the sensory spinal or cranial nerve ganglia since the time that the primary infection resulted in varicella.

When the nasociliary branch of the ophthalmic division of the trigeminal nerve is involved, the typical papulo-vesicular rash appears on the tip of the nose and this is almost always accompanied by keratitis. The corneal lesions vary in type and severity. In some cases there are discrete superficial stromal opacities or grouped vesicular ulcerative lesions of the corneal epithelium. Such lesions commonly heal without sequelae. More serious lesions comprise neurotrophic keratitis often with severe ulceration, and chronic disciform keratitis which almost always results in severe corneal scarring. Zoster keratitis may be accompanied by iritis and there is evidence that chronic persistent iritis sometimes occurs in the absence of corneal involvement.

Laboratory aid in the diagnosis of either zoster or varicella is rarely required, but if it is then the demonstration of nuclear inclusions in giant cells in scrapings from the vesicles similar to those seen in herpes simplex is of value. During the first week of zoster keratitis, V-Z virus may be demonstrated by fluorescent antibody staining in corneal epithelial cells obtained by scraping.

Varicella

Crusting vesicles occur on the lids as elswhere in the skin. They may also affect the conjunctiva and cornea. Such vesicles normally heal without scarring. A serious occasional complication is disciform keratitis which may persist for months and result in stromal vascularization and permanent scarring.

Vaccinia

Vaccinial infection of the eye usually results from transfer of virus from a vaccination site. Alternatively, the virus may lodge in pre-existing lesions of the lids (e.g. blepharitis), conjunctiva or cornea (e.g. vernal keratoconjunctivitis) during the viraemic period following vaccination.

The evolution of the lid lesions through papule, vesicle, pustule, crust and scar is accompanied by local cellulitis and regional lymphadenitis.

Corneal infection, which rarely occurs without lid lesions, is manifest as marginal keratitis or corneal pustules or occasionally as central disciform keratitis. Marginal keratitis usually heals satisfactorily but may result in astigmatism. Pustular keratitis has a tendency to destroy the corneal stroma and may perforate the globe while disciform keratitis commonly results in severe stromal scarring.

The viruses of vaccinia and variola are members of the poxvirus group to which the viruses of fowlpox, myxomatosis and molluscum contagiosum also belong. Vaccinial elementary bodies, like those of variola, are brick-shaped structures with electron-dense centres. Vaccinia and variola inclusions (Guarnieri bodies) are weakly eosinophilic bodies found in epithelial cells obtained from vesicles.

Variola

Catarrhal or purulent conjunctivitis is a common complication of the prodromal and eruptive phases of smallpox. Very occasionally pustules develop in the bulbar conjunctiva and cornea leading to corneal perforation. Alternatively, the cornea may display disciform keratitis with marked vascularisation resulting in dense scarring.

Measles

Conjunctivitis: acute catarrhal conjunctivitis is part of the prodromal catarrhal phase of measles and precedes the appearance of the typical skin rash. Pathognomonic Koplik's spots consisting of leucocytes and giant cells often appear on the caruncle a day or two before they appear in the mouth. Minute fluorescein-staining punctate opacities in the corneal and conjunctival epithelium can be observed and these are accompanied by severe photophobia beginning in the prodromal phase of the disease and often persisting for many weeks. An interesting feature of the pathology of measles is the formation of Warthin–Finkeldey syncytial cells measuring up to 100 μm and containing as many as 100 nuclei. They first appear in the incubation period and can be demonstrated in nasal secretions before the skin rash appears. Similar cells with eosinophilic, haloed nuclear inclusions develop in measles-infected tissue cultures.

Keratomalacia: in much of sub-Saharan Africa, acute corneal ulceration following measles is the commonest cause of childhood blindness. Specific measles keratitis and secondary herpes simplex infection may be local contributory infections, but there is nearly always a background of protein calorie malnutrition. Tissue vitamin A deficiency may also be a factor.

Mumps

Painful and usually bilateral dacryoadenitis is a frequent complication of mumps. The inflammation usually subsides spontaneously but occasionally results in abscess formation. Dacryoadenitis is accompanied by conjunctival hyperaemia and occasionally by episcleritis. During the course of the disease keratitis may develop as a unilateral dense stromal opacity either limited to one segment or involving the whole cornea and accompanied by iritis. Spontaneous resolution without sequelae is the rule.

Mumps virus is a member of the myxovirus group to which the viruses of influenza and Newcastle disease of fowls also belong. Infection with Newcastle disease virus most commonly causes a follicular conjunctivitis of short duration with preauricular adenitis and less often an upper respiratory infection or an influenzal type illness. A history of exposure to fowls or laboratory virus may be available.

Interstitial keratitis

Most cases of diffuse interstitial keratitis occur in congenital syphilitics. It is usually associated with an anterior uveitis. In the acute stage there is necrosis usually of the deeper stromal lamellae associated with massive lymphocytic infiltration and followed by ingrowth of vessels. Resolution of the inflammatory process and subsequent stromal scarring result in a characteristic pathological picture with fine vessels persisting in the deep stroma, often adjacent to Desçemet's membrane which is irregularly thickened and may, in longstanding cases, show secondary guttate changes (Fig. 5.6).

NON-INFECTIVE CONJUNCTIVITIS

Allergic conjunctivitis

Except in cases obviously related to airborne pollens and animal dander and associated with other allergic manifestations such as hay fever, the specific causes of allergic conjunctivitis are difficult to identify with certainty.

Vernal conjunctivitis

Spring catarrh is a chronic recurrent bilateral inflammation which often shows seasonal exacerbations, though not always in spring. Clinically the condition is characterised by flat-topped papillae in the upper tarsal conjunctiva or a gelatinous or waxy roll of inflammatory

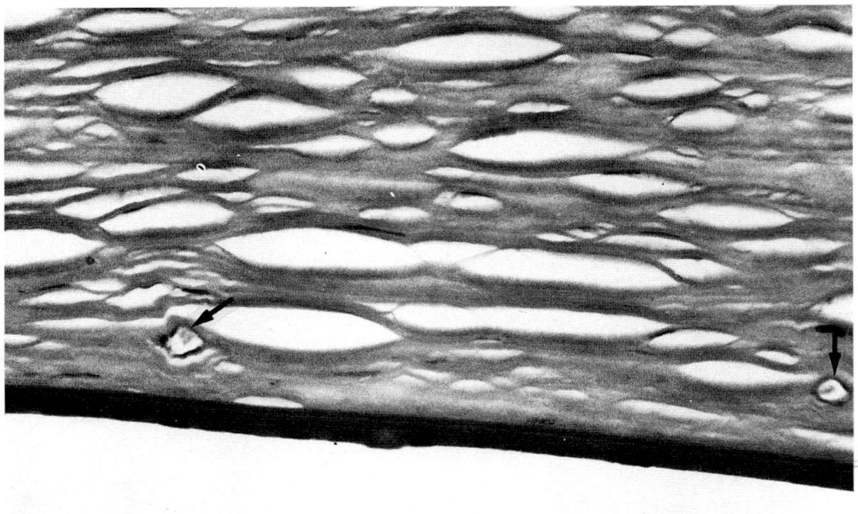

Fig. 5.6 Old interstitial keratitis. Small vessels present in deep stroma (arrows) which contain red cells. Desçemet's membrane is slightly thickened. PAS/ tartrazine (×320).

tissue beneath the limbal epithelium. The papillae develop because the conjunctival epithelium is anchored at intervals to the tarsal plate; accumulation of exudate and granulation tissue between these fixed points pushes the epithelium upwards forming papillae within which the conjunctival vessels are visible (Fig. 5.7). Shallow ulcers in the upper half of the cornea are also described in association with opacification of the underlying Bowman's membrane. A dense deposit may form in the ulcer base, the removal of which is necessary before re-epithelialisation can occur.

The disease commences with epithelial and goblet cell proliferation, hyperaemia and stromal infiltration by mononuclear cells and eosinophils. Lymph follicle formation is minimal. Later the stroma becomes thickened by granulation tissue and eventually much hyaline fibrous tissue is formed. An excess of eosinophils is found in the stringy mucous discharge in the conjunctival sac and in scrapings from the upper tarsal conjunctiva.

A giant papillary conjunctivitis of the upper tarsal conjunctiva resembling vernal conjunctivitis can result from wearing both hard and soft contact lenses.

Phlyctenular conjunctivitis

This condition occurs as a complication of tuberculosis or staphylococcal blepharitis and is thought to be an expression of hypersensitivity to bacterial proteins. It is characterised by whitish nodules surrounded by a zone of hyperaemia, most frequently at the limbus and some-

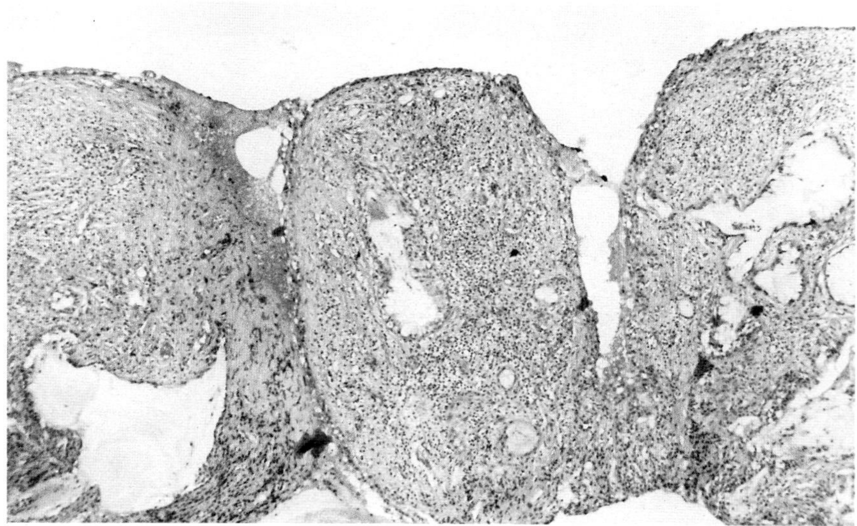

Fig. 5.7 Allergic conjunctivitis. Swollen conjunctiva exhibiting pseudopapillary appearance. H & E (×64).

times in the cornea. The nodules, composed of neutrophils and small lymphocytes, ulcerate, discharge their contents and heal by fibrosis.

Progressive phlyctenular disease may lead to marginal corneal ulceration or a creeping invasion of the cornea by ulcerative inflammation accompanied by a leash of vessels (fascicular ulcer). Corneal phlyctens may induce pannus formation from the corresponding limbal segment. Occasionally, Salzmann's nodular corneal degeneration develops in eyes previously affected by phlyctenular conjunctivitis.

Ligneous conjunctivitis

This is a rare pseudomembranous conjunctivitis of unknown aetiology which often begins in childhood and persists for months or even years. The disease is commonly bilateral and it is characteristic that the pseudomembrane rapidly reforms after removal. In the course of time the eyelids suffer woody induration as a result of the formation in the palpebral conjunctivae of granulation tissue containing masses of hyaline substances rich in hyaluronic acid. Occasionally corneal involvement leads to perforation. The abnormal masses contains plasma proteins and abnormal blood vessels with endothelial gaps have recently been described (Hidayat & Riddle, 1987).

NON-INFECTIVE CORNEAL ULCERATION

Small recurrent marginal ulcers accompanying conjunctivitis or blepharitis may be an expression of hypersensitivity to staphylococcal toxin. Extensive circumferential ulceration of the corneal periphery (gutter ulcer) sometimes occurs in association with rheumatoid arthritis, polyarteritis nodosa, systemic lupus erythematosus and Wegener's granulomatosis or as a complication of influenza or bacillary dysentery.

Mooren's ulcer (corneal melting syndrome)

This chronic serpiginous ulcer is an uncommon, slowly progressive bilateral disease of unknown aetiology occurring in otherwise healthy, but usually elderly persons. It begins as a grey peripheral infiltrate which breaks down into a furrow ulcer. This spreads both circumferentially and towards the centre of the cornea, undermining the surface layers as it goes, to form an overhanging lip (Fig. 5.8). The margin of the ulcer is infiltrated with lymphocytes and plasma cells. Hypopyon and perforation rarely occur in the absence of secondary infection, and in contradistinction to corneal melting associated with 'connective tissue diseases' such as rheumatoid arthritis, the sclera is never invaded.

The reported pathological changes have been variable, particularly as to the nature and severity of the inflammatory infiltrate. Some cases apparently show little inflammatory reaction while others exhibit a heavy infiltrate of lymphocytes and polymorphs. Destruction of the corneal stroma has been attributed to liberation of collagenase from the latter. The conjunctiva is another possible source of collagenase. Recent observations have associated corneal melting with fibroblastic activity (Young & Watson, 1982).

Keratoconjunctivitis sicca (KCS)

In KCS there is a deficiency in aqueous tear secretion so that the tear film does not cover the corneal surface

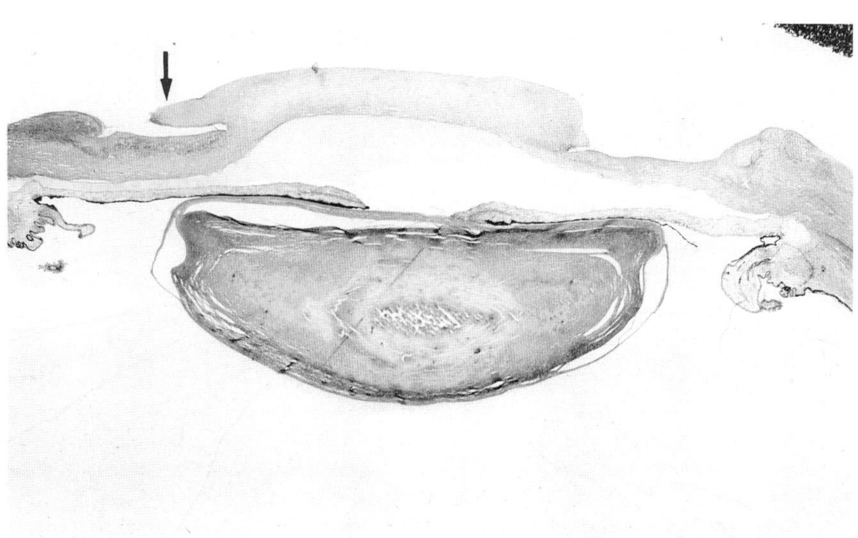

Fig. 5.8 Mooren's ulcer. Note deep stromal ulceration at periphery on both sides with overhanging lip on one side (arrow). Masson's trichrome stain. (Specimen by courtesy of Dr J.L. S. Smith.)

evenly. Electrophoresis of tears shows a constant early decrease or absence of lysozyme.

Microscopic studies have shown that the conjunctival epithelium becomes increasingly stratified while the population of goblet cells is reduced. The epithelial cells tend to separate in sheets which may contribute to the filaments observed on the cornea in these cases. Susceptibility to secondary infection, especially by *Staphylococcus aureus*, is high.

The salivary and lacrimal glands exhibit intense lymphocytic infiltration which almost entirely replaces the secreting acini. The gland may not be substantially enlarged and the normal lobular pattern is often well preserved. Sometimes the histological picture is that of a benign lymphoepithelial lesion (Chapter 16).

KCS is frequently part of a more generalised disorder and the combination of xerostomia, polyarthritis and KCS is referred to as Sjögren's syndrome. This condition, which affects principally women over the age of 40, is the expression of an autoimmune disorder. In a majority of patients, autoantibodies to salivary duct antigens are present in the serum. There is also a high incidence of serum antinuclear antibody and more than one third of patients have positive LE cell tests. The rheumatoid factor can be demonstrated in a majority of patients although only 50% have clinical manifestations of rheumatoid arthritis. It is by far the commonest ocular complication of this disease, eventually affecting from 10 to 30% of longstanding cases. It may also occur less commonly in related disorders.

EPISCLERITIS AND SCLERITIS

Episcleritis

In this condition there is oedema and intense congestion of the superficial episcleral vascular network. The inflammation is usually sectorial and affects the interpalpebral area preferentially. Microscopically the inflamed area is densely infiltrated with lymphocytes, but few other inflammatory cells are seen. True rheumatoid nodules have been reported, but serious destructive changes in the sclera do not occur. About a third of cases suffer from a variety of associated systemic diseases, including rheumatoid arthritis.

Scleritis

By contrast with episcleritis, scleritis is a destructive process which takes various forms such as brawny scleritis, rheumatoid nodule of the sclera, nodular scleritis, scleromalacia perforans and massive granuloma of the sclera. The term necrogranulomatous scleritis seems appropriate for all these.

Typically, necrogranulomatous scleritis is an acute anterior scleritis characterised by exacerbations and remissions which may ultimately result in the formation of a sequestrum of necrotic sclera lying at the base of a punched out conjunctival ulcer. Although scleral perforation and uveal prolapse may occur (scleromalacia perforans), eventual healing leaving a slate-blue spot is not uncommon.

When the scleritis is diffuse (brawny scleritis), the sclera becomes greatly thickened and the inflammation tends to spread into the uvea. These cases run a protracted course, often with severe pain and loss of vision. If the inflammation is located posteriorly and there is no history of rheumatoid arthritis or other connective tissue disorder, they may be misdiagnosed clinically as malignant melanomata.

Approximately one third of patients with with necrogranulomatous scleritis have rheumatoid arthritis, especially those with scleromalacia perforans. Other associations include polyarteritis nodosa, Wegener's granulomatosis, systemic lupus erythematosus and herpes zoster. However, many patients present no evidence of generalised disease.

Microscopically, the nodular lesions consist of a central focus of fibrinoid necrosis circumscribed by a ring of histiocytes which may be elongated and form a radial palisade together with neutrophils, eosinophils, lymphocytes, plasma cells and a variable number of giant cells. Scleral collagen fibres undergoing necrosis become frayed and lose their birefringence under polarised light. If there is extensive destruction, as in brawny scleritis, extensive fibrosis occurs with massive thickening of the sclera.

The scleral changes appear to resemble closely those seen in the nodules which develop subcutaneously or in joint capsules and fascias in rheumatoid arthritis. The necrosis, in both cases, is thought to be initiated by immune complex deposition.

EFFECTS OF NOXIOUS AGENTS

Chemical injuries

While the precise manner in which the tissues are damaged may vary, common features exist between the effects of chemicals such as strong acids and alkalis on the cornea and conjunctiva. Limited exposure will result in intense hyperaemia and oedema of the conjunctiva and lacrimation. If this is sufficient to flush the irritant from the eye without significant tissue destruction, the condition will rapidly resolve without ill-effects. If exposure is severe enough to result in extensive tissue necrosis, the results are likely to be catastrophic. Necrotic conjunctiva will slough off and subsequent fibrosis obliterate the conjunctival sac to a greater or lesser extent. Similarly, if damage to the cornea is confined to the epithelium, no ill-effects will ensue, but heavy exposure with extensive destruction of corneal stroma must result in severe scarring and vascularization. The latter is a conspicuous feature of chemical burns of the cornea and occurs at both superficial and deep levels.

Acid burns

Strong acids precipitate the tissue proteins and this tends to limit penetration.

Alkali burns

Alkalis destabilise tissue proteins, break down cell membranes and react with the lipids of these structures to form soluble compounds that penetrate rapidly. Classically, three stages have been recognised (Lemp, 1974):

1 *Acute stage.* There is ischaemic necrosis of the conjunctiva and sloughing of the corneal epithelium with opacification of the deeper tissues and iritis. Polymorphs infiltrate the necrotic tissues. The infiltration by polymorphs may be heavy and is probably at least partly accounted for by breakdown product(s) in alkali-burned collagen that are chemotactic and can also activate a respiratory burst (Pfister *et al.*, 1987).

2 *Reparative stage.* The epithelium regenerates, the cornea is vascularised and the iritis subsides.

3 *Stage of late complications.* These include symblepharon, the appearance of a vascular membrane on the cornea, recurrent corneal ulceration, uveitis, cataract and glaucoma.

Collagenase activity is high in rabbit corneas subjected to alkali burns and it has been suggested that collagenase derived from the ingrowing epithelium and from leucocytes 'melt' the damaged tissues.

The end result of an alkali burn depends critically on the extent of conjunctival involvement, limbal ischaemia and necrosis (see Fig. 5.9). The densely scarred vascularised cornea which only too often ensues is difficult to treat successfully by keratoplasty. Dryness due to destruction of goblet cells often aggravates the problem.

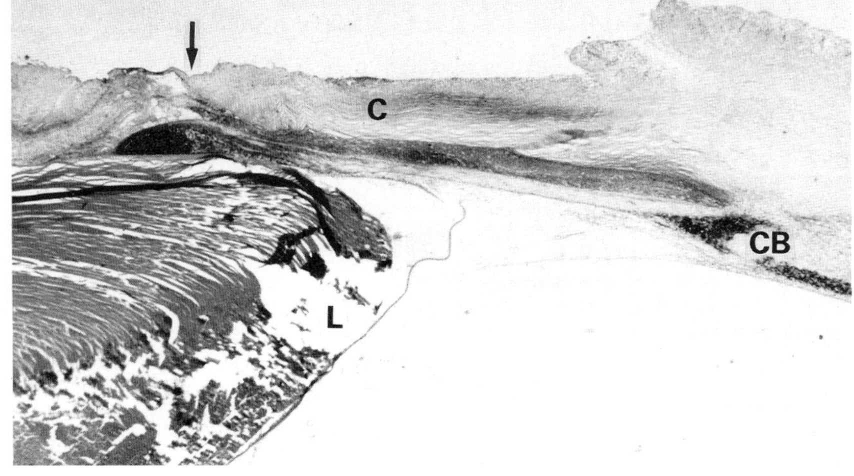

Fig. 5.9 Alkali burn caused by the explosion of a non-rechargeable alkali–managanese battery during an attempt to recharge it. (a) The epithelium of the cornea and conjunctiva is completely denuded and there has been substantial stromal erosion with a large central corneal perforation the margin of which is indicated by an arrow. The iris and ciliary body (CB) are also necrotic. The dark areas are inflammatory infiltrate. The lens (L) has become disrupted during cutting. (C = corneal stroma) (×20).

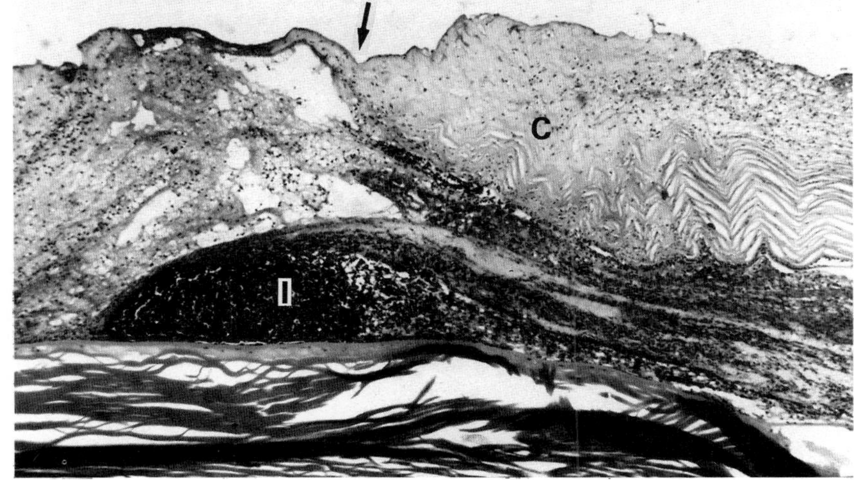

Fig. 5.9 (b) Central part showing margin of perforation in more detail. (I = iris) (×160).

Reaction to foreign material

In general, matter such as sutures, glass splinters, vegetable fibres, etc. excites a typical granulomatous foreign body reaction in the conjunctiva. Two particular types of foreign matter deserve special mention:

1 *Golf ball cores*. These contain a suspension of barium sulphate crystals under high pressure and if the core is pierced the fluid spurts out with considerable force. The crystals are apparently forced through the conjunctival epithelium without causing detectable surface damage to form a pasty yellow mass in the bulbar conjunctiva. Microscopically, pools of birefringent crystals are seen in the substantia propria surrounded by macrophages and foreign body giant cells (Fig. 5.10).

2 *Caterpillar bristles*. The bristles of certain hairy caterpillars not only contain irritant secretion, but are covered in spines so that if they become embedded in the cornea or conjunctiva they cause intense local irritation and tend to work their way into the eye where they excite granulomatous nodules (see Chapter 18).

Effects of ionising radiation

Conjunctiva

The immediate effect of a significant dose of ionising radiation is hyperaemia and oedema. This is followed eventually by the appearance of telangiectasia and crumbly keratin plaques may form on the tarsal conjunctiva. High dosage will result in scarring, distortion and symblepharon.

Cornea

Corneal complications may arise following radiotherapy either through decreased lacrimal secretion causing dryness or through direct damage. The immediate effect of irradiation is the appearance of punctate epithelial erosions. Later corneal sensitivity decreases and intractable ulceration ensues. A not infrequent outcome of radiotherapy for malignancies such as antral carcinoma is loss of the eye because of a perforated corneal ulcer.

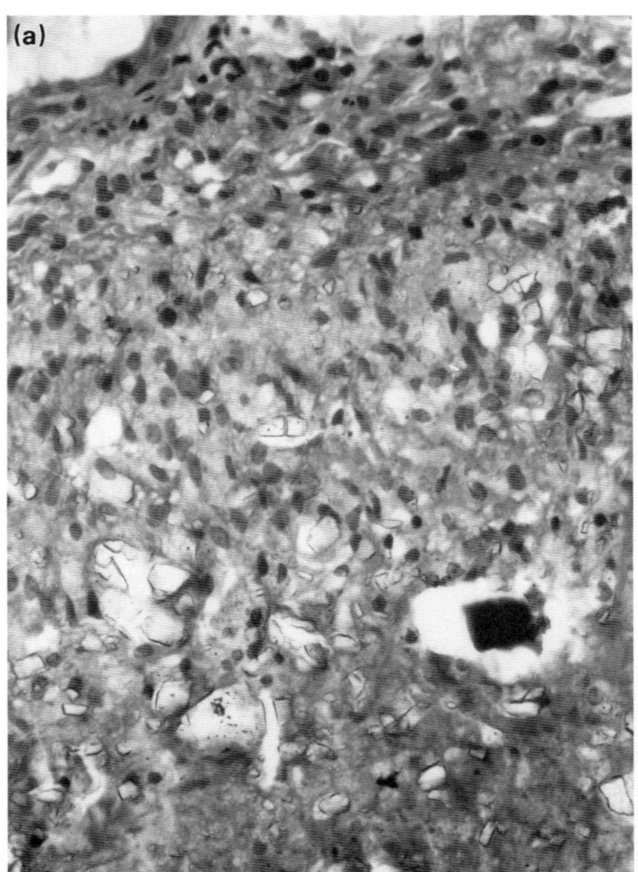

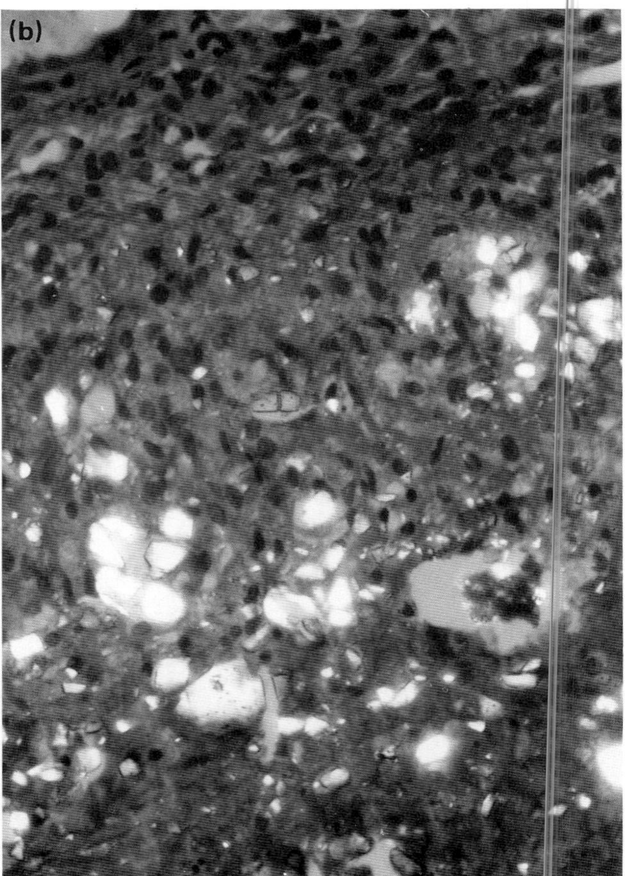

Fig. 5.10 Golf ball injury. Conjunctival deposit of barium sulphate crystals. (a) Under normal illumination showing palisade-like arrangement of crystal-containing macrophages around the deposit. (Reproduced with permission from Lucas *et al.* 1976.) (b) Same field under polarised light. H & E (×250).

DEGENERATIONS

Degenerations of cornea and conjunctiva are conveniently considered together. They fall into two categories: firstly those promoted by particular climatic conditions, especially exposure to ultraviolet (UV) light, namely pinguecula, pterygium and spheroidal degeneration of the cornea; and secondly those associated with chronic ocular or systemic disease, namely band keratopathy, amyloidosis and lipid keratopathy.

Degenerations (1)

Pinguecula

A pinguecula is a localised elevated area close to the limbus in the interpalpebral fissure. Its elevation and colour are the result of degenerative changes in the subepithelial collagen. This breaks into short, often basophilic curled fragments which stain positively for elastin (elastosis). Later this degenerative product is transformed into an eosinophilic granular or glassy mass in which calcium granules may be deposited. Fibrovascular proliferation is less prominent than in a pterygium and there is no invasion of the cornea.

Elastosis similar to that seen in pingueculae and pterygia also occurs in the skin after excessive exposure to sunlight. Though it has always been doubted that the fibres staining for elastin were actually elastin because they resisted digestion by elastase, recent electron microscopic studies have indicated that abnormal elastin fibres are apparently formed (Austin *et al.*, 1983).

Pterygium

A pterygium (wing) is a wedge of conjunctival tissue ploughing across the limbus into the superficial cornea in the interpalpebral fissure commonly on the nasal side.

Although the pathogenesis of pterygium is not fully understood, it is probable that the drying of the interpalpebral tear film is an important factor. This exposes the peripheral corneal epithelium, Bowman's membrane and the underlying corneal stroma to the destructive effects of ultraviolet (UV) light, and the tissue damage thus sustained stimulates the advance of the limbal vessels into the cornea. That other factors may operate in some situations is suggested by the observation of a high incidence of pterygia among indoor sawmill workers.

Drying of the interpalpebral film occurs most readily in the medial third of the interpalpebral fissure because this part of the conjunctiva is farthest from the lacrimal glands and nearest to the puncta and because, with the eyes partially closed against glare or wind, the medial third of the the conjunctiva remains relatively more exposed than the lateral. Drying of the tear film occurs not only when atmospheric humidity is low, but also when there is exposure to constant wind.

In the genesis of pterygium, pinguecula and spheroidal degeneration of the cornea the most damaging solar radiation is UV light, especially when reflected from snow, water or ice. High doses of UV light cause nuclear fragmentation and cell death. In the corneal epithelium this results in punctate epithelial erosions stainable by 1% rose bengal. Recovery is rapid and complete after limited exposure, but repeated daily exposures result in the formation of punctate ulcers which uncover Bowman's membrane.

After prolonged exposure to UV light, holes appear in Bowman's membrane (colander degeneration) beneath the areas of epithelial necrosis, and the underlying corneal stroma becomes oedematous. These peripheral corneal changes appear to stimulate invasion by blood vessels and fibroblasts from the limbus, hastened by such factors as chronic infection or dust which increase corneal vascularity. Subsequent organisation of this fibrovascular tissue causes traction which draws the characteristic wing of conjunctival tissue onto the cornea. The presence of colander degeneration of Bowman's membrane and oedema of the underlying stroma at the apex of the pterygium indicate that the degenerative process is still active and that the pterygium is progressing.

Microscopically a pterygium consists of fibrovascular tissue, the collagen fibres of which often exhibit elastosis. Except at its apex, the pterygium is covered by conjunctival epithelium. The microscopic apex, consisting of avascular fibroblastic tissue, can be seen spearing its way into the cornea along the cleavage planes between the epithelium, Bowman's membrane and the substantia propria. It is covered by corneal epithelium. Bowman's membrane is thinned and fragmented and the gaps in it are filled with fibrous tissue (Fig. 5.11). Older pterygia become densely fibrous with areas of hyaline degeneration and sometimes granular calcification. Dysplastic changes may also appear in the overlying epithelium.

Spheroidal degeneration of the cornea

This condition, which is also known as climatic droplet or Labrador keratophy is also prevalent in conditions of high exposure to UV light. It is characterised by the deposition of rounded proteinaceous matter in Bowman's membrane and the superficial corneal stroma. The material does not stain for elastin and is rich in tryptophane, tyrosine, cysteine and cystine. Its source is unknown.

The interrelationship of pterygium, pinguecula and spheroidal degeneration is of interest. It is widely believed, but nevertheless doubtful, that pterygia arise from pingueculae. Spheroidal deposits similar to those seen in

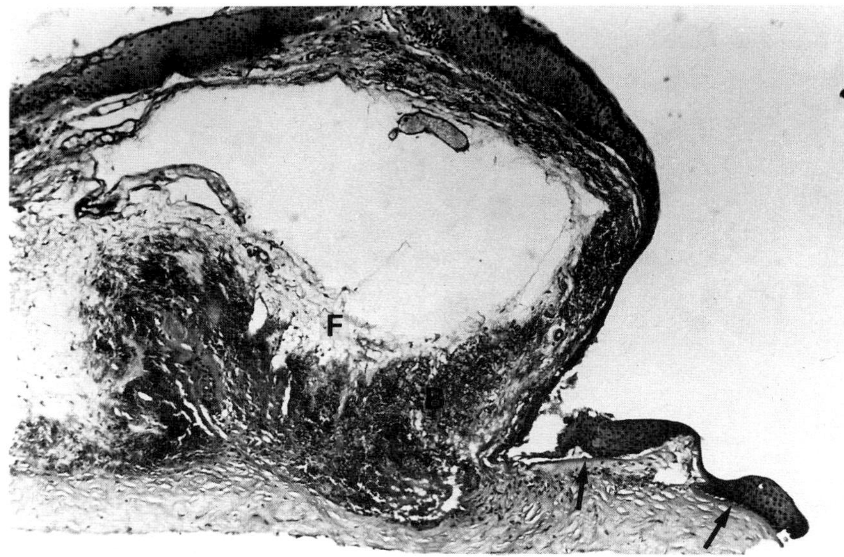

Fig. 5.11 Pterygium. (a) Low power view showing fibrovascular tissue (F) with a large underlying mass of basophilic material (B) in *substantia propria*. Encroachment onto the corneal margin with consequent disruption of Bowman's membrane (arrows) is clearly seen. H & E (×64).

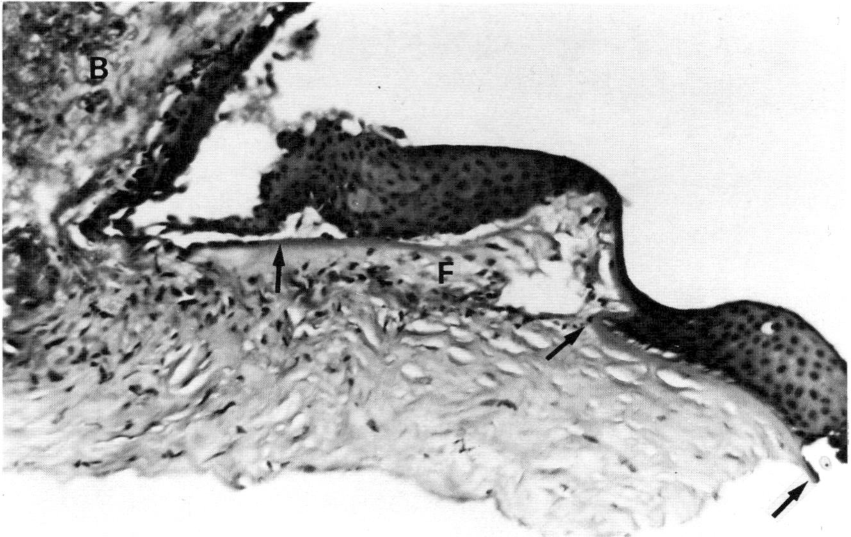

Fig. 5.11 (b) Higher power view of corneal margin. H & E (×125).

the cornea may be seen in pingueculae, but rarely in pterygia. Spheroidal degeneration of the cornea is often associated with pingueculae, but rarely with pterygia.

Degenerations (2)

Band keratopathy

This type of degeneration is seen mainly as a complication of chronic iridocyclitis or longstanding glaucoma. It also occurs as a complication of hypercalcaemia in such conditions as vitamin D poisoning, sarcoidosis, hyperparathyroidism and severe renal disease.

Microscopically (Fig. 5.12), there is an extracellular deposition of calcium phosphate in the epithelial basement membrane, Bowman's membrane and the superficial stromal lamellae imparting a fine basophilic stippling. In time, Bowman's membrane becomes densely calcifed and fragmented. These changes are accompanied by an ingrowth of degenerative pannus and the replacement of superficial corneal lamellae by an avascular scar in which refractile hyaline globules are deposited.

Amyloidosis

Small nodules of amyloid are occasionally found in the conjunctiva. Larger more widespread deposits may cause cause swelling of the lids and conjunctiva. In routine sections, amyloid appears as eosinophilic amorphous deposits in connective tissue and in the walls of blood vessels. It is stained red by congo red and shows apple green dichroism under polarised light. With thioflavine-

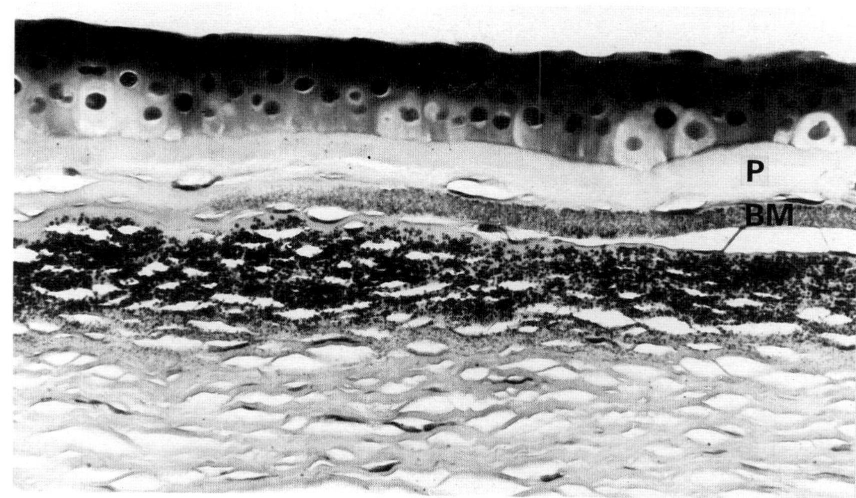

Fig. 5.12 Band keratopathy. Fine hyaline fibrous pannus (P) between epithelium and Bowman's membrane (BM) with basophilic calcific stippling of Bowman's membrane and anterior stromal lamellae. Masson's trichrome (×320).

T it gives a greenish fluorescence under UV illumination. The cause of these deposits is obscure. Some may represent 'burned out' local plasmacytomata.

Amyloid may occasionally be deposited in the cornea, usually between the epithelium and Bowman's membrane in a wide variety of chronic eye diseases. This must not be confused with lattice dystrophy.

Lipid keratopathy

Lipid plaques sometimes form in or near areas of stromal vascularisation due, for example, to herpes simplex and herpes zoster. They result from haemorrhage or exudation of plasma from the stromal vessels. The fat deposits, which consist predominantly of cholesterol and fatty acids are accompanied by a granulomatous inflammatory reaction (Fig. 5.13).

Salzmann's nodular degeneration of the cornea

In this rare and usually unilateral condition, large bluish-white opacities appear successively in corneas showing evidence of past keratitis. The opacities form at the ends of vascular loops and are consequently arranged in an arc or circle concentric with the limbus. They consist of nodules of hyaline collagen lying between the epithelium and Bowman's membrane which is often focally destroyed.

ABNORMAL PIGMENTATIONS

Endogenous or exogenous local or systemic factors may cause abnormal pigmentation of the cornea, conjunctiva or sclera. The pigmentation may be due to melanin or melanin-like pigments or metallic deposits.

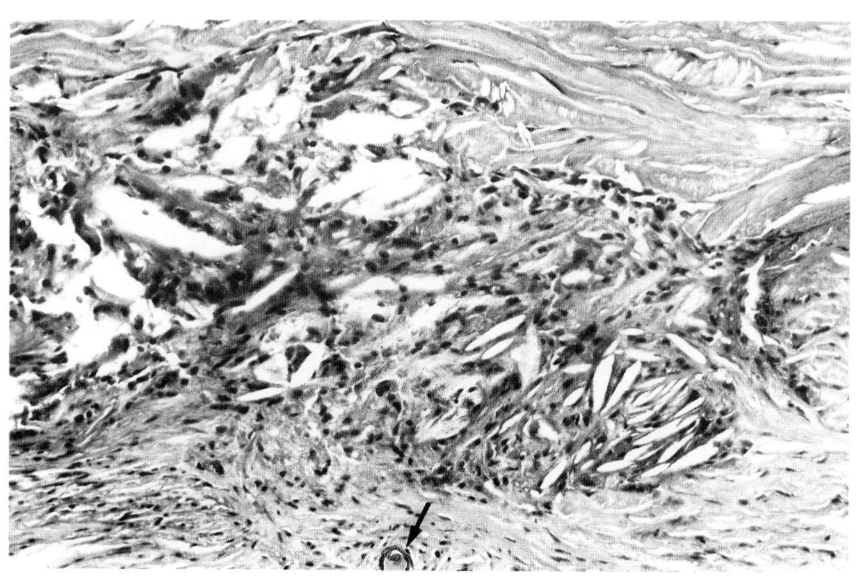

Fig. 5.13 Lipid keratopathy. Cholesterol crystal profiles in stromal granulomatous infitrate. A small blood vessel can be seen (arrow). H & E (×160).

Pigmentation due to local factors

Hudson–Stahli line

This is a horizontal line across the cornea at the line of lid closure which is due to deposition of iron in the epithelium, mainly the basal layer. It is seen mostly in late middle age. The precise local factors responsible are not known.

Epinephrine

Deposits of melanin or melanin-like substance derived by oxidation of epinephrine occur in the conjunctiva and cornea after prolonged topical use of this drug. In the conjunctiva the pigment is most commonly found in small crypts in the epithelium of the lower palpebral conjunctiva (Fig. 5.14), while in the cornea it is located either between the epithelium and Bowman's membrane or mainly in the latter (black cornea).

Foreign bodies

Local pigmentation may occur in relation to retained metallic foreign bodies containing iron (siderosis) or copper (chalcosis).

Haemorrhage

Siderotic staining of the corneal stroma occurs after hyphaema, haemorrhage from ruptured new vessels or after a large subconjunctival haemorrhage and may be slow to clear.

Pigmentation due to systemic disease

Addison's disease

The conjunctival melanosis of Addison's disease is due to increased cytocrine activity of the epithelial melanocytes, possibly as a result of unopposed production of pituitary melanocyte stimulating hormone.

Ocular ochronosis

Alkaptonuria results from an inborn inability to metabolise phenylalanine and tyrosine beyond the stage of homgentisic acid (hydroquinone acetic acid) which is excreted in the urine where it undergoes oxidation to a melanin-like substance. In middle age, most alkaptonurics develop deposits of brown oxidation products of homogentisic acid, especially in cartilages and connective tissue including the sclera, where semilunar or V-shaped brown areas appear midway between the corneal margin and the inner or outer canthus. The pigment is found in macrophages or encrusted on coiled fragments of degenerate collagen fibres in the vicinity of the insertions of the rectus muscles.

Kinnier Wilson's disease

One of the most striking pigment rings (Kayser–Fleischer) is seen in this condition. It is due to the deposition of copper in the periphery of Desçemet's membrane.

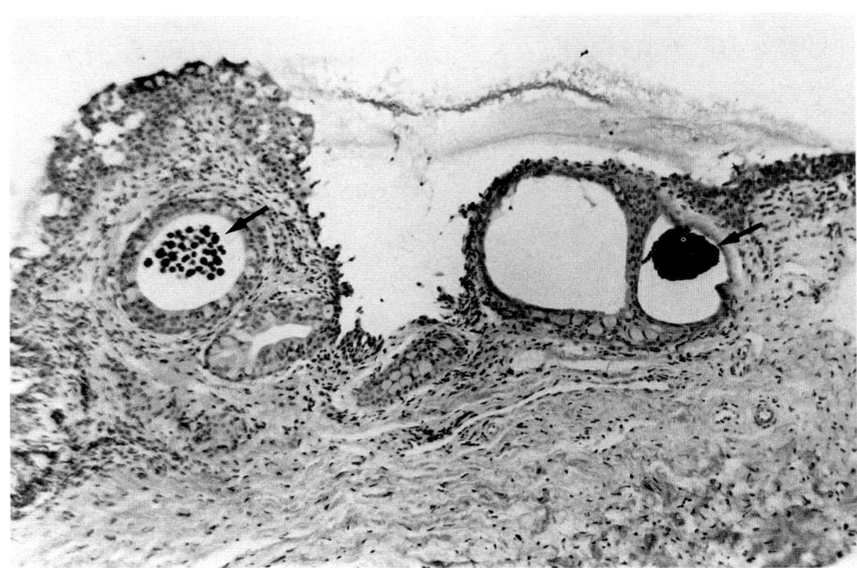

Fig. 5.14 Conjunctival epinephrine deposits (arrows) in epithelial cysts. Masson fontana (×94).

Haemolytic anaemia

Deposits of iron in the deeper layers of the cornea have been reported.

Exogenous systemic causes of pigmentation

Argyrosis

Silver staining of the tissues results from prolonged therapeutic (argyrol, silver nitrate) or industrial (silver plating and polishing) exposure. In sections of the conjunctiva, fine black granules of reduced silver are found mainly in the elastic and reticulin fibres of blood vessels and the basement membrane of the epithelium (which is itself pigment-free).

Chrysiasis

A purple or red deposit may be seen in the superficial stroma after prolonged administration of gold salts for rheumatoid arthritis.

Phenolic compounds

Prolonged absorption of phenol compounds such as carbolic or picric acids due to industrial or therapeutic exposure, may result in a similar syndrome. In these cases the melanin-like pigment results from the oxidation of phenolic substances in the body.

Quinone

Keratitis and yellow staining of the cornea and conjunctiva in the interpalpebral fissure occur after long exposure to quinone, an intermediate product in the manufacture of hydroquinone photographic developer.

Phenothiazines

These and related drugs may cause deposition of melanin granules at the level of Desçemet's membrane and sometimes in the stroma and Bowman's membrane.

Chloroquine

With long-term oral administration deposition of chloroquine occurs in the epithelium and superficial stroma. These appear as fine yellowish-white dots arranged in whorls. The corneal deposits are of minor importance compared to the effect on the retina (Chapter 10).

A brownish-olive line may appear in the lower half of the cornea due to the deposition of melanin spots at the level of Desçemet's membrane.

Amiodarone

Deposition of amiodarone may occur in similar manner to that of chloroquine and produce a similar appearance.

CORNEAL DYSTROPHIES

The cornea is subject to a variety of of dystrophies which may be classified topographically into three groups according to the primary site of origin of the early pathological changes:

1 *Anterior*: these involve the epithelium and Bowman's membrane. This group includes epithelial basement membrane dystrophy, Meesmann's epithelial dystrophy and Reis–Bückler's dystrophy).
2 *Stromal*: this group includes granular, macular, lattice and crystalline dystrophies. After keratoplasty, these dystrophies may eventually recur in the graft.
3 *Posterior*: these involve the endothelium and Desçemet's membrane and comprise cornea guttata, Fuchs' combined, congenital hereditary endothelial and posterior polymorphous dystrophies.

In general, the dystrophies are rare, bilateral disorders which progress slowly without the cornea becoming vascularised. They show an autosomal dominant mode of inheritance with the main exception of macular dystrophy, in which the mode is autosomal recessive. In certain other forms, which will be noted in the descriptions below, the mode is variable.

Anterior dystrophies

Epithelial basement membrane dystrophy (Cogan)

This is the commonest anterior dystrophy and presents after the age of 30 with transient blurring of vision and recurrent corneal erosions. There are three components to the pathology:

1 Thickening of the basement membrane with the formation of extensions into the epithelium. Thickened areas of basement membrane appear as 'maps' clinically.
2 Epithelial microcysts containing desquamated cell debris form in the epithelium. These are seen clinically as dots or blebs.
3 Fibrillary material is laid down between the basement membrane and Bowman's membrane.

Meesmann's epithelial dystrophy

In this dystrophy, the epithelial changes may commence in infancy and progress with age, resulting in mild ocular discomfort and some loss of visual acuity. Wth appropriate magnification, minute opacities are seen studding the corneal epithelium of both eyes. These are intra-epithelial cysts measuring 10–15 μm and containing PAS-positive debris derived from the degeneration of abnormal epithelial cells. The debris also stains for glycosaminoglycans with colloidal iron. In general the epithelial cells contain an abundance of glycogen and exhibit frequent mitotic figures and the basement membrane is thickened and multilaminar. By electron microscopy, the epithelial cells are seen to contain 'peculiar substance' which is fibrillogranular material of unknown composition, but characteristic of the condition.

Reis–Bückler's dystrophy

Patients with this dystrophy suffer prolonged and painful recurrent epithelial erosions from childhood until the age of about 20 years. These are accompanied by progressive diffuse scarring at the level of Bowman's membrane which in time produces a characteristic clinical appearance of numerous interwoven ring-like figures.

Microscopically, Bowman's membrane is extensively replaced by scar tissue of variable thickness (Fig. 5.15). Where Bowman's membrane is absent, there is a corresponding loss of epithelial basement membrane and associated hemidesmosomes. This loss may well account for the recurrent desquamations or erosions of the epithelium.

The characteristic ultrastructural finding is the accumulation beneath the epithelium of non-banded microfibrils approximately 8 nm in diameter.

Stromal dystrophies

Granular dystrophy (Groenouw I)

Opacities appear in the first decade deep to Bowman's membrane in the central area of the cornea. Later they spread more deeply, but the peripheral cornea is always spared. The opacities are discrete and the cornea between them remains clear, so that patients retain useful vision until late in life.

Microscopically the opacities consist of nodular accumulations of hyaline substance which stains bright red with Masson's trichrome stain (Plate 1). Under the electron microscope the deposits are seen to consist of masses of electron-dense rods or plates of variable length. They are 100–500 nm in width and usually appear to have fractured ends (Fig. 5.16). Histochemical studies have shown the deposits to be a protein which contains tyrosine, tryptophane, arginine and sulphur-containing amino-acids. The material is unlikely, therefore, to originate from degenerated collagen which is deficient in such amino-acids. Staining for phospholipids by luxol fast blue is also positive and it has been suggested (Rodrigues *et al.*, 1983) that the material may represent an early genetic alteration in the assembly of, or processing of, membrane-derived corneal epithelial proteins and phospholipids.

Macular dystrophy (Groenouw II)

This first appears in the first or second decade as a diffuse cloudiness of the stroma which gradually spreads outwards to the periphery and deeply to Desçemet's membrane. Ill-defined opacities develop in the general haze

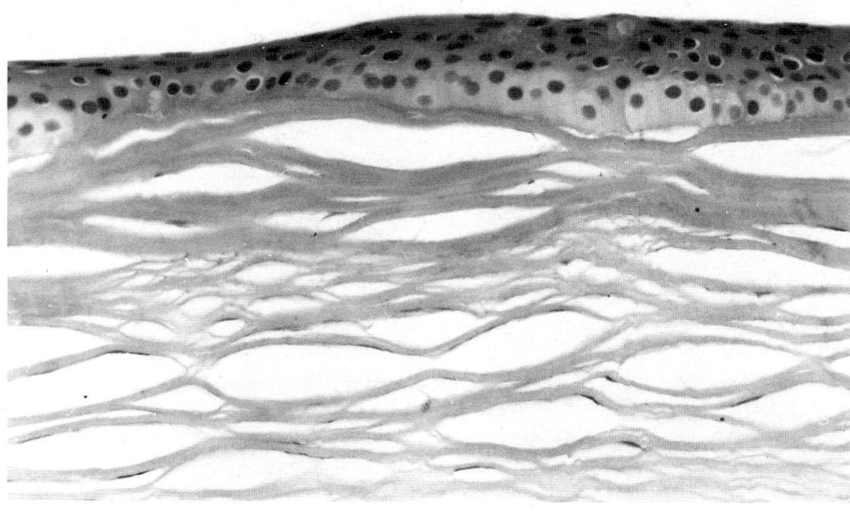

Fig. 5.15 Reis–Bückler's dystrophy. Epithelium irregular with some loss of normal stratification and Bowman's membrane replaced by a layer of hyaline fibrous tissue. H & E (×320).

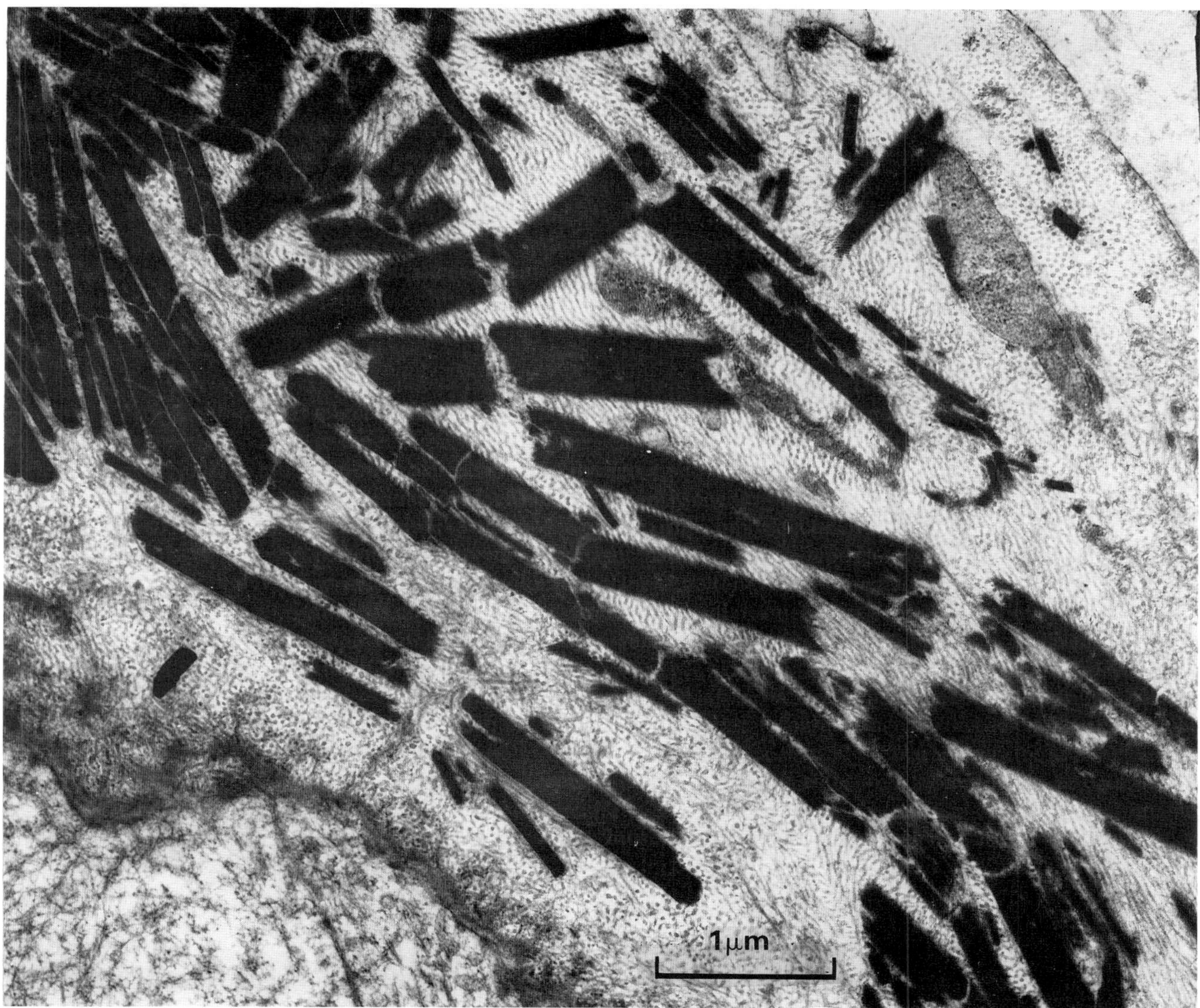

Fig. 5.16 Granular dystrophy. Electron micrograph showing the fractured rods characteristic of the condition. (×26 950).

and vision is often seriously impaired by the age of 30.

Clouding is due to the accumulation within keratocytes and endothelial cells and in the corneal stroma and Desçemet's membrane of material originally thought to consist mainly of keratan sulphate proteoglycan (see Appendix III) which stains with PAS (Plate 2), crystal violet, alcian blue and Hale's colloidal iron. Deposition is heaviest in the anterior stroma in the axial region. By electron microscopy (Fig. 5.17), the material is seen to consist of rounded, membrane-bound aggregates of fibrillary material. It was not clear whether macular dystrophy was the result of a genetic enzyme defect in the keratocytes and endothelial cells rendering them unable to metabolise the glycosaminoglycan which they produce or whether the glycosaminoglycan was itself an abnormal product. However, recurrence had occasionally been observed after keratoplasty and, in such cases, deposition of the glycosaminoglycan in the graft endothelium was found. Since host endothelium is not thought to be able to re-populate grafts in man, this implied that the glycosaminoglycan was an abnormal metabolite which the donor endothelium was unable to metabolise.

It has now been established that the abnormal material may consist of abnormal proteoglycan containing undersulphated keratan sulphate proteoglycan and oversulphated chondroitin sulphate proteoglycan as well as abnormal glycoproteins (see Panjwani *et al.*, 1986).

Lattice dystrophies

Lattice dystrophy Type 1 (Biber–Haab–Dimmer): this relatively common form of lattice dystrophy first appears

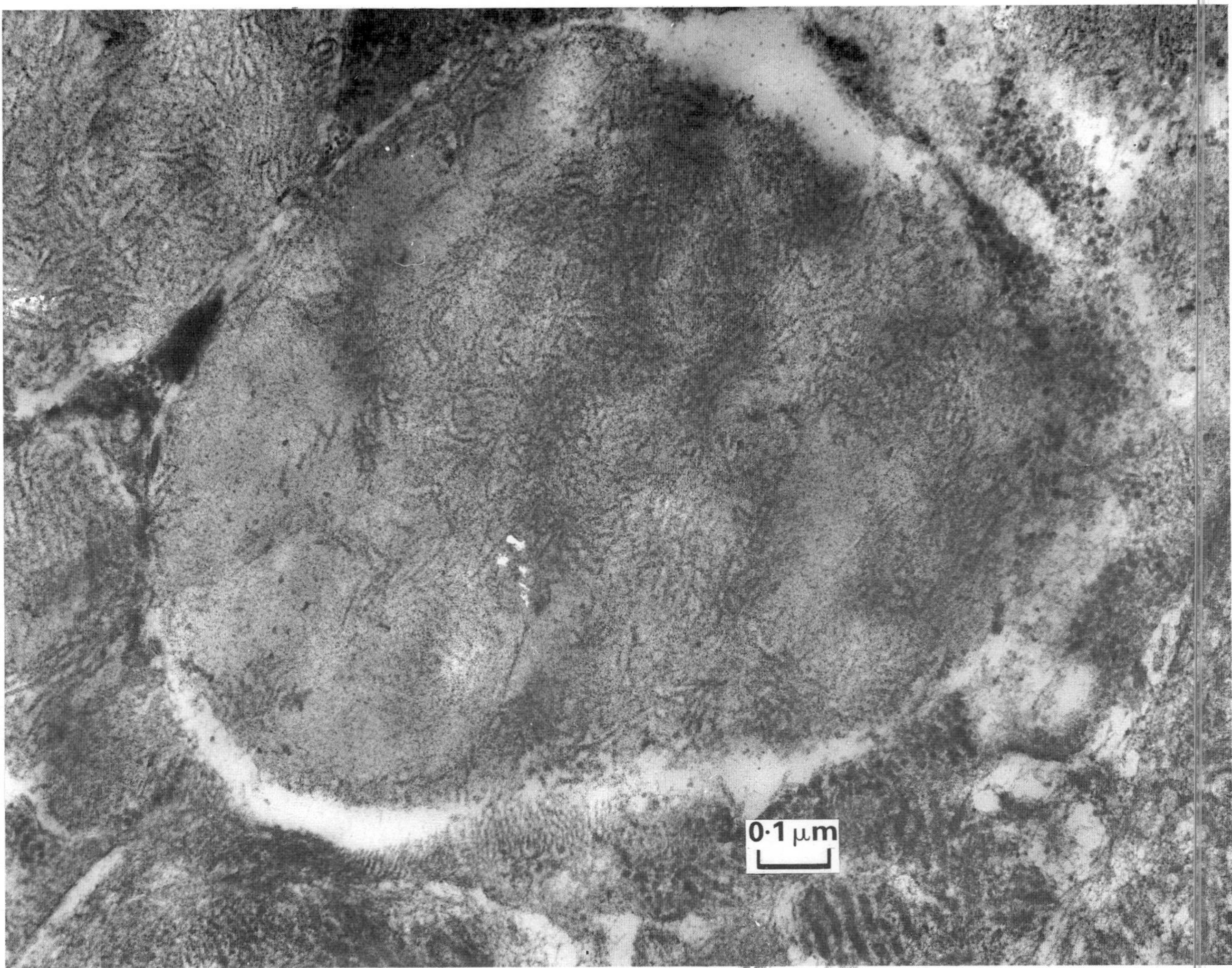

Fig. 5.17 Macular dystrophy. Electron micrograph showing the filamentous character of the material which is enclosed in membrane-bound vesicles. (×113 700).

towards the end of the first decade. By the age of 40, vision is seriously impaired, partly because of stromal opacities but mainly by dense hyalinised fibrous tissue which develops between the epithelium and Bowman's membrane (Plate 3a), possibly as a result of epithelial inflammatory attacks to which these patients are prone. The stromal opacities form a lattice pattern throughout most of the stromal depth, but do not reach the periphery.

In sections, the stromal opacities are often fusiform in profile, non-granular and PAS-positive. They stain positively for amyloid with Congo red, crystal violet and thioflavine-T. Under polarised light they show an apple-green dichroism with Congo red (Plate 3b). By electron microscopy, the material consists of felt-like masses of non-branching, non-banded fibrils 8–10 nm in diameter.

The condition presumably represents a hereditary form of primary localised amyloidosis. Amyloid is a fibrous protein whose characteristics depend on the fact that the polypeptide chains are arranged in sheets at right angles to the long axis of the filaments (β-pleated configuration). Two main types are recognised:

1 AL amyloid in which the polypetides are derived from the light chains of immunoglobulins. Systemic deposition of this type of amyloid is of the primary type often associated with multiple myelomatosis.

2 AA amyloid in which the polypeptide chains show sequence identity with the N-terminal end of a plasma protein. Systemic deposition of this type of amyloid is of the secondary type.

In addition, about 5% of all types of amyloid consist of soluble P protein.

When the type of amyloid in Type 1 lattice dystrophy has been identified, it has been of the AA type. The amyloid material may be a product of abnormal keratocytes or may be derived indirectly from stromal glycosaminoglycans or collagen by the action of lysosomal enzymes released by abnormal keratocytes.

Keratoplasty is effective, but recurrence may eventually occur in the graft, presumably as a result of repopulation by host cells.

Lattice dystrophy Type 2 occurs in association with familial systemic amyloidosis. In this type the amyloid deposits in the corneal stroma tend to be deeper and more peripheral. The skin and conjunctiva are involved and there is a progressive cranial neuropathy.

Gelatinous drop-like dystrophy is a third rare type of amyloid deposition in which inheritance is thought to be autosomal recessive and deposition of amyloid is entirely subepithelial.

Crystalline dystrophy (Schnyder)

As well as showing a dominant mode of inheritance, this dystrophy occasionally occurs sporadically. It is characterised by the deposition of cholesterol crystals in Bowman's membrane and the anterior stroma. These may be observed soon after birth, but rarely cause serious opacification until the third or fourth decade. There is an inconstant association with hyperlipidaemia.

Posterior dystrophies

Cornea guttata

An inheritance pattern cannot always be demonstrated in cornea guttata, but the disease may occur as an autosomal dominant or show a familial distribution.

Excrescences, warts or guttae appear on the posterior surface of Desçemet's membrane. By specular microscopy they are seen as dark spots which are at first confined to the central cornea, but later extend to the periphery. The excrescences are assumed to be the product of dystrophic corneal endothelium, the cells of which are irregular in size and shape and contain brown pigment, but retain their barrier and pumping functions since there is no oedema of the corneal stroma. The excrescences are composed of Desçemet's membrane material and are very similar to Hassall–Henle warts which develop as an expression of ageing in the peripheral cornea. Secondary cornea guttata may complicate other degenerative conditions, especially longstanding interstitial keratitis.

Fuchs' combined dystrophy

This endothelial dystrophy is of late onset and is commoner in females. There is normally no consistent pattern of inheritance, but transmission through consecutive generations has been recorded. It is bilateral and the earliest change is indistinguishable from cornea guttata. Gradual failure of endothelial function, however, leads to stromal and epithelial oedema, subepithelial bullae and the formation of a thin layer of fine subepithelial fibrous tissue (Fig. 5.18a). These changes are localised according to the severity of the changes in Desçemet's membrane and associated attenuation of the endothelium in a particular area.

Microscopically, the corneal endothelium is intact, but its cells are variable in size and thinner and fewer in number than normal. Desçemet's membrane is irregularly thickened and typically bears hemisperical or flat-topped warts on its posterior surface (Fig. 5.18b). These are composed of basement membrane material. They are sometimes buried in the thickened membrane (Fig.

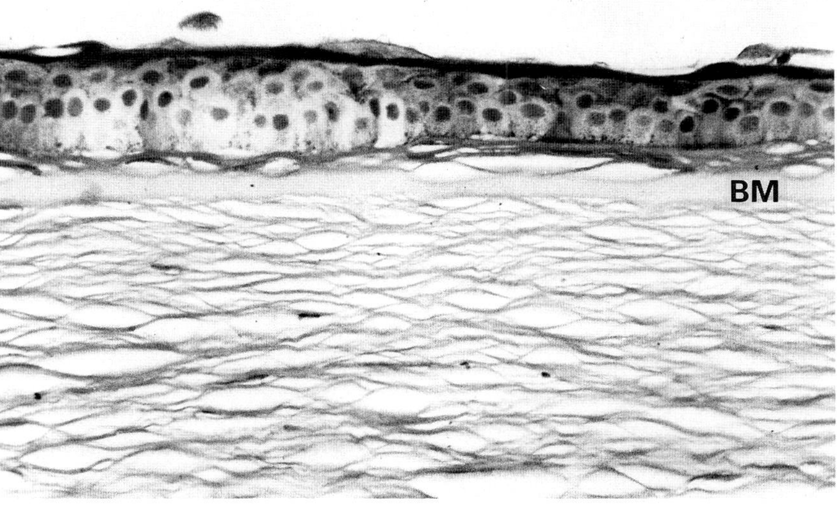

Fig. 5.18 Fuchs' dystrophy. (a) Epithelial oedema with degenerative pannus between epithelium and Bowman's membrane (BM). PAS/tartrazine (×320).

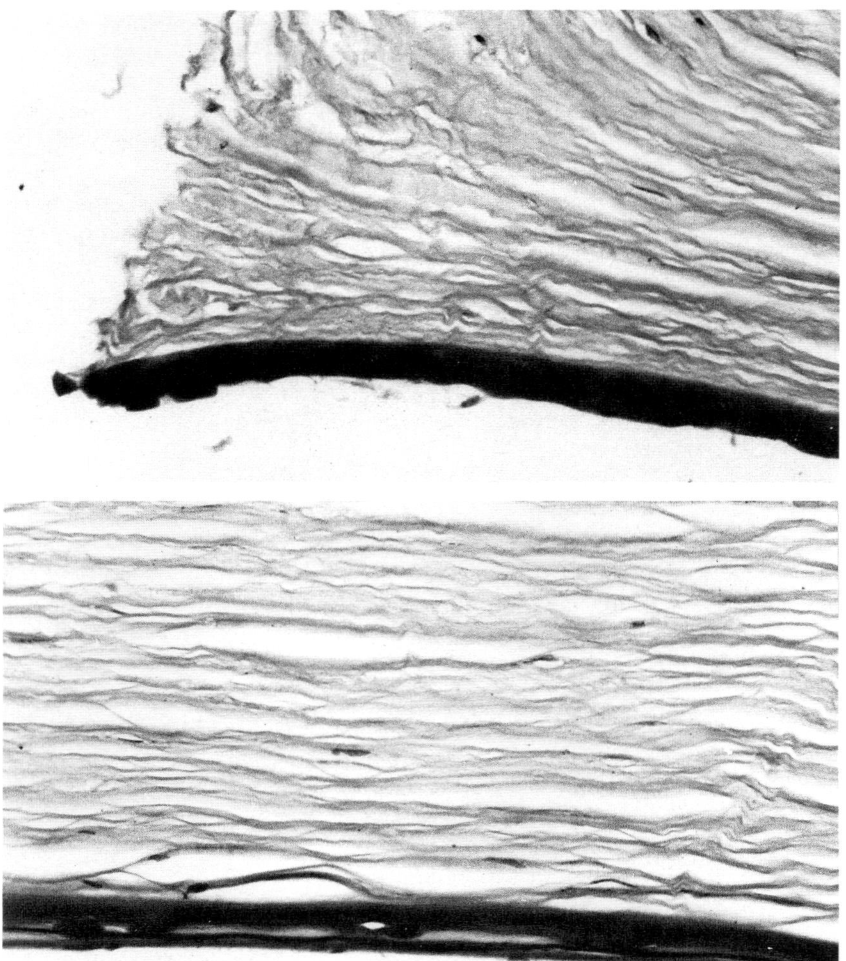

Fig. 5.18 (b) Periphery of corneal disc showing thickening of Desçemet's membrane and posterior excrescences of variable profile. PAS/tartrazine (×320).

Fig. 5.18 (c) Central cornea. In this area, the 'warts' appear buried. PAS/tartrazine (×320).

5.18c), and may then be demonstrable only by phase contrast or electron microscopy. Thickening of Desçemet's membrane is due to the deposition on its posterior surface of additional layers composed of basement membrane material and collagen, both normal and long-banded fibrils.

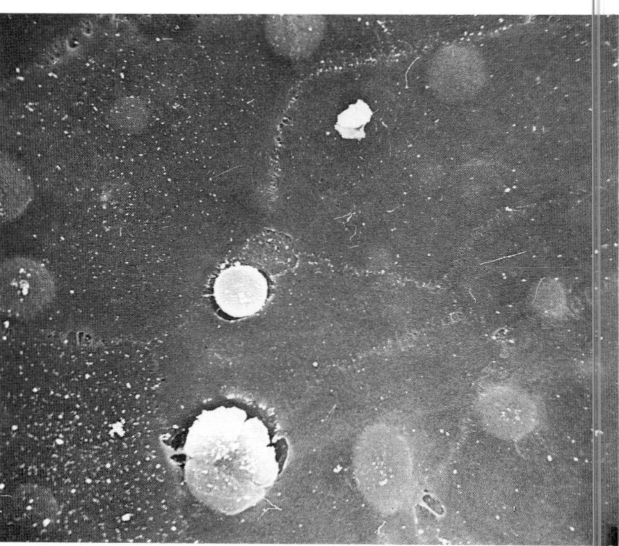

Fig. 5.18 (d) Scanning electron micrograph showing excrescence in various stages of development. Two appear to have ruptured the endothelium, but this may be factitious. (×900).

Posterior polymorphous dystrophy (Schlichting)

This is a slowly progressive dystrophy first becoming evident in childhood. The characteristic pathological features are:

1 Desçemet's membrane becomes irregular in thickness and multilaminar due to the deposition of layers of basement membrane material interspersed with layers of collagen (Figs 5.19a & b) including collagen fibrils showing long (55–110 nm) banding. Breaks in Desçemet's membrane occur. These probably correspond with the lacunae observed clinically.

2 The endothelial cells acquire epithelial-like properties.

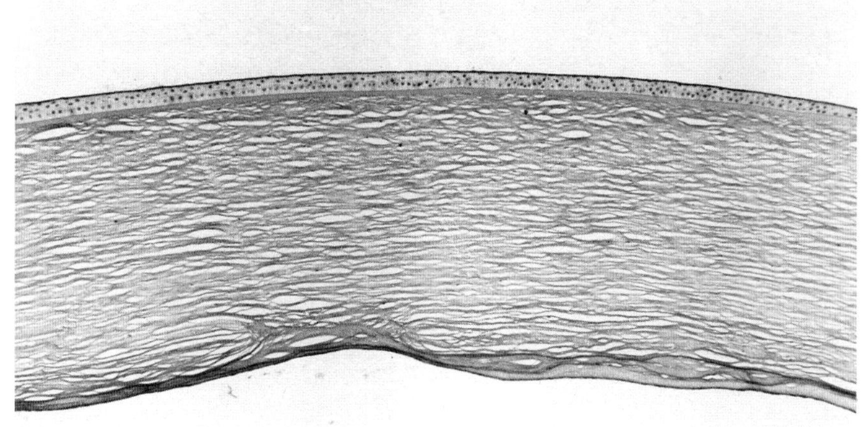

Fig. 5.19 Posterior polymorphous dystrophy. (a) Showing the irregular, but widespread thickening of Desçemet's membrane. PAS/tartrazine (×64).

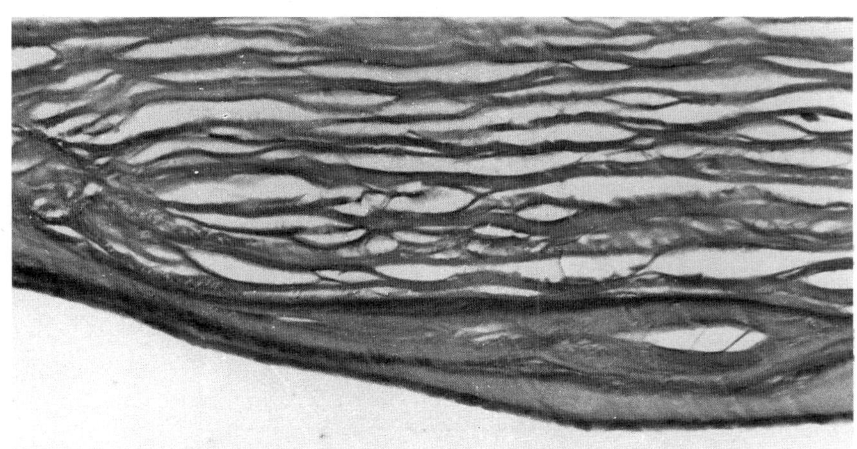

Fig. 5.19 (b) Detail of grossly thickened area showing lamination. PAS/tartrazine (×320).

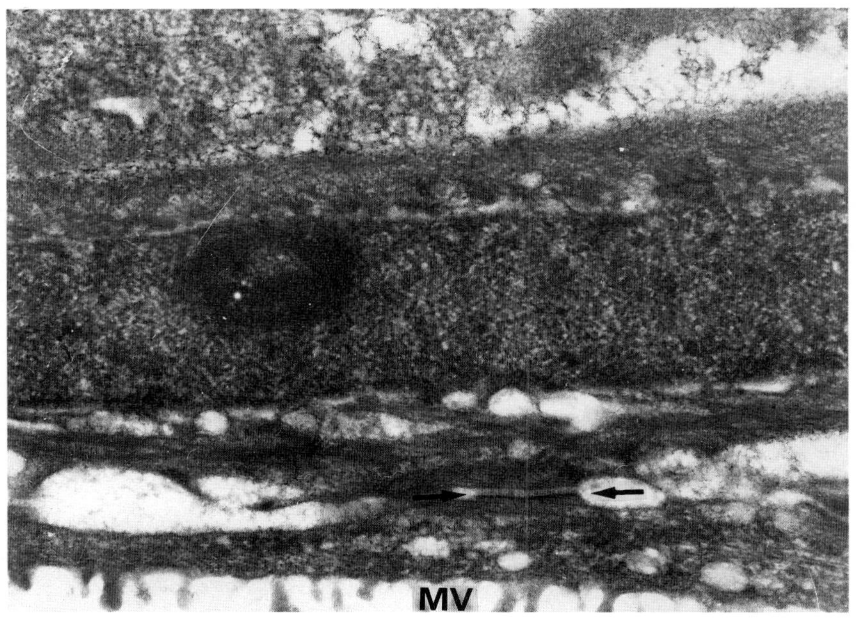

Fig. 5.19 (c) Electron micrograph showing desmosome (arrows) between the overlying cytoplasm of two endothelial cells. Microvilli (MV) are present on the surface of the superficial cell. (×29 250).

They become irregular in shape and develop numerous microvilli. Thin layers of cells with desmosomes between the overlying cells are formed (Fig. 5.20c).

3 Band keratopathy is a common association. Stromal and epithelial oedema occur late.

Congenital hereditary corneal dystrophy

Inheritance of this dystrophy may be dominant or recessive. There is bilateral haziness of the cornea from birth due to stromal and epithelial oedema.

Microscopically, the epithelium shows basal oedema and often partial loss of Bowman's membrane and subepithelial fibrosis. The endothelium is attenuated centrally and may even be absent or replaced by fibroblast-like cells. The anterior part of Desçemet's membrane is normal, but lamination results from the deposition of layers of collagenous tissue containing randomly orientated collagen filaments (about 35 nm diameter) and fibrils (about 35 nm diameter) together with basement membrane material and some keratocytes.

KERATOCONUS

Keratoconus is conveniently considered with the corneal dystrophies. The condition predominantly affects those in the second and third decades. No consistent pattern of inheritance is seen, but it has been described in association with a variety of systemic diseases, particularly atopy and Down's syndrome. The condition is characterised by progressive corneal ectasia and cone formation which result in blurring of vision, irregular astigmatism and corneal scarring.

Microscopically, dehiscences are seen in the epithelial basement membrane and Bowman's membrane (Fig. 5.20a) which correspond to anterior clear spaces observed clinically under the slit lamp. These become filled by downgrowths of the oedematous epithelium or upgrowths of scar tissue generated by underlying keratocytes. Reduction in the number of lamellae results in thinning of the corneal stroma (Fig. 5.20b), while the epithelium and basement membrane are thickened. Iron derived from tear secretion is deposited in epithelial cells around the base of the cone. This may be observed clinically as Fleischer's ring. In advanced cases, normal lamination is disturbed and ruptures in Desçemet's membrane lead to disturbances of corneal hydration resulting in either chronic stromal oedema or the more dramatic corneal hydrops of sudden onset (acute keratoconus) (Fig. 5.20c & d), a rare condition most likely to be encountered in adult mongoloids.

Refractive errors due to keratoconus respond well to treatment with hard contact lenses. When this fails and the cornea is opaque, keratoplasty is usually successful.

OCULAR CICATRICIAL PEMPHIGOID

Pemphigoid is a rare condition associated with an increased prevalence of HLA B12 in those affected. Involvement of the conjunctiva is serious because progressive shrinkage and cicatrisation result in entropion, trichiasis, xerosis and corneal opacification. The conjunctival blisters are subepithelial and there is no acantholysis as in pemphigus. The epithelium undergoes squamous metaplasia with loss of goblet cells and it may keratinise. Granulation tissue forms in the substantia propria and there is an inflammatory infiltrate predominantly of lymphocytes and plasma cells, though in the acute stage polymorphs may be numerous. Later, intense fibrosis occurs.

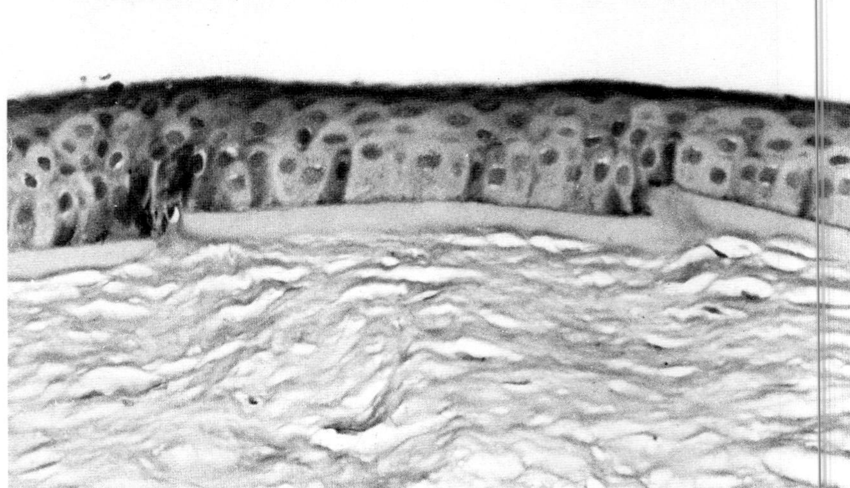

Fig. 5.20 Keratoconus. (a) Breaks in Bowman's membrane. PAS/tartrazine (×320).

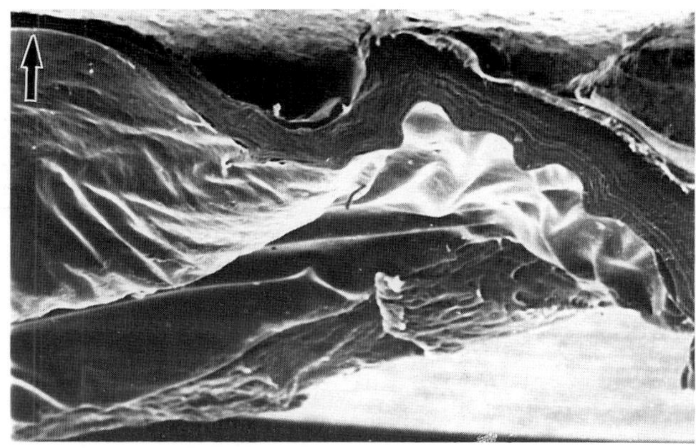

Fig. 5.20 (b) Scanning electron micrograph showing central stromal thinning (arrow). The peripheral stroma appears thickened and Desçemet's membrane thrown into a series of folds. (×37).

Immunoglobulins and the C3 component of complement are found bound to the basement membrane in about half the cases, though this is not diagnostic. Immunoglobulins may also be bound to conjunctival epithelium (see Mondino & Brown, 1980). The oral mucosa is involved in 50% of cases and a biopsy of oral mucosa may be preferable to provide adequate material for diagnostic purposes.

In pemphigus, which occasionally affects the conjunctiva, there is acantholysis and the bullae are intraepithelial. Immunoglobulins, particularly IgG, and the C3 component of complement are bound to the tonofibrils of the epithelial cells. The bullae usually heal without scarring.

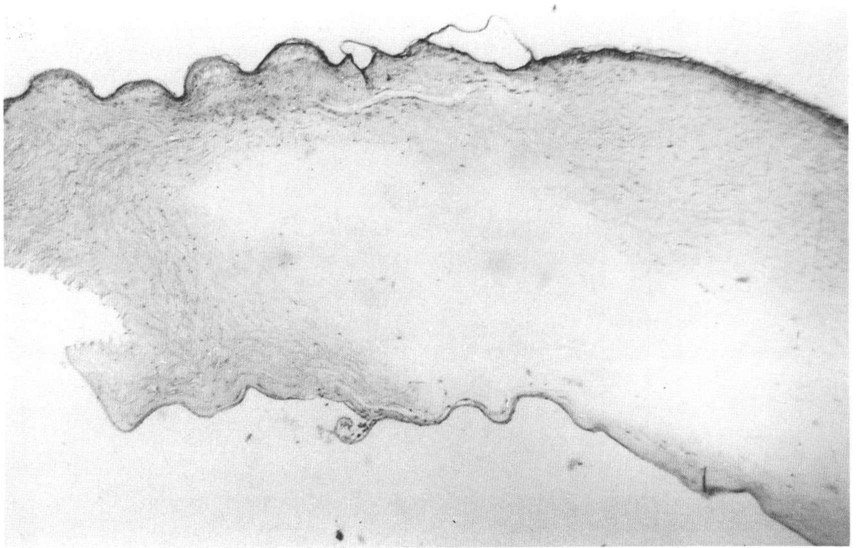

Fig. 5.20 (c) & (d) Hydrops. Gross central stromal oedema with break in Desçemet's membrane (arrows). PAS/tartrazine. (c) (×41); (d) (×18).

(c)

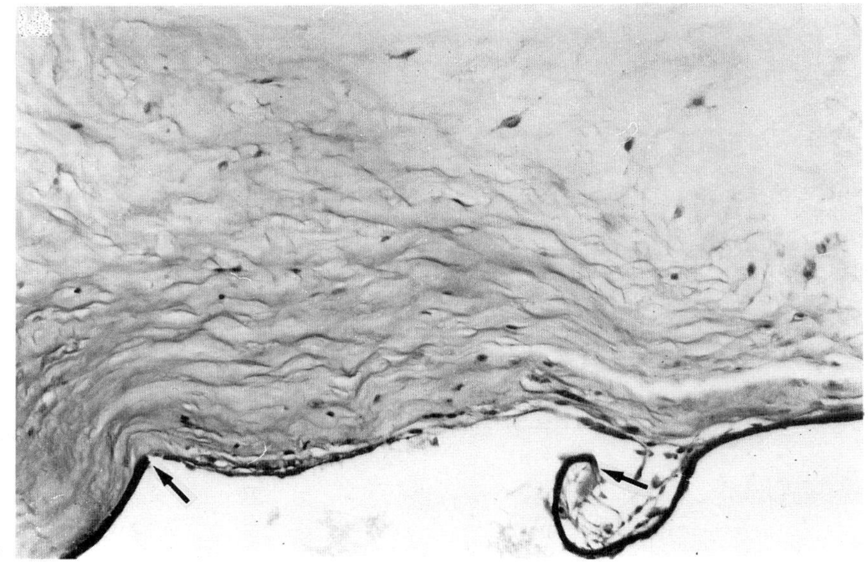

(d)

CHAPTER 5

TUMOURS OF THE CONJUNCTIVA

Choristomata

These tumours arise from the continued growth of normal tissue displaced (*choristos* = separated) from its normal situation as the result of a developmental error. The best known examples of ocular choristomata are orbital dermoid cysts (Chapter 14) and the following solid conjunctival and epibulbar tumours.

1 Dermoid tumours most frequently form smooth, white hairy tumours astride the limbus consisting of fibrofatty tissue covered by epidermis complete with pilosebaceous follicles and sweat glands (Fig. 5.21). These growths are usually unilateral, but may be bilateral or multiple. They are sometimes associated with internal malformations of the eye (Chapter 17).

2 Dermolipoma (dermofibrolipoma) is a malformation which occurs in the fornices, especially at the outer canthus. It is composed of fibrofatty tissue and covered by conjunctival epithelium or occasionally by epidermis. Adnexal structures are often difficult to demonstrate.

3 Complex choristomata resemble either of the above tumours, but contain other ectopic tissues such as lacrimal gland, cartilage, smooth muscle and nerve fibres.

4 Epibulbar osseous choristomata consist of a nodule or plaque of bone lying in the subconjunctival tissues.

More serious degrees of anomalous differentiation may result in replacement of the whole cornea by dermoid tissue.

Benign epithelial lesions

Conjunctival papillomata

Conjunctival papillomata occur most often in the second and third decades. They may arise anywhere on the conjunctiva, but the lid margin near the inner canthus, the limbus and the caruncle are the chief sites. Those arising at the limbus tend to become flattened, while those arising at the lid margin or on the caruncle are exuberant fleshy growths.

Microscopically, the individual papillae consist of a delicate fibrovascular core covered by thick stratified non-keratinising epithelium containing goblet cells (Fig. 5.22). A variable degree of epithelial dysplasia may be seen. Some papillomata recur repeatedly after removal, but malignant transformation is rare.

The demonstration of cells with a small hyperchromatic nucleus surrounded by clear cytoplasm (koilocytes) which are associated with papillomavirus-induced tumours and actual serological evidence of the presence of viral antigen indicate that some conjunctival papillomata are virus-induced.

Keratotic plaques

Keratotic plaques are characterised by acanthosis and variable hyperkeratosis or parakeratosis. There is no cellular atypia and maturation from basal cell to prickle cell is normal. Occasional heavily keratinised crateriform lesions resembling keratoacanthoma have been reported.

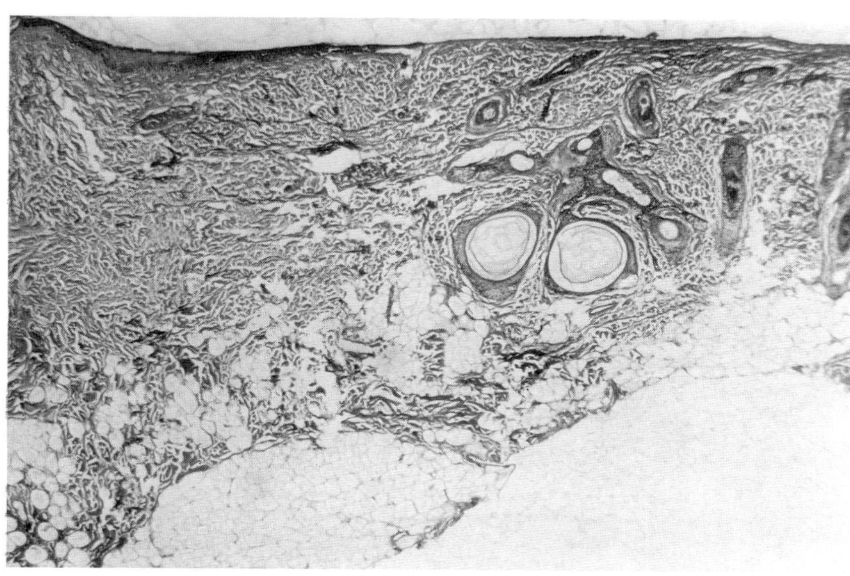

Fig. 5.21 Choristoma. Limbal dermoid showing pilary complexes and subcutaneous fat. H & E (×24).

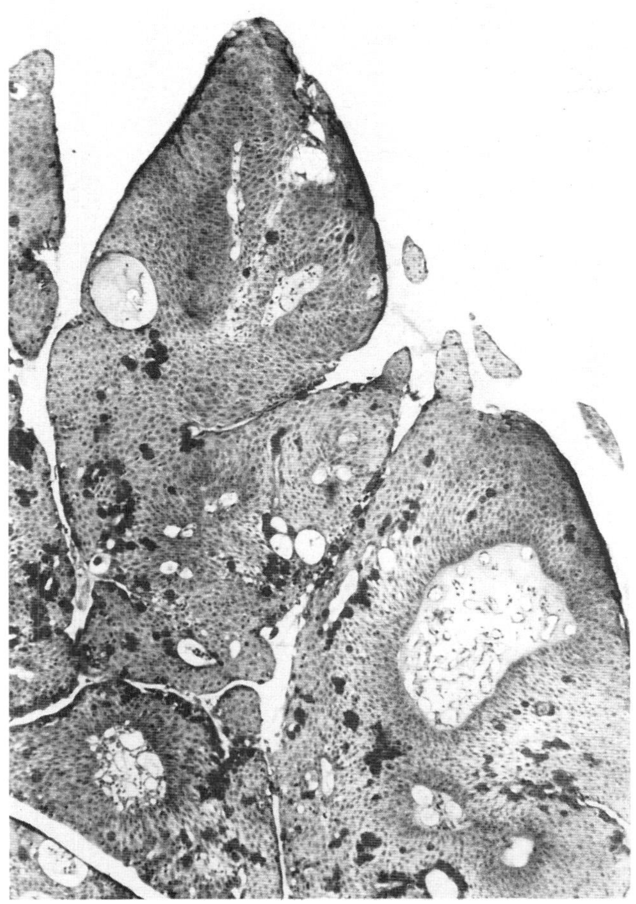

Fig. 5.22 Conjunctival papilloma. Goblet cells in papillae picked out by PAS staining. (×71).

Pre-cancerous epithelial lesions

Epithelial dysplasia

In this condition, the orderly progression of cells from the basal layer of the epithelium to the surface is disturbed. The cells appear uneven in size, shape and staining and cells in mitosis may be seen at all levels. Such changes are commonly seen in relation to pingueculae and pterygia and the condition may be related to actinic keratosis.

Carcinoma in situ

Carcinoma *in situ* commonly presents as a limbal plaque in the interpalpebral fissure which may well be described clinically as leucoplakia, though it should be emphasised that the term does not carry any specific pathological connotation. Spread onto the cornea may occur. The plaques show severe dysplastic changes of the type described above. In addition, the epithelium is thickened, there is complete loss of stratification, abnormal mitoses appear at all levels and the substantia propria is infiltrated with lymphocytes (Fig. 5.23). Usually there is little surface keratin, but sometimes there is overlying hyperkeratosis so that the lesions resemble cutaneous actinic keratosis.

Recurrence after removal is common, but transformation into invasive squamous cell carcinoma is rare. Such transformation, which must be carefully sought, is indicated by transgression of the epithelial basement membrane by elements of malignant epithelium.

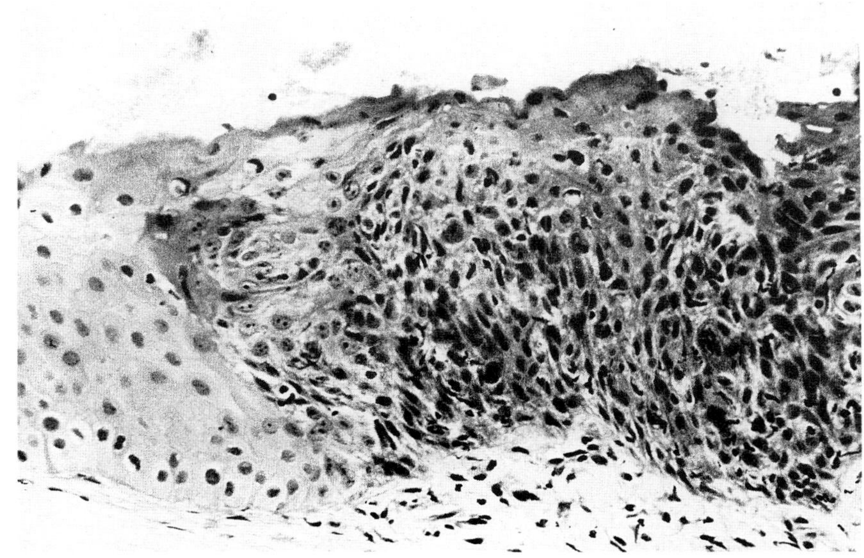

Fig. 5.23 Conjunctiva. Carcinoma *in situ*. Boundary of neoplastic area with normal epithelium on left hand side. H & E (×260).

Malignant epithelial tumours

Squamous cell carcinomata

Invasive squamous cell carcinomata are uncommon. Like the pre-cancerous lesions from which they may arise, the limbus is the commonest site (Fig. 5.24). The sclera tends to limit deep invasion. These carcinomata thus tend to form a large papillary mass which may spread over the cornea as well as into the fornix. Regional and distant metastases and invasion of the orbit are late and rare events. It may thus be possible to control the condition with local excision. Squamous cell carcinoma of the conjunctiva may appear as a complication of xeroderma pigmentosum and involve both eyes at at early age.

Mucoepidermoid carcinomata

These rare tumours contain mucus-secreting cells in addition to the epidermoid component. They are more aggressive locally and have a worse prognosis than squamous cell carcinomata.

Adnexal tumours

Adnexal tumours in the caruncle include adenomata of sweat gland and sebaceous gland origin similar to those which occur in the lids (Chapter 6). Malignant counterparts of these tumors are very rare.

Adenomata originating from the accessory lacrimal glands of the caruncle include pleomorphic adenomata similar to those of the salivary glands and the rare, but

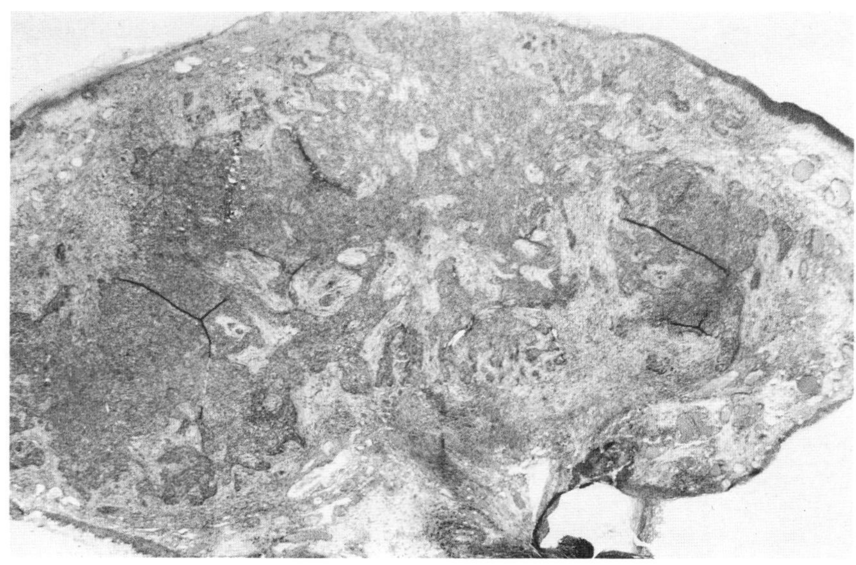

Fig. 5.24 Limbal carcinoma of conjunctiva. (a) Low power H & E (×20).

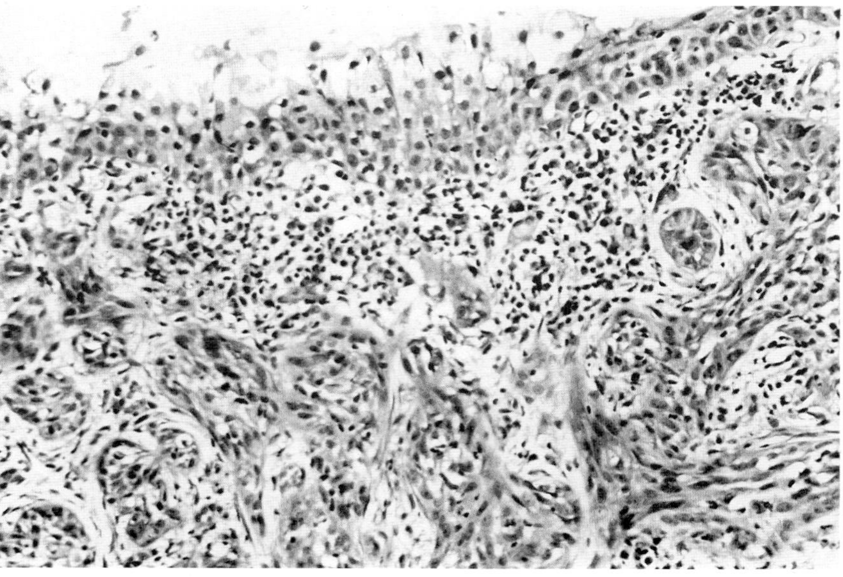

Fig. 5.24 (b) Higher power showing spindly appearance of cells. The epithelial surface is seen at top of picture. There is a dense stromal infiltrate, mainly of lymphocytes, but many eosinophils were also present as is sometimes noted in squamous cell carcinomata. H & E (×160).

interesting oxyphil adenoma or oncocytoma. The cells of the latter exhibit a striking granular eosinophilia, which is due to the presence of an excess of large mitochondria in their cytoplasm. The origin of the cells and the reason for the mitochondrial abnormality are unknown.

MISCELLANEOUS LESIONS

Haemangiomata, lymphangiomata, neurofibromata, neurilemmomata, fibroxanthomata and nodular fasciitis occur in the conjunctiva, but are rare. Lymphangiomata consist of thin walled endothelial-lined vessels containing lymph. No clearcut distinction can be made from lymphangiectasia. Spontaneous or post-traumatic haemorrhage may first draw attention to their presence.

Telangiectasia: affects the conjunctival blood vessels as part of the ataxia-telangiectasia syndrome of Louis–Barr and of hereditary haemorrhagic telangiectasia (Rendu–Osler–Weber disease) (see Chapter 15).

BIBLIOGRAPHY

General

Bahn, C. F., Falls, H. F., Varley, G. A., Meyer, R. F., Edelhauser, H. F. & Bourne, W. M. (1984) Classification of corneal endothelial disorders based on neural crest origin. *Ophthalmology* **91**, 558–563.

Bron, A. J. & Seal, D. V. (1986) The defences of the ocular surface. *Transactions of the Ophthalmological Society of the UK* **105**, 18–25.

Easty, D. L. (1986) Infection in the compromised eye. *Transactions of the Ophthalmological Society of the UK* **105**, 61–68.

Grayson, M. (1983) *Diseases of the Cornea*. C. V. Mosby Co., St Louis.

Maurice, D. M. (1957) The structure and transparency of the cornea. *Journal of Physiology* **136**, 263–286.

Pierce, J. M., Ward, M. E. & Seal, D. V. (1982) Ophthalmia neonatorum in the 1980's: incidence, aetiology and treatment. *British Journal of Ophthalmology* **66**, 728–731.

Scott, J. E. & Haigh, M. (1988) Keratan sulphate and the ultrastructure of cornea and cartilage: a 'stand-in' for chondroitin sulphate in conditions of oxygen lack? *Journal of Anatomy* **158**, 95–108.

Setala, K. (1979) Corneal endothelial cell density after an attack of acute glaucoma. *Acta Ophthalmologica* **57**, 1004–1013.

Shamsuddin, A. K. M., Nirankari, V. S., Purnell, D. M. & Chang, S. H. (1986) Is the corneal posterior cell layer truly endothelial? *Ophthalmology* **93**, 1298–1303.

Watt, P. J. (1986) Pathogenic mechanisms of organisms virulent to the eye. *Transactions of the Ophthalmological Society of the UK* **105**, 26–31.

Williamson, J. & Brown, L. R. (1978) *The Eye in Connective Tissue Disease*. Arnold, London.

Wilson, L. A. ed. (1979) *External Diseases of the Eye*. Harper & Row, New York.

Mycotic infections

Jones, B. R. (1975) Principles in the management of oculomycosis. *Transactions of the American Academy of Ophthalmology and Otolaryngology* **79**, 15–53.

McClean, J. M. (1963) Oculomycosis. *American Journal of Ophthalmology* **56**, 537–549.

Chlamydial infections

Jones, B. R. (1980) Changing concepts of trachoma and its control. *Transactions of the Ophthalmological Society of the UK* **100**, 25–29.

Amoebic keratitis

Hirst, L. W., Green, W. R., Merz, W., Kaufmann, C, Visvesvara, G. S., Jensen, A. & Malin, H. (1984) Management of acanthamoeba keratitis. A case report and review of the literature. *Ophthalmology* **91**, 1105–1111.

Wright, P., Warhurst, D. & Jones, B. R. (1985) Acanthamoeba keratitis successfully treated medically. *British Journal of Ophthalmology* **69**, 778–782.

Viral infections

Baringer, S. R. (1976) The biology of herpes simplex infections in humans. *Survey of Ophthalmology* **21**, 171–174.

Dawson, C. R. & Togni, B. (1976) Herpes simplex eye infections: clinical manifestations, pathogenesis and management. *Survey of Ophthalmology* **21**, 121–135.

Dawson, C. R., Togni, B. & Moore, T. E. (1968) Structural changes in chronic herpetic keratitis studied by light and electron microscopy. *Archives of Ophthalmology* **79**, 740–747.

Easty, D. L. (1985) *Virus Disease of the Eye*. Lloyd-Luke, London.

Easty, D. L., Maini, R. N. & Jones, B. R. (1973) Cellular immunity in herpes simplex keratitis. *Transactions of the Ophthalmological Society of the UK* **93**, 171–180.

Ghosh, M., Dixon, W. S. & Hunter, W. S. (1986) Herpes simplex keratitis: a clinicopathogic case report. *Canadian Journal of Ophthalmology* **21**, 175–177.

Hedges, T. R. & Albert, D. M. (1982) The progression of the ocular abnormalities of herpes zoster. Histopathologic observations of nine cases. *Ophthalmology* **89**, 165–176.

Knopf, H. L. S. & Hierholzer, J. C. (1975) Clinical and immunologic responses in patients with viral keratoconjunctivitis. *American Journal of Ophthalmology* **80**, 661–672.

Martinet, A. C. (1981) Herpes simplex. *Transactions of the Ophthalmological Society of the UK* **101**, 308–311.

Metcalf, J. F. & Kaufman, H. E. (1976) Herpetic stromal keratitis — evidence for cell-mediated pathogenesis. *American Journal of Ophthalmology* **82**, 827–834.

Meyers-Elliott, R. H., Pettit, T. H. & Maxwell, A. (1980) Viral antigens in the immune ring of herpes simplex stromal keratitis. *Archives of Ophthalmology* **98**, 879–904.

Ostler, H. B. (1976) Herpes simplex: the primary infection. *Survey of Ophthalmology* **21**, 91–99.

Ostler, H. B. & Thygeson, P. (1976) The ocular manifestations of herpes zoster, varicella, infectious mononucleosis and cytomegalovirus disease. *Survey of Ophthalmology* **21**, 148–159.

Pavan-Langston, D. & Hettinger, M. E. (1980) Ocular herpes: an update. *Annals of Ophthalmology* **13**, 1213–1216.

Polack, F. M., Habash, N., Zam, S. & Burdette, M. G. (1982) Cell-mediated immunity in herpetic keratitis measured by leukocyte migration inhibition. *Annals of Opthalmology* **14**, 825–827.

Sandford-Smith, J. H. & Whittle, H. C. (1979) Corneal ulceration following measles ulceration. *British Journal of Ophthalmology* **63**, 720–724.

Schwartz, H. S., Vastine, D. W., Yamashiroya, H. & West, C. E. (1975) Immunofluorescent detection of adenovirus antigen in epidemic keratoconjunctivitis. *Investigative Ophthalmology and Visual Science* **15**, 199–297.

Tullo, A. B. (1980) Clinical and epidemiological features of adenovirus keratoconjunctivitis. *Transactions of the Opthalmological Society of the UK* **100**, 263–264.

Tullo, A. B., Easty, D. L., Shimeld, C., Stirling, P. E. & Darville, J. M. (1984) Isolation of herpes simplex virus from corneal discs of patients with chronic stromal keratitis. *Transactions of the Opthalmological Societies of the UK* **104**, 159–165.

Van Rij, G., Klepper, L., Perperkamp, E. & Schaap, G. J. P. (1982) Immune electron microscopy and a cultural test in the diagnosis of adenovirus ocular infection.

Weiner, J. M., Carrol, N. & Robertson, I. F. (1985) The granulomatous reaction in herpetic stromal keratitis. Immunological and ultrastructural findings. *Australia and New Zealand Journal of Ophthalmology* **13**, 365–372.

Non-infective corneal ulceration

Abdel-Khalek, L. M. R., Williamson, J. & Lee, W. R. (1978) Morphological changes in human conjunctival epithelium. II. In keratoconjunctivitis sicca. *British Journal of Ophthalmology* **62**, 800–806.

Kassan, S. S. & Gardy, M. (1978) Sjögren's syndrome: an update and overview. *The American Journal of Medicine* **64**, 1037–1046.

Williamson, J., Gibson A. A. M., Wilson, T., Forrester, J. V., Whaley, K. & Dick, W. C. (1973) Histology of the lacrimal gland in keratoconjunctivitis sicca. *British Journal of Ophthalmology* **57**, 852–858.

Young, R. D. & Watson, P.G. (1982) Light and electron microscopy of corneal melting syndrome. *British Journal of Ophthalmology* **66**, 341–356.

Non-infective conjunctivitis

Allansmith, M. R., Korb, D. R. & Greiner, J. V. (1978) Giant papillary conjunctivitis induced by hard or soft contact lens wear: quantitative histology. *Ophthalmology* **88**, 766–788.

Chamber, J. D., Blodi, F. C., Golden, B. & McKee, A. P. (1969) Ligneous conjunctivitis. *Transactions of the American Academy of Ophthalmology and Otolaryngology* **73**, 996–1004.

Hidayat, A. A. & Riddle P. J. (1987) Ligneous conjunctivitis. A clinicopathologic study of 17 cases. *Ophthalmology* **94**, 949–959.

Interstitial keratopathy

Wolter, J. R. (1960) Secondary cornea guttata: a late change in luetic interstitial keratopathy. *American Journal of Ophthalmology* **50**, 17–25.

Pingueculae and pterygia

Austin, P., Jakobiec, F. A. & Iwamoto, T. (1983) Elastodysplasia and elastodystrophy as the pathological bases of ocular pterygia and pingueculae. *Ophthalmology* **90**, 96–109.

Norn, M. S. (1979) Prevalence of pinguecula in Greenland and its relation to pterygium and spheroid degeneration. *Acta Ophthalmologica* **57**, 96–105.

Degenerations

Croxatto, J. O., Dodds, C. M. & Dodds, R. (1985) Bilateral and massive lipoidal infiltration of the cornea (secondary lipoidal degeneration). *Ophthalmology* **92**, 1686–1690.

Jensen, O. A. & Norn, M. S. (1982) Spheroid degeneration of the conjunctiva. Histochemical and ultrastructural examination. *Acta Ophthalmologica* **60**, 79–82.

Johnson, G. J. & Overall, M. (1978) Histology of spheroidal degeneration of the cornea in Labrador. *British Journal of Ophthalmology* **62**, 53–61.

Lucas, D. R., Knox, F. & Davies, S. (1982) Apparent monoclonal origin of lymphocytes and plasma cells infiltrating ocular adnexal amyloid deposits: report of two cases. *British Journal of Ophthalmology* **66**, 600–606.

Scleritis

Barr, C. C., Davis, H. & Culbertson, W. W. (1981) Rheumatoid scleritis. *Ophthalmology* **88**, 1269–1273.

Ferry, A. P. (1969) The histopathology of rheumatoid episcleral nodules. *Archives of Ophthalmology* **82**, 77–78.

Fraunfelder, F. T. & Watson, P. G. (1976) Evaluation of eyes enucleated for scleritis. *British Journal of Ophthalmology* **60**, 227–230.

McGavin, D. D. M., Williamson, J., Forrester, J. V., Foulds, W. S., Buchanan, W. W., Dick, W. C., Lee, P., MacSween, R. N. M. & Whaley, K. (1976) Episcleritis and scleritis. A study of their clinical manifestations and association with rheumatoid arthritis. *British Journal of Ophthalmology* **60**, 192–226.

Lyne, A. J. & Pitkeathley, D. A. (1968) Episcleritis and scleritis. *Archives of Ophthalmology* **80**, 171–176.

Sevel, D. (1965) Rheumatoid nodule of the sclera. *Transactions of the Ophthalmological Society of the UK* **85**, 357–367.

Watson, P. G. & Hazleman, B. L. (1976) *The Sclera and Systemic Disorders*. Saunders, Philadelphia.

Noxious agents

Blodi, F. C. (1958) The late effects of X-radiation on the cornea. *Transactions of the American Ophthalmological Society* **66**, 413–449.

Klingele, T. G., Alves, L. E. & Rose, E. P. (1984) Amiodarone keratopathy. *Annals of Ophthalmology* **16**, 1172–1176.

Lemp, M. A. (1974) Cornea and sclera. Annual review devoted to alkali burns. *Archives of Ophthalmology* **92**, 158–170.

Lucas, D. R., Dunham, A. C., Lee, W. R., Weir, W. & Wilkinson, F. C. F. (1976) Ocular injuries from liquid golf ball cores. *British Journal of Ophthalmology* **60**, 740–747.

O'Grady, R. & Schoch, D. (1973) Golf ball granuloma of the eyelids and conjunctiva. *American Journal of Ophthalmology* **76**, 148–151.

Pfister, R. R., Haddox, J. L., Dodson, R. W. & Harkins, L. E. (1987) Alkali-burned collagen produces a locomotory and metabolic stimulant to neutrophils. *Investigative Ophthalmology and Visual Science* **28**, 295–304.

Steele, C., Lucas, D. R. & Ridgway, A. E. A. (1984) Endophthalmitis due to caterpillar setae: surgical removal and electron microscopic appearance of the setae. *British Journal of Ophthalmology* **68**, 284–288.

Abnormal pigmentations

Barraquer-Somers, E., Chan, C. C. & Green, W. R. (1983) Corneal epithelial iron deposition. *Ophthalmology* **90**, 729–734.

Brodrick, J. D. (1979) Pigmentation of the cornea. Review and case history. *Annals of Ophthalmology* **11**, 855–861.

Dalgleish, R. (1965) Ring-like corneal deposits in a case of congenital spherocytosis. *British Journal of Ophthalmology* **49**, 40–42.

Corneal dystrophies

Cogan, D. G., Kuwabara, T., Donaldson, D. D. & Collins, E. (1974) Microcystic dystrophy of the cornea. A partial explanation for its pathogenesis. *Archives of Ophthalmology* **92**, 470–474.

Fine, B. S., Yanoff, M., Pitts, E. & Slaughter, F. D. (1977) Meesmann's epithelial dystrophy of the cornea. *American Journal of Ophthalmology* **83**, 633–642.

Garner, A. (1969a) Histochemistry of corneal macular dystrophy. *Investigative Ophthalmology* **8**, 475–483.

Garner, A. (1969b) Histochemistry of corneal granular dystrophy. *British Journal of Ophthalmology* **53**, 799–807.

Ghosh, M. & McCulloch, C. (1986) Recurrent corneal erosion, microcystic epithelial dystrophy, map configurations and fingerprint lines in the cornea. *Canadian Journal of Ophthalmology* **21**, 246–252.

Hori, S. & Tanishima, T. (1982) Transmission and scanning electron microscopic studies on endothelial cells in macular corneal dystrophy. *Japanese Journal of Ophthalmology* **26**, 190–198.

Johnson, B. L., Brown, S. I. & Zaidman, G. W. (1981) A light and electron microscopic study of recurrent granular dystrophy. *American Journal of Ophthalmology* **92**, 49–58.

Kirkness, C. M., McCartney, A., Rice, N. C., Garner, A. & Steele, McG. (1987) Congenital hereditary corneal oedema of Maumenee: its clinical features, management and pathology. *British Journal of Ophthalmology* **71**, 130–144.

Klintworth, G. K. (1980) Corneal dystrophies. In *Ocular Pathology Update*, ed. D. H. Nicholson. Masson, New York.

Klintworth, G. K., Ferry, A. P., Sugar, A. & Reed, J. (1982) Recurrence of lattice corneal dystrophy type I in the corneal grafts of two siblings. *American Journal of Ophthalmology* **94**, 540–546.

Klintworth, G. K., Reed, J., Stainer, G. A. & Binder, P. S. (1983) Recurrence of macular corneal dystrophy within grafts. *American Journal of Ophthalmology* **95**, 60–72.

Lanier, J. D., Fine, M. & Togni, B. (1976) Lattice corneal dystrophy. *Archives of Ophthalmology* **94**, 921–924.

Mondino, B. J., Cholappadi, V. S. R., Skinner, M., Cohen, A. S. & Brown, S. J. (1980) Protein AA and lattice dystrophy. *American Journal of Ophthalmology* **89**, 377–380.

Panjwani, N., Rodrigues, M. M., Alroy, J., Albert, D. M. & Baurn, J. (1986) Alterations in stromal glycoconjugates in macular corneal dystrophy. *Investigative Ophthalmology and Visual Science* **27**, 1211–1216.

Polack, F. M., Bourne, W. M., Forstot, S. L. & Yamaguchi, T. (1980) Scanning electron microscopy of posterior polymorphous corneal dystrophy. *American Journal of Ophthalmology* **89**, 575–584.

Purcell, J. J., Rodrigues, M., Chishti, M. I., Riner, R. N. & Dooley, J. M. (1983) Lattice corneal dystrophy associated with familial systemic amyloidosis (Meretoja's syndrome). *Ophthalmology* **90**, 1512–1517.

Rice, N. S. C., Ashton, N., Jay, B. & Blach, R. K. (1968) Reis–Bücklers' dystrophy. A clinico-pathological study. *British Journal of Ophthalmology* **52**, 577–603.

Rodrigues, M. M., Krachmer, J. H., Hackett, J., Gaskins, R. & Halkias, A. (1986) Fuchs' corneal dystrophy. A clinicopathologic study of the variation in corneal oedema. *Ophthalmology* **93**, 789–796.

Rodrigues, M. M., Streeten, B. W., Krachmer, J. H., Laibson, P. R., Salem, N., Passoneau, J. & Chock, S. (1983) Microfibrillar protein and phospholipid in granular corneal dystrophy. *Archives of Ophthalmology* **101**, 802–810.

Takahashi, T., Kondo, T, Isobe, T. & Okada, S. (1983) A case of corneal amyloidosis. *Acta Ophthalmologica* **61**, 150–156.

Tripathi, R. C. & Garner, A. (1970) Corneal granular dystrophy. A light and electron microscopical study of its recurrence in a graft. *British Journal of Ophthalmology* **54**, 361–372.

Waring, G. O., Laibson, P. R. & Rodrigues, M. (1974) Clinical and pathologic alterations of Desçemet's membrane: with emphasis on endothelial metaplasia. *Survey of Ophthalmology* **18**, 325–368.

Waring, G. O., Rodrigues, M. M. & Laibson, P. R. (1978) Corneal dystrophies. I. Dystrophies of the Bowman's layer, epithelium and stroma. II. Endothelial dystrophies. *Survey of Ophthalmology* **23**, 71–122, 147–168.

Weber, F. L. & Babel, J. (1980) Gelatinous drop-like dystrophy. A form of primary corneal amyloidosis. *Archives of Ophthalmology* **98**, 144–148.

Weller, R. O. (1980) Crystalline stromal dystrophy: histochemistry and ultrastructure of the cornea. *British Journal of Ophthalmology* **64**, 46–52.

Witsche, H., Sundmacher, R., Theopold, H. & Jaeger, W. (1980) Posterior polymorphous dystrophy of the cornea (Schlichting). *von Graefes Archiv fur Ophthalmologie* **214**, 15–25.

Yamaguchi, T., Polack, F. M. & Valenti, J. (1980) Electron microscopic study of recurrent Reis–Bucklers' dystrophy. *American Journal of Ophthalmology* **90**, 95–101.

Yanoff, M., Fine, B. S., Colosi, N. J. & Katowitz, J. S. (1977) Lattice corneal dystrophy. Report of an unusual case. *Archives of Ophthalmology* **95**, 651–655.

Wheeler, G. E. & Eiferman, R. A. (1983) Immunohistochemical identification of the AA protein in lattice dystrophy. *Experimental Eye Research* **36**, 181–186.

Keratoconus

Ihailainen, A. (1986) The clinical and epidemiological features of keratoconus. Genetic and external factors in the pathogenesis of the disease. *Acta Ophthalmologica* **64**, Supplement 178.

Shapiro, M. B., Rodrigues, M. M., Mandel, M. R. & Krachmer, J. M. (1986) Anterior clear spaces in keratoconus. *Ophthalmology* **93**, 1316–1319.

Pemphigoid

Franklin, R. M. & Fitzmorris, C. T. (1983) Antibodies against conjunctival basement membrane zone. Occurrence in cictracial pemphigoid. *Archives of Ophthalmology* **101**, 1611–1613.

Mondino, B. J. & Brown, S. I. (1981) Ocular cicatricial pemphigoid. *Ophthalmology* **88**, 95–100.

Tumours

Erie, J. C., Campbell, R. J. & Liesegang, T. J. (1986) Conjunctival and corneal intra-epithelial neoplasia. *Ophthalmology* **93**, 176–183.

Greer, C. H. (1969) Oxyphil cell adenoma of the lacrimal caruncle. *British Journal of Ophthalmology* **53**, 198–202.

Lass, J. H., Jenson, A. B., Papale, J. J. & Albert, D. M. (1983) Papillomavirus in human conjunctival papillomas. *American Journal of Ophthalmology* **95**, 364–368.

Rao, N. A. & Font, R. L. (1976) Mucoepidermoid carcinoma of the conjunctiva. *Cancer* **38**, 1699–1709.

Rennie, I. G. (1980) Oncocytomas (oxyphiladenomas) of the lacrimal caruncle. *British Journal of Ophthalmology* **64**, 935–939.

Robertson, M. C. (1984) Corneal epithelial dysplasia. *Annals of Ophthalmology* **16**, 1147–1150.

Chapter 6 The eyelids

NORMAL STRUCTURE

The eyelids are structurally complex. The external surface is covered by skin which is thin and normally lacks subcutaneous fat. Well-developed pilary complexes form the eyelashes. The sebaceous glands of Zeis are part of these complexes while the Meibomian glands, which reside in the tarsal plate, are the enlarged sebaceous glands of a non-existent posterior row of cilia. The tarsal plate is a thick layer of collagen which stiffens the lids. There are also eccrine sweat glands, apocrine sweat glands (glands of Moll) and the accessory lacrimal glands of Krause.

This structural complexity results in a diversity of pathological lesions. Lesions derived from components such as blood and lymphatic vessels and nerves are identical to those described under orbit (Chapter 14) and some of those relating to the tarsal conjunctiva have been dealt with in Chapter 5.

ACUTE SUPPURATIVE LESIONS

Hordeolum internum

This is an acute staphylococcal infection of a Meibomian gland which progresses to the formation of an abscess and usually discharges through the conjunctiva. The inflammation frequently produces pre-auricular adenitis, but spread of the infection is fortunately rare.

Hordeolum externum

An external hordeolum or stye is a localised staphylococcal infection of a lash follicle, its accessory glands and the immediately surrounding tissue. It is thus a small boil at the lid margin. After discharge of pus at the lid margin, healing is prompt, but spread of the infection to adjacent follicles frequently occurs.

GRANULOMATOUS INFLAMMATIONS

Chalazion

A chalazion is a mass of granulomatous inflammatory tissue induced by the exposure of retained Meibomian secretion to the action of phagocytic cells. It is similar to the tuberculoid reaction sometimes seen in the superficial dermis in acne vulgaris and to that induced in animals by the subcutaneous injection of sterile fat or wax.

Chalazia occur most commonly in the upper lids of adults. They are not infrequently multiple and, although usually arising without apparent cause, may be preceded by chronic meibomianitis, blepharitis or acne rosacea. Repeated recurrences should arouse suspicion of a sebaceous carcinoma.

Chalazia may resolve and disappear, remain stationary, fibrose into a hard nodule, liquefy to form a thin fibrous sac containing glairy fluid, suppurate or even calcify. Usually, they increase in size and burst through the conjunctiva to present as a fleshy mass. Less often they track forwards to form a flat subcutaneous tumour or along a Meibomian duct to appear at the lid margin.

Microscopic appearances vary according to the stage of development reached before removal, but characteristically the lesion is a granuloma rich in epithelioid and giant cells orientated to sebaceous acini or their remains. Small lymphocytes, neutrophils, plasma cells and eosinophils are often plentiful and small lymphoid foci may be present. Clear rounded spaces left by lipids dissolved out in processing are frequently seen. Staining frozen sections for fat may help to confirm the diagnosis. The granulomatous foci become confluent and eventually destroy not only the secretory acini, but also the gland duct and surrounding structures (Fig. 6.1a & b).

OTHER GRANULOMATOUS INFLAMMATIONS

Although chalazion is by far the commonest granuloma encountered in the lids, the possibility of other causes of granulomatous inflammation such as sarcoidosis, tuberculosis, fungal infections or the presence of foreign matter must be kept in mind.

Sarcoid granulomata

Sarcoid granulomata consist of discrete, non-caseating foci of epithelioid and giant cells. The foci are uniform in size and often sharply circumscribed by lymphocytes and

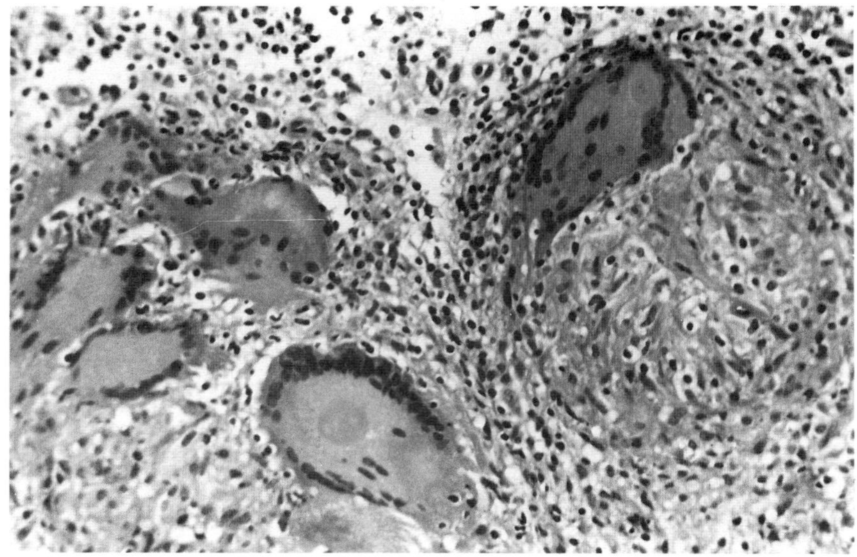

Fig. 6.1 Chalazion. (a) Cluster of giant cells and epithelioid follicle giving a sarcoid-like picture. H & E (×260).

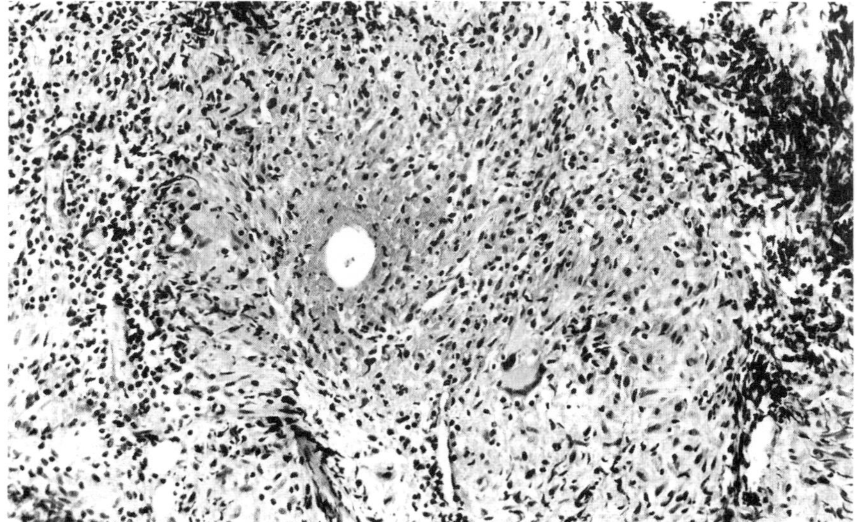

Fig. 6.1 (b) Fat vacuole surrounded by macrophages. H & E (×160).

plasma cells. In chalazia, on the other hand, the granulomata are confluent and may contain micro-abscesses and stainable fat.

Dermal tuberculosis

Many clinical forms of dermal tuberculosis are described, the commonest of which, lupus vulgaris, sometimes spreads to the eyelids from the cheeks or nasal mucosa. Microscopically, there are typical tubercles in which acid-fast bacilli can be demonstrated.

Fungal infections

Fungal infections are rare. Possible infecting organisms include *Blastomyces dermatidis* and *Coccidioides immitis*. Most fungal infections show a combination of granulomatous inflammation and micro-abscesses in which the Grocott–Gomori and PAS stains (Appendix IV) may serve to pinpoint the causative organisms.

Foreign matter

Foreign material and the mouth parts of biting insects, the spines of sea urchins and cacti can all occasionally induce sarcoid-like granulomata when accidentally implanted in the skin.

Palisading granulomata

Palisading granulomata occasionally affect the subcutaneous tissue of the lids. Histologically, these granu-

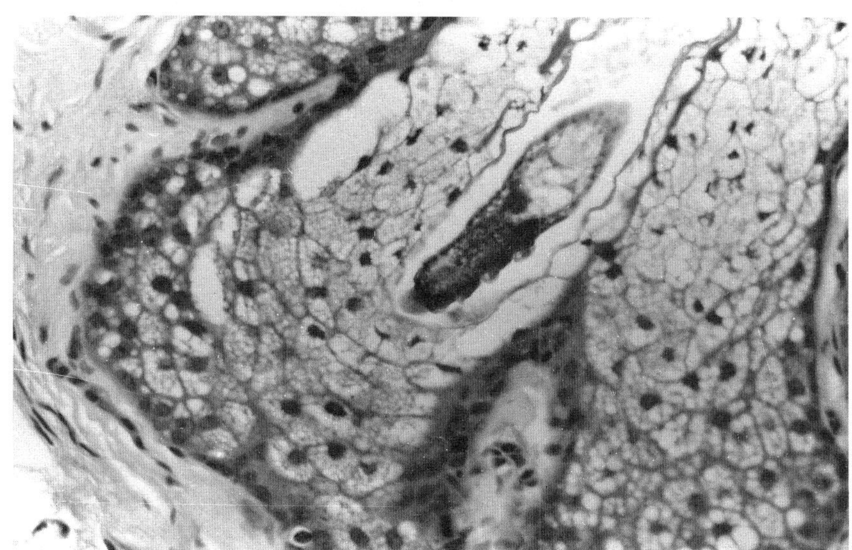

Fig. 6.2 Profile of head of a *Demodex* mite in a Meibomian gland, in a wedge resection for basal cell carcinoma. H & E (×320).

lomata are characterised by a core of necrotic collagen surrounded by a palisade of fibroblasts and histiocytes. Although they resemble the nodules of rheumatoid arthritis and rheumatic fever, no cause is usually found.

Nodular fasciitis

Nodular fasciitis occasionally involves the eyelids.

DEMODEX INFESTATION

Two species of demodectic mites may infest the eyelids in man, *Demodex folliculorum* in the eyelash and hair follicles and *Demodex brevis* in the sebaceous and Meibomian glands. In the hair follicle, the mite lies along the hair shaft with its tail at the surface and thus produces a characteristic collar of faeces, epithelial and lipid debris. Infestation is easily demonstrated by mounting epilated lashes in oil. Several parasites may infest one follicle. The rate of infestation increases with age. Light infestation may be symptom-free, while heavy infestation may cause a blepharitis. In the sebaceous glands, heavy infestation may result in destruction of the gland, blockage of the ducts and both acute and granulomatous inflammation. The picture resembles a chalazion and *Demodex* has been thought to be implicated in the pathogenesis of chalazia.

The parasites may occasionally be identified as an incidental finding in paraffin sections of biopsy specimens (Fig. 6.2).

BENIGN EPIDERMAL LESIONS

Viral

Verrucae

Verrucae (warts) are common on the eyelids. They are caused by a virus or viruses of the *Papova* group. The virus is transferred by autoinoculation by scratching and can also be spread directly or indirectly to other persons. The incubation period ranges from several weeks to several months. Warts on the lid margin may induce conjunctivitis which is sometime complicated by painful keratitis and even corneal ulceration.

All types of verrucae have a papillary structure and the papillae characteristically appear to radiate outwards and upwards from the base (Fig. 6.3a). There is a corresponding displacement of the dermal papillae and adnexal structures in the adjacent skin. The papillae are short in plane warts and long and slender in digitate warts.

Microscopically there is acanthosis and vacuolation of the cells in the granular and upper prickle cell layers. Large granular masses of keratohyalin are often present in the granular layer (Fig. 6.3b). Cells in mitosis may be numerous and not confined to the basal layer, but there is never any loss of polarity or other evidence of dysplasia. Parallel funnels of hyperkeratosis and parakeratosis are seen on the surface of common warts while plane warts show a characteristic basket-weave arrangement of the stratum corneum. Eosinophilic and basophilic intranuclear bodies have been reported in the prickle cells of plantar and palmar warts, but are rare in other types.

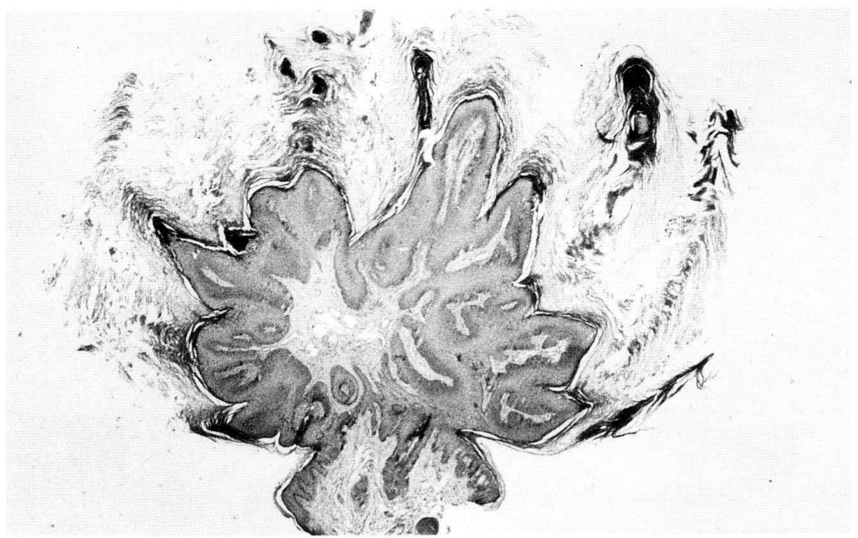

Fig. 6.3 Viral wart. (a) Low power to show radial array of spiky papillae. Masson (×20).

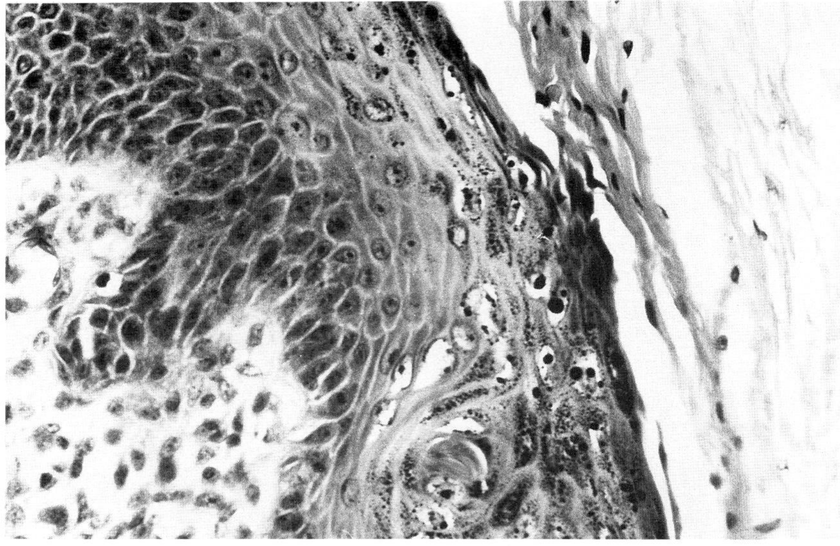

Fig. 6.3 (b) High power showing acanthosis, coarse basophilic granules in vacuolated cells and rounded nuclei being shed in the keratin scale. H & E (×420).

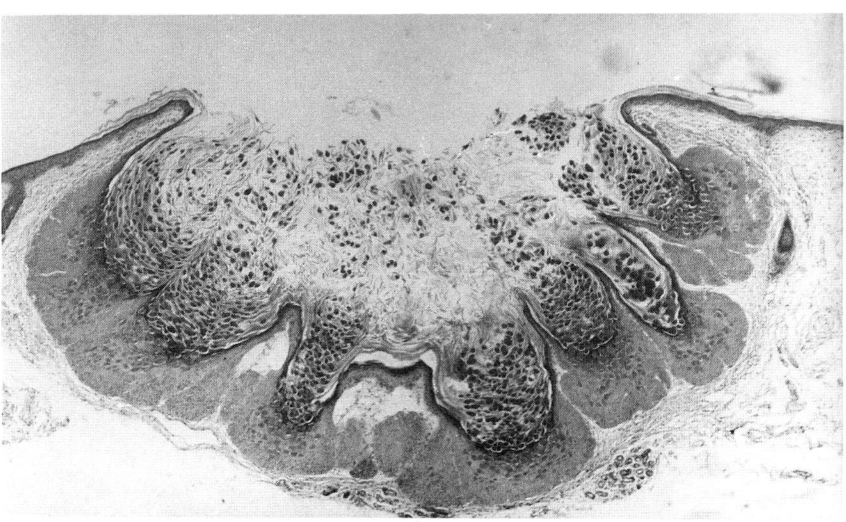

Fig. 6.4 *Molluscum contagiosum*. The centre of the nodule is occupied by inclusion bodies originating in and discharged from surrounding epidermal lobules.

Mollucum contagiosum

The virus of molluscum contagiosum belongs to the pox virus group. It is spread by direct contact or by fomites. The incubation period is 2 weeks or more.

The virus parasitises epidermal cells inducing the formation of small painless grey-white nodules which are umbilicated. Although the virus does not infect the conjunctiva, necrotic material discharged from nodules on the lid margin sometimes causes a follicular conjunctivitis which may progress to pannus formation and even corneal scarring.

The virus elementary bodies are rectangular in shape and contain DNA. They multiply in the cytoplasm of epidermal cells to form eosinophilic inclusions 20–40 μm in length. Micro-dissection has shown these inclusions to be operculated sachets divided by internal septa into compartments packed with elementary bodies. As the inclusion bodies increase in size they displace and finally destroy the cell nuclei. The infected epidermis exhibits increased mitotic activity and proliferates to form a compact lobulated tumour projecting above the surrounding skin. Its constituent lobules converge to form a central cavity packed with inclusion bodies (Fig. 6.4).

Other hyperkeratotic papillomata

Basal cell papillomata (seborrhoeic wart)

These common benign keratoses form brown excrescences covered by an unctuous scale which can be removed by light rubbing. They are sharply circumscribed and rise abruptly from the epidermal surface as though stuck on the skin. Microscopically, seborrhoeic keratoses consist of mature basal and squamous cells in variable proportions enclosing islands of connective tissue. Horny cysts are formed by endokeratinisation and retention of keratin within hair follicles and sweat ducts traversing the tumour (Fig. 6.5a). Sometimes cysts dominate the picture while at other times they are inconspicuous in the

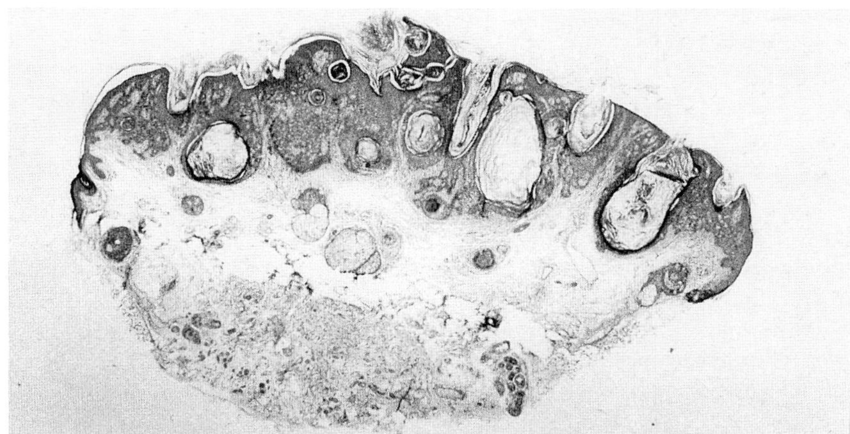

Fig. 6.5 Basal cell papilloma (seborrhoeic wart). (a) Low power to show typical gross form with flat papillae and horny microcysts. H & E (×20).

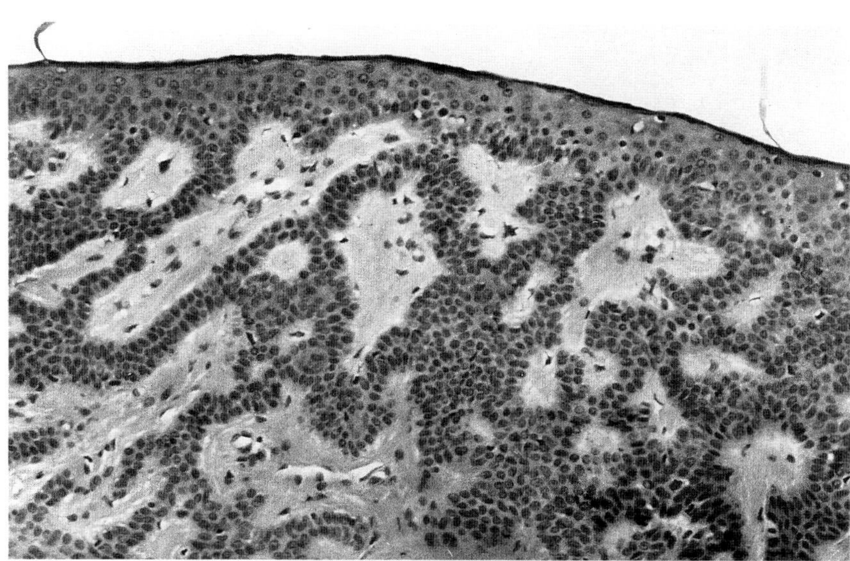

Fig. 6.5 (b) Higher power showing the reticular pattern produced by strands of proliferating basaloid cells. H & E (×160).

broad masses of epidermal cells. The lesions may be papillary, but are often solid with a domed surface. There is also a distinctive variant composed of thin anastomosing strands of basaloid cells extending down into the dermis (Fig. 6.5b). The dark colour of the lesions is due to melanin which is most conspicuous in the basal cells.

Though these lesions are commonly slow growing, activation may occur. With accelerated growth, the proportion of squamous to basal cells increases and the stroma becomes densely infiltrated with lymphocytes.

Squamous cell papillomata

These are simple papillomata which consist of fibrovascular cores clothed by hyperplastic and often heavily keratinised epidermis showing normal cell maturation. They are similar to verrucae, but do not show any of the features by which verrucae may be recognised.

Keratoacanthomata

Typically keratoacanthoma forms a solitary hemispherical nodule with a central keratin-filled crater on the exposed skin of elderly persons. It grows rapidly to attain a size of 1–2 cm in a few weeks or months, after which it may spontaneously regress leaving only a small scar.

Sections through the centre of the tumour show a bowl-shaped lesion filled with keratin bordered by acanthotic epidermis. The margin of the bowl has a characteristically tapering edge (Fig. 6.6a). The epidermal squames have prominent intercellular bridges and a 'washed-out' appearance. Necrotic epidermal pearls infiltrated by polymorphs are also a common feature.

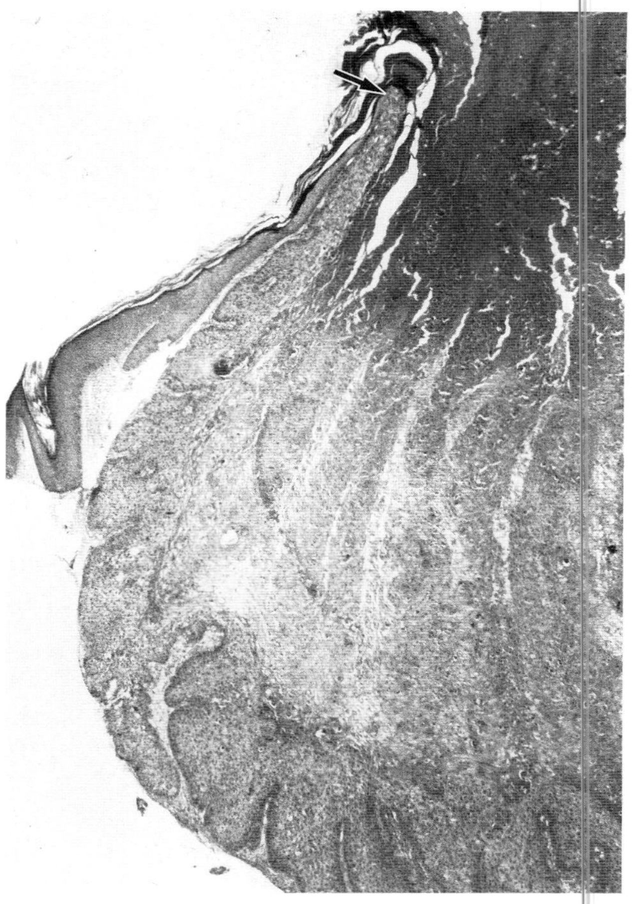

Fig. 6.6 Keratoacanthoma. (a) Low power to show the typical bowl-shaped profile with tapering shoulder (arrow). H & E (×20).

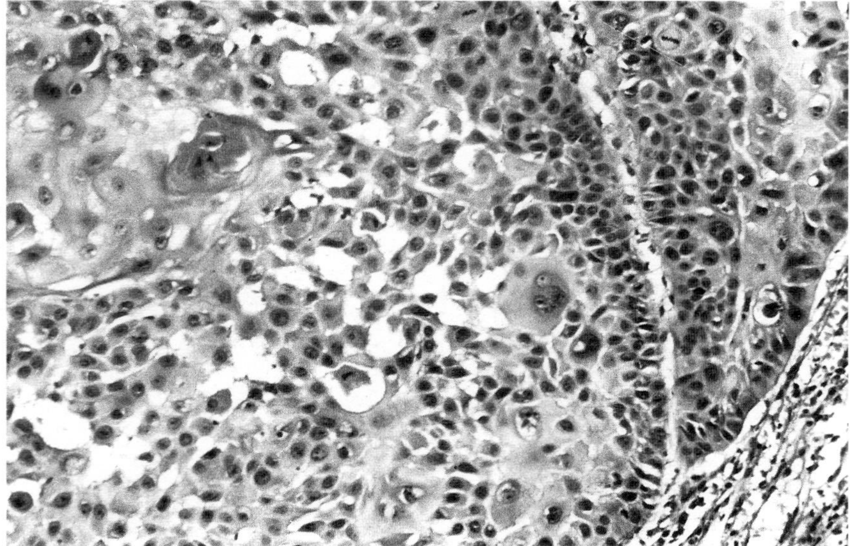

Fig. 6.6 (b) Higher power to show well marked dysplasia along the lower boundary of the lesion. H & E (×320). This lesion was incompletely excised and recurred. The dysplastic changes were much less marked in the recurrence.

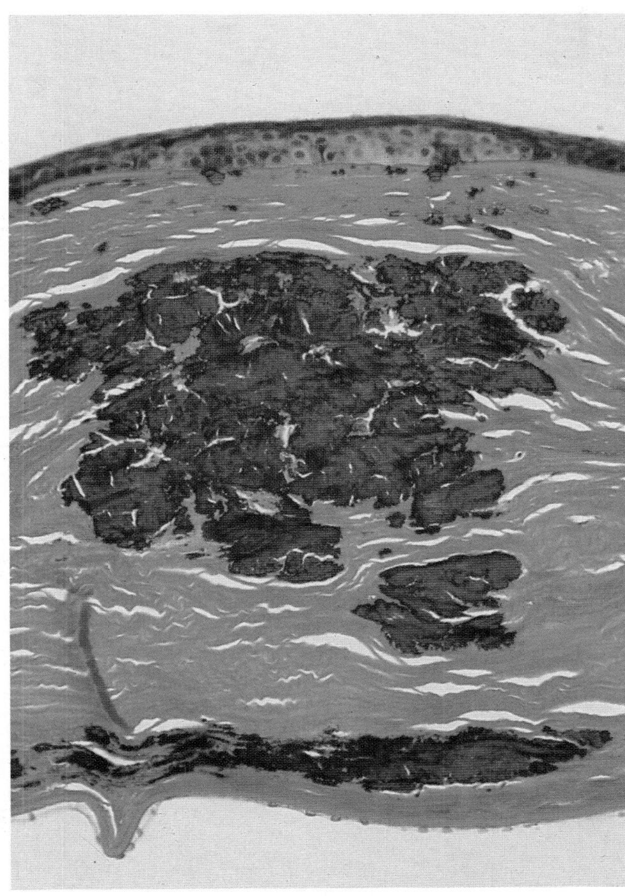

Plate 1 Granular dystrophy. Massive stromal deposits of the abnormal material heavily stained by the red component of Masson's trichrome stain. (× 230.)

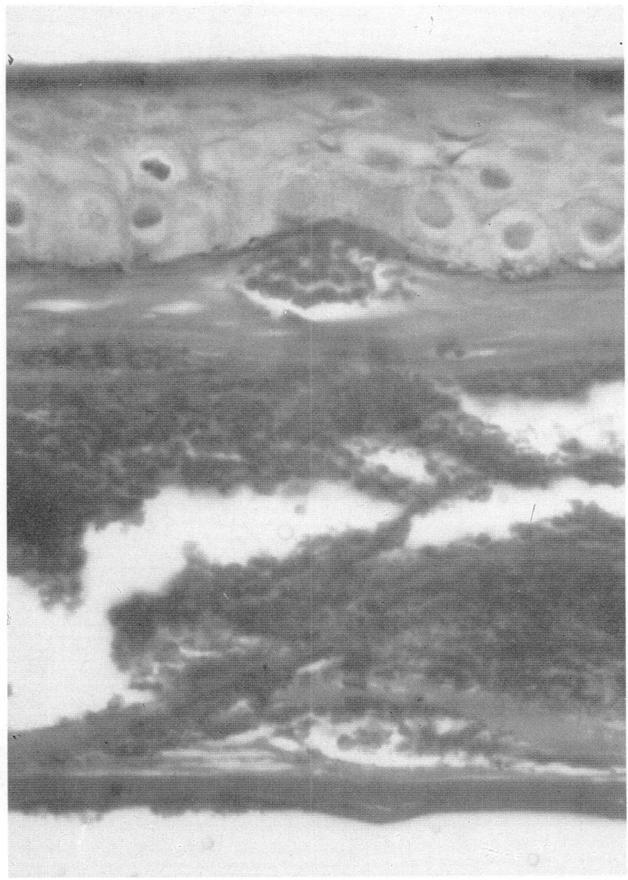

Plate 2 Macular dystrophy. Deposit of granular material heavily stained by the PAS method deep to the epithelium. There has been some subepithelial fibrosis and Bowman's membrane is difficult to identify in this area (× 460.)

(a) 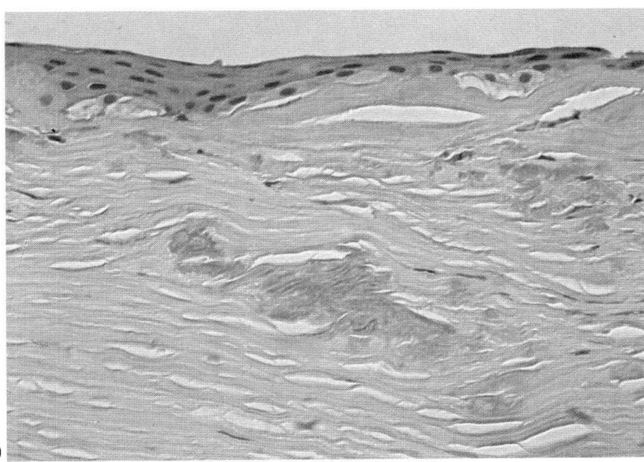

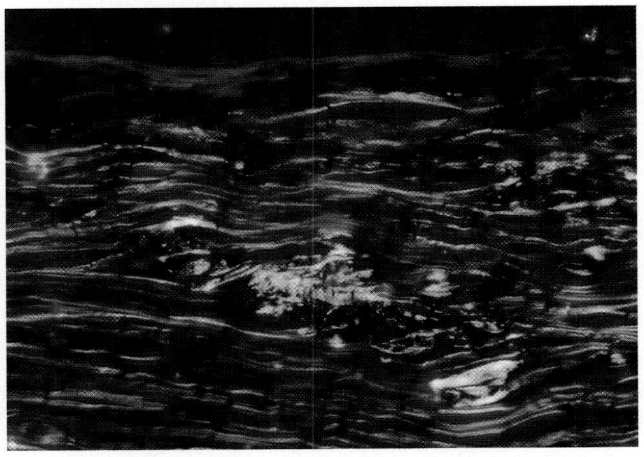 (b)

Plate 3 Lattice dystrophy. (a) Showing gross scarring deep to the epithelium and deposits of amyloid stained by Congo red in the stroma (× 230); (b) corresponding field viewed under polarised light showing the birefringence of the deposits which appear green (dichroism). (× 230.)

[*facing page 86*]

Well-marked cellular atypia suggestive of carcinoma is often seen (Fig. 6.6b). At the base of the tumour, cores of epidermal cells extend irregularly into the dermis. There is usually a dense dermal infiltrate of lymphocytes and plasma cells with a sprinkling of eosinophils. The infiltrate often extends into the base of the lesion.

Differentiation from squamous cell carcinoma depends principally on the configuration of the lesion and may, if the dysplasia and dermal infiltration are prominent, be difficult. A biopsy of the lesion may readily result in the mistaken diagnosis of squamous cell carcinoma unless care is taken to remove a wedge-shaped slice which will enable the characteristic configuration of the lesion to be recognised.

Cutaneous horn

This is a clinical term for a keratinous pillar which may have different pathological causes. Probably the commonest is actinic keratosis, but squamous cell carcinomata, unresolved keratoacanthomata and trichilemmomata may all give rise to cutaneous horns.

Pseudocarcinomatous hyperplasia

Epidermal hyperplasia at the edges of persistent ulcers or overlying chronic inflammatory conditions of the dermis such as lupus vulgaris or fungal infections may simulate well-differentiated squamous cell carcinomata. Distinguishing features are that cellular atypia is never pronounced while inflammatory infiltration of the hyperplastic epidermis is. Pseudocarcinomatous hyperplasia may undergo conversion to squamous cell carcinoma if the inflammatory process lasts long enough.

PRECANCEROUS EPIDERMAL LESIONS

Actinic (solar or senile) keratosis

Actinic keratoses which form scaly plaques in areas of exposed skin should be viewed with suspicion because they sometimes develop into squamous cell carcinomata. Those actinic keratoses in which the surface layer of keratin is overabundant and adherent may, as already noted, present clinically as a cutaneous horn.

The pathological basis of the lesion is dysplasia and irregular proliferation of the epidermis, and hyperplasia of the pilary adnexal epithelium. The abnormal epidermal keratinocytes form layers of parakeratin while the adnexal keratinocytes form layers of keratin at the adnexal ostia. This gives rise to the characteristic picture of alternating columns of orthokeratosis and parakeratosis seen in histological sections. Suprabasal splitting in the epidermis due to degeneration of the intercellular bridges and consequent loss of cohesion between prickle cells is a useful diagnostic sign when present (Fig. 6.7).

Cellular atypia and disorderly cellular arrangement similar to that seen in squamous cell carcinoma are present but less advanced, and there is no invasive growth into the dermis. Actinic keratosis has been termed developing or incomplete carcinoma. There is dense infitration of the subjacent dermis with lymphocytes and plasma cells and often a sprinkling of eosinophils. The dermal collagen shows degenerative changes evidenced by hyalinisation, increased basophilia and the appearance of coarse fibres which stain for elastica.

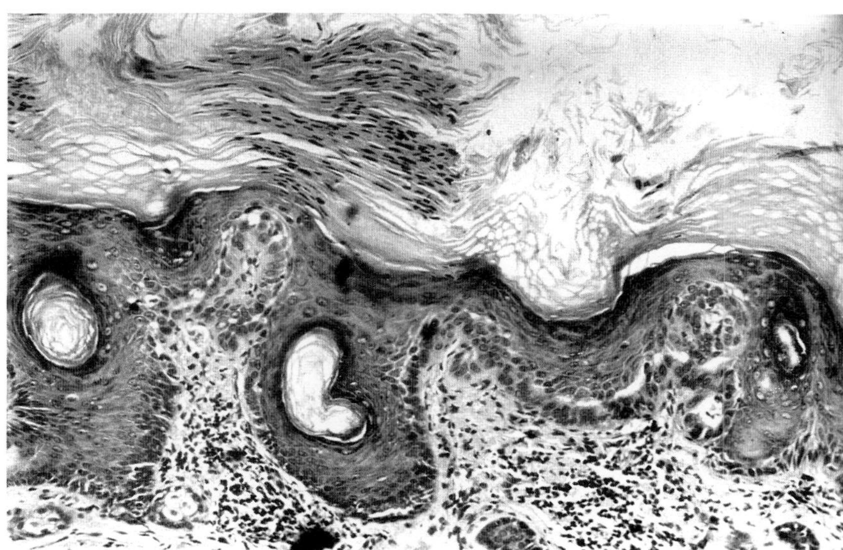

Fig. 6.7 Actinic (senile) keratosis. Alternating hyperkeratosis and parakeratosis is seen on the surface of the epidermis. Suprabasal splitting is clearly visible and there is chronic inflammatory infiltration in the superficial dermis.

Bowen's disease

This lesion presents clinically as indolent scaly plaques which enlarge slowly.

Microscopically, there is hyperkeratosis and parakeratosis on the surface of the much thickened epidermis, the rete ridges of which are elongated and widened. Throughout the whole thickness of the epidermis the cells lie in complete disarray. Striking cellular pleomorphism and hyperchromasia are seen and mitotic figures, which are often abnormal, are present at all levels. Many of the cells show bizarre giant nuclei or clusters of nuclei. Premature keratinisation of individual cells is a common and characteristic feature, the keratinised cells having pyknotic nuclei in homogeneous and strongly eosinophilic cytoplasm. The basement membrane remains intact and the upper dermis usually contains a moderate infiltrate of lymphocytes and plasma cells. Though the picture is the prototype of carcinoma *in situ*, invasive carcinoma rarely develops.

Arsenic ingestion may cause identical lesions, but these are often multiple and show considerable numbers of cells with clear cytoplasm.

Radiation dermatosis

The cutaneous lesions induced by ionising radiation are similar to those of actinic keratosis, but additional degenerative changes are observed in the dermis including an increase in, and irregular, staining and hyalinisation of the collagen fibres of the dermis, superficial telangiectasia and the appearance of bizarre fibroblasts. The deeper blood vessels may be thrombosed. The hair follicles are destroyed, but the sweat glands survive.

MALIGNANT EPIDERMAL LESIONS

Basal cell carcinomata

Basal cell carcinomata are the commonest malignant tumours of the eyelids and occur most frequently in the lower lids in older patients. They are usually single and present as slowly growing, firm pearly nodules or typical ulcers with rolled edges at or near the lid margin. The tumours show variable degrees of local invasiveness, but only very rarely metastasise. Basal cell carcinomata originate from the basal layer of the epidermis or the hair follicle and are composed of basaloid-type cells. These sometimes show transition to a squamous type which has a larger paler nucleus and more abundant eosinophilic cytoplasm and areas of sebaceous differentiation may also occur. Some basal cell carcinomata contain considerable amounts of melanin both in the constituent cells and in the stroma. According to the predominant pattern of growth, the following histological types of basal cell carcinomata are recognised:

1 The solid type is composed of irregularly shaped islands of neoplastic cells within the dermis. Cells at the perimeter of these masses are columnar and form distinct palisades (Fig. 6.8a & b). Cells within the palisades are haphazardly arranged and are usually smaller with hyperchromatic nuclei and relatively little cytoplasm. For this reason, such growths appear basophilic in H & E sections.

2 The cystic type of basal cell carcinoma is a variant of the solid type. Necrosis of cells in the centre of the tumour islands results in substantial pseudocysts lined by neoplastic cells and containing cell debris.

3 The adenoid variety of basal cell carcinoma is composed of ribbons of neoplastic basal cells enclosing islands

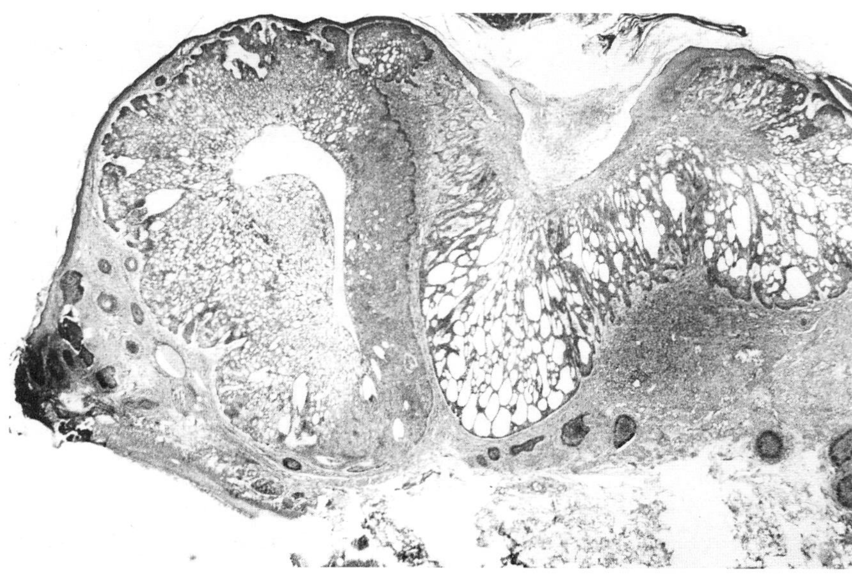

Fig. 6.8 Basal cell carcinoma, adenoid cystic with solid areas. (a) Low power. Note central ulceration. H & E (×20).

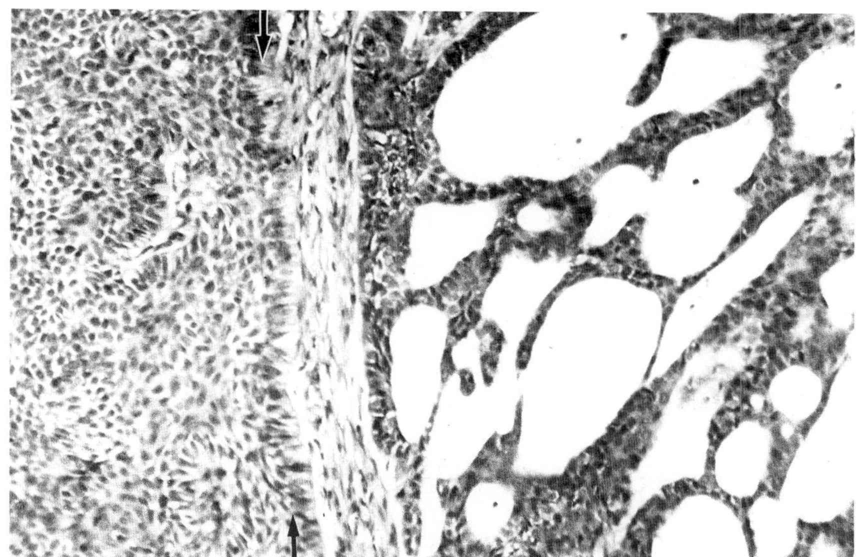
Fig. 6.8 (b) Higher power to show solid area (left) and adenoid cystic area (right). Note palisade of cells along the boundary of solid area (arrows).

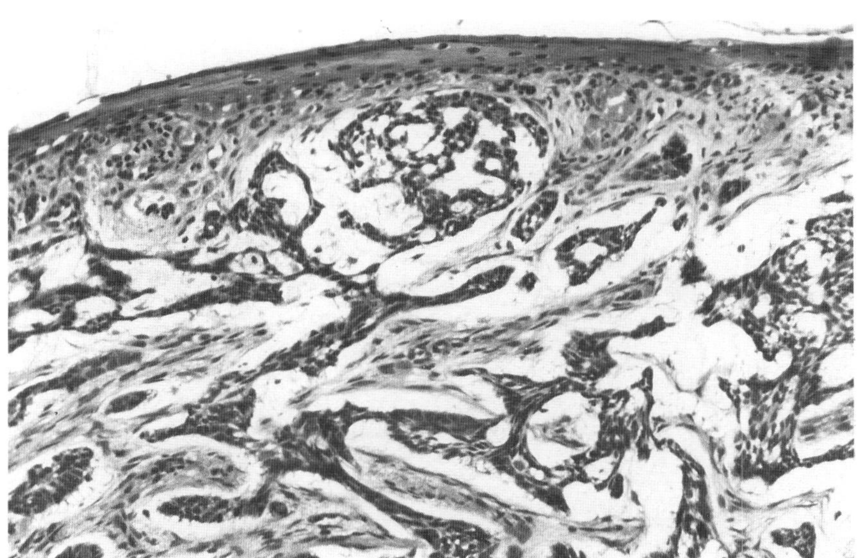
Fig. 6.8 (c) Morphoea type. Note irregular strands of flattened cells with abundant cellular stroma between them.

of connective tissue. Gland-like formations are frequently present, but there is no evidence of true secretory activity (Fig. 6.8a & b). Connective tissue within and around the growth is prone to mucoid degeneration.

4 Keratotic basal cell carcinoma is so called because it contains keratotic whorls and horn cysts as a result of squamous differentiation of the neoplastic basal cells.

5 The morphoea or fibrosing type of basal cell carcinoma is characterised by innumerable nests and thin strands of neoplastic cells embedded in a dense cellular fibrous (desmoplastic) stroma (Fig. 6.8c). Tumours of this kind may invade deeper structures and are frequently incompletely excised because their margins are difficult to define.

Recurrence after treatment

Primary treatment by radiotherapy or surgery is successful in over 90% of cases. Except in the case of morphoea-type tumours, histological evidence of incomplete excision does not imply that recurrence is inevitable, though it is obviously likely. Control of excision by frozen sections has been shown to give excellent results.

Squamous cell carcinomata

Squamous cell carcinoma of the eyelids is a more serious condition than basal cell carcinoma and is fortunately much less common. It rarely arises in normal skin being usually preceded by solar keratosis, carcinoma *in situ* or keratosis due to arsenic, tar or ionising radiation. It usually presents as as a hard nodule or indurated crusted ulcer, but occasionally produces an exuberant papillary outgrowth or a cutaneous horn. In contrast to basal cell carcinoma, spread to the regional lymph nodes may occur, though this is usually late.

Microscopically, squamous cell carcinomata arise from the prickle or squamous cells of the epidermis, but the degree of squamous differentiation varies greatly so that a wide variety of histological patterns is found, ranging from well-differentiated keratinising carcinomata to anaplastic spindle cell growths resembling sarcomata. Normal squamous cells have large pale nuclei and relatively abundant opaque eosinophilic cytoplasm. They are linked by desmosomes, the sites of which are seen in routine preparations as spines or bridges crossing the intercellular spaces. Well differentiated squamous carcinomata retain many of these features and tend to form cell nests and keratin pearls. Such growths are less malignant than those in which evidence of differentiation is minimal. In poorly differentiated carcinomata, the finding of a few intercellular bridges may be the only light microscopic evidence of their squamous cell origin. Squamous cell carcinoma is an invasive growth which evokes a dense cellular infiltrate in the stroma and underlying dermis. This comprises lymphocytes, plasma cells and often eosinophils.

Basisquamous cell or metatypical carcinoma is a tumour in which the cell type or cellular arrangement makes it difficult to decide between basal cell or squamous cell carcinoma. Such tumours normally behave like basal cell carcinomata and do not metastasise to the regional lymph nodes.

BENIGN TUMOURS OF SEBACEOUS GLANDS

Benign tumours of the sebaceous glands may originate in the Meibomian glands, the glands of Zeis or the sebaceous glands of the lacrimal caruncle. Some benign growths are strictly hyperplasias, while others are true adenomata. Both occur in middle or old age.

Hyperplasias

The lesions consist of wide central ducts around which are crowded numerous mature sebaceous nodules composed of normal cells. They are often multiple and may be associated with acne rosacea and rhinophyma.

Adenomata

These are larger and less differentiated and show progressive growth. Incomplete removal may be followed by recurrence.

'Adenoma sebaceum'

The dermal component of tuberose sclerosis (Chapter 15) is inappropriately named since the facial nodules are fibrovascular hamartomata in which the sebaceous glands are only passively involved.

SEBACEOUS CARCINOMATA

This rare neoplasm occurs more often in the eyelids than anywhere else in the body and arises more frequently in the upper than in the lower lid. Though it most commonly arises from the Meibomian glands, origin from the gland of Zeis and from the caruncular sebaceous glands is also well recognised. Patients are usually elderly, but this carcinoma occasionally develops in adolescents and young adults, sometimes as a consequence of irradiation of a retinoblastoma in early childhood.

The lesion most commonly presents as an atypical or recurrent chalazion, but may resemble a basal cell carcinoma or form yellow nodules at the lid margin with loss of cilia. Among its more deceptive presentations are diffuse thickening of the eyelid and unilateral blepharoconjunctivitis or keratoconjunctivitis. These manifestations may be complicated by carcinoma *in situ* of the overlying epidermis or pagetoid invasion by the adenocarcinoma of neighbouring epidermis and conjunctiva to produce a chronic eczematoid lesion.

Microscopically, the neoplasm is made up of bulky lobules composed of poorly differentiated epithelial cells with hyperchromatic nuclei and sebaceous cells with abundant vacuolated lipid-containing cytoplasm (Fig. 6.9a). Foci of squamous cells may sometimes be seen. Numerous cells in mitosis are usually present. Necrosis in the centre of the lobules results in the accumulation of fatty debris and pyknotic nuclear fragments. Frozen sections stained for fat (Fig. 6.9b) can be helpful in establishing the diagnosis in difficult cases.

Presumptive evidence of origin from the glands of Zeis is provided by infiltration of the tumour within the hair sheath (Fig. 6.9c).

Intra-epithelial spread is characterised by the presence of clusters or larger groups of tumour cells in the epithelium bordering the tumour (Fig. 6.9d)

Prognosis

Comparison of older with more recent series shows that, with early recognition and adequate treatment, the outcome with these tumours has improved.

Size is an important prognostic factor. In a recent

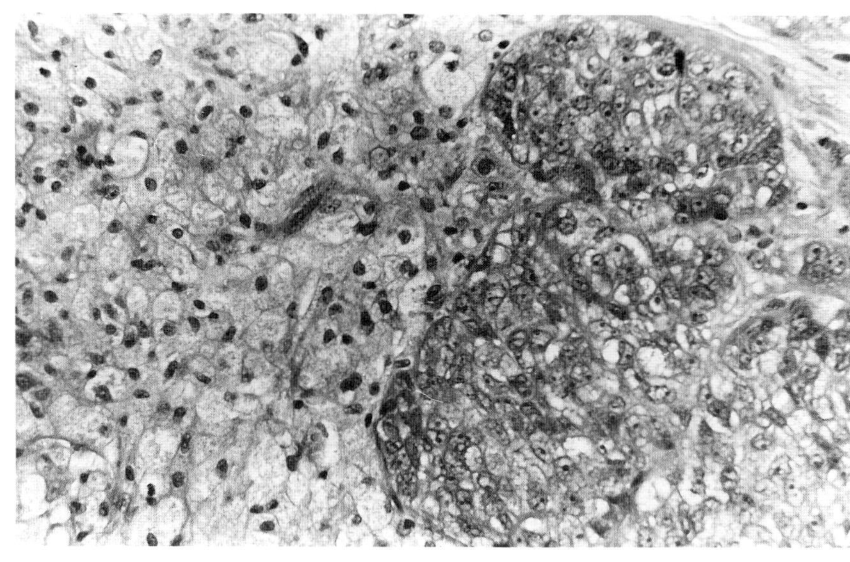

Fig. 6.9 Sebaceous carcinoma. (a) Showing poorly differentiated area (right) and well-differentiated area (left) in which the resemblance of the cells to those of normal sebaceous glands is obvious. H & E (×260).

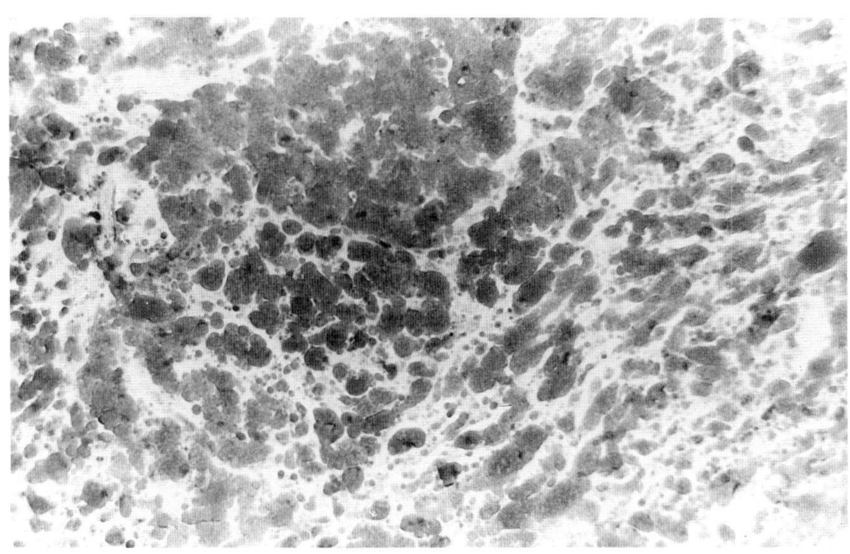

Fig. 6.9 (b) Frozen section stained by oil red 'o' to show large content of fat. (×260).

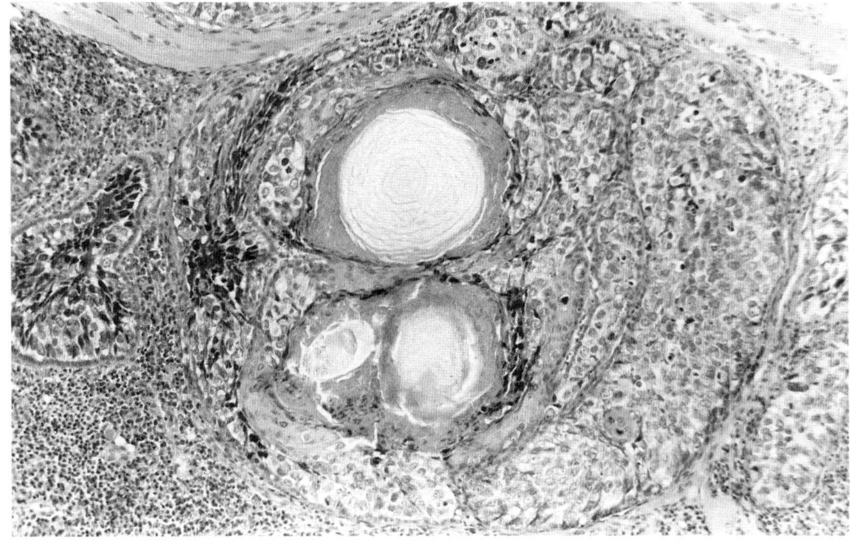

Fig. 6.9 (c) Tumour growing along hair sheaths from glands of Zeis. H & E (×94).

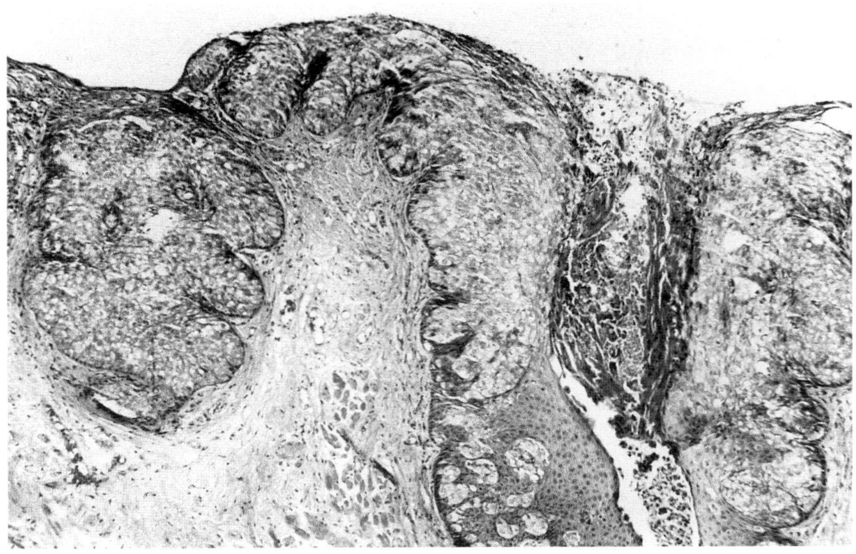

Fig. 6.9 (d) Intraepithelial spread involving aperture of the canaliculus. Masson (×160).

series (Rao *et al.*, 1978), no tumour smaller than 6.0 mm in greatest dimension had a fatal outcome, while the mortality with tumours greater than 20 mm was 60%.

Unfavourable histological features are:

1 Multicentric origin.
2 Poor sebaceous differentiation.
3 An infiltrative growth pattern.
4 Carcinomatous invasion of the overlying epithelium.

TUMOURS OF THE HAIR FOLLICLE

Trichoepitheliomata

Trichoepithelioma is an uncommon benign neoplasm showing differentiation towards hair follicles. It forms a firm nodule at the lid margin in adults. Distributed through the dermis there are multiple small squamous cell cysts containing keratin. Around these cysts are mantles of small basal cells which often branch at random to connect with adjacent hair follicles and the basal layer of the epidermis. Poorly differentiated trichoepitheliomata merge imperceptibly with basal cell carcinomata of the keratotic type.

Trichofolliculomata

Trichofolliculoma is a hamartoma consisting of a central cystic space opening to the surface and lined by squamous epithelium from which branch an array of abortive hair follicles in various stages of development. It is benign and usually solitary.

Trichilemmomata

Trichilemmomata are benign tumours consisting of masses of glycogen-rich clear cells with sharply defined borders enclosing thin cores of keratin suggestive of hair shafts. The cell masses are continuous with the epidermis and are well demarcated from the surrounding dermis by a peripheral palisade of cells reminiscent of that seen in basal cell carcinomata. As already noted there may be a substantial overlying cap of keratin so that the lesion presents as cutaneous horn. More than one tumour is not uncommonly present.

The tumours are easily misdiagnosed as basal cell or squamous cell carcinoma.

Inverted follicular keratosis

Inverted follicular keratosis is a small benign circumscribed keratotic tumour which usually becomes manifest as a solitary nodule projecting from the skin surface. The lesion is sometimes warty and may accumulate sufficient keratin to form a horn. Inverted follicular keratosis often develops rapidly over a few months and is sometimes accompanied by itching, burning, oozing and repeated scab formation.

Microscopically, the tumour is a mass of epidermal cells sharply delineated from the underlying dermis without any evidence of the infiltrative epithelial strands seen in kerato-acanthoma, pseudocarcinomatous hyperplasia or squamous cell carcinoma. Some lesions have a crater filled with keratin at their summit. The mass is composed of basal and squamous cells and the junction between the two types of cell is often marked by highly characteristic eddies of concentrically arranged squamous cells, usually without keratin formation. Cellular atypia is not evident and cellular infiltration of the underlying dermis is minimal or absent.

Pilomatricomata (benign calcifying epithelioma of Malherbe)

Pilomatricoma is an uncommon tumour thought to be derived from the germinal matrix cells of the hair bulb. Approximately 10% of all pilomatricomata occur in the eyebrow or upper lids. Many of the patients are under 20 years of age and present with a small solitary, freely movable and often cystic subcutaneous nodule. Pilomatricomata are benign, but occasionally recur if incompletely excised.

The tumour commences as a small cyst, the wall of which is composed of basophilic cells strongly resembling those of the hair root matrix. As the cells proliferate, the cyst enlarges and its wall becomes infolded. Later the cells undergo progressive keratinisation during which they enlarge and become eosinophilic while their nuclei shrink and disappear. Masses of keratin in which the cell outlines persist ('shadow' or 'ghost' epithelium) are produced (Fig. 6.10a). These masses evoke a vigorous foreign body giant cell reaction (Fig. 6.10b) and commonly become calcified. Bone may also occasionally be laid down.

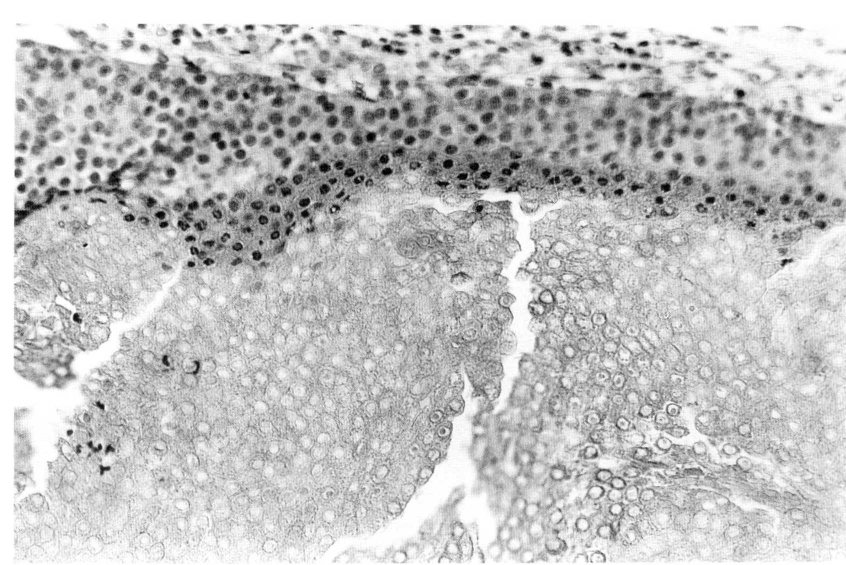

Fig. 6.10 Pilomatricoma. (a) Showing 'ghost' epithelium arising from a layer of hair matrix-like epithelium. H & E (×260).

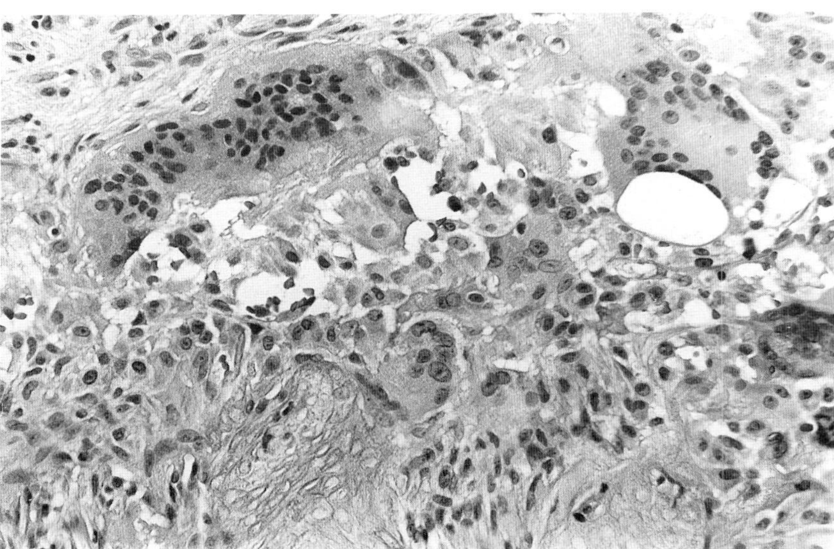

Fig. 6.10 (b) Massive giant cell reaction to the 'ghost' epithelium. H & E (×260).

CHAPTER 6

TUMOURS OF SWEAT GLANDS

The generic term for a sweat gland tumour is hidradenoma. The terms spiradenomata and syringomata were originally used to describe tumours arising from the secretory coil and duct respectively. While the epithelium of the secretory parts of the gland is distinctive, both eccrine and apocrine glands have ducts lined by two-tiered epithelium. Syringomata and retention cysts arising from these ducts are thus very similar. The eccrine duct terminates in a spiral which passes through the epidermis. The apocrine duct is shorter and opens into the pilary antrum.

Papillary syringadenomata (syringocystadenoma papilliferum)

The papillary syringadenoma consists of a warty plaque from which channels of two-tiered epithelum extend downwards into cystic spaces in the dermis and often form villus-like structures around which there is dense infiltration with plasma cells.

Hydrocystomata

A hydrocystoma consists of uni- or multilocular cysts lined by two-tiered apocrine-type epithelium which sometimes contains pigment granules and may show papillary infolding.

Eccrine spiradenomata

An eccrine spiradenoma is a solitary, often painful, circumscribed dermal nodule structurally resembling eccrine sweat gland coils.

Eccrine acrospiromata (clear cell or nodular hidradenoma)

An eccrine acrospiroma is a well demarcated multilocular tumour structurally resembling an eccrine sweat duct and containing numerous cells rich in glycogen (clear cells).

Dermal cylindromata

Dermal cylindromata are commonly encountered as multiple nodules of variable size on the face and scalp (turban tumour). The nodules are composed of lobules of epithelial cells surrounded by a thick hyaline (PAS positive) membrane.

Syringomata

Syringoma takes the form of single or multiple nodules, sometimes confined to the eyelids, composed of ductular formations or epithelial cells.

Chondroid syringomata (mixed tumours)

A chondroid syringoma is a tumour composed of epithelial and mesenchymal elements resembling a mixed salivary or lacrimal tumour (Chapter 14).

METASTATIC TUMOURS

Metastatic deposits of carcinoma occur much less frequently in the eyelids than in the eye itself. The source is usually lung in men and breast in women and the lesion in the eyelid may be the presenting symptom of the primary disease.

CYSTS

Sudoriferous cysts

Sudoriferous cysts present as transparent vesicles at the lid margin, particularly of the lower lid. The majority are retention cysts of the glands of Moll. They are commonly multilocular and, if not ruptured during excision, contain thin amorphous secretion. They are lined by two tiers of cells. The cells of the inner layer are columnar or cuboidal, while those of the outer myoepithelial layer are smaller and flatter (Fig. 6.11b). The inner cells may show adherent globules of secretion and sometimes form small fronds projecting into the lumen of the cyst. With rising intracystic pressure, the lining cells become stretched and may eventually be reduced to a single layer of flattened cells.

Keratinous cysts

Epidermal cysts

Epidermal cysts are extremely common and result from the accumulation of laminated keratin and sebaceous secretion in obstructed hair follicles. The mixture forms a soft greasy paste. The cysts are lined by keratinising epithelium (Fig. 6.11a), but there is no dermal collagen. No associated adnexal structures or remnants thereof are identifiable, thus distinguishing epidermal from dermoid cysts. Epidermal cysts have been known for years as sebaceous cysts, but, although they usually contain sebaceous material, they are not derived from sebaceous glands.

Milia

Milia are histologically similar, but much smaller and often multiple. Distension of the infundibulum of the pilary follicle may also involve the apocrine sweat duct, the lining of the cyst may thus consist partially of two-tiered epithelium.

Pilar cysts

Pilar cysts are much less common. They are lined by layers of squamous-like cells which, however, lack intercellular bridges. These undergo keratinisation without the formation of keratohyalin granules and, instead of laminated keratin, an amorphous eosinphilic mass of keratin builds up the lumen (Fig. 6.11c).

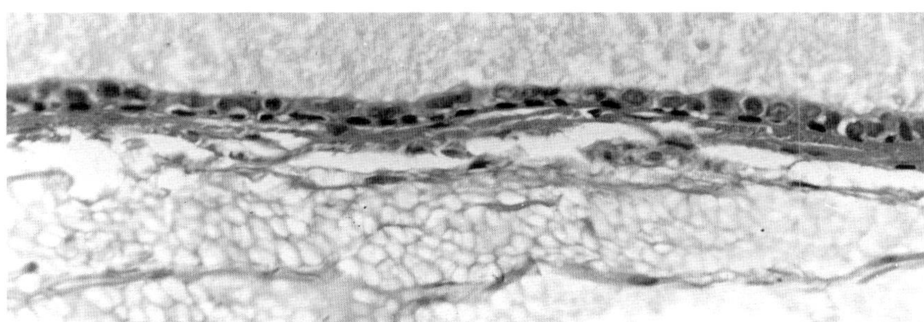

Fig. 6.11 (a) Wall of sudoriferous cyst. Note cubical inner layer and outer flat myoepithelial layer.

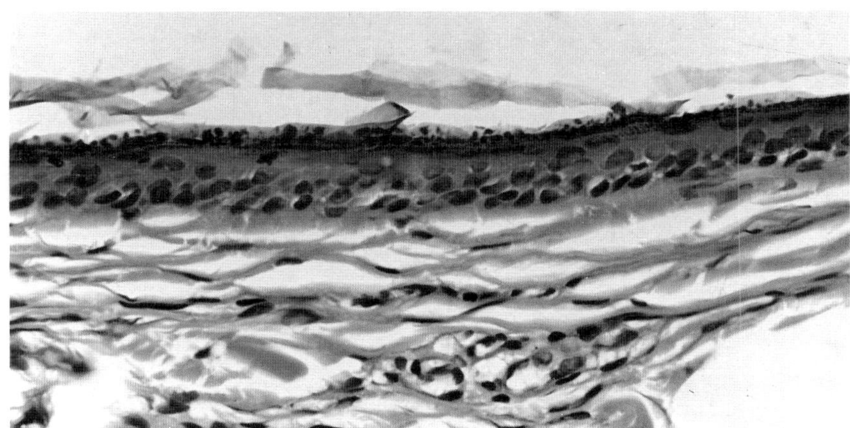

Fig. 6.11 Cysts. (b) Wall of epidermal cyst. Note granular layer and flakes of keratin.

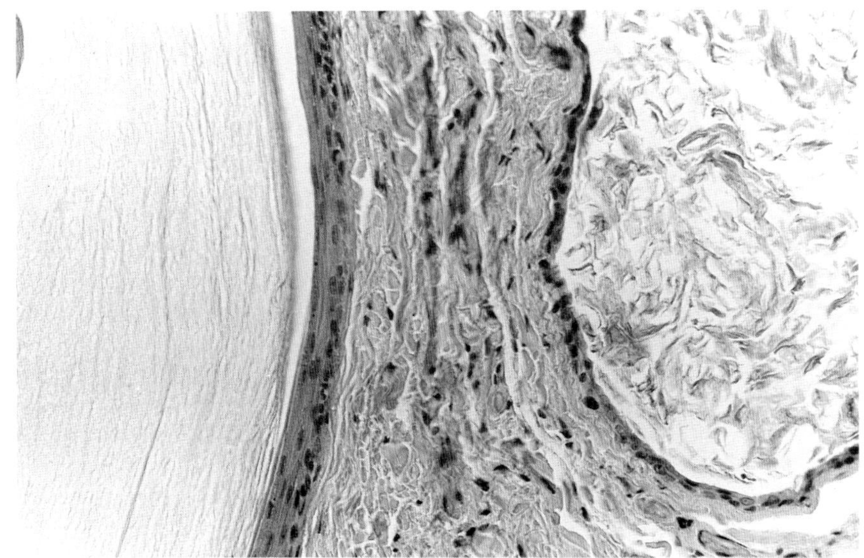

Fig. 6.11 (c) Small adjacent keratinous cysts. The left hand cyst contains a mass of pilary keratin. The right hand cyst is a milium forming in the pilary antrum. In the part shown the wall is lined by two-tiered epithelium, but the cyst contains flaky keratin.

Rupture of the wall of any type of keratinous cyst results in a foreign body giant cell reaction to the cyst contents.

Dermoid cysts

Dermoid cysts are described in Chapter 14.

XANTHOMATA

Xanthelasmata

Xanthelasma is by far the commonest xanthoma to occur in the eyelids. Beginning as a soft flat yellowish plaque at the inner canthus of the upper lid, it tends to become bilaterally symmmetrical in all four lids. Most of the patients are females in middle age or older, often with elevated serum levels of cholesterol and lipid. Microscopically, the plaque consists of massed lipophages in the dermis and subcutaneous tissues (Fig. 6.12). The cells tend to form lobules around blood vessels and adnexal structures. There is no inflammatory reaction and fibrosis is minimal.

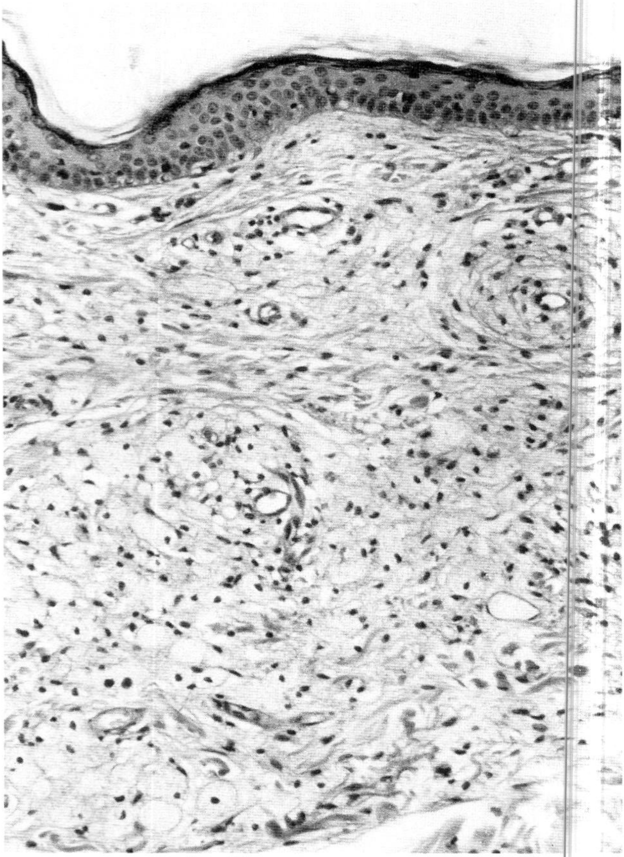

Fig. 6.12 Xanthelasma. Massive aggregation of foam cells in dermis. Most dense in lower part. PAS/tartrazine (×175).

Juvenile xanthogranulomata

Although the most frequent ocular expression of this uncommon disease of infants and children is histiocytic infiltration of the anterior uvea which may present clinically as hyphaema (see Chapter 8), it is occasionally manifest by lesions in the lids or beneath the bulbar conjunctiva or in the orbit. Juvenile xanthogranuloma in the eyelid may be a solitary lesion or part of a more extensive skin eruption over the head and neck. Blood lipids are normal and spontaneous regression is the rule.

The microscopic appearance of juvenile xanthogranuloma varies with the age of the lesion. In the early stages, it consists mainly of histiocytes with a minimum of giant cells and no demonstrable lipid. In the second and characteristic phase, abundant lipid is present in lipophages and giant cells, many of which are of the Touton type, and fibroblasts and eosinophils appear. Finally the lesion becomes progressively more fibrotic and loses its characteristic cytology.

Fibrous histiocytomata

These uncommon benign growths form small unencapsulated fibrous nodules composed of histiocytes and fibroblasts with a variable, but usually small number of lipophages and giant cells.

Dermatofibroma is a somewhat similar benign growth composed of histiocytes and fibroblasts among which numerous small blood vessels are often present. Frequently, lipophages and siderophages form a prominent component and impart a yellowish-brown or bluish-black colour to the lesion.

VASCULAR TUMOURS

Haemangiomata are described in detail in Chapter 14, but the following observations are relevant to haemangiomata occurring in the eyelids.

Telangiectatic haemangiomata

Telangiectatic haemangiomata are not true haemangiomata. They consist of dilated, thin-walled vessels of varying size and endothelial proliferation is not seen. In the eyelids, they are usually part of a more extensive lesion following the approximate facial distribution of the trigeminal nerve. Such lesions may be part of the Sturge–Weber syndrome (see Chapter 15).

Infantile haemangiomata

The great majority of infantile haemangiomata are either present at birth or appear in the first month of life. They start to regress by the time the patient is a year old, but the process may take several years to complete. The tumour consists of solid masses of primitive endothelial cells in which, however, evidence of differentiation into capillary channels is usually seen in some areas. Such differentiation can be accentuated by silver staining for reticulin.

Cavernous haemangiomata

In the eyelids, cavernous haemangiomata form soft subcutaneous tumours composed of large, thin-walled vessels and a variable complement of capillaries. Like other vascular tumours, they are prone to undergo involution by sclerosis.

Cirsoid aneurysms

Cirsoid aneurysms predominantly affect the elderly. They consist of a convoluted knot of vessels of medium size which is, in fact, an arteriovenous shunt. In section, the convolutions are seen as a series of profiles of thick-walled vessels. Haemorrhage and thrombosis not uncommonly occur in these lesions.

Granuloma pyogenicum

Macroscopically, granuloma pyogenicum forms a rounded sessile or pedunculated growth varying in colour from red to dark brown which bleeds easily when injured. The precise nature of the lesion is controversial, but it is probably neither a true tumour nor a granuloma. It consists essentially of inflammatory granulation tissue. Thus sections show a mass of capillaries of quite variable character in an oedematous collagenous stroma. There is often an epidermal collarette at the base of the growth which causes the pedunculation. Feeder vessels may be seen entering the base. In older lesions, ulceration of the surface leads to infiltration by inflammatory cells of all types.

NEURAL TUMOURS

Neurofibromata and neurilemmomata may occur in the eyelids. Their microscopic appearances are described in Chapter 14.

BIBLIOGRAPHY

Ahluwalia, B. K., Khurana, A. K., Chugh, A. D. & Mehtani, V. G. (1986) Eccrine spiradenoma of the eyelid. *British Journal of Ophthalmology* **70**, 580–583.

Beard, C. (1981) Management of malignancy of the eyelids. *American Journal of Ophthalmology* **92**, 1–6.

Bek, K. & Jensen, O. A. (1978) *External Ocular Tumours, A Clinicopathologic Study of 300 Cases.* W. B. Saunders & Co., Philadelphia & George Thieme Publishers, Stuttgart.

Boniuk, M. & Zimmerman, L. E. (1968) Sebaceous carcinoma of the eyelid, eyebrow, caruncle and orbit. *Transactions of the American Academy of Ophthalmology and Otolaryngology* **72**, 619–642.

Callahan, M. A. & Callahan, A. C. (1978) Sebaceous carcinoma of the eyelids. In *Ocular and Adnexal Tumours*, ed. F. A. Jakobiec, pp 477–483. Aesculapius Publishing Co., Birmingham, Ala.

Chalfin, J. & Putterman, A. M. (1979) Frozen section control in surgery of basal cell carcinoma of the eyelid. *American Journal of Ophthalmology* **87**, 802–809.

Collin, J. R. O. (1976) Basal cell carcinoma in the eyelid region. *British Journal of Ophthalmology* **60**, 806–809.

Coston, T. O. (1967) *Demodex folliculorum* blepharitis. *Transactions of the American Ophthalmological Society* **65**, 361–392.

Doxanas, M. T. & Green, W. R. (1984) Sebaceous gland carcinoma: review of 40 cases. *Archives of Ophthalmology* **102**, 245–249.

Doxanas, M. T., Green, W. R. & Iliff, C. E. (1981) Factors in the successful management of basal cell carcinoma of the eyelids. *American Journal of Ophthalmology* **91**, 726–736.

English, F. P. & Cohn, D. (1983) *Demodex* infestation of the sebaceous gland. *American Journal of Ophthalmology* **95**, 843–844.

English, P. & Nutting, W. B. (1981) Demodicosis of ophthalmic concern. *American Journal of Ophthalmology* **91**, 362–372.

Farmer, E. R. & Helwig, E. B. (1980) Metastatic basal cell carcinoma: a clinicopathologic study of seventeen cases. *Cancer* **46**, 748–757.

Jacobs, G. H., Rippey, J. J., Altini, M. & Dent, M. (1982) Prediction of the aggressive behaviour in basal cell carcinoma. *Cancer* **49**, 533–537.

Lahav, M., Albert, D. M., Bahr, R. & Craft, J. (1981) Eyelid tumours of sweat gland origin. *Graefes Archiv für Klinische und Experimentelle Ophthalmologie* **216**, 301–311.

Lever, W. F. & Schaumburg-Lever, G. (1983) *Histopathology of the Skin*, 6th Edn. J. B. Lippincot & Co., Philadelphia.

MacKie, R. M. (1984) *Milne's Dermatopathology*. Edward Arnold, London.

Morgan, L. W., Linberg, J. V. & Anderson, R. L. (1987) Metastatic disease first presenting as eyelid tumours: a report of two cases and review of the literature. *Annals of Ophthalmology* **19**, 13–18.

Ni, C., Dryja, T. P. & Albert, D. M. (1981) Sweat gland tumours in the eyelids: a clinicopathological analysis of 55 cases. *International Ophthalmology Clinics* **22**, 1–22.

Ni, C., Kimball, G. P., Craft, J. L., Wang, W. J., Chong, C. S. & Albert, D. M. (1982) Calcifying epithelioma: a clinicopathological analysis of 67 cases with ultrastructural study of 2 cases. *International Ophthalmology Clinics* **22**, 62–86.

Ni, C., Searl, S. S., Kuo, P. K., Chu, F. R., Chomg, C. S. & Albert, D. M. (1982) Sebaceous cell carcinomas of the ocular adnexa. *International Ophthalmology Clinics* **22**, 23–61.

Ni, C., Wagoner, M., Kieval, S. & Albert, D. M. (1984) Tumours of Moll's glands. *British Journal of Ophthalmology* **68**, 502–506.

Pinkus, H. & Mehregan, A. M. (1981) *A Guide to Dermatohistopathology*, 3rd Edn. Appleton Century Crofts, New York.

Rao, N. A., Hidayat, A. A. & McLean, I. W. (1982) Sebaceous carcinoma of the ocular adnexa: a clinicopathologic study of 104 cases, with five-year follow-up data. *Human Pathology* **13**, 113–122.

Rao, N. A., McLean, I. W. & Zimmerman, L. E. (1978) Sebaceous carcinoma of eyelids and caruncle: correlation of clinicopathologic features with prognosis. In *Ocular and Adnexal Tumours*, ed. F. A. Jakobiec, pp 461–476. Aesculapius Publishing Co., Birmingham, Ala.

Reifler, D. M., Ballitch II, H. A., Kessler, D. L., Stawiski, M. A. & O'Gawa, G. M. (1987) Tricholemmoma of the eyelid. *Ophthalmology* **94**, 1272–1275.

Sassani, J. W. & Yanoff, M. (1979) Inverted follicular keratosis. *American Journal of Ophthalmology* **87**, 810–813.

Straatsma, B. R. (1956) Meibomian gland tumours. *Archives of Ophthalmology* **56**, 71–93.

Ten Seldam, R. E. J., Helwig, E. B., Sobin, L. H. & Torloni, H. (1974) *Histological Typing of Skin Tumours*. World Health Organisation, Geneva.

Wesley, R. E. & Collins, J. W. (1982) Basal cell carcinoma of the eyelid an indicator of multifocal malignancy. *American Journal of Ophthalmology* **94**, 591–593.

Chapter 7 Pigmented lesions of the eyelids and conjunctiva

INTRODUCTION

Melanin

Melanin is the pigment responsible for most of the physiological and pathological colour variations in the skin and ocular tissue. It comprises a variety of related pigments varying in hue from tan to black. Melanin can be bleached by hydrogen peroxide, potassium permanganate and ferric chloride. Ammoniacal silver nitrate turns melanin black and, therefore, makes fine granules more conspicuous, especially if they are scanty. Haemosiderin, with which melanin may be confused, cannot be bleached or blackened by the above reagents, but is stained blue by Perls' method (see Appendix IV).

Melanocytes

Melanocytes are mature melanin-forming cells. The term melanoblast implies an immature cell and should be used only in this sense. Macrophages which have ingested melanin are known as melanophages, or sometimes as chromatophores. The term melanophore has become almost valueless through misuse. It means melanin-carrier and refers either to melanophages or to contractile cells found in lower animals.

The DOPA (3,4-dihydroxyphenylalanine) reaction is used to identify melanocytes by demonstrating the presence of tyrosinase (DOPA-oxidase) in their cytoplasm. This enzyme converts the DOPA-'reagent' to black DOPA-melanin. Only cells actively forming melanin give this reaction.

Melanocytes, being derived from neural crest, contain neuron-specific enolase and S100 protein which can be identified by the use of specific anti-sera. This may be of value in confirming the diagnosis of derivative amelanotic tumours. However, it must be said, that the more anaplastic a tumour is, the less likely it is to betray its origin by expressing such markers.

In the human body melanocytes are normally found in the following locations:

1 Epidermis.
2 Juxtacutaneous epithelia, e.g. conjunctiva, nose, mouth, rectum and vagina.
3 Within the globe — uveal melanocytes, the retinal pigmented epithelium and the pigmented epithelium of the ciliary body and iris.
4 Pia mater. These melanocytes are the source of the rare primary malignant melanomata of the meninges and brain which are notable for the fact that they rarely, if ever, metastasise outside the brain.

Melanocytes may be found in abnormal situations, e.g. the dermis and episclera as a developmental abnormality. With the exception of the retinal pigmented epithelium and the pigmented epithelium of the iris and ciliary body, which are derived fromn the optic cup, all melanocytes are thought to originate in the neural crest.

CLASSIFICATION OF PIGMENTED LESIONS

To try to circumvent the confusion sometimes experienced in trying to relate melanotic lesions of the eyelids and conjunctiva to one another and to those which occur elsewhere in the body, they have been classified according to the type of melanocyte from which they are derived:

Epidermal melanocytes

1 Cutaneous pigmented naevi.
2 Ephelis (freckle).
3 Lentigo.
4 Primary acquired melanosis (including Hutchinson's melanotic freckle).
5 Malignant melanoma.

Dermal melanocytes

1 Oculodermal melanocytosis.
2 Blue naevus.

Epithelial melanocytes of the conjunctiva

1 Pigmented naevi.
2 Ephelis (congenital pigmented spot).
3 Primary acquired epithelial melanosis.
4 Malignant melanoma.

Subconjunctival melanocytes

1 Episcleral melanosis.
2 Blue naevus.

LESIONS DERIVED FROM EPIDERMAL MELANOCYTES

Epidermal melanocytes are found insinuated between the basal cells of the epidermis where they maintain their position by numerous dendritic processes extending between neighbouring cells and into the dermis. These processes, which either join those from other melanocytes or end in blunt expansions on the surfaces of neighbouring epidermal cells, are the channels through which melanin is transferred from the melanocytes to the epidermal cells.

In routine preparations of formalin-fixed tissue the cytoplasm of epidermal melanocytes often shrinks away from the surrounding cells and collapses around the nucleus leaving an empty unstained space. Such cells are known as 'clear cells' (Fig. 7.1). For a proper appreciation of the number of melanocytes in the epidermis and the complexity of their ramifying processes, special preparations are necessary.

Pigmented naevi

Cutaneous pigmented naevi are malformations composed mainly of naevus cells. The majority of pigmented naevi are either present at birth or become apparent during early life. The constituent naevus cells are derived by proliferation from epidermal dendritic melanocytes which, as previously noted, are interposed at intervals between the cells of the basal layer. Since this layer is at the interface between the epidermis and the dermis it is referred to as the junctional zone and proliferation of melanocytes in this plane is called junctional proliferation.

Evolution

Naevi originating by junctional proliferation develop in three stages:

1 *Junctional naevi:* the proliferating melanocytes at first produce nests or theques of multiplying cells within the junctional zone (Fig. 7.2a). These nests tend to be discrete and separated by small or large tracts of normal epidermis. As the nests enlarge they are extruded from the epidermis into the dermis. This is a normal process in the evolution of naevi and does not signify malignant invasion. Naevi in which the proliferating cells are either in the epidermis or closely adjacent to its deep surface are termed junctional naevi. The constituent naevus cells are either large with pale cytoplasm which may be clear or stippled with finely granular melanin or are small, compact and angular in outline with opaque cytoplasm and hyperchromatic oval nuclei. Mitotic figures are never numerous, but may occasionally be seen especially in naevi in children. Junctional activity tends to be more active in children and the newly formed intra-epidermal nests give an impression of anaplasia. Allowance must be made for this since malignant melanomata are very rare before puberty.

2 *Compound naevi:* continuing junctional proliferation may be observed (Fig. 7.2b) with substantial accumulation of naevus cells in the dermis, often extending to a considerable depth. As the naevus cells move away from the epidermis, they lose their melanin and the ability to form it.

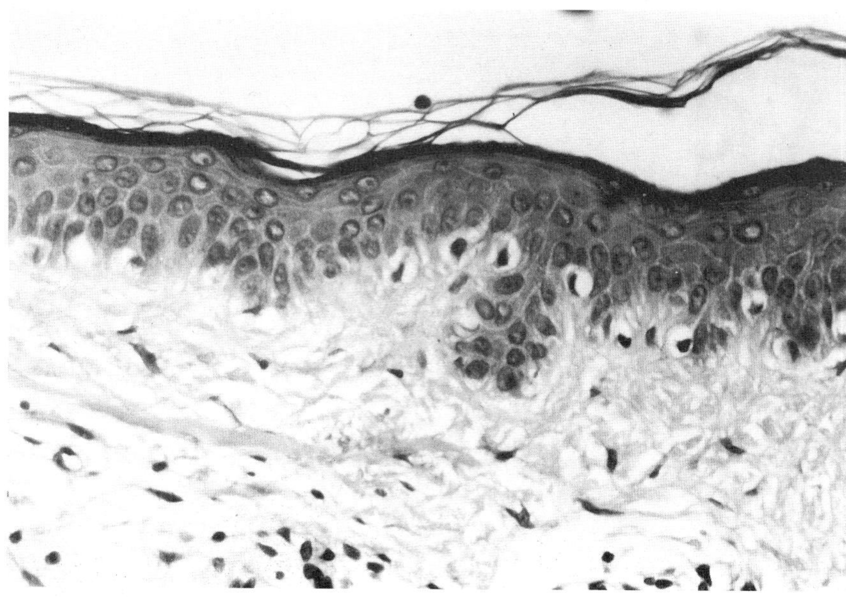

Fig. 7.1 Epidermal melanocytes as usually seen in routine preparations.

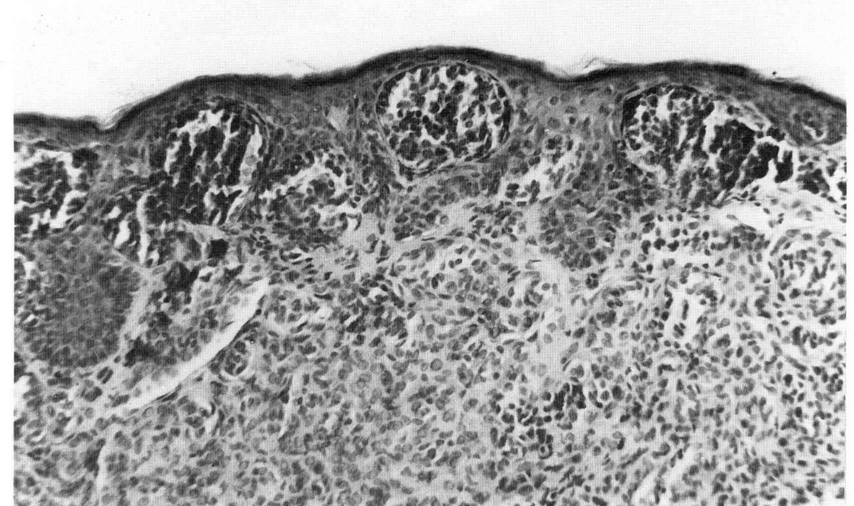

Fig. 7.2 Evolution of naevi. (a) Nests of naevus cells are seen in nests in the dermo-epidermal junctional region.

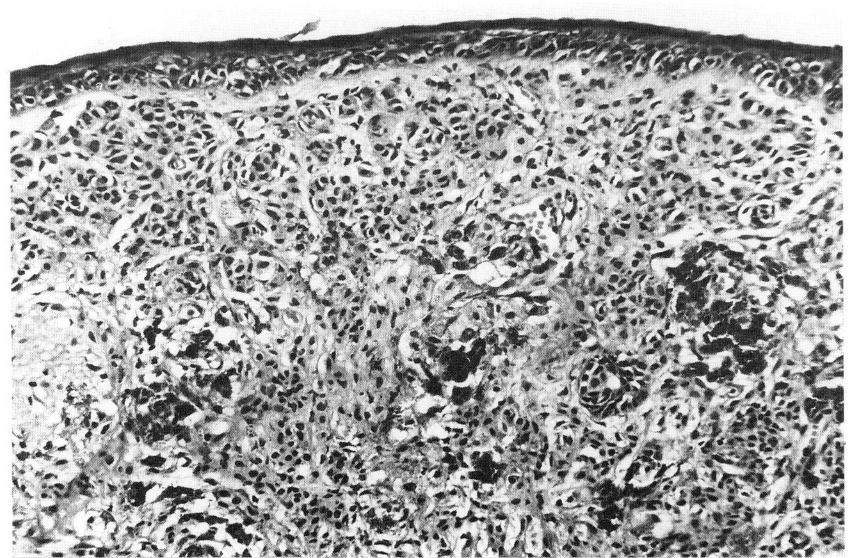

Fig. 7.2 (b) Intradermal naevus with increased number of melanocytes in overlying epidermis indicative of persistent junctional activity.

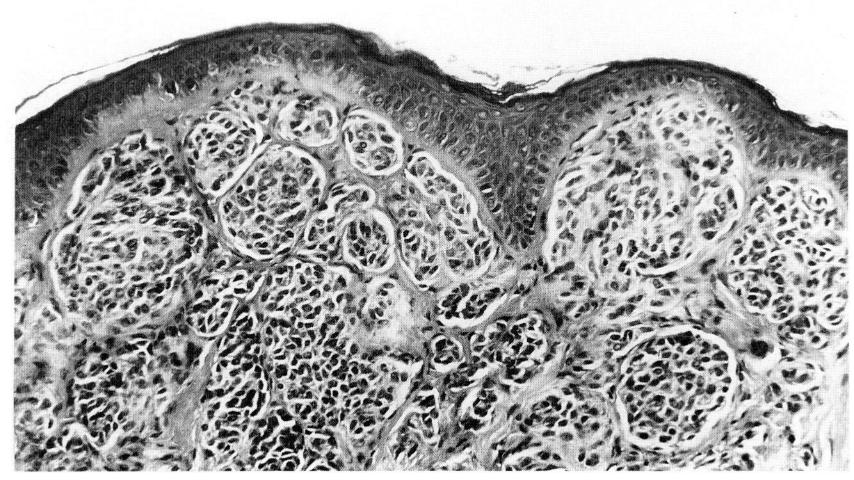

Fig. 7.2 (c) Deep intradermal naevus with no junctional proliferation evident in the overlying epidermis. The naevus cells in the dermis are arranged in more clearly defined theques than in (b) or (c). H & E (×160).

Naevi in which both junctional proliferation and dermal accumulations of naevus cells are present are known as compound naevi. In the eyelid extensive infiltrations of naevus cells around adnexal structures are not infrequent and may be mistaken for malignant infiltration. Junctional activity may persist in the Meibomian ducts after it is no longer seen in surface epidermis.

3 *Deep (intradermal) naevi:* these are mature naevi which have completed their growth (Fig. 7.2c). The epidermis no longer exhibits junctional proliferation and is often separated from the naevus cells in the dermis by a layer of collagen. The naevus cells often appear cuboidal or angulated and multinucleated cells are sometimes seen. Progressive fibrosis occurs starting in the deeper part of the naevus and the arrangement of the cells into nests and theques is gradually lost, though it usually persists superficially. Often only these superfical cells retain pigment.

Although the evolution of naevi through three stages is widely accepted, Masson (1951) proposed the important alternative concept that deep naevus cells are derived from the Schwann cells of cutaneous nerves and migrate upwards to mingle with naevus cells from the epidermis.

Juvenile melanoma (Spitz naevus)

Children and young adults are subject to a peculiar rare melanotic tumour of the skin sometimes called a spindle-cell and epithelioid naevus, which may mimic a malignant melanoma, but does not metastasise and is curable by local excision. The lesion is commonly dome-shaped, and may grow rapidly. It consists of large compact spindle cells arranged in interlacing bundles which appear to 'rain down' from the epidermis. These cells are intermingled with a variable proportion of large epithelioid cells with clearly defined opaque cytoplasm (Fig. 7.3). Bizarre cell forms also occur and giant cells with 10–20 nuclei grouped in a peripheral ring may be present. Pigment is usually scanty. The overlying epidermis may show pseudoepitheliomatous hyperplasia.

Ephelis (freckle)

Genetic factors, certain hormonal stimuli and exposure to ultraviolet light and ionising radiations induce hyperactivity of the epidermal melanocytes which distribute their excess melanin to surrounding epidermal cells. This process of melanin transfer accounts for freckles, *café au lait* spots, racial differences in skin colour and sun tan. In all these conditions, the epidermal cells, especially those of the basal layer, contain abundant melanin granules. The number of melanocytes is not increased and may, indeed, be decreased.

Lentigo

1 *Senile lentigo:* in older people, multiple macules of irregular size and shape appear in areas exposed to the sun. The rete ridges are elongated and expanded and exhibit basal cell hypermelanosis. The number of melanocytes is increased, but nests of naevus cells are not formed. In time, flattening of the rete ridges may occur and differentiation from primary acquired melanosis then becomes difficult. The dermal collagen is replaced by short, wavy basophilic fibres which accept elastic tissue stains (actinic elastosis).

2 *Lentigo simplex:* this form of lentigo shows only slight

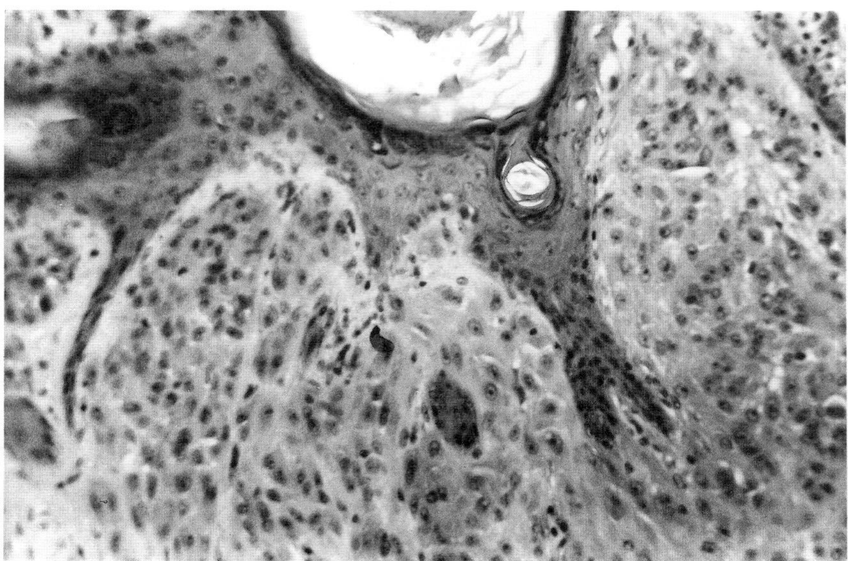

Fig. 7.3 Spitz-type naevus. Large epithelioid cells with conspicuous nucleoli are present in the dermis and there is some pseudoepitheliomatous hyperplasia of the epidermis. H & E (×160).

elongation of the rete ridges, but a marked increase in the number of melanocytes in the basal layer of the epidermis and even an occasional nest of naevus cells in the junctional zone. The ocular interest of this lesion is that it may present as dark brown macules in the periorbital and peri-oral regions, on the palms and soles, the lips and oral mucosa and occasionally on the conjunctivae.

Primary acquired melanosis

There has been much confusion over the nomenclature and prognosis of this lesion and two distinct types have been recognised:

1 A lesion which typically occurs on the face of older people as a slowly spreading brown, flat area with an irregular border. After many years it may develop into invasive melanoma which experience has shown to have a better survival rate than other cutaneous melanomata.

Microscopically there is extensive junctional proliferation of pleomorphic abnormal melanocytes which infiltrate into the overlying layer of prickle cells. The dermal collagen characteristically shows marked elastotic degeneration (synonyms include Hutchinson's melanotic freckle, lentigo maligna and precancerous melanosis).

2 In other cases, which are usually more rapidly progressive, the melanocytes have a balloon-like or 'pagetoid' aspect with eosinophilic or vacuolated cytoplasm. In the basal layer of the epidermis the melanocytes sometimes assume a spindle form and tend to obscure the dermo-epidermal junction so that it may be difficult to decide if early invasion of the dermis has occurred. Mitotic figures may be seen, but are not numerous. The subjacent dermis is infiltrated by lymphocytes and melanophages, but elastotic degeneration of the collagen is not a prominent feature.

The stage of intra-epithelial spread is termed the 'radial growth phase'. Invasion of the dermis by tumour melanocytes signals the onset of invasive malignant melanoma and is termed the 'vertical growth phase'.

Malignant melanomata

Malignant melanomata in the eyelids may arise in areas of primary acquired melanosis or *de novo* in the absence of any antecedent spreading pigmentation. The former are referred to as lentigo maligna melanomata or superficial spreading melanomata according to the category of acquired melanosis from which they are derived, and the latter as nodular melanomata. Nodular melanomata may also occasionally arise in association with a pre-existing junctional naevus. Superficial spreading melanomata differ from lentigo maligna melanomata in that they arise at an earlier age, run a shorter time course and have a less favourable prognosis. The 5 year survival rate for the lentigo maligna melanomata may be as high as 90%.

Nodular melanomata occur at all ages, but are rare before puberty. They invade the dermis at an early stage, but do not spread widely in the adjacent epidermis (Fig. 7.4). Lymphatic drainage channels may also consequently be invaded early. These features presumably account for the poor prognosis, the 5 year survival rate being 40%.

Established melanomata are infiltrative destructive growths characterised by cellular pleomorphism and varied growth patterns. The constituent cells range from cuboidal or polygonal with abundant rose-pink cytoplasm to spindly forms with scanty cytoplasm. Bizarre giant forms and abnormal mitoses may occur. Pigment formation is variable and some melanomata are amelanotic. Fontana staining (Appendix IV) is necessary to expose very fine melanin granules which may be extremely inconspicuous in H & E sections. In anaplastic tumours the cells grow in solid masses which appear as sheets in sections, while in more differentiated tumours the cells may be arranged in interlacing fascicles or an alveolar pattern may be simulated.

Prognosis: the occurrence of metastasis has been shown to be related to the interconnected factors of depth of dermal invasion and tumour thickness, blood-borne metastases being rare with tumours with a dermal component of less than 1.5 mm in thickness.

The manner in which any particular tumour metastasises is unpredictable. Some may spread by lymphatic channels to produce local satellite growths, while others show little local spread, but produce early metastases in the regional lymph nodes. Others may disseminate mainly by the bloodstream (cf. ocular melanomata Chapter 8).

By contrast with intraocular melanomata, the constituent cell type does not appear to be an important factor in determining prognosis.

MELANOTIC LESIONS DERIVED FROM DERMAL MELANOCYTES

Dermal melanocytes are elongated branching cells packed with melanin granules which, as their names implies, are confined to the dermis. They are seen in large numbers only in Mongolian spots, blue naevi and areas of aberrant dermal melanosis, of the kind which occasionally develop in the lids and adjacent areas of the face (oculodermal melanocytosis).

Oculodermal melanocytosis (naevus of Ota)

In this rare usually unilateral condition of hypermelanosis, ocular melanocytosis is accompanied by ipsilateral melanocytosis of the dermis of the periorbital skin and

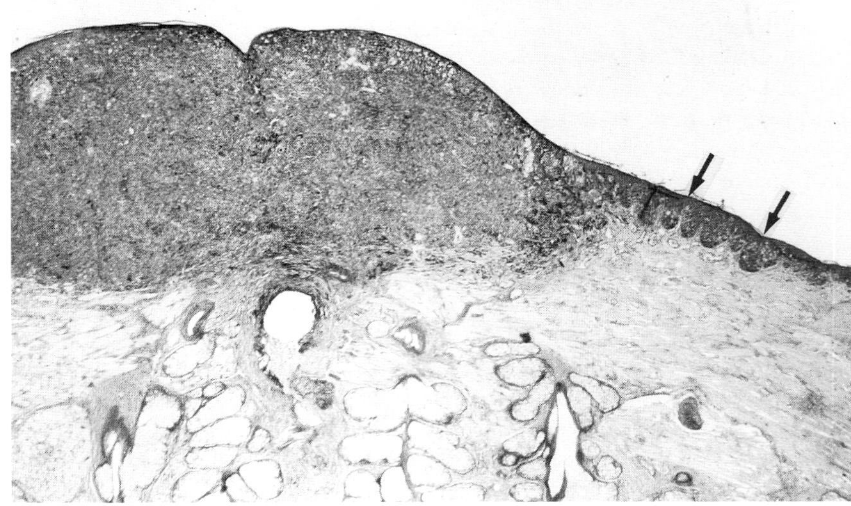

Fig. 7.4 Melanoma of lid margin. Section parallel to lashline to show lateral limits (arrows). (a) Low power includes one margin showing spread into the adjacent epidermis. PAS/tartrazine.

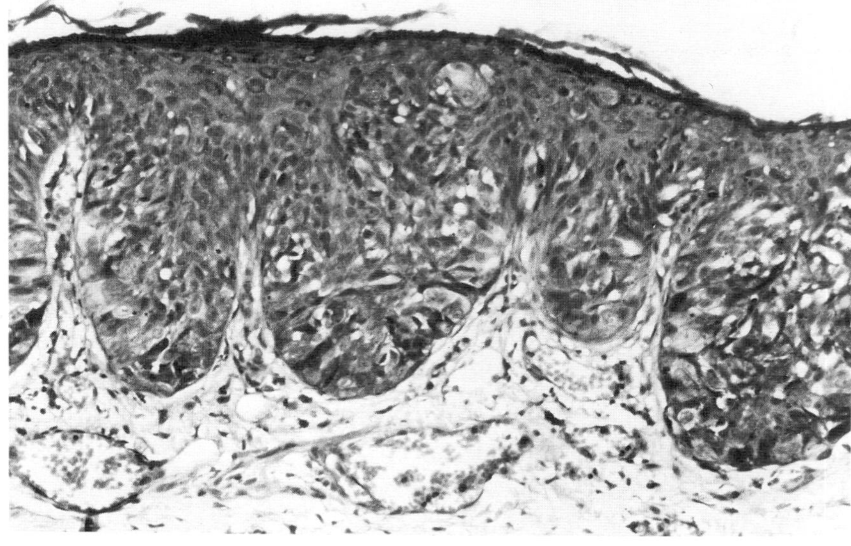

Fig. 7.4 (b) Higher power of area between arrows. (×160).

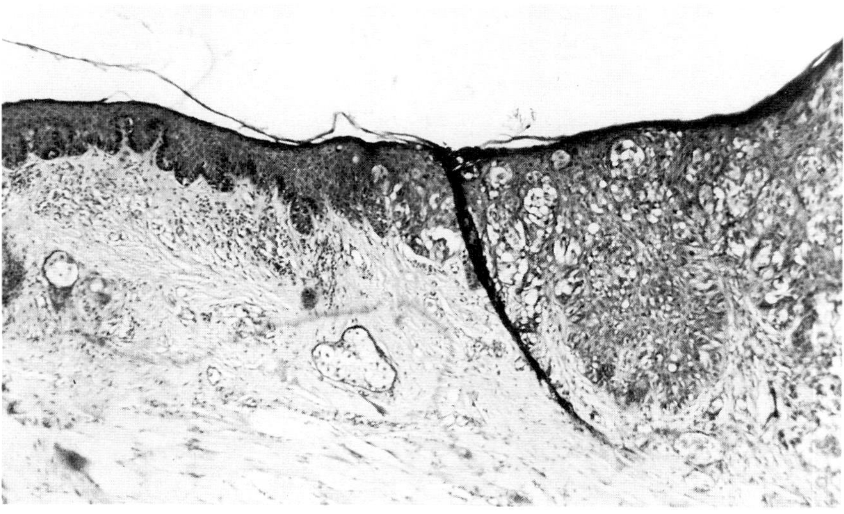

Fig. 7.4 (c) Other margin showing rather less extensive spread. Though nodular in appearance, the amount of spread just qualifies for classification as a superficial spreading melanoma. (×160).

eyelids and frequently of the substantia propria of the nasal and oral mucosa as well. In addition, the orbital tissues and leptomeninges of the frontal lobe are occasionally involved. The condition, which is much commoner in dark-skinned races, especially Asiatics, is usually present at birth, but may not develop until puberty or early adult life. Once established it persists unchanged or slowly progresses. Skin colour varies from dark brown to slate-grey. Malignant change is very rare, but malignant melanomata in the choroid, iris or orbit have occasionally been reported in association with this naevus.

Elongated branching and strap-like melanocytes are scattered through the dermis where they often gather round blood vessels, sweat ducts and hair follicles. The structure of the dermis is not disturbed and the epidermis is not involved. The DOPA reaction is mostly negative or only weakly positive.

An excess of similar branching melanocytes accounts for the hyperpigmentation of the episclera, sclera and uvea.

Blue naevus

Blue naevi are uncommon, benign melanocytic tumours in the deep or superficial dermis which appear blue because of the filtering effect of the tissues overlying them. Although usually congenital, they may not appear until adult life. Once established, they normally remain unchanged for life, although sometimes more cellular variants may continue to enlarge slowly and very occasionally undergo malignant change.

Microscopically, the interstices of the dermal connective tissue are packed with heavily pigmented elongated branching and strap-like melanocytes forming a tumour with ill-defined margins (Fig. 7.5). This distinctive microstructure is thus quite different from that of the deep or intradermal naevi of epidermal origin with which they may, however, sometimes be associated.

CONJUNCTIVAL LESIONS DERIVED FROM EPITHELIAL MELANOCYTES

Interspersed between the basal cells of the conjunctival epithelium there are dendritic melanocytes comparable in every way to those in the epidermis. Except in dark-skinned races, they are inconspicuous and require special preparations to render them clearly visible (DOPA or Fontana's silver).

Pigmented naevi

The evolution of pigmented naevi of the conjunctiva is the same as that described for cutaneous naevi.

Pigmented naevi are the commonest conjunctival tumours and are usually visible from an early age. They occur most frequently at the limbus and inner canthus where junctional naevi appear as a circumscribed pigmented spot and compound or sub-epithelial naevi as a flat plaque varying in colour from fleshy or light tan to black. Flecks of pigment are frequently present in the surrounding conjunctiva when the naevus is heavily pigmented.

Microscopically the structure is similar to that already described for cutaneous naevi, but complicated by the fact that cryptic downgrowths of conjunctival epithelium are usually present in the naevus (Fig. 7.6). Junctional activity may be present in the epithelium of these down-

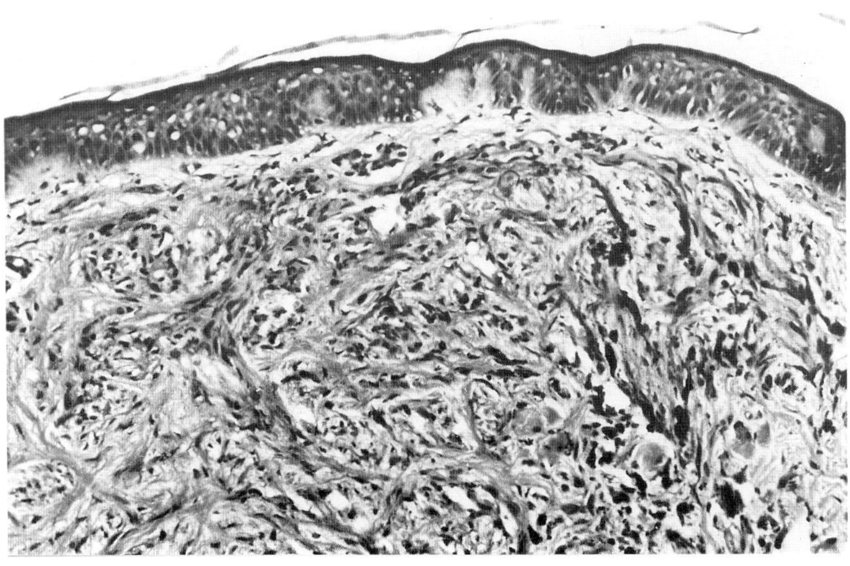

Fig. 7.5 Blue naevus. Note spindly appearance of cells, many of which are heavily pigmented. H & E (×160).

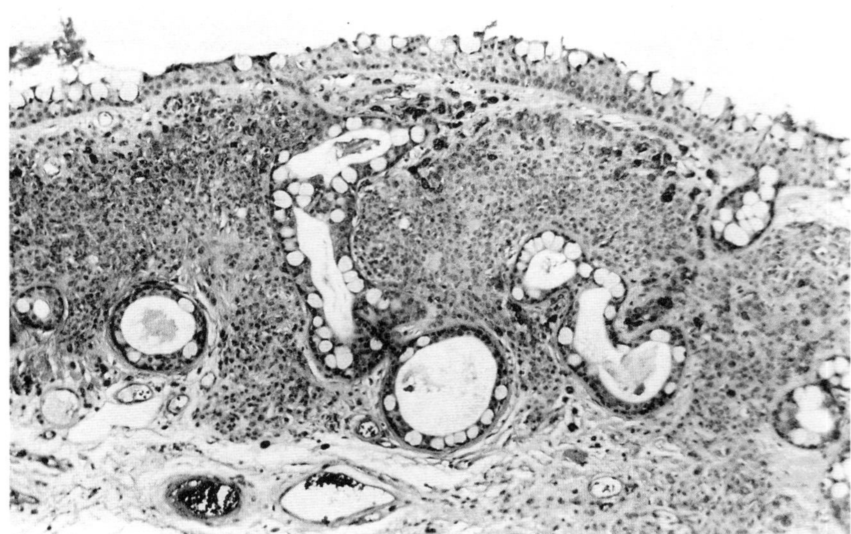

Fig. 7.6 Conjunctival naevus. Arrangement of the naevus cells into theques is not marked. There is superficial pigmentation, most of the pigment being in macrophages. Note the cryptic downgrowths of conjunctival epithelium which characterise these naevi. H & E (×94).

growths as well as in the surface epithelium. Blockage of the crypts may lead to the formation of cysts containing mucus and simulate growth. Focal accumulations of lymphocytes in the substantia propria around naevi are common.

Junctional and compound naevi of the conjunctiva have a limited capacity for malignant change which is indicated clinically by attacks of inflammation, enlargement and deepening pigmentation. However, these signs are more often due to other causes such as formation of epithelial cysts, puberty, pregnancy or infection.

In children, the presence of cells in mitosis in conjunction with widespread junctional activity may present a somewhat alarming appearance, but malignant melanomata are very rare before puberty.

Ephelis (congenital pigmented spot)

This pigmented lesion is comparable in appearance and histological structure to a skin freckle or *café au lait* spot. The pigmented area which is usually at or near the limbus, is flat and circumscribed and moves with the conjunctiva. It may show white striae due to the presence of pigment-free epithelial downgrowths. By contrast with acquired melanosis, the pigmented area is present from an early age and remains static. Racial pigmentation of the conjunctiva is similar in all respects, but more extensive.

Microscopically, the basal cells in the pigmented area are full of melanin granules acquired by transfer from the local epithelial melanocytes. There is no melanocytic proliferation and the conjunctiva is otherwise normal.

Congenital epithelial melanosis does not predispose to melanoma formation, presumably because of the absence of junctional proliferation.

Primary acquired epithelial melanosis

Primary acquired melanosis usually develops insidiously in middle age or later life. It is typically unilateral and may appear anywhere in the conjunctiva and be associated with a similar melanosis of adjacent parts of the lids. Progress is variable. Some cases remain almost static; some progress slowly over the years and may wax and wane while others progress rapidly to involve the whole conjunctiva.

At least three histological stages of increasing atypia can be recognised:

1 *Simple epithelial melanosis*

There is an excess of melanin in the conjunctival epithelium which is often not confined to the basal cells, but also affects the overlying prickle cells (Fig. 7.7a). Sometimes there is a minor degree of junctional proliferation, but no atypia.

2 *Epithelial melanosis with moderate atypia (precancerous melanosis)*

Clinically this commences as a flat pigmented macule which gradually spreads until eventually the whole of the bulbar and palpebral conjunctiva, caruncle and adjacent skin of the lids may be involved in a flat, finely granular pigmentation. Occasionally, the melanosis develops simultaneously over a large area of the conjunctiva.

Invasion of the substantia propria occurs in only a minority of cases (17% according to Reese) and often only after several years. In the remaining cases, the melanosis may fluctuate in size, become quiescent, or

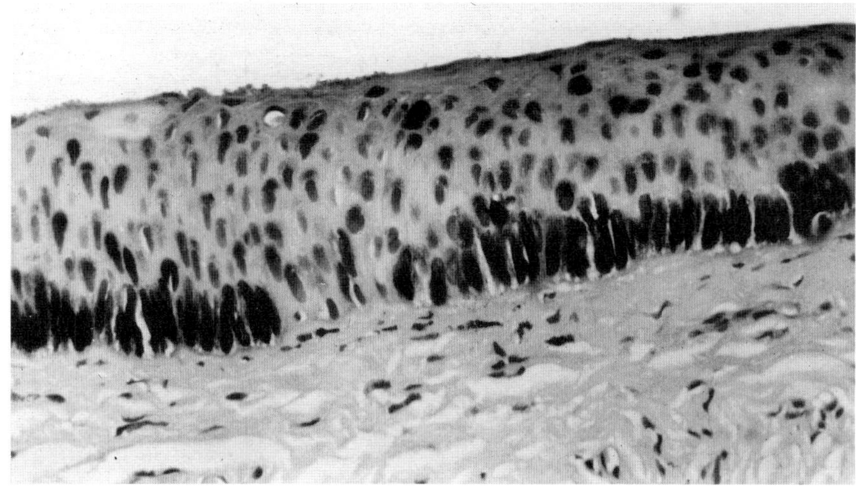

Fig. 7.7 Acquired melanosis of the conjunctiva. (a) Simple epithelial melanosis in an adult.

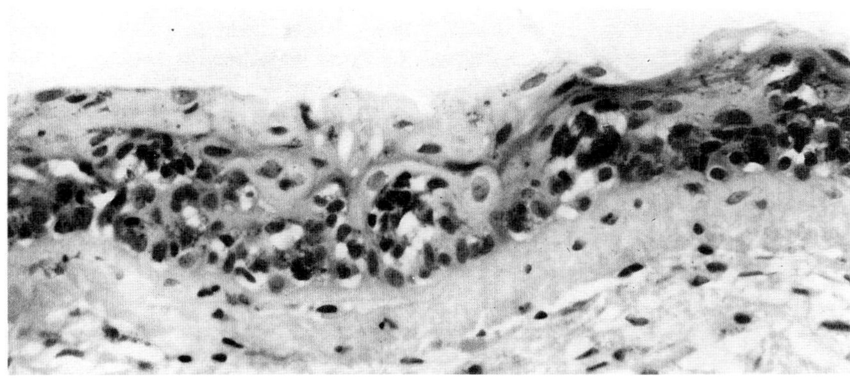

Fig. 7.7 (b) Area with atypia confined mainly to the deeper part of the epithelium. H & E (×320).

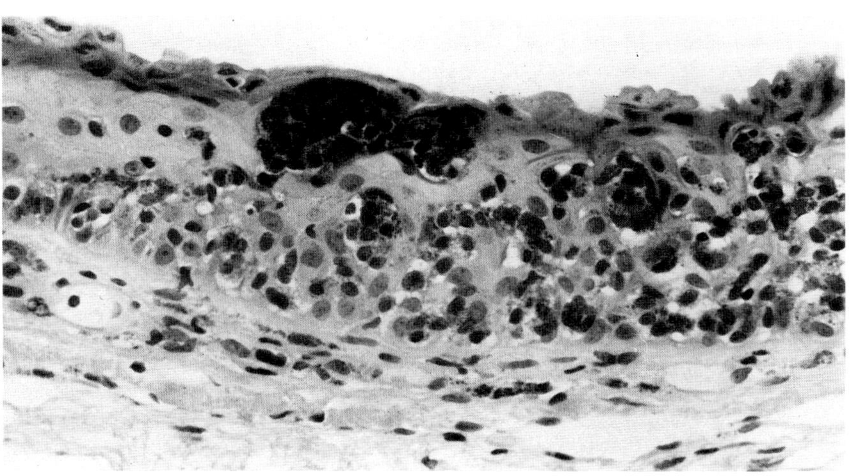

Fig. 7.7 (c) Area with atypia in which there is migration of cells towards the surface. H & E (×320).

even undergo spontaneous regression.

Microscopically, the intra-epithelial melanocytes multiply diffusely in the junctional zone (Fig. 7.7b) and segregate to form intra-epithelial nests which impart a characteristic pigmented granularity to the surface of the lesion. Neoplastic melanocytes also migrate upwards towards the surface of the epithelium either singly or in clumps (Fig. 7.7c). This is the exact opposite of what happens in naevi.

Because the proliferation is intra-epithelial and extends in continuity in a centrifugal manner, the area of melanosis resembles a slowly spreading stain.

3 *Epithelial melanosis with marked atypia*

The normal epithelial cells are extensively replaced by pleomorphic melanocytes and the lesion assumes a 'pagetoid' appearance and is, in effect, a superficial spreading melanoma in 'radial growth phase'. Thereafter, malignant infiltration of the substantia propria may occur and the lesion has become an invasive melanoma.

Malignant melanomata

Malignant melanomata of the conjuctiva are rare, about twenty times less common than malignant melanomata of the choroid. They may arise *de novo*, in a pre-existing naevus or, as already described, in an area of acquired melanosis.

As in the case of cutaneous melanomata, melanomata arising in areas of acquired melanosis have been differentiated into lentigo maligna melanomata, which have a prolonged intra-epithelial phase and metastasise late, and superficial spreading melanomata in which the intra-epithelial phase is short and metastasis occurs early. In practice, however, the distinction may not always be easy to make. In about 50% of melanomata it is impossible on histological grounds to establish any pre-existing lesion.

The common sub-sites are the bulbar conjunctiva, the fornices and the caruncle. On the bulbar conjunctiva, the tumour may appear as a small well-defined pigmented nodule at the limbus. Sometimes the growth is more diffuse and may involve more than 25% of the bulbar conjunctiva. Because of anatomical constraints, those that arise in the fornices or on the caruncle, tend to be polypoid. Local spread is to the pre-auricular lymph nodes.

As with cutaneous melanomata, prognosis appears to

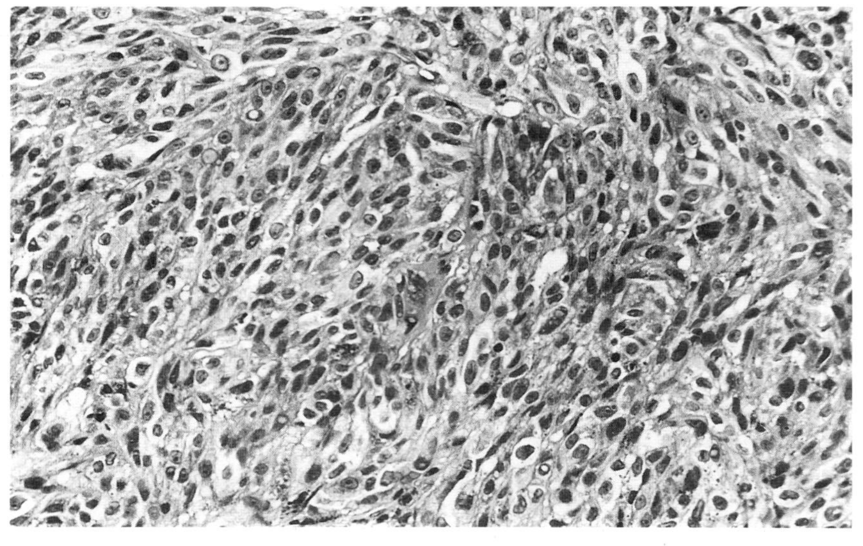

Fig. 7.8 Malignant melanoma of the conjunctiva. (a) Spindle cell type. H & E (×260).

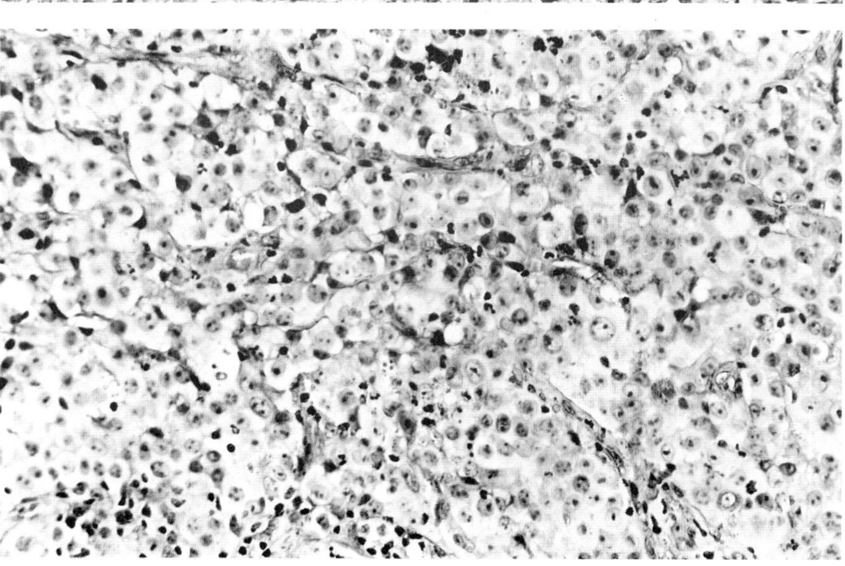

Fig. 7.8 (b) Small epithelioid type. H & E (×260). (Reproduced with permission from Jeffrey *et al.*, 1986.)

be related to tumour thickness. In some cases of localised limbal melanomata repeated excisions of local recurrences have been made over a period of years without blood-borne metastases appearing. With more diffuse growths and those arising on the caruncle or in the fornix, prognosis is poor. Exenteration is usually effective in controlling local recurrence, but, because of deaths from blood-borne metastases the 5 year survival rate is less than 50%.

The constituent cells are similar in types (Fig. 7.8) to those already described for cutaneous melanomata and the predominant type also appears unimportant prognostically.

MELANOTIC LESIONS DERIVED FROM SUBCONJUNCTIVAL MELANOCYTES

Elongated branching melanocytes packed with melanin granules are found in large numbers beneath the conjunctiva in episcleral melanosis, ocular melanocytosis, oculodermal melanocytosis and very occasionally in the conjunctival membrane itself where it constitutes a blue naevus which is sometimes associated with a junctional naevus in the overlying conjunctival epithelium. Multiple blue naevi in the bulbar and tarsal conjunctiva have been reported.

Episcleral melanosis is nearly always congenital and unilateral and often associated with ocular melanocytosis. Viewed through the bulbar conjunctiva the colour varies from pinkish-grey to slate-blue. Characteristically, the pigmentation is flat, lies beneath the insertions of the recti muscles and stops short of the limbus leaving a pigment-free circumcorneal band. Cuffs of melanocytes round the anterior perforating vessels may be seen in darker spots. The conjunctival epithelium moves over the pigmented area. Microscopically, the episcleral tissues contain abundant branching and spindle-shaped melanocytes resembling those of the uvea. Malignant change rarely, if ever, occurs.

Pigmented spots 3–4 mm from the limbus sometimes occur in the absence of widespread episcleral melanosis. These spots, which may not appear until adult life, are composed of uveal melanocytes clustered in the perforating channels of the anterior ciliary vessels or around an intrascleral nerve loop.

BIBLIOGRAPHY

Bernadino Jr., V. B., Naidoff, M. A. & Clark Jr., W. H. (1976) Malignant melanomas of the conjunctiva. *American Journal of Ophthalmology* **82**, 383–394.

Breslow, A. (1970) Cross-sectional area and depth of invasion in the prognosis of cutaneous melanoma. *Annals of Surgery* **172**, 902–908.

Brownstein, S., Henry, M. & Bernardo, A. I. (1979) Malignant melanoma of the conjunctiva after 11 years. *Canadian Journal of Ophthalmology* **14**, 142–146.

Clark Jr., W. H., From, L., Bernadino, E. A. & Mihm M. C. (1969) The histogenesis and biologic behaviour of primary malignant melanoma of the skin. *Cancer Research* **29**, 705–727.

Clark, W. H. & Mihm, M. C. (1969) Lentigo maligna and lentigo maligna melanoma. *American Journal of Pathology* **55**, 39–67.

Folberg, R., McLean, I. W. & Zimmerman, L. E. (1984) Conjunctival melanosis and melanoma. *Ophthalmology* **91**, 673–678.

Gonder, J. R., Wagoner, M. D. & Albert, D. M. (1980) Ocular pathology for clinicians. 4. Idiopathic acquired melanosis. *Ophthalmology* **87**, 835–840.

Greer, C. H. (1954) Precancerous melanosis. *Proceedings of the Royal Society of Medicine* **47**, 26–29.

Heakind, P. (1978) Conjunctival melanocytic lesions: natural history. In *Ocular and Adnexal Tumours*, ed. F. A. Jakobiec, pp 572–582. Aesculapius Publishing Co., Birmingham, Ala.

Jakobiec, F. A. (1984) The ultrastructure of conjunctival melanocytic tumours. *Transactions of the American Ophthalmological Society* **82**, 599–752.

Jay, B. (1965) Naevi and melanomata of the conjunctiva. *British Journal of Ophthalmology* **49**, 169–204.

Jeffrey, I. J. M., Lucas, D. R., Lee, W. R. & McEwan, C. (1986) Malignant melanoma of the conjunctiva. *Histopathology* **10**, 363–378.

Jeffrey, I., Royston, P., Sowter, C., Slavin, G., Pomerance, A., Goolamali, S. & Pinto, D. (1983) Prognostic value of tumour thickness in cutaneous malignant melanoma. *Journal of Clinical Pathology* **36**, 51–56.

Liesegang, T. J. & Campbell, R. J. (1980) Mayo clinic experience with conjunctival melanomas. *Archives of Ophthalmology* **98**, 1385–1389.

McGhee, C. N., Ni, C., Albert, D. M. & Chu, F. R. (1982) Conjunctival melanoma. *International Ophthalmology Clinics* **22**, 35–56.

McGovern, V. J., Mihm, M. C., Bailey, C., Booth, J. C., Clark Jr., W. H., Cochran, A. J., Hardy, E. G., Hicks, J. D., Levene, A., Lewis, M. G., Little, J. H. & Milton, G. W. (1973) The classification of malignant melanoma and its histological reporting. *Cancer* **32**, 1442–1457.

McGovern, V. J. (1976) *Malignant Melanoma: Clinical and Histological Diagnosis*. John Wiley & Sons, New York.

McGovern, V. J. (1982) *Melanoma: Histological Diagnosis and Prognosis*. Raven Press, New York.

Masson, P. (1951) My conception of cellular naevi. *Cancer* **4**, 9–38.

Naidoff, M. A., Bernardino Jr., V. B. & Clark Jr., W. H. (1976) Melanocytic lesions of the eyelid skin. *American Journal of Ophthalmology* **82**, 371–382.

Rodriguez-Sains, R. S., Jakobiec, F. A. & Iwamoto, T. (1981) Lentigo maligna of the lateral canthal skin. *Ophthalmology* **88**, 1186–1192.

Silvers, D. N., Jakobiec, F. A., Freeman, T. R., Lefkowitch, J. H. & Klie, R. C. (1978) Melanoma of the conjunctiva: a clinicopathologic study. In *Ocular and Adnexal Tumours*, ed. F. A. Jakobiec, pp 583–599. Aesculapius Publishing Co., Birmingham, Ala.

Zimmerman, L. E. (1978) The histogenesis of conjunctival melanomas. The first Algernon Reese lecture. In *Ocular and Adnexal Tumours*, ed. F. A. Jakobiec, pp 600–631. Aesculapius Publishing Co., Birmingham, Ala.

Chapter 8 Pigmented and other tumours of the uveal tract

BENIGN MELANOCYTIC TUMOURS

Uveal melanocytes

Most melanocytes within the globe are located in the uveal tract where the majority of the tumours to which they give rise are also found. The uveal melanocyte is a comparatively large cell with branching processes which are packed to their tips with melanin granules. Like other melanocytes it is derived from the neural crest.

Naevi

The term naevus strictly means a birth-mark and is commonly applied to pigmented cutaneous 'moles'. The term is also widely, if inappropriately, applied to uveal lesions which are not normally present at birth, but commonly appear in adult life. Both cutaneous and uveal lesions are said to be composed of 'naevus cells', but notwithstanding their common origin, uveal naevus cells differ considerably both in appearance and properties from epidermal naevus cells. However, the term has been used so widely to describe certain uveal lesions, some of which infiltrate locally, but do not metastasise, that it has been retained here.

Though the predominant type and relative proportions vary considerably, the same types of cell occur in all intraocular naevi. The following basic types may be recognised:

1 Plump polyhedral or elongated cells with voluminous cytoplasm are so densely packed with melanin granules as to obscure the nucleus. Bleaching the melanin reveals cells, sometimes indistinctly outlined, with a small nucleus usually lacking a nucleolus though small peripherally located nucleoli may be present. Naevi in which such cells predominate are known as 'magnocellular naevi' (Fig. 8.1). Electron microscopic studies have shown that the cells contain giant melanomsomes, but few cytoplasmic organelles. An unpigmented 'epithelioid' variant of this type of cell also occurs.

2 Slender spindle cells with dense elongated nuclei and little or no pigment.

3 Fusiform or dendritic cells which are less heavily pigmented than the first type and contain relatively larger nuclei.

Iris naevi

Iris freckles may be regarded as small naevi. They consist of small aggregations of flattened cells deep to the an-

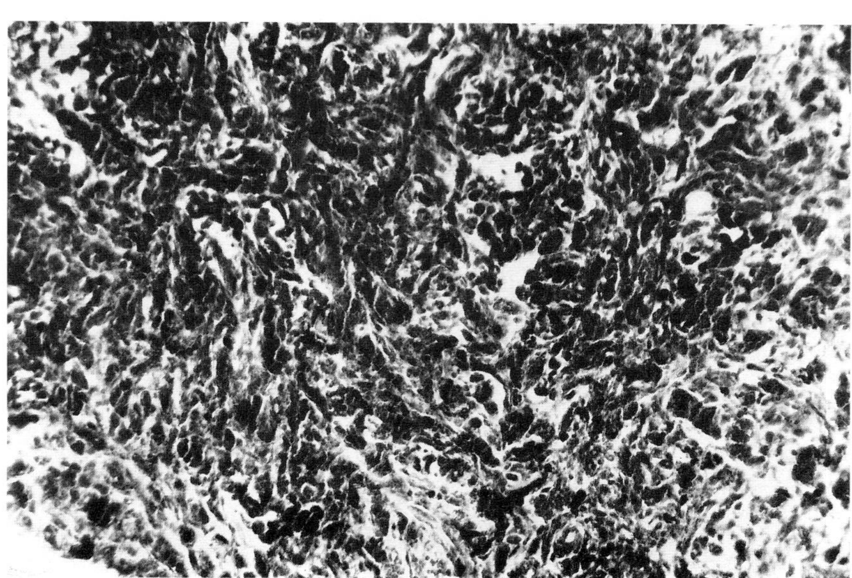

Fig. 8.1 Cells in a magnocellular naevus of ciliary body. (a) Before bleaching.

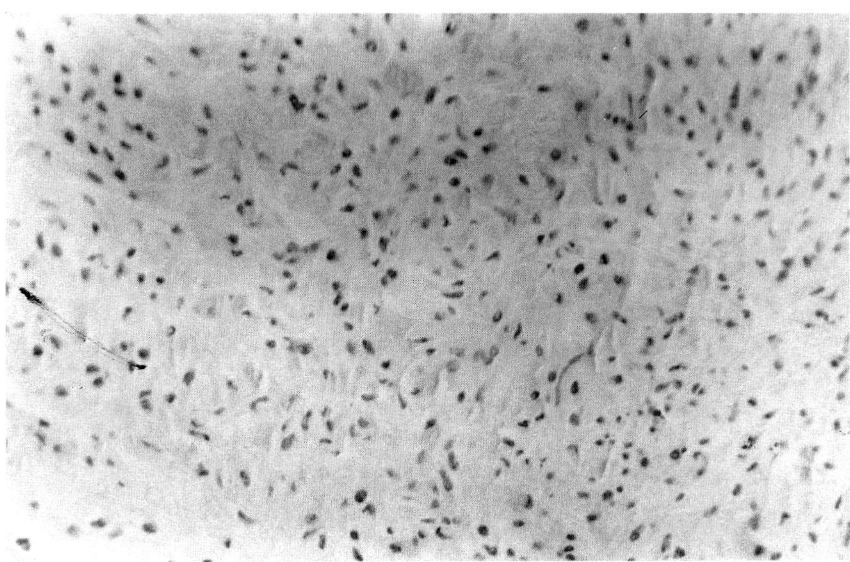

Fig. 8.1 (b) After bleaching. The cell outlines in the bleached preparation are indistinct, but the smallness of their nuclei can be appreciated. H & E (×260).

terior surface of the iris. More extensive naevi (Fig. 8.2a) usually appear in middle age, though they may occasionally be seen in childhood. About 40% arise in the inferotemporal quadrant and are often located peripherally. The commonest type is composed predominantly of small spindle and dendritic cells which proliferate in the anterior stroma. Plaques are formed on the anterior surface of the iris (Fig. 8.2b). Later extension occurs to the posterior surface (Fig. 8.2c & d) and through the root of the iris into the ciliary body which may make complete resection difficult. However, it is noteworthy that, even after apparently incomplete resection, recurrence does not necessarily occur. Such infiltrating growths have long been regarded as malignant melanomata, but, since they rarely if ever metastasise, this diagnosis cannot be accepted without reservation and the term 'progressive naevus' has been applied to them.

Obstruction of the outflow apparatus by pigment debris, cells or haemorrhage may cause secondary glaucoma. Some diffuse superficial naevi are associated with anterior synechiae and extension of Desçemet's membrane over the trabecular meshwork. These present clinically with heterochromia and unilateral glaucoma (Cogan–Reese syndrome, see Chapter 12).

Naevi composed predominantly of other types of cells are uncommon, but 'magnocellular' and 'epithelioid' naevi have been described. These are intrastromal and do not form surface plaques.

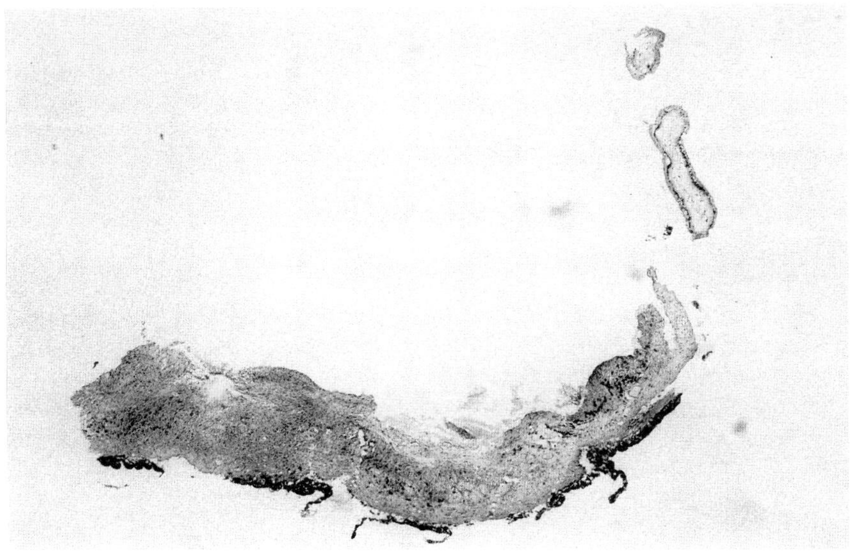

Fig. 8.2 Iris naevi. (a) Low power showing diffuse involvement of iris extending on the right hand side into ciliary processes.

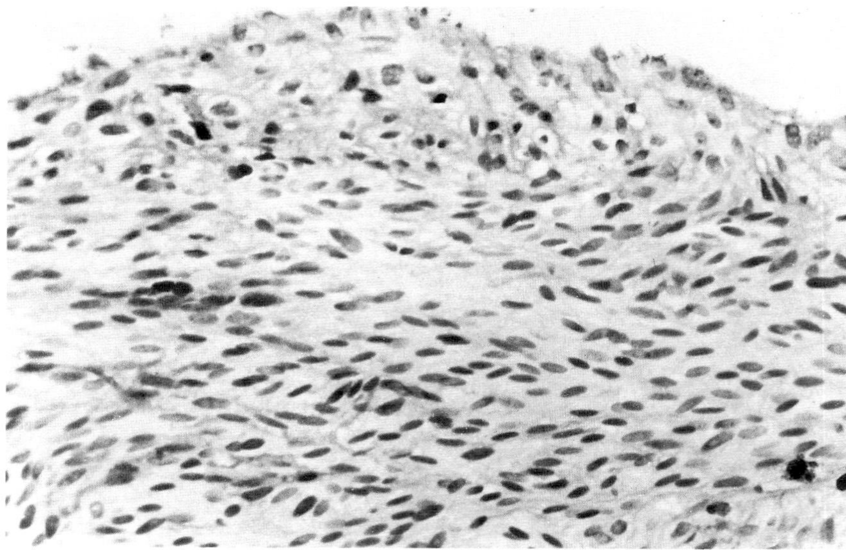

Fig. 8.2 (b) Spindle cells in plaque on surface. H & E (×320).

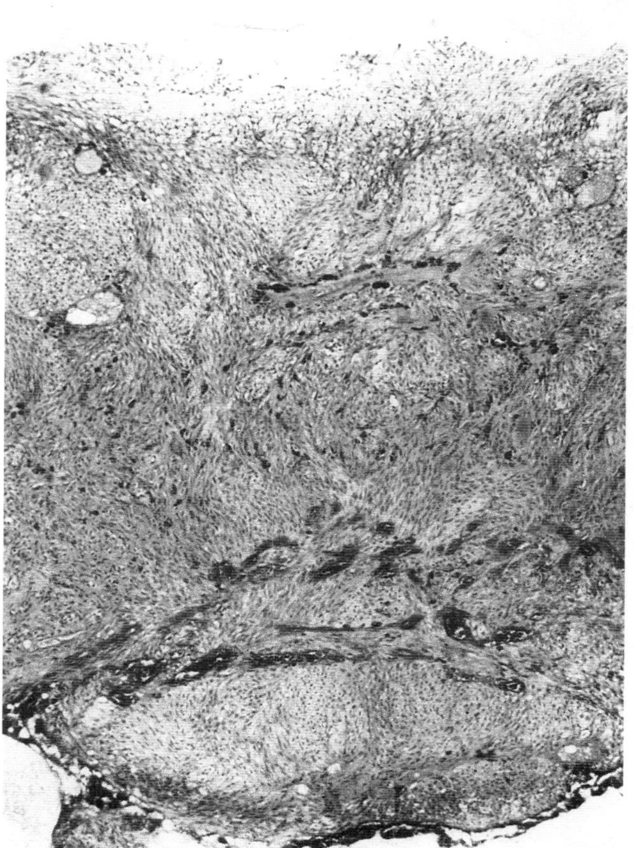

Fig. 8.2 (c) Naevus involving stroma diffusely and forming plaques on both anterior and posterior surfaces of iris. H & E (×70).

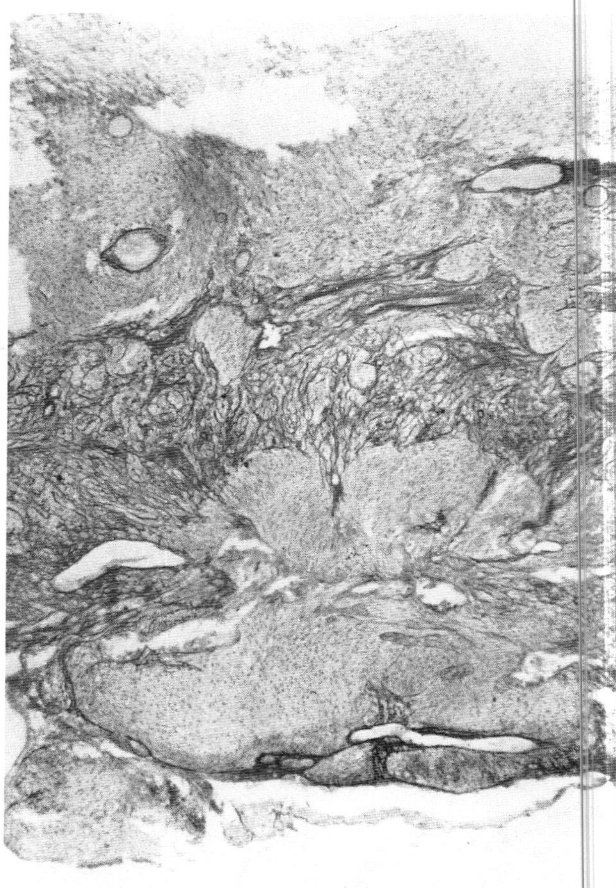

Fig. 8.2 (d) Similar area after staining by silver for reticulin fibres. Note dense reticulin stroma where the iris is infiltrated, but lack of argyrophilic fibres in surface plaque (×70).

Choroidal naevi

Choroidal naevi also appear in adult life. Ninety per cent are located posterior to the equator where half of all choroidal melanomata occur. They consist of flat, circumscribed aggregations of cells which are usually more variable in appearance than those in iris naevi.

Choroidal naevi lie in the outer choroidal layer and may extend along underlying neurovascular channels into the sclera. Most naevi cause some thickening of the choroid and larger naevi compress the choriocapillaris and sometimes obliterate it. Interference with the local microcirculation may be responsible for degeneration of the retinal pigmented epithelium and the drüsen formation often seen over the surface of naevi. In time this may lead to atrophy of the rods and cones (Fig. 8.3) and result in a limited scotoma. At its perimeter, a naevus blends imperceptibly into the choroidal stroma and, unlike a malignant melanoma, does not compress or displace the stroma.

Unless heavily pigmented, choroidal naevi are difficult to see and may be discovered only on macroscopic or microscopic examination of eyes enucleated for other reasons. Most choroidal naevi probably remain unchanged throughout life, but malignancy does sometimes supervene. Although increasing visual impairment and enlargement of a naevus will always excite suspicion of malignant change, they are not always entirely reliable signs. The frequency with which naevi undergo malignant change is unknown, but is a rare event.

Magnocellular naevi, which are always benign, sometimes enlarge, infiltrate locally and produce visual disturbance.

MALIGNANT MELANOMATA

Incidence

Although malignant melanoma is the commonest malignant primary intraocular tumour, it is rare. The incidence has been estimated as 2–6 cases per 10 000 eye patients. Males and females are about equally affected. Uveal melanomata are 15 times as common in Caucasians as in non-white races. The average age at presentation is approximately 50 years for cilio-choroidal and 40 years for those affecting the iris. Seventy per cent of all cases present between the ages of 40 and 70 and first presentation before the age of 25 and after the age of 80 years is uncommon. The neoplasm is nearly always single, primary and unilateral, but a melanoma may be accompanied by one or more naevi, usually in the iris. Approximately 85% of melanomata originate in the choroid, 10% in the ciliary body and 5% in the iris. There is little evidence of hereditary influence, although transmission through three generations has been recorded (Walker *et al.*, 1979).

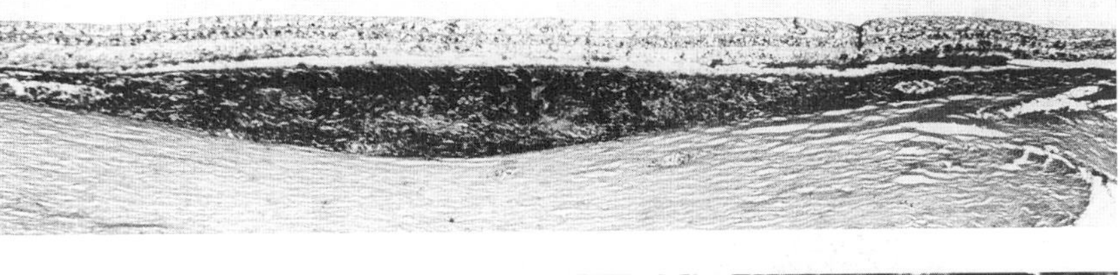

Fig. 8.3 Choroidal naevus. (a) Low power showing expansion of choroid and partial atrophy of overlying retina.

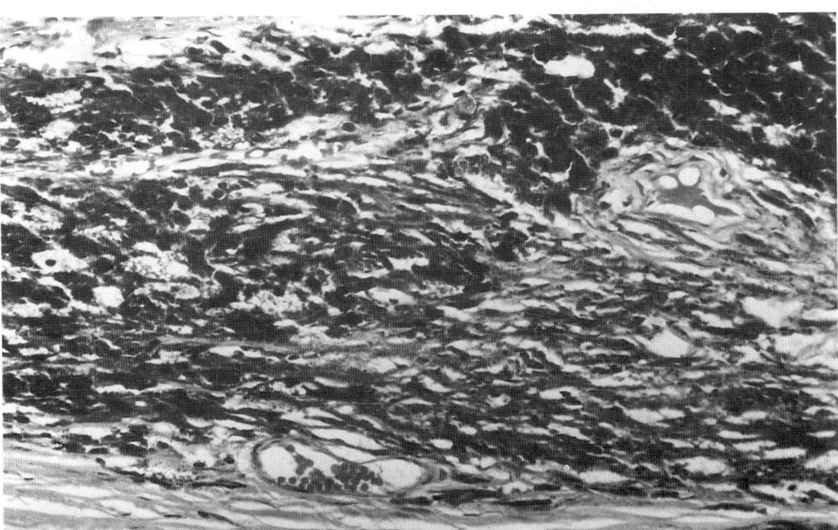

Fig. 8.3 (b) Higher power showing naevus is composed of large rounded heavily pigmented cells with an admixture of more spindly forms. H & E (×260).

Malignant uveal melanomata occasionally occur as a second primary malignancy and may also complicate rare congenital disorders such as oculodermal melanocytosis (Chapter 7) or the dysplastic naevus syndrome.

Origin from naevi

It has been suggested that many, perhaps the majority, of uveal melanomata are derived from pre-existing naevi and that careful examination will reveal 'naevoid' areas in many tumours. While it is clear that naevi may progress to malignancy, no firm estimate can at present be given of what proportion of malignant melanomata arise in this way.

Iris

The problem of differentiating 'naevi' from 'malignant melanomata', or, put another way, of saying whether a given tumour has metastatic potential, arises with small spindle cell tumours in both the iris and choroid, but more often with iris tumours because they are normally small when excised. In borderline cases, the need to ensure careful follow-up by labelling them 'melanomata' has to be weighed against the possibility of causing needless alarm.

Sub-site

The majority of iris melanomata arise in the same subsite as the naevi, that is peripherally in the lower half. They may be circumscribed or diffuse.

Microscopical features

Most are composed of spindle cells, a proportion of which will be plump and contain conspicuous nucleoli. Intranuclear pseudo-inclusions are common (Fig. 8.4). Epithelioid cells are rarely seen. In contradistinction to 'epithelioid' naevus cells, malignant epithelioid cells are not embedded in dense stroma. Pigmentation is variable and amelanotic lesions occur.

Reticulin is present in variable amounts in these tumours and may be useful in distinguishing progresssive naevi from melanomata in that the surface plaque of a naevus does not contain reticulin while a superficial melanoma invariably does.

Special types

The term 'tapioca melanoma' has been applied to tumours that present as multiple translucent nodules on the surface of the iris. Most are low-grade spindle cell tumours, but one malignant case which metastasised has been reported.

Complications

As with naevi, obstruction of the meshwork by pigment, cellular debris and haemorrhage may cause secondary glaucoma.

Spread and metastasis

Local spread occurs into the trabecular meshwork and ciliary body, sometimes circumferentially around the root of the iris and trabecular meshwork giving rise to secondary glaucoma. Such cases are called 'ring melanometa'. Metastasis to distant organs occurs in $<5\%$ of cases. It may be promoted by exceptional factors such as drainage surgery or trauma (Jakobiec & Silbert, 1981).

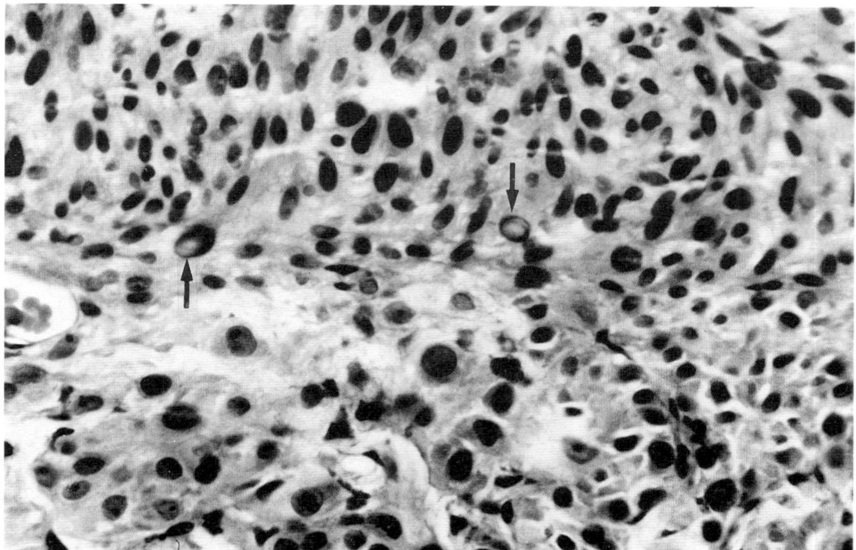

Fig. 8.4 Iris melanoma. (a) Cell detail showing several pseudonuclear inclusions (arrows). H & E (×410).

Fig. 8.4. (b) (*Opposite*) Electron micrograph showing cytoplasm apparently enclosed within a rim of nucleus (N) (×11 500).

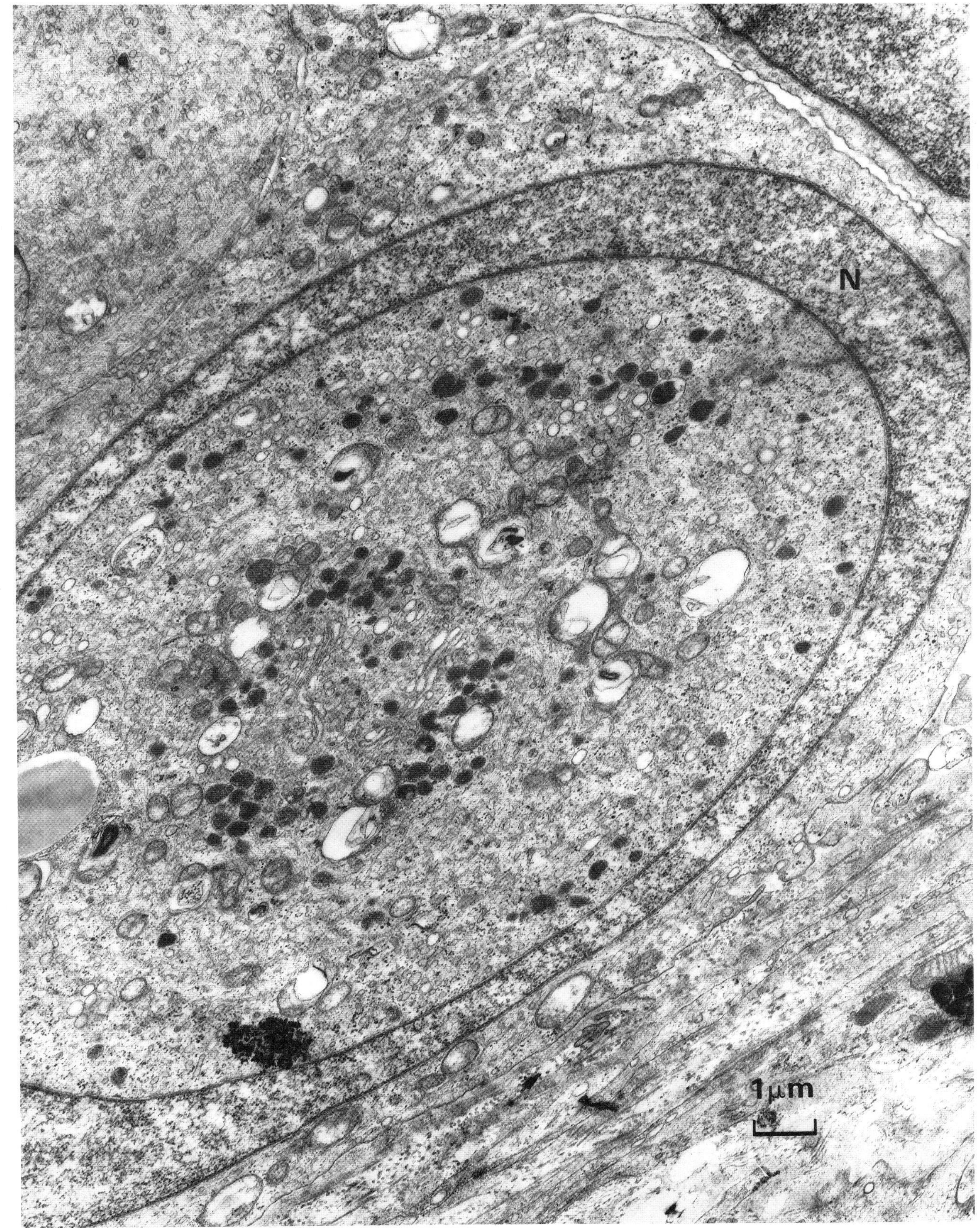
N
1 μm

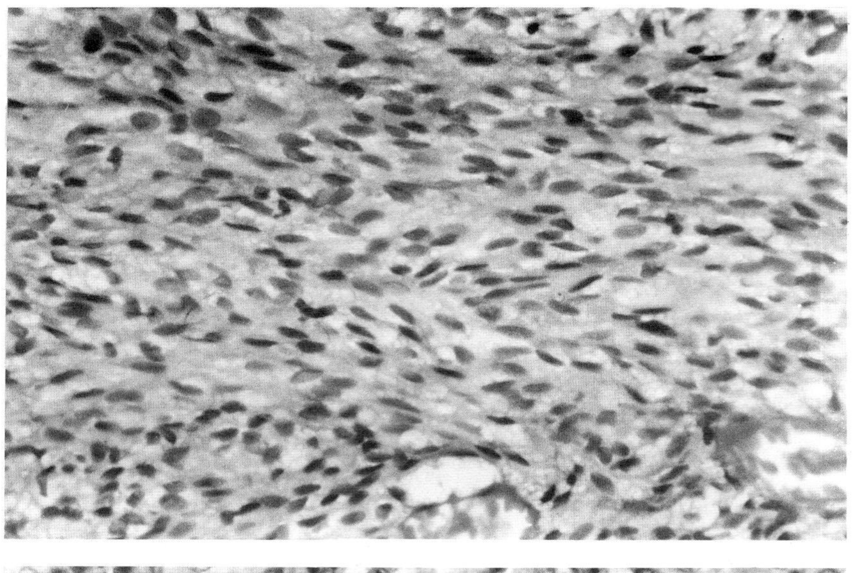

Fig. 8.5 Cell types in choroidal melanoma. (a) Spindle A. H & E (×410).

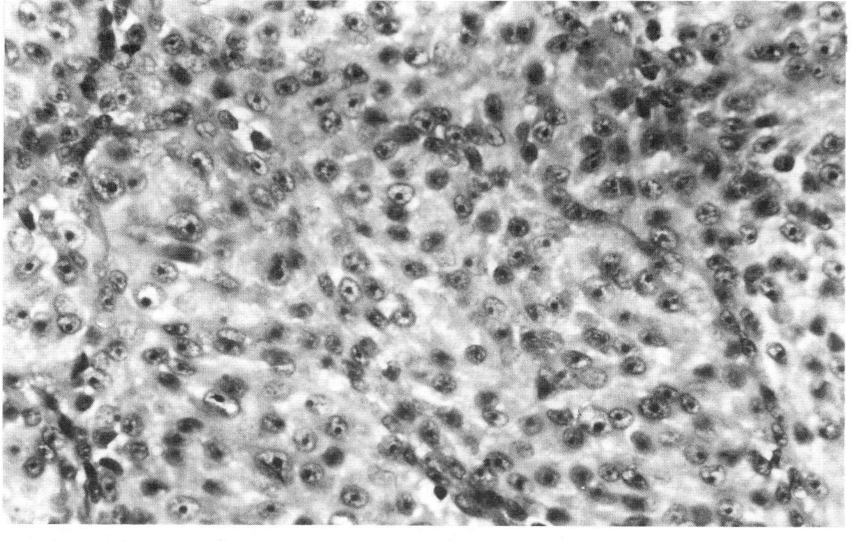

Fig. 8.5 (b) Spindle B. H & E (×410).

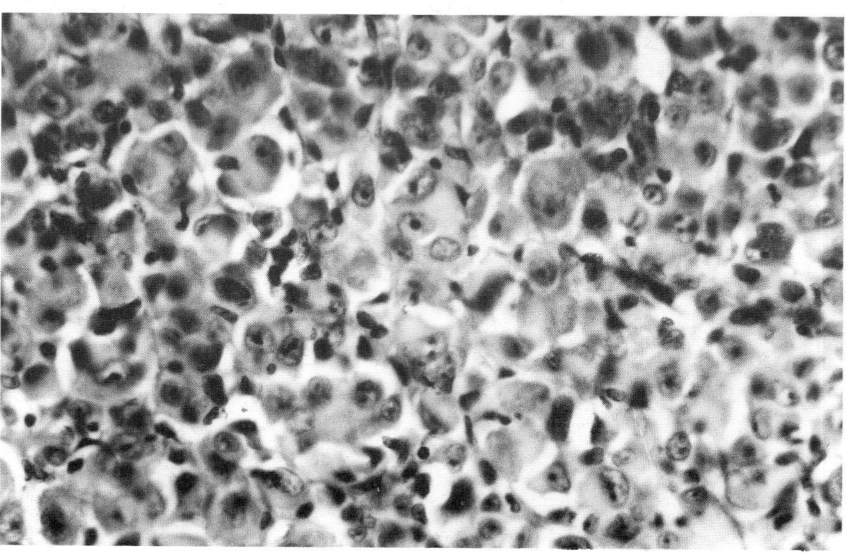

Fig. 8.5 (c) Epithelioid. Masson trichrome (×410).

Prognosis

The low rate of metastasis means that prognosis for life is excellent and vision can usually be preserved by local resection.

Choroid and ciliary body

Sub-site

Fifty per cent of ciliochoroidal melanomata are situated posteriorly, and the posterior superior temporal quadrant is the commonest sub-site.

Microscopical features

The prototypical cells of which melanomata are composed were first categorised in a now classical paper by Callender (1931). Classification by these cell types has stood the test of time as a simple, if subjective, method of grading.

Callender recognised two basic cell types:

1 *Spindle cells:* subtype A is slender and usually contains little pigment. The nucleus is elongated and has a delicate reticular structure. Nuclear material is not well defined and a longitudinal crease is present in the nuclear membrane. As already mentioned these cells are not clearly distinguishable from spindle-type naevus cells (Fig. 8.5a).

Subtype B spindle cells are plumper, their nuclei are ovoid and contain coarse chromatin and a conspicuous central nucleolus. Cytoplasmic pigment content is variable (Fig. 8.5b).

2 *Epithelioid cells:* these cells have large rounded eosino-

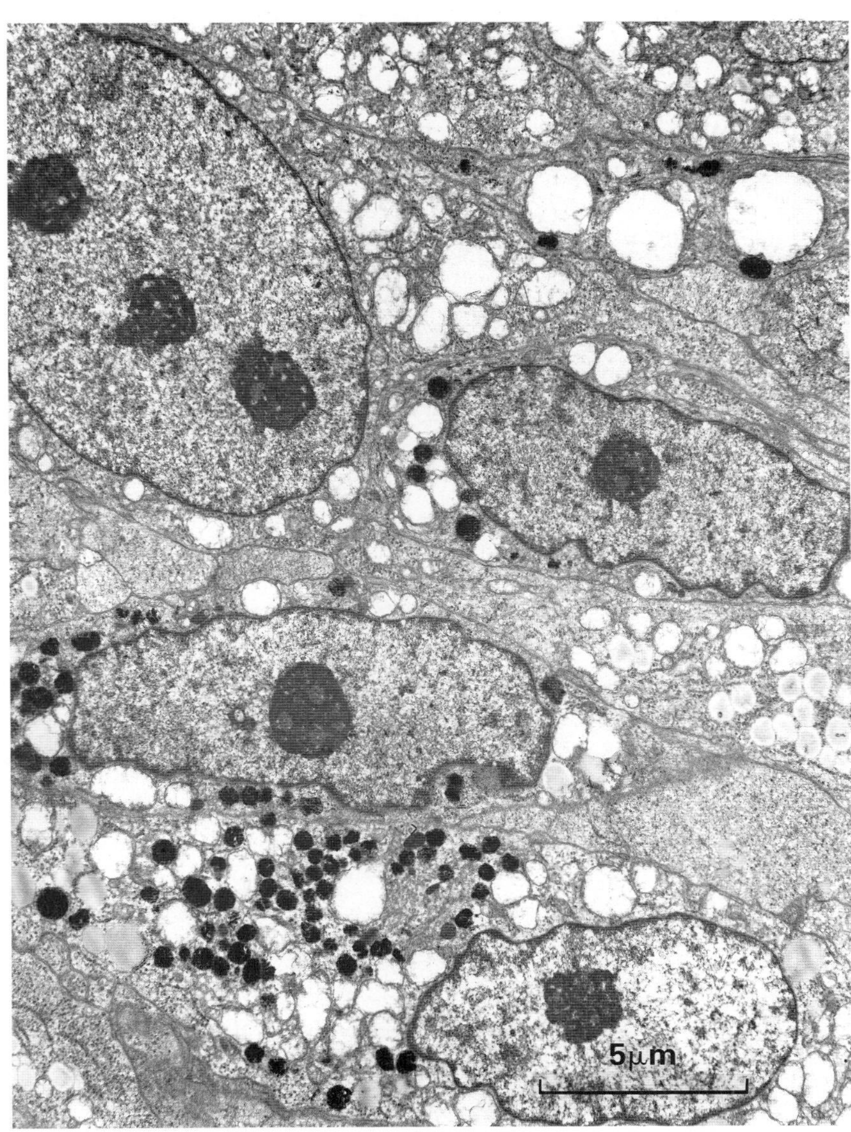

Fig. 8.6 EM spindle B. (a) Group of cells containing variable numbers of melanosomes. Note large nucleoli. The mitochondria are swollen. Other intracellular organelles are difficult to identify (×5610).

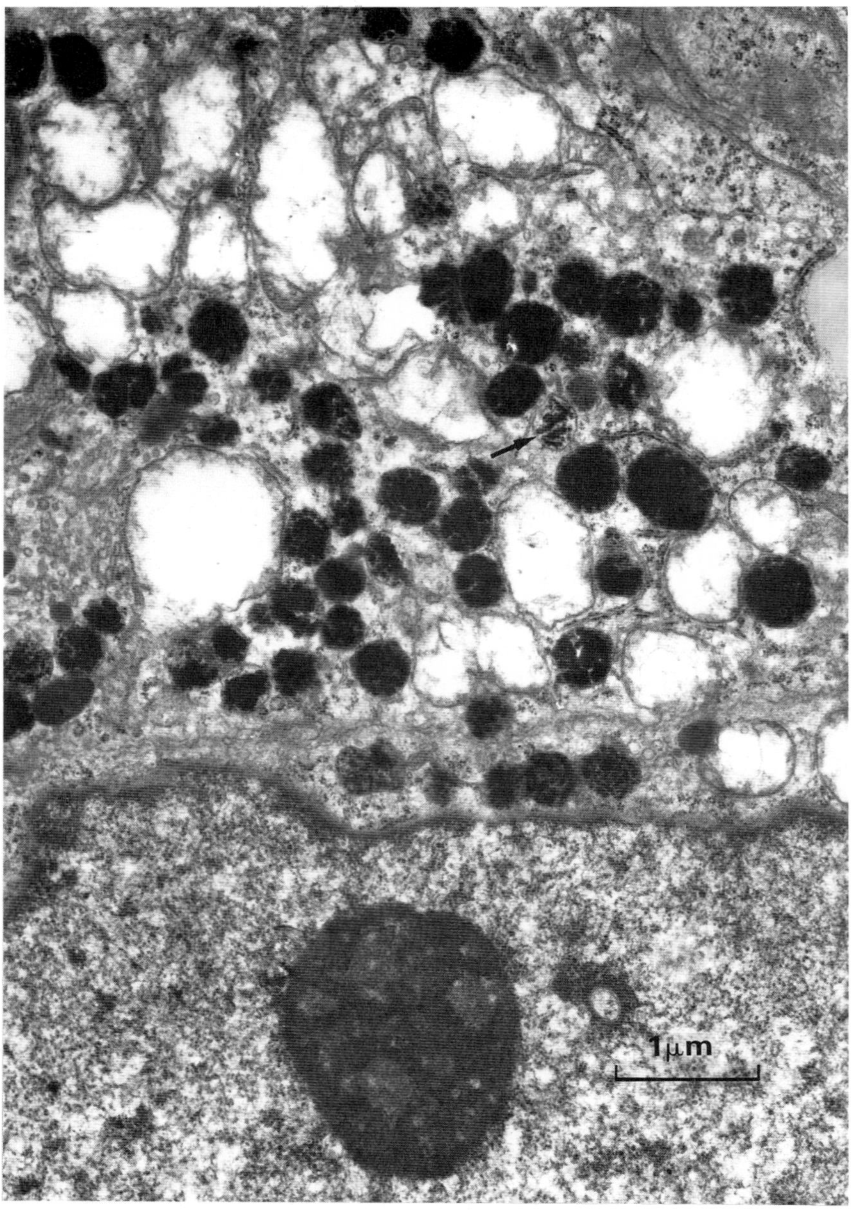

Fig. 8.6 (b) Detail of primary melanosomes. Poorly melanised melanosome indicated by arrow (×19 300).

philic cytoplasm with an eccentrically situated rounded nucleus containing coarse chromatin and a large nucleolus. Multinucleate forms are sometimes seen. Pigment content is variable (Fig. 8.5c).

Electron microscopy has shown that the cytoplasm of spindle A cells contains numerous fine filaments, but scanty rough endoplasmic reticulum (RER) and a few mitchodria. Spindle B cells contain fewer filaments, but more RER and mitochondria (Fig. 8.6a), while in epithelioid cells there are no filaments, but abundant RER and numerous mitochondria. Melanosomes are present in variable numbers (Fig. 8.6b & c) and the poorly melanised pre-melanosomes may be useful in identifying apparently amelanotic metastases.

Electron microscopy has also shown that foam or ballon cells, which are not uncommonly seen particularly in the base of melanomata (Fig. 8.7), are tumour cells with large lipid vacuoles. Melanosomes are seen between the vacuoles.

Cells in mitosis are seldom numerous in melanomata, even rapidly growing epithelioid melanomata rarely show mitotic figures comparable in number to those seen in an anaplastic carcinoma. Most melanomata contain a mixture of cell types usually with spindle B predominating. Not infrequently, there are anaplastic areas where the cells are more epithelioid in character. Pure spindle A melanomata are uncommon, but some spindle B melanomata may also contain an admixture of spindle A cells.

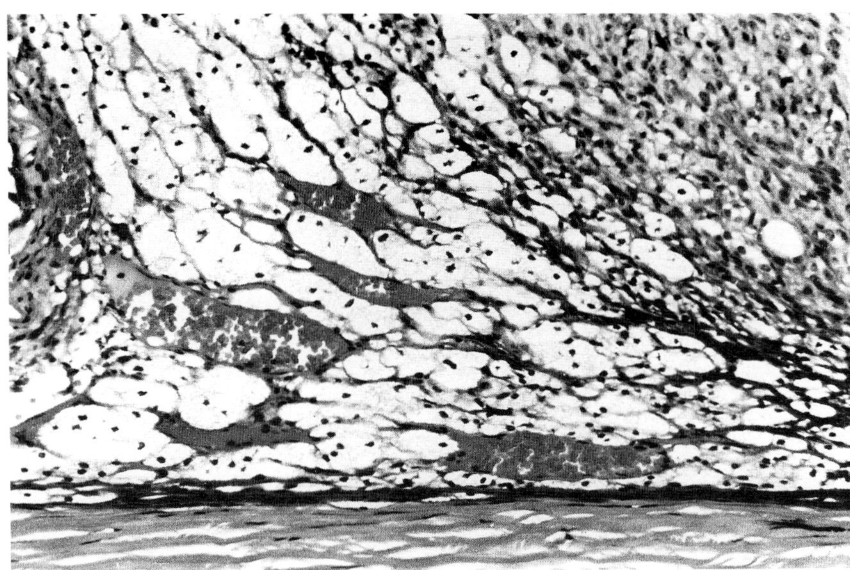

Fig. 8.7 Balloon cells in base of choroidal melanoma. H & E (×260).

As a general rule, spindle cells predominate in small tumours, but as the tumour enlarges, its cell population appears to become more heterogenous — the multiclonal proliferation theory. The spindle cells are usually arranged in compactly woven bundles, but the more anaplastic the tumour, the less orderly is this arrangement.

Reticulin: an argyrophil collagenous stroma — reticulin (see Appendix II) — is laid down in malignant melanomata and the amount has been claimed to have prognostic significance. It is most abundant in low-grade spindle cell areas and scanty in anaplastic areas. It may vary considerably in different parts of the tumour and tends to be abundant in the base which is the oldest and least rapidly growing part of the tumour (Fig. 8.8).

Lymphocytic infiltration: about 15% of choroidal melanomata show some lymphocytic infiltration, though it is heavy in less than 5%. However, such cases do not have a better prognosis, as would be expected if the infiltration represented a defensive immunological response by the host.

Types

Circumscribed: most choroidal melanomata form circumscribed masses which gradually expand the choroid (Fig. 8.9a). Bruch's membrane is at first pushed inwards and then ruptured so that the tumour assumes a 'collar-stud' or 'mushroom' shape with a nodular subretinal head connected by a narrow neck to a wider choroidal

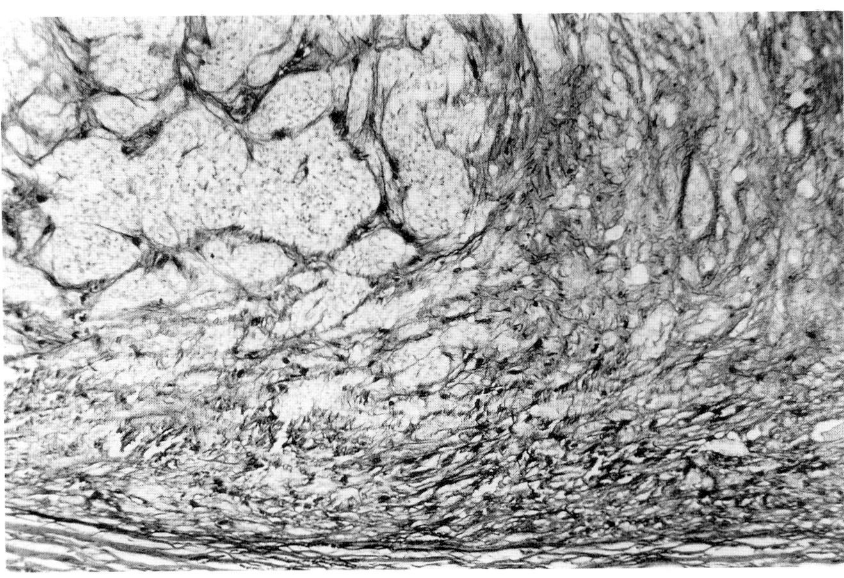

Fig. 8.8 Choroidal melanoma stained for reticulin fibres. Note great variation in the density of the fibres even within this relatively small field (×64).

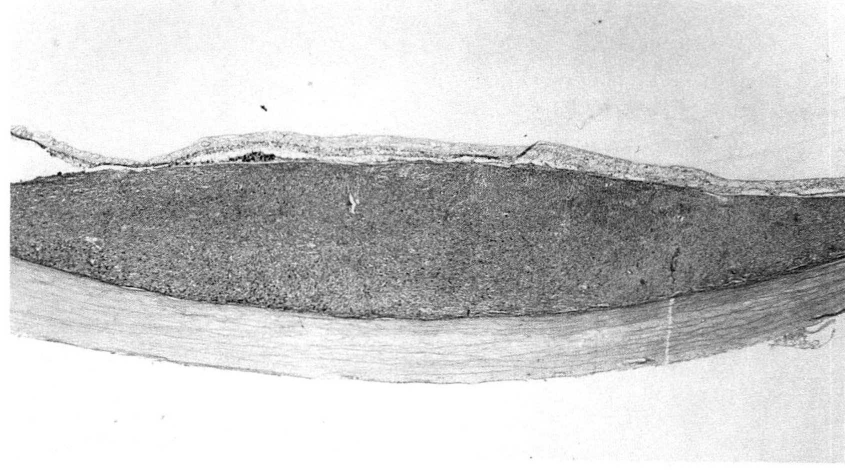

Fig. 8.9 Tumour profiles. (a) Small flat posteriorly situated tumour with no detachment of overlying retina.

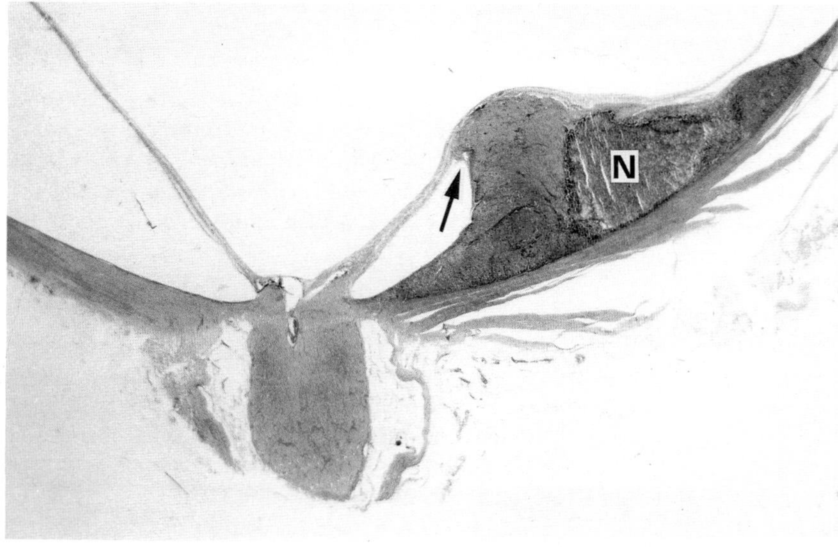

Fig. 8.9 (b) 'Collar-stud' profile. Posteriorly situated tumour which has just ruptured Bruch's membrane (arrow). Large area of necrosis present (N). The retinal detachment is factitious.

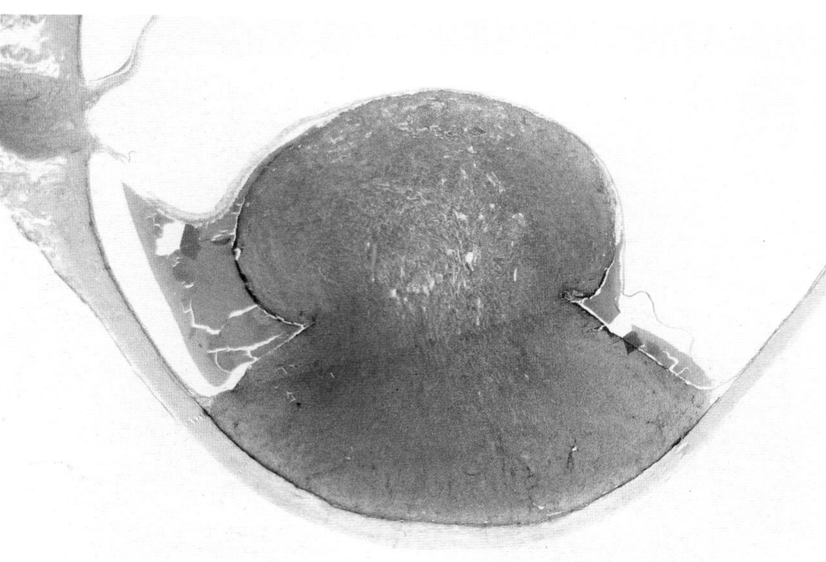

Fig. 8.9 (c) 'Cottage-loaf' profile. Note serous exudate around tumour.

base (Fig. 8.9b & c). The size which the tumour reaches before rupturing Bruch's membrane is very variable. It is tacitly assumed that rapid growth results in early rupture because the membrane has no time to stretch. Thereafter, the head may outgrow the base. Strangulation of the neck of the tumour in the aperture may result in congestion and haemorrhage in the head. The overlying retina is progressively detached and the subretinal space filled with serous exudate which may gravitate downwards causing remote and often extensive detachment inferiorly. The pigmented epithelium over the tumour is usually disrupted, though reactive proliferation may occur. The retina overlying the tumour shows secondary changes in the outer layers due to the detachment and may also exhibit cystic disruption, but rarely contains haemorrhages in the early stages. Occasionally a tumour may break through into the vitreous without detaching the retina (Fig. 8.10) (see Knapp–Rønne type). Detached viable neoplastic cells are rarely found in the subretinal fluid of an associated retinal detachment, because the majority of choroidal melanomata are compact and well-knit.

If the eye is retained for several years, a melanoma may grow large enough to fill it, but usually the globe is enucleated long before this because visual deterioration, glaucoma, endophthalmitis, or intraocular haemorrhage have drawn attention to the presence of the neoplasm and made enucleation unavoidable.

Juxta-papillary melanomata may either infiltrate round the margin of Bruch's membrane into the space between the retina and pigmented epithelium and then lobulate over the optic nerve head, or may surround it in an annular manner (Fig. 8.11). Since the nerve head is relatively fixed, such melanomata infiltrate its substance and discrete black spidery deposits of malignant cells may then appear in the surrounding retina lying immediately beneath the internal limiting membrane. However, unlike retinoblastomata, they seldom grow down the optic nerve towards the brain.

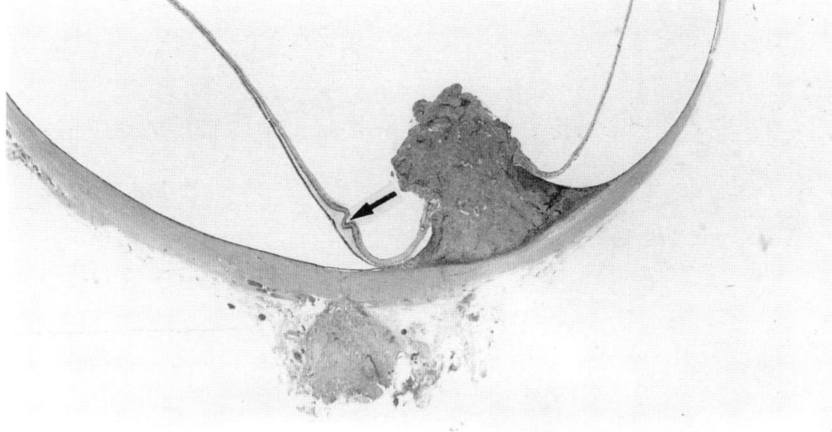

Fig. 8.10 Rupture of retina. Posteriorly situated tumour close to fovea (indicated by arrow) which has ruptered retina before attaining a large size. The detachment is factitious.

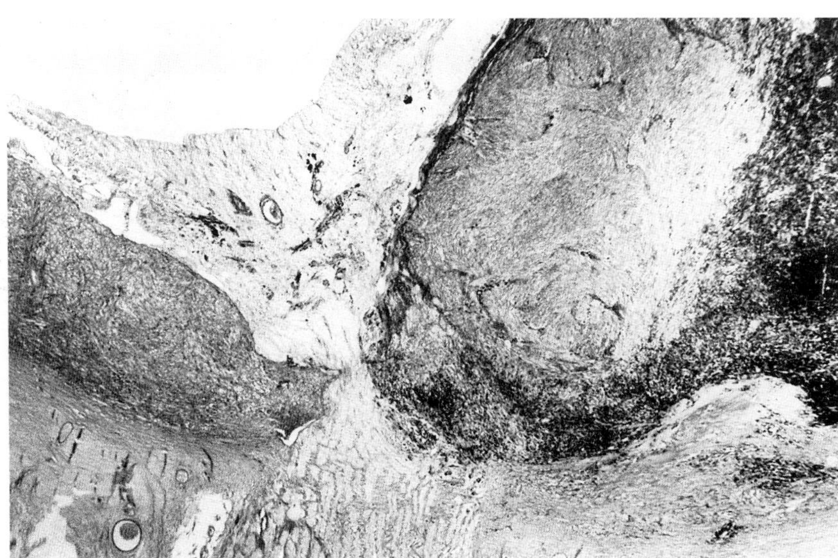

Fig. 8.11 Constriction of optic nerve by large posteriorly situated melanoma. PAS/tartrazine (×20).

Cilio-choroidal melanomata commence in the outer layers of the ciliary body or anterior choroid and, due to the relative spaciousness of the tissue, tend to form large lenticular or globular tumours which encroach on the posterior chamber and may press upon the lens causing displacement and cataract. The growth may infiltrate backwards into the choroid and forwards into the root of the iris and angle to form a tongue of tumour visible in the anterior chamber. Later it may partially fill the anterior chamber and incorporate iris (Fig. 8.12). Penetration of the sclera is common (see below). Retinal detachment may not occur. When it does, it is often late in appearance and mainly posterior to the tumour. Tumour seeding via the aqueous can occur on the iris and posterior corneal surface and these deposits may be the presenting sign.

Necrotic melanomata: focal necrosis and haemorrhage are not uncommon in melanomata and may be the cause of cystic spaces which are occasionally noted. Some melanomata undergo massive necrosis. Usually islands of viable cells can be found, but occasionally only the reticulin stroma of the tumour perists. Extensive necrosis results in an inflammatory reaction in the uvea and sclera which sometimes involves orbital fat. There is often considerable intraocular haemorrhage with necrosis of the retina, iris and ciliary processes and opacification of the lens. Eventually the globe may shrink.

While it has been suggested that the necrosis occurred as a result of immunological rejection, little evidence exists to support the idea. Moreover, the prognosis is not good for necrotic melanomata, as would be expected if this were the case. Most cases must presumably be due to

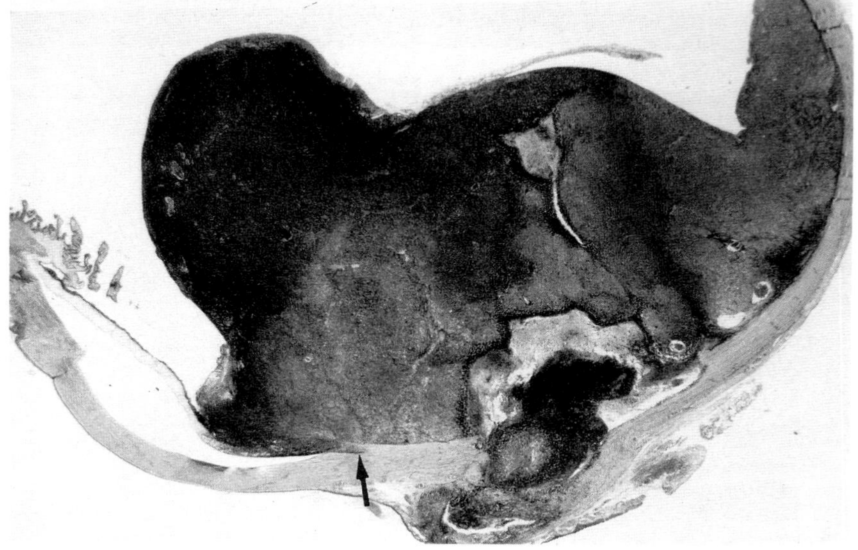

Fig. 8.12 Ciliochoroidal melanoma. (a) Low power showing large ciliochoroidal melanoma which has infiltrated trabecular meshwork (arrow) and root of iris and perforated sclera to form a subconjunctival mass.

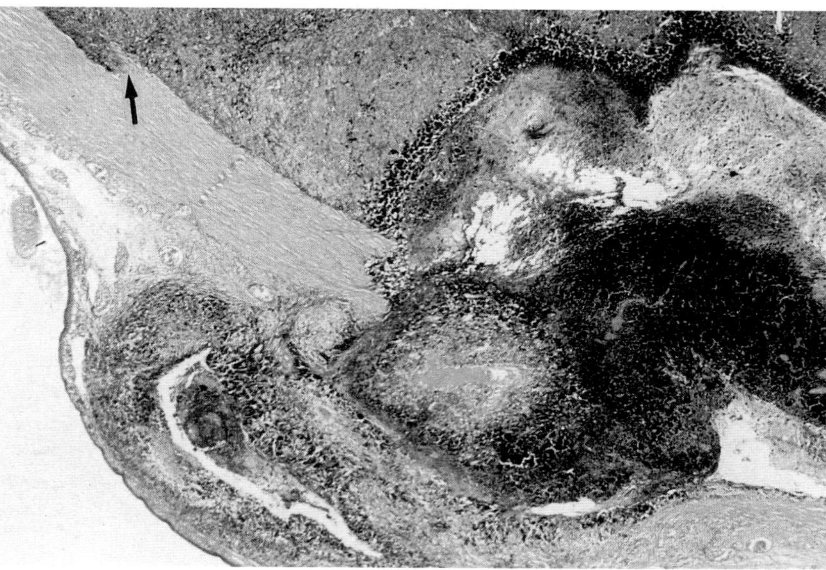

Fig. 8.12 (b) Higher power showing scleral perforation and subconjunctival mass in more detail.

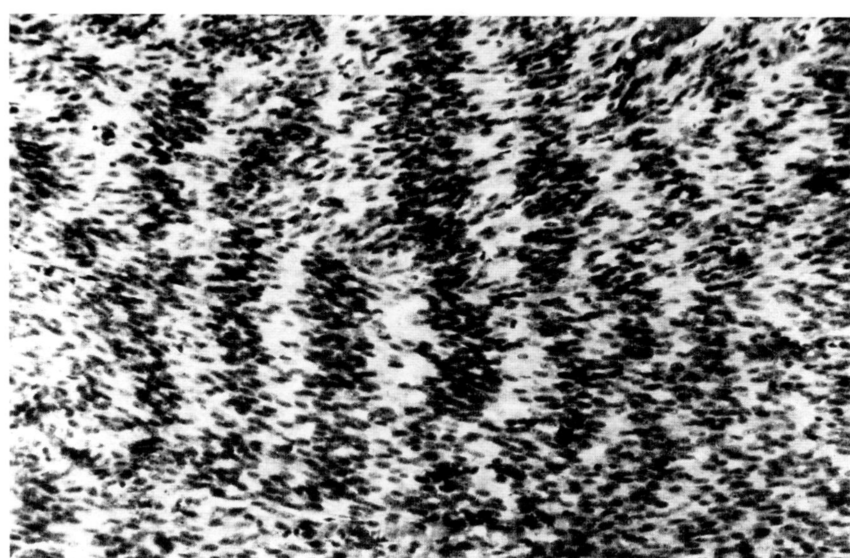

Fig. 8.13 Melanoma of choroid showing a well-marked fascicular structure. Masson trichrome (×160).

failure of the blood supply. Necrotic melanomata may present clinically as uveitis or even orbital cellulitis.

Fascicular: this uncommon type has a predominantly spindle B cell population and is usually lightly pigmented or amelanotic. The tumour cells are arranged in columns with their nuclei perpendicular to the axis of the column (Fig. 8.13). The appearance is reminscent of the palisading seen in neurilemmomata.

Diffuse: these melanomata constitute about 5% of uveal melanomata. They infiltrate at least 25% of the uvea without forming a mass thicker than 7.0 mm at any point. They are thus likely to be confused with deposits of secondary carcinoma or leukaemic infiltrates.

The majority are of the more anaplastic types, i.e mixed, epithelioid or necrotic. Extrasceral extension is present in 40% of cases at the time of enucleation and is often found to have occurred through more than one emissary canal. Intravascular invasion of the choroidal vessels may also be present.

There is often a long delay before the eye is enucleated because clinical recognition of this type is difficult. This is reflected in a higher 5 year metastatic death rate.

Knapp–Rønne: true 'Knapp–Rønne' melanomata constitute less than 1% of all uveal melanomata. They are located near the optic nerve head and have an anaplastic cell structure. Characteristically, they invade the retina early and form a spongy mass in the vitreous. Cavernous spaces within the tumour may or may not contain blood. Dilated vascular spaces are thought to be caused by

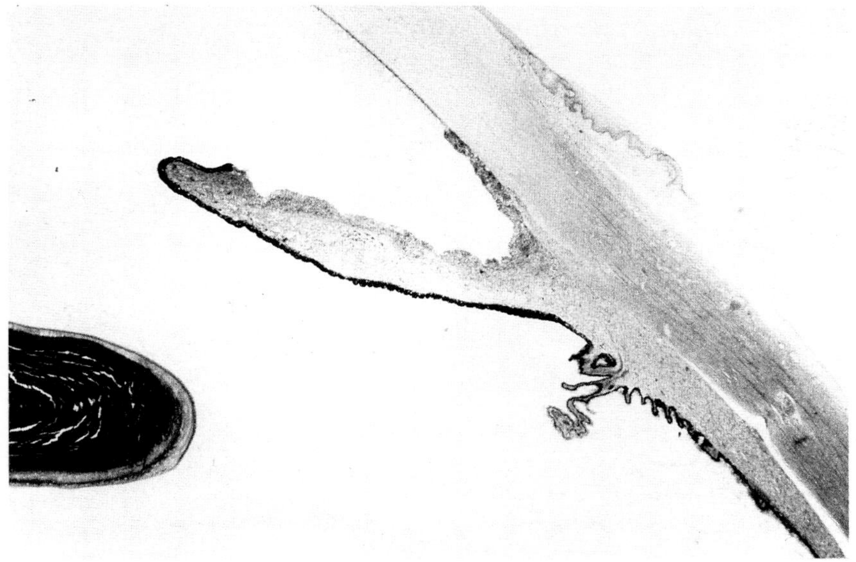

Fig. 8.14 Ring melanoma. (a) Low power to show the extent of the growth on the surface of the iris and cornea. H & E (×20).

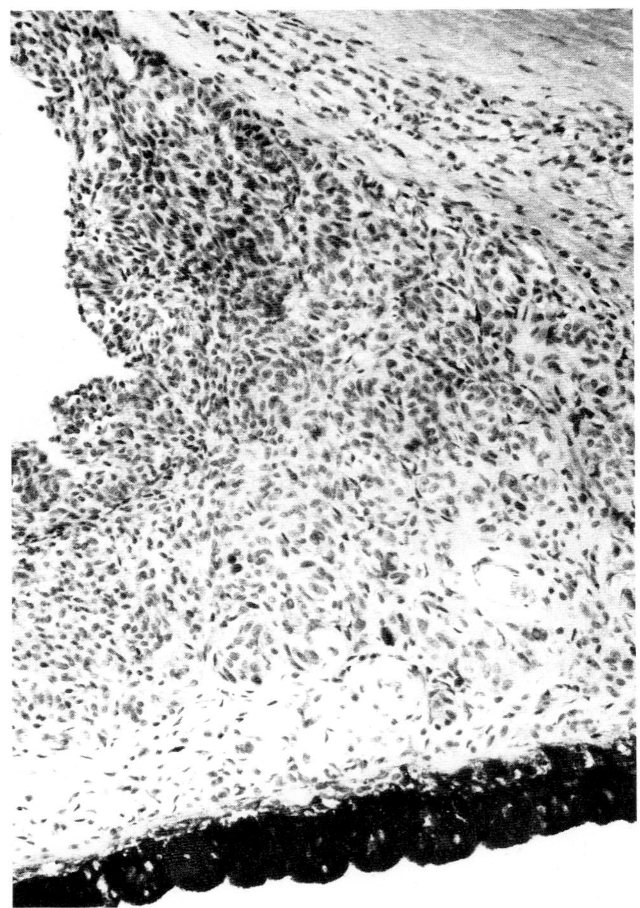

Fig. 8.14 (b) Higher power showing infiltration of the deeper tissues in the chamber angle. H & E (×170).

strangulation of vessels where the tumour passes through Bruch's membrane. The mechanism by which the bloodless spaces are formed is not known. They may possibly, as already suggested, be post-necrotic. Clinical presentation is typically with a vitreous haemorrhage.

Ring melanoma: this uncommon type results from circumferential diffuse infiltration of the anterior ciliary body, root of iris and trabecular meshwork usually by a relatively low grade tumour. Tumour cells are shed into the aqueous (Fig. 8.14). Such tumours present with glaucoma.

Complications

Some complications such as massive necrosis, vitreous haemorrhage and secondary glaucoma due to neoplastic infiltration of the trabecular meshwork have already been mentioned. Glaucoma may also result from angle closure which is due to the formation of vascular synechiae. Neovascular proliferation on the iris is noted to occur with some melanomata. Sometimes no obvious pathological mechanism for secondary glaucoma is demonstrable.

Growth, spread and metastasis

As the tumour grows it gradually occupies more and more space within the globe, but the rate at which this occurs varies greatly (Fig. 8.15). Spontaneous regression is rare, but has been recorded (Lambert *et al.*, 1986).

Extrascleral extension may occur early but is uncommon in small tumours. Published figures from older series indicate that up to 15% of enucleated globes containing melanomata show extrascleral extension.

Choroidal melanomata invade the sclera directly to a variable extent (Fig. 8.16) and grow along the emissary canals. If left untreated, such extensions fill up the orbit

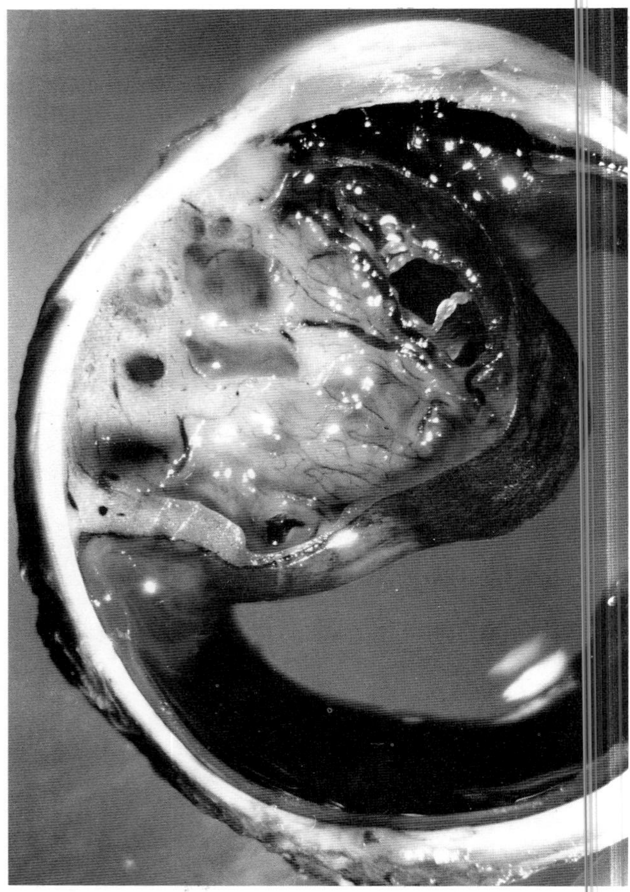

Fig. 8.15 Two cases which illustrate the extreme variation in the rate of growth of different tumours. (a) The patient was first seen 12 years before enucleation when she was 37 and told she had a 'cyst'. The eye subsequently became blind and painful and was enucleated. It shows a large highly cystic melanoma of the ciliary body. A small episcleral plaque not visible in the photograph was present posterior to the limbus.

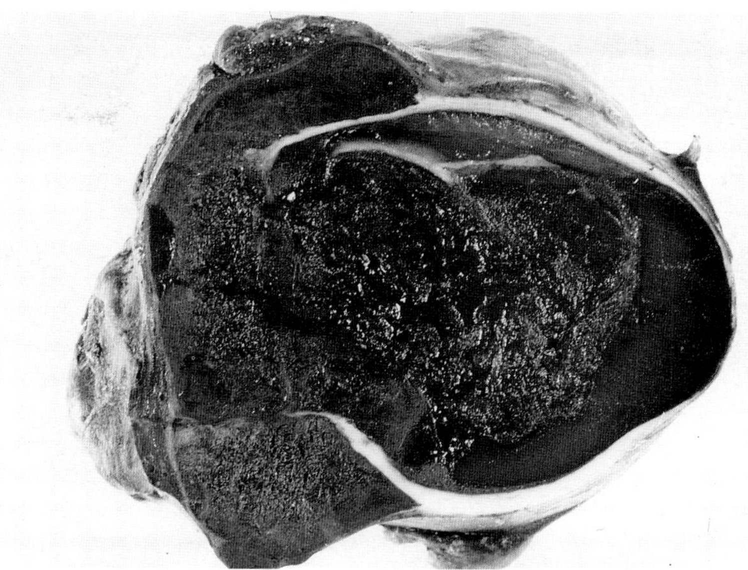

Fig. 8.15 (b) The patient was first seen 5 years before enucleation. He was then aged 42 and had failing vision in his left eye. An inferonasal choroidal mass with a retinal detachment was found and removal of the eye recommended. However, he repeatedly failed to attend for treatment.

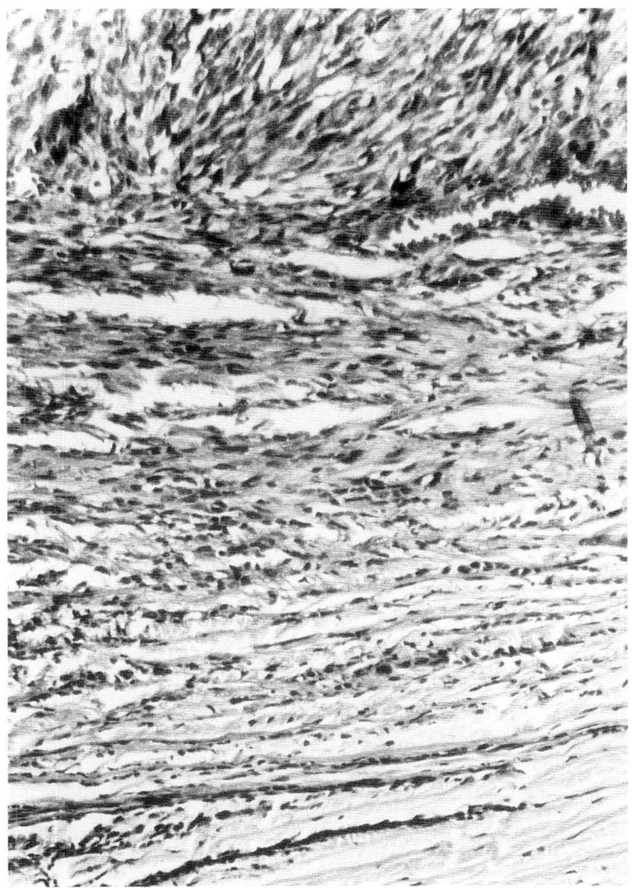

Fig. 8.16 Scleral invasion. Boundary zone between a choroidal melanoma and the sclera (lower half) showing infiltration of the tumour between the scleral lamellae. Masson trichrome (×170).

and may extend into the cranium, nose and nasal sinuses.

Melanomata in the ciliary body traverse the channels transmitting the the anterior ciliary vessels and form visible episcleral nodules at their points of exit. Tumours involving the angle may infiltrate along the perivascular spaces of the limbal vascular plexus to appear at the limbus where they may form large superficial growths. In addition, extraocular extension sometimes occurs directly through the sclera. This is facilitated by necrosis of the growth and neighbouring sclera or by the presence of an area of local weakness such as an old drainage or cataract operation scar (Fig. 8.17). Extension along the long posterior ciliary nerve into the orbit has also been reported.

Haematogenous metastasis: by contrast with cutaneous melanomata, uveal melanomata do not have direct access to lymphatics and thus cannot initially spread to regional lymph nodes. However, the tumours are frequently very vascular and, when in emissary canals, are in intimate contact with thin-walled veins. Occasionally tumour emboli may be seen within blood vessels (Fig. 8.18). To minimise the risk of dislodging tumour cells into the vascular system, recent publications have stressed the importance of handling tumour-containing eyes with the utmost care during diagnostic procedures and subsequent enucleation. About 2.5% of cases have established metastases at the time of enucleation.

Distant metastases from intraocular growth or from its extrascleral extension are the cause of death from melanomata. One unsolved mystery is the appearance of distant metastases many years after the enucleation of the tumour-bearing eye. The average time interval between enucleation and the appearance of metastases is 2 to 3 years, but intervals of 20 to 25 years have been

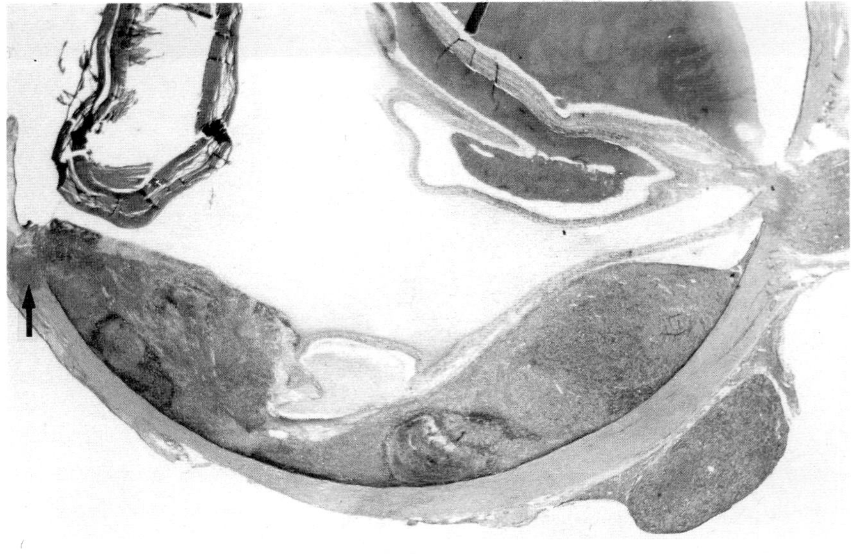

Fig. 8.17 Invasion of a trabeculectomy site. (a) Low power showing a large ciliochoroidal melanoma with extrascleral extension posteriorly and invasion of a trabeculectomy site anteriorly (arrow).

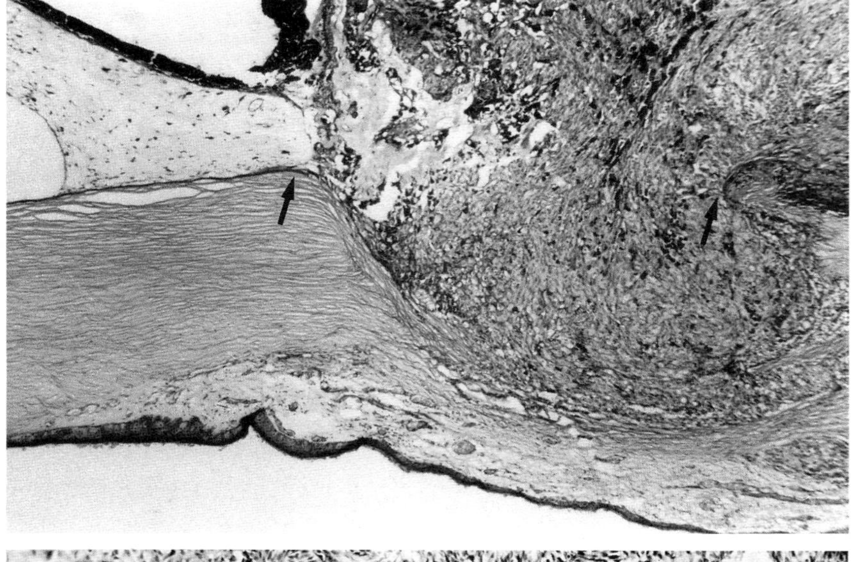

Fig. 8.17 (b) Higher power showing invasion of trabeculectomy site (margins indicated by arrows) in more detail. PAS/tartrazine (×43).

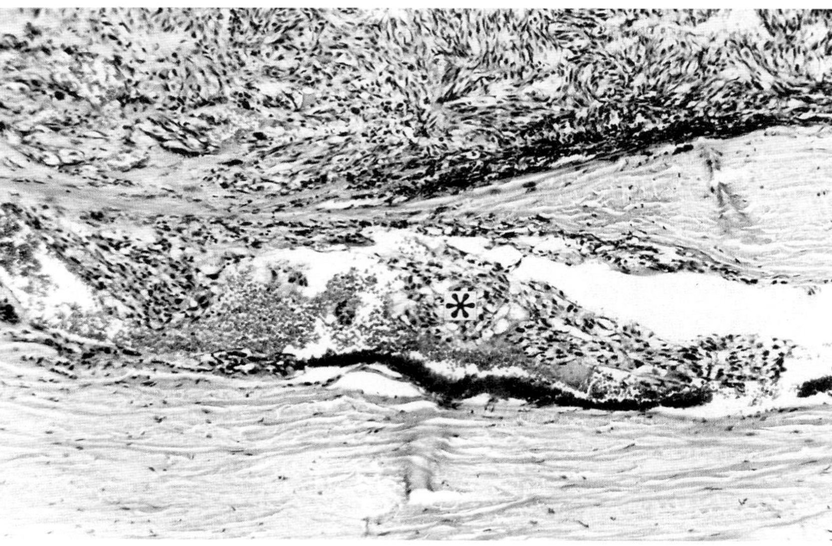

Fig. 8.18 Vascular invasion. Substantial clump of tumour cells (asterisk) in vein passing through a posterior scleral emissary canal. H & E (×95).

recorded. The liver is the commonest site for secondary deposits, but few tissues are exempt. Metastatic deposits may differ from the primary growth in microscopic structure.

Patients with melanomata may excrete colourless melanogen in their urine, but this rarely occurs until the disease is far advanced and liver metastases are established. The urine darkens on standing or on the addition of ferric chloride due to the oxidation of melanogen to melanin. On the addition of sodium nitroprusside, the urine turns green and blue as a result of the formation of ferric ferrocyanide.

Recent studies (Donoso *et al.*, 1983) have suggested that serum levels of sialic acid and hepatic cell-surface enzymes and isoenzymes may be useful in detecting early metastatic disease from malignant melanomata.

Prognosis

Mortality after enucleation has been estimated in many different series. After 5 years mortality ranged from 16 to 86% and after 10 years from 27 to 64% in different series (see Zimmerman, 1980).

Actuarial mortality rates taken from a comprehensive survey (Paul *et al.*, 1962) are given in Table 8.1. This method takes account of patients not followed for a specific time or who died during the study and gives a lower mortality rate than direct calculation.

Table 8.1 Actuarial mortality rate (%) after enucleation for melanoma of choroid and ciliary body (from Paul *et al.*, 1962).

	5 years	10 years	15 years
All cases	29	40	46
Spindle A	5	15	19
Spindle B and fascicular	11	20	26
Mixed and necrotic	40	54	59
Epithelioid	57	66	72

Factors affecting the prognosis have been studied exhaustively:

Cell type: In contrast to experience with cutaneous and conjunctival melanomata, it is well established that the prognosis of uveal melanomata is clearly related to the predominant tumour-cell type. As can be seen from Table 8.1, spindle A tumours have the best prognosis and epithelioid tumours the worst. There is indeed some doubt as to whether pure spindle A tumours have ever metastasised. However, grading by cell type suffers from two limitations:

1 Sections necessarily only sample the cell population of the tumour and a small anaplastic area may be missed.

2 While the basic cell types are easily identified, intermediate forms occur and many tumours have a mixed population. Classification of a given tumour, even by experienced ophthalmic pathologists, may thus vary. In an attempt to make a more objective assessment, an index has been devised relating the variability of nucleolar size to the size of the tumour itself (Gamel & McLean, 1984).

Size is probably the single most reliable prognostic indicator. Small tumours have a better prognosis than large. 'Small' has been defined differently in various series, but, in practice, can be taken to mean tumours with a greatest dimension of less than 10.0 mm. Two other factors which affect prognosis are related size, as follows:

1 Rupture of Bruch's membrane is an adverse prognostic factor which is more likely to occur in large tumours.

2 Posteriorly located tumours have a better prognosis than anteriorly located tumours. However, posteriorly located tumours often cause symptoms while still small. By contrast, anteriorly located tumours may reach a large size before causing any symptoms.

Pigment content: heavily pigmented tumours have a worse prognosis than lightly pigmented or amelanotic tumours.

Extrascleral extension: as would be expected, the prognosis is poor when extension into the orbit has occurred.

The enucleation controversy

Provoked by the observation by Zimmerman, McLean and Foster (1978 and in numerous subsequent papers) based on a re-examination of earlier mortality figures published by Paul *et al.* (1962) that a peak mortality occurs between 2 and 3 years after enucleation, a great deal of discussion has taken place in recent years as to the value of enucleation as a therapeutic measure. Several different interpretations have been placed on the significance of these observations:

1 *Uveal melanomata tend to metastasise late, but dissemination of malignant cells is promoted by enucleation.* At the same time, the patient's physiological or immunological response to the tumour may be decreased (Zimmerman *et al.* 1978). Although the ability of showers of tumour cells liberated into the blood to develop into metastases is in some doubt, careful handling of tumour-containing eyes during diagnostic procedures and enucleation is clearly prudent. Some have advocated such measures as freezing or irradiating the tumour prior to enucleation. There is little evidence to support the proposition that any effective immunological reaction to melanomata normally occurs let alone that it would be jeopardised by removal of the tumour.

2 *Uveal melanomata typically metastasise before they*

become symptomatic. Enucleation probably does not, therefore, influence survival, but should be carried out as soon as possible to save those cases in which it has not occurred (Manschot & van Peperzeel, 1980). Some eyes with useful vision will thereby be sacrificed.

3 *Post-operative deaths result from slowly growing tumour cells that have metastasised before enucleation*. Enucleation, although relatively ineffective, remains the treatment of choice, but little is to be lost by delaying the enucleation of eyes which retain good vision. Small slowly growing or static benign tumours which cannot at present be distinguished clinically from small malignant tumours could thus be kept under observation and some useful eyes containing essentially benign tumours might be saved (Gass, 1980).

4 *Haematogenous dissemination occurs when tumour growth accelerates and becomes clinically manifest* (see Albert, 1978). The implications of this view appear to be the same as those of the previous proposition.

For a review of this controversy, the reader is referred to Apple and Blodi (1980), Gass (1980) and Zimmerman and McLean (1980).

Errors in diagnosis

Unsuspected melanomata: in up to 10% of enucleated eyes, a melanoma which was not suspected clinically may be found. Occasionally, the secondary detachment due to a melanoma (or even a secondary carcinoma — see Fig. 8.19), is mistakenly treated as primary, but most errors result from opacification of the media caused by:

1 Dense cataract.

2 Necrosis of the tumour with secondary endophthalmitis, scleritis and phthisis bulbi.

3 Factors unrelated to the tumour such as a previous injury.

4 Secondary glaucoma.

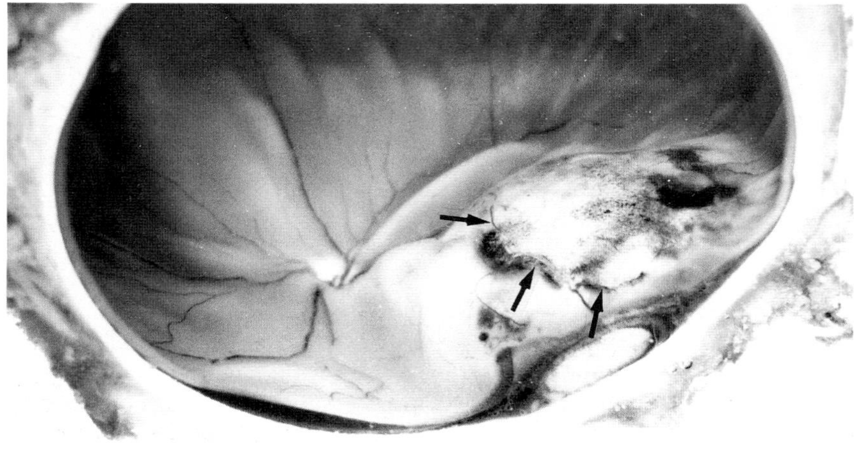

Fig. 8.19 Effects of laser treatment. (a) Macroscopic picture of treated tumour showing destruction of retina over the tumour. Margin of retina indicated by arrows.

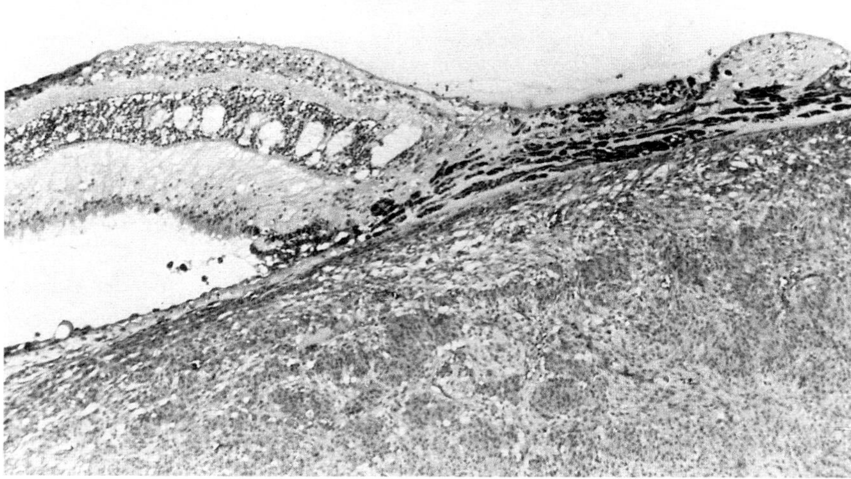

Fig. 8.19 (b) Photomicrograph showing margin of retina sealed to tumour by layers of proliferating glia and pigmented epithelium. H & E (×64).

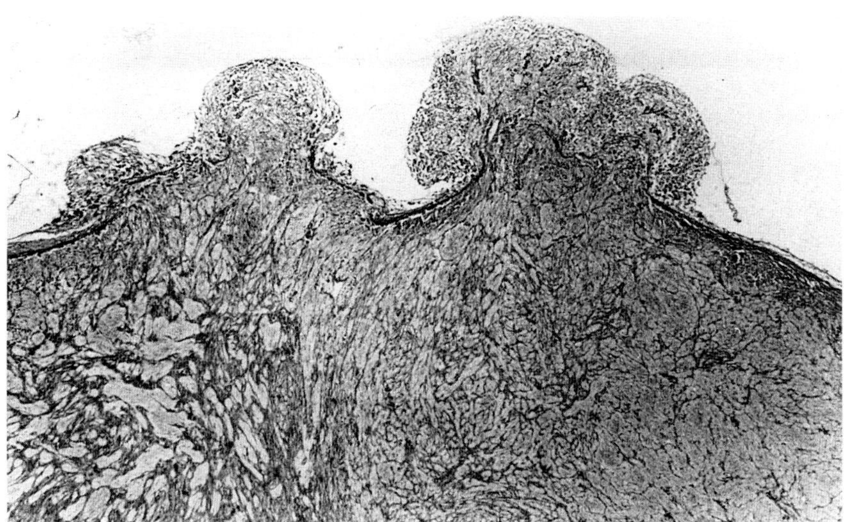

Fig. 8.19 (c) Multiple ruptures in Bruch's membrane (silver stain) (reproduced with permission from Duvall & Lucas, 1981).

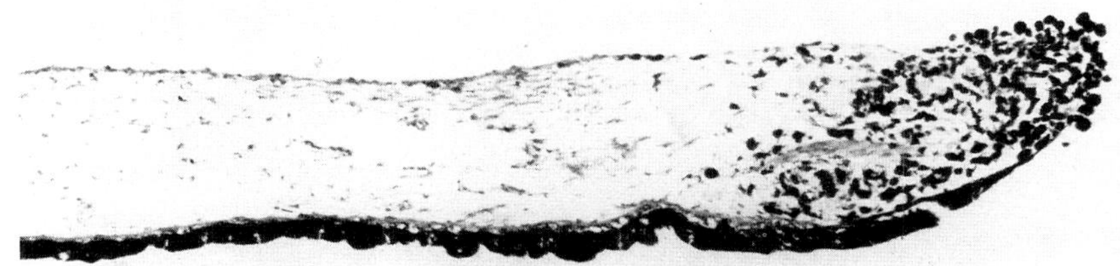

Fig. 8.19 (d) Post-necrotic atrophy of pupillary border of iris. H & E (×64).

Lesions mistaken for melanomata: with the widespread use of more sophisticated diagnostic techniques such as fluorescein angiography and ultrasonography, far fewer eyes are now being enucleated with an erroneous clinical diagnosis of malignant melanoma.

The lesions, other than choroidal naevi, which have been mistaken for malignant melanoma include:

1 Rhegmatogenous detachment, especially if large degenerative cysts are present.
2 Macular disease, especially if subretinal bleeding occurs.
3 Posterior uveitis.
4 Retinoschisis.
5 Choroidal or ciliochoroidal detachment.
6 Metastatic carcinoma.
7 Haemangioma.
8 Melanocytoma of optic nerve head.
9 Proliferative or hypertrophic lesions of the pigmented epithelium.
10 Lymphoid or lymphomatous deposits.

Effects of local treatments

Radiotherapy: melanomata are not particularly radiosensitive, but regression can be induced by large doses of γ or β-rays administered by inserting applicators containing the appropriate emitter (^{60}cobalt, ^{60}ruthenium, ^{106}rhodium or radon). Eyes that have been examined histologically have been enucleated because of complications and failure of the tumour to regress. Necrosis may be seen in the tumour, but is not necessarily attributable to the radiotherapy. This promotes melanomacrophagic activity. Although cytological evidence of 'dormancy' has been described following treatment by a ^{60}ruthenium plaque (Lee, 1987), when regression of the tumour occurs ischaemia is probably an important factor. While no direct effect on the tumour may be demonstrable, radiation damage may be seen in the adjacent ocular tissues, namely retina, optic nerve and sclera.

Apart from the dubious value of radiotherapy, the risk of death from metastatic disease is probably increased by the use of such treatment in preference to enucleation (Manschot & Van Strik, 1987).

Photocoagulation: argon laser or xenon arc beams are used to treat small melanomata primarily by interfering with their blood supply and later by direct destruction of the tumour. Again, only unsuccessfully treated cases have been examined histologically, usually some time after treatment, when direct damage to the tumour is difficult to demonstrate. However, the retina overlying the tumour is destroyed (Fig. 8.20a). This is associated with pigment proliferation (Fig. 8.20b) and rupture of the tumour through Bruch's membrane which may result in tumour cells being shed into the vitreous. Vitreous haemorrhage is common.

If the iris is exposed to the beam necrosis occurs. Post-necrotic atrophy of the pupillary border is a not uncommon finding (Fig. 8.20d).

Surgical excision: small tumours can be treated by local excision, usually after ringing the tumour by laser burns to compromise its blood supply. The tumour is removed with a plaque of underlying sclera. Recurrence at the original site may occur and sometimes tumour cells are disseminated around the globe (Fig. 8.21).

Other complications include vitreous haemorrhage and retinal detachment. Unusual forms of organisation of subretinal haemorrhages and hypertrophy, hyperplasia and metaplasia of the pigmented epithelium may give rise to 'pseudomelanomata' (Lee, 1987).

OTHER PRIMARY TUMOURS

Leiomyomata

Leiomyomata are rare benign tumours of the iris which usually arise in the sphincter or dilator pupillae, but occasionally in other sites where smooth muscle is not present. They have been estimated to comprise 4–33% of primary iris tumours (Sunba *et al.*, 1980). This wide

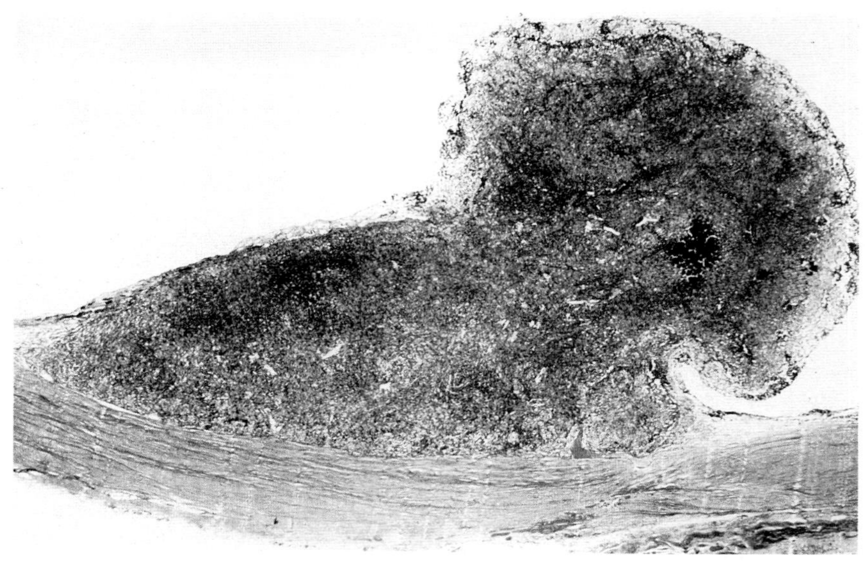

Fig. 8.20 Recurrence after surgery. (a) On sclera at site of excision. H & E (×64).

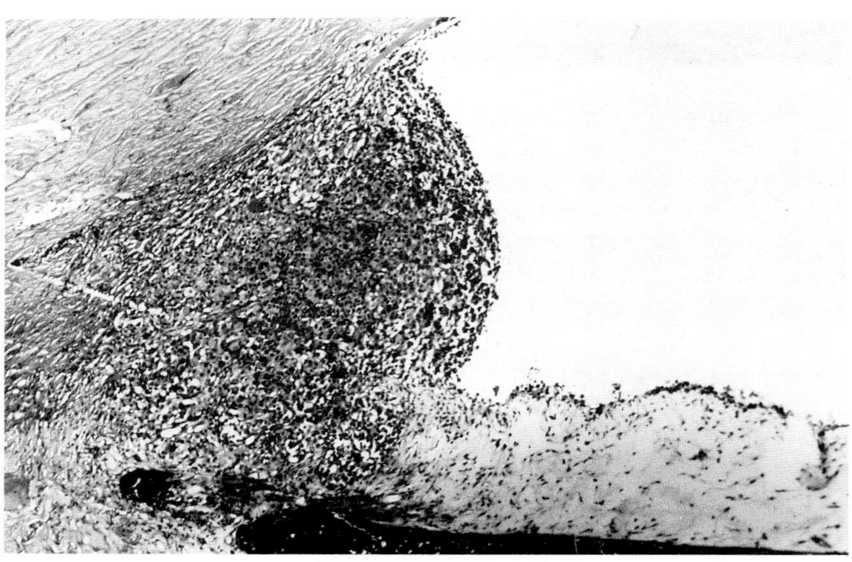

Fig. 8.20 (b) In anterior chamber angle. Note spread of tumour along anterior surface of iris. Tumour cells were widely disseminated in the eye.

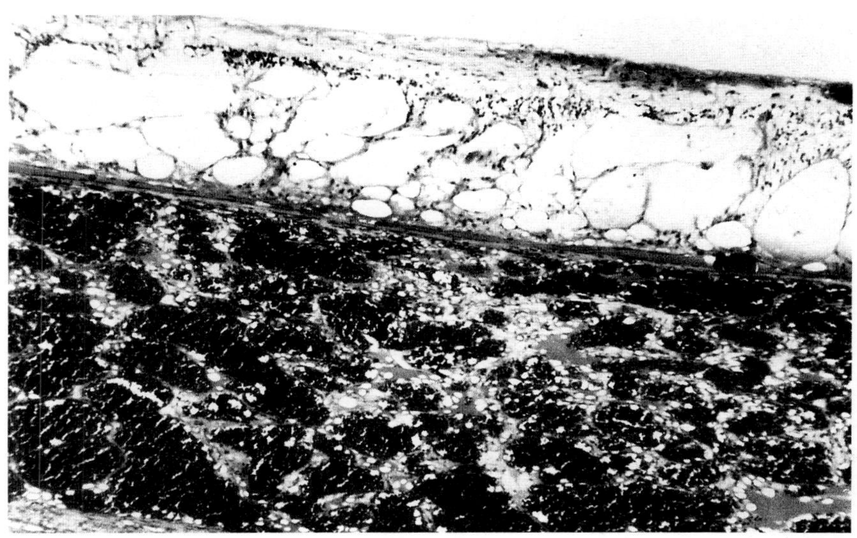

Fig. 8.21 Haemangioma of choroid. The full thickness of the choroid is replaced by the haemangioma and the overlying retina shows advanced microcystic degeneration. Masson trichrome (×64).

range reflects the fact that they are often difficult to differentiate from lightly pigmented melanocytic tumours.

Typically they are well vascularised tumours composed of elongated spindle cells which often show nuclear palisading. Pigmentation is absent or light. Myoglial fibrils are normally seen after with phosphotungstic acid haematoxylin, and electron microscopy reveals the presence of intracytoplasmic actinomysin filaments. However, these criteria are not absolute since cells may be found in typical melanocytic tumours which contain myoglial fibrils and actinomysin filaments.

The presence and distribution of oxytalan fibres (see Appendix II), which form part of the normal elastic fibre system, has recently been found useful in distinguishing leiomyomata from melanocytic tumours (Sunba *et al.*, 1980). They are more plentiful in the former.

Neurofibromata and neurilemmomata

Neurofibromata and neurilemmomata occur very occasionally in the choroid. Involvement of the uvea in neurofibromatosisis is much commoner (Chapter 15). Uveal neurofibromata may be pigmented.

Haemangiomata

Haemangiomata are typically located at the posterior pole. They are thought to be congenital, but may not become manifest until adult life.

Histologically, choroidal haemangiomata are of cavernous type. They consist of wide, thin-walled channels with little intervening stroma (Fig. 8.22). The overlying retina undergoes local cystoid degeneration and sometimes becomes completely detached. Reactive proliferation of the pigment epithelium may also occur. An epichoroidal membrane of collagen and basement membrane material from the retinal pigment epithelium sometimes forms over the surface of the tumour and, in time, bone may develop in this membrane and in the haemangioma itself. The drainage angle may be normal, but is sometimes narrowed or even closed by adhesions. As a result, secondary glaucoma may occur. Glaucoma may also occur in the absence of any obvious morphological cause, presumably as a result of circulatory disturbance.

In Sturge–Weber disease (Chapter 15), a choroidal haemangioma with glaucoma of either infantile or adult type is accompanied by a homolateral flat cutaneous angioma and a homolateral meningeal haemangioma or capillary-venous malformation with 'tram-line' calcification of the underlying cerebral cortex. Many incomplete forms of the disease are described and the whole subject is riddled with eponyms.

Juvenile xanthogranuloma

Although juvenile xanthogranuloma is characteristically a benign cutaneous disorder of infants and young children, it sometimes involves the eye and ocular tissues. It may present as a nodule in the eyelids or a limbal tumour resembling a solid dermoid, or even as an orbital tumour causing proptosis, but its commonest ocular manifestation is focal or diffuse infiltration of the iris which sometimes extends into the ciliary body. Microscopically, the infiltrate consists of polygonal and spindle shaped histiocytes with a variable admixture of Touton-type giant cells, eosinophils and plasma cells in a highly vascular stroma. Hyphaema is a frequent and important presenting sign. In other cases, the infiltrate induces heterochromia or simulates uveitis. Cells are shed into the aqueous, occasionally in sufficient numbers to block aqueous outflow. Suspected cases should be examined carefully for cutaneous nodules which can be biopsied to confirm diagnosis.

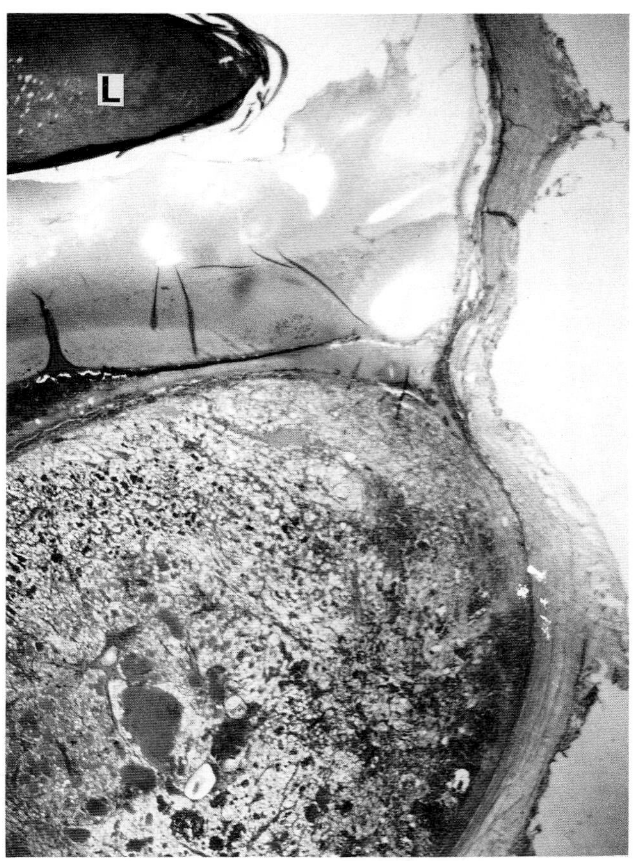

Fig. 8.22 Secondary from a hypernephroma. (a) Low power. The scleral indentation at the top is where a plomb had been applied (L = lens).

SECONDARY TUMOURS

Carcinomata form by far the largest group of metastatic intraocular tumours. About 40% are derived from carcinoma of the female breast and about 40% from carcinoma of the lung. The remainder arise from carcinomata of the gut, pancreas, thyroid, prostate, kidney (Fig. 8.19), uterus and testis.

The malignant emboli nearly always enter the eye via the short posterior ciliary arteries to lodge in the posterior choroid, frequently deep to the macula. There may be more than one metastatic deposit in one eye and asynchronous involvement of both eyes is not uncommon. The usual interval between detection of the primary growth and evidence of intraocular metastasis is 2 years, but much longer intervals have been recorded. Often intraocular deposits are merely part of a terminal carcinomatosis, but in nearly half the cases coming to enucleation, visual disturbance is a presenting symptom which draws attention to an unsuspected primary growth. The average age at enucleation is 50 to 55 years and the duration of life thereafter rarely exceeds 12 months in untreated cases.

A typical secondary appears as a flat, slightly yellowish plaque over which there is a shallow retinal detachment. Only rarely do carcinomata rupture Bruch's membrane or invade the retina or optic nerve and extrascleral extension is uncommon and late.

Metastatic deposits of any kind in the anterior uvea, retina or optic nerve are very rare. In the iris, secondaries tend to form fleshy nodules. Metastatic carcinomata of

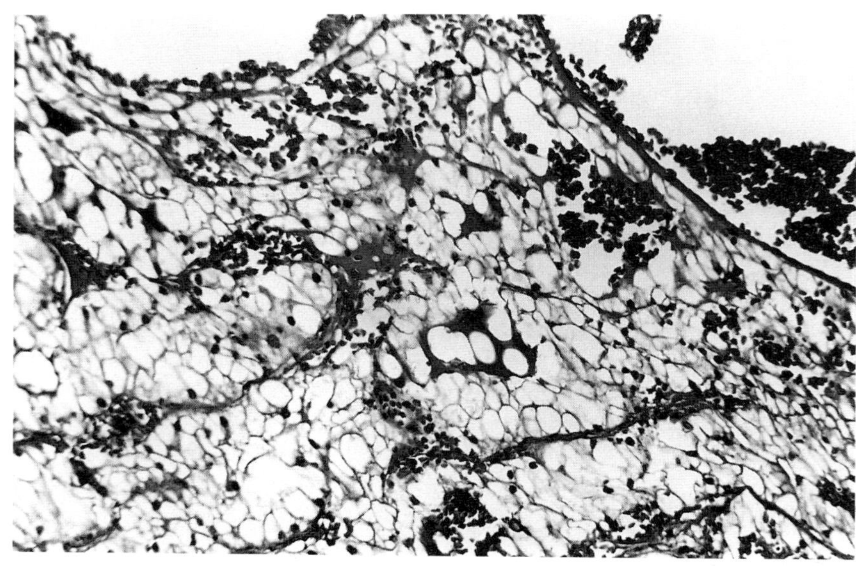

Fig. 8.22 (b) Higher power showing typical structure of tumour. H & E (×95).

the ciliary body may be confused with melanotic tumours arising from the pars ciliaris retinae (see Chapter 11), but these usually have a large extra-uveal portion projecting towards the lens. Their derivation from ciliary epithelium can normally be established. Metastatic carcinomata in either the iris or ciliary body may simulate iridocyclitis clinically. In such cases, examination of aspirated aqueous fluid may help to establish the diagnosis.

Invasion of the inner eye by an epibulbar squamous cell carcinoma or orbital neoplasm is no more than a rare curiosity.

The histology of a metastasis is naturally related to that of the primary tumour, but the following types are those most commonly encountered:

Spheroidal cell carcinomata

Most of these are intra-duct carcinomata originating in the female breast and consist of solid lobules and columns of rounded or polygonal cells with indistinct cytoplasmic outlines and oval nuclei with fine, uniformly dispersed chromatin. Sometimes tubules and acini lined by columnar cells are seen. Stroma varies from fine interlobular strands to coarse intersecting fibrous trabeculae stained with melanin or haemosiderin. Mitotic activity is marked and the growth exhibits a characteristic uniformity in nuclear size, shape and staining intensity. Choroidal melanomata, by contrast, contain few mitotic figures, but show much more cellular pleomorphism. They rarely invoke much stromal reaction and are usually pigmented to some extent.

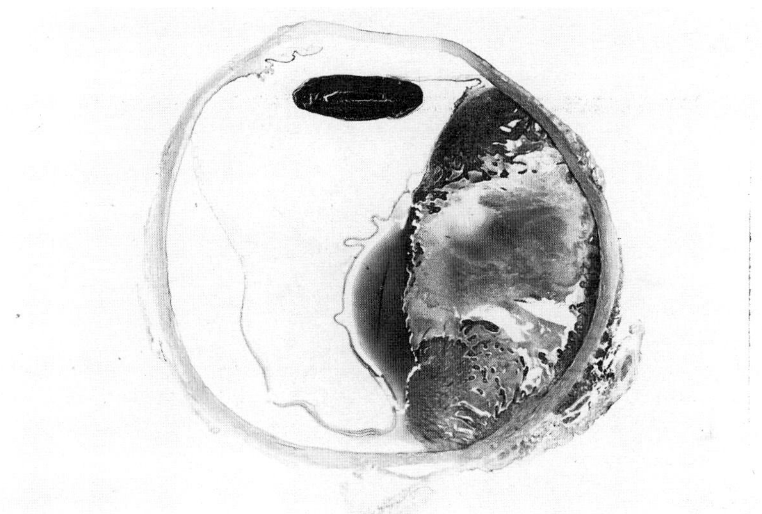

Fig. 8.23 Secondary from an 'oat cell' carcinoma of lung. (a) Low power showing extensive deposit in choroid and smaller plaque on episclera.

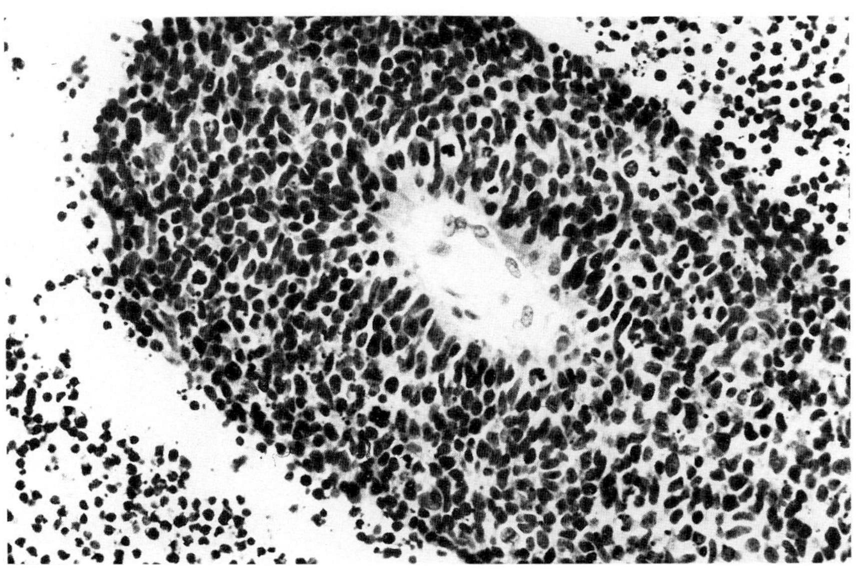

Fig. 8.23 (b) Higher power showing perivascular mantle of typical small hyperchromatic cells. H & E (×320).

Oat cell carcinomata

These occur most commonly in men and are derived from primary carcinomata of similar structure in the lung. They are composed of small, hyperchromatic cells which lack cohesion and are arranged in shoals, drifts and irregular lobules within an open fibrovascular spongework. Areas of necrosis in which residual viable cells form mantles around blood vessels are common (Fig. 8.23). The appearance can simulate that of a retinoblastoma and vascular staining with DNA salts also occurs occasionally as in retinoblastomata.

Adenocarcinomata

These are less common and are usually derived from sources other than breast such as gut, lung or thyroid. They are cystic papilliferous growths with columnar and cubical cells clothing slender branching connective tissue trabeculae and are thus unlike any other choroidal tumour. Their histological structure seldom provides any exact indication of their source (Fig. 8.24).

Cutaneous melanomata

Clinically evident metastases to the eye from cutaneous melanomata are rare. However, microscopic evidence of metastasis to the eye involving retina and choroid and associated with metastases in brain was noted in 30% of superficial spreading melanomata (Fishman *et al.*, 1976).

Lymphoma

Deposits of lymphoma, especially the large cell varieties formerly classified as 'reticulum cell sarcomata' (Chapter 16), are occasionally seen in the eye. Choroidal involvement usually occurs in association with involvement of the retina and brain.

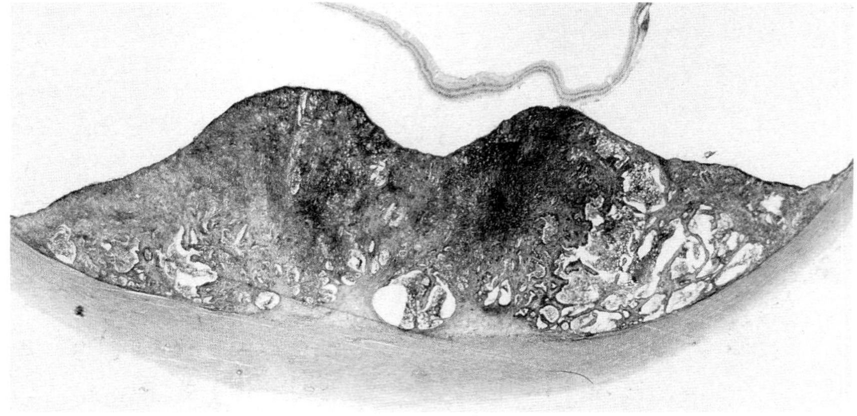

Fig. 8.24 Secondary from adenocarcinoma of lung. (a) Low power showing rather flat profile of growth.

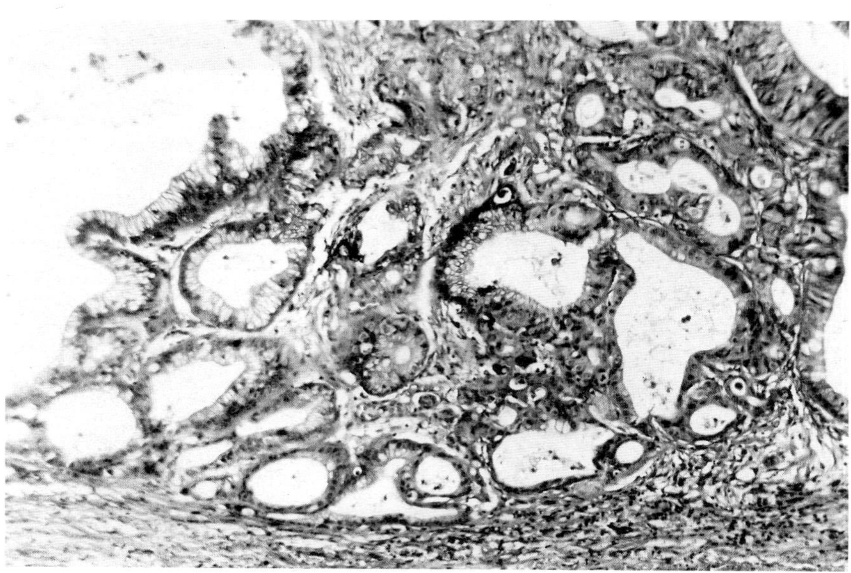

Fig. 8.24 (b) Higher power to show typical adenoid differentiation. H & E (×94).

BIBLIOGRAPHY

General

Andersen, S. R. (1976) Tumours of the eye and its adnexa. *Acta Ophthalmologica* **54**, 1–16.

Ashton, N. (1964) Primary tumours of the iris. *British Journal of Ophthalmology* **48**, 650–668.

Boniuk, M., ed. (1964) *Ocular and Adnexal Tumours*, Section III. C. V. Mosby Co., St Louis.

Jakobiec, F. A., ed. (1978) *Ocular and Adnexal Tumours*. Aesculapius Publishing Co., Birmingham, Ala.

Reese, A. B. (1976) *Tumours of the Eye*, 3rd Edn. Harper & Row, New York.

Benign melanocytic lesions

Albert, D. M., Searl, S. S., Forget, B., Lavin, P. T., Kirkwood, J. & Nordlund, J. J. (1983) Uveal findings in patients with cutaneous melanoma. *American Journal of Ophthalmology* **95**, 474–479.

Deutsch, T. A. & Jampol, L. M. (1985) Large drüse-like lesions on the surface of choroidal nevi. *Ophthalmology* **92**, 73–76.

Gamel, J. W., McLean, I. W. & Zimmerman, L. E. (1978) Melanocytic lesion of the posterior uvea: the impact of new pathologic concepts on prognosis and management. In *Ocular and Adnexal Tumours*, ed. F. A. Jakobiec, pp 19–30. Aesculapius Publishing Co., Birmingham, Ala.

Gonder, J. R., Augsburger, J. J., McCarthy, E. F. & Shields, J. A. (1982) Visual loss associated with choroidal nevi. *Ophthalmology* **89**, 961–965.

Gonder, J. R., Shields, J. A. & Augsburger, J. J. (1982) A study to determine the prevalence rate of ocular melanocytosis. *Ophthalmology* **89**, 950–952.

Haas, B. D., Jakobiec, F. A., Iwamoto, T., Cox, M., Bernacki, E. G. & Pokorny, K. L. (1986) Diffuse choroidal melanocytoma in child. A lesion extending the spectrum of choroidal hamartomas. *Ophthalmology* **93**, 1632–1638.

Jakobiec, F. A., Moorman, L. T. & Jones, I. S. (1979) Benign epithelioid cell naevi of the iris. *Archives of Ophthalmology* **97**, 917–921.

Jakobiec, F. A. & Silbert, G. (1981) Are most iris 'melanomas' really naevi? *Archives of Ophthalmology* **99**, 2117–2132.

Juarez, C. P. & Tso, M. O. M. (1980) An ultrastructural study of melanocytomas (magnocellular naevi) of the optic disk and uvea. *American Journal of Ophthalmology* **90**, 48–62.

Lee, J. S., Smith, R. E. & Minckler, D. S. (1982) Scleral melanocytoma. *Ophthalmology* **89**, 178–182.

MacIlwaine IV, W. A., Anderson Jr., B. & Klintworth, G. K. (1979) Enlargement of a histologically documented choroidal naevus. *American Journal of Ophthalmology* **87**, 480–486.

Naumann, G. O. H., Hellner, K. & Naumann, L. (1971) Pigmented nevi of the choroid. Clinical study of secondary changes in the overlying tissues. *Transactions of the American Academy of Ophthalmology and Otolaryngology* **75**, 110–122.

Naumann, G., Yanoff, M. & Zimmerman, L. E. (1966) Histogenesis of malignant melanoma of the uvea. I. Histopathologic characteristics of naevi of the choroid and ciliary body. *Archives of Ophthalmology* **76**, 784–796.

Rosen, E. S. & Garner, A. (1969) Benign melanoma of the choroid. Recognition of malignant change using clinical photographic techniques. *British Journal of Ophthalmology* **53**, 621–626.

Samuels, S. L. (1965) Juvenile melanoma of iris and ciliary body. *Transactions of the American Academy of Ophthalmology and Otolaryngology* **69**, 1061–1063.

Scheie, H. G. & Yanoff, M. (1979) Iris naevus (Cogan–Reese) syndrome. *Archives of Ophthalmology* **93**, 963–970.

Shields, J. A. & Annesley Jr., W. H. (1977) Necrotic melanocytoma of iris with secondary glaucoma. *American Journal of Ophthalmology* **84**, 826–829.

Shields, J. A., Karan, D. S., Perry, H. D. & Donoso, L. A. (1985) Epithelioid cell naevus of the iris. *Archives of Ophthalmology* **103**, 235–237.

Thomas, C. I. & Purnell, E. W. (1970) Ocular melanocytoma. *American Journal of Ophthalmology* **67**, 79–86.

Malignant melanomata

General

Albert, D. M., Chang, M. A., Lamping, K., Weiter, J. & Sober, A. (1985) The dysplastic nevus syndrome. A pedigree with primary malignant melanomas of the choroid and skin. *Ophthalmology* **92**, 1728–1734.

Barr, C. C. (1978) Small melanomas of the choroid. In *Ocular and Adnexal Tumours*, ed. F. A. Jakobiec, pp 12–18. Aesculapius Publishing Co., Birmingham, Ala.

Barr, C. C., McLean, I. W. & Zimmerman, L. E. (1981) Uveal melanoma in children and adolescents. *Archives of Ophthalmology* **99**, 2133–2136.

Barry, D. R. (1973) Malignant melanoma of the choroid. A review of the histopathology of 100 cases. *Transactions of the Ophthalmological Society of the UK* **93**, 647–664.

Brown, G. C. & Shields, J. A. (1981) Mechanisms of optic disc swelling with diffuse choroidal melanomas: clinicopathologic correlations. *British Journal of Ophthalmology* **88**, 77–82.

Brownstein, S., Sheikh, K. M. & Lewis, M. G. (1976) Tumor-associated antibodies in the serum of patients with uveal melanoma. *Canadian Journal of Ophthalmology* **11**, 147–154.

Callender, G. R. (1931) Malignant melanotic tumours of the eye: a study of histologic types in 111 cases. *Transactions of the American Academy of Ophthalmology and Otolaryngology* **36**, 131–142.

Donoso, L. A., Nagy, R. M., Brockman, R. J., Augsburger, J. J., Shields, J. A., Berd, D. & Mastrangelo, M. J. (1983) Metastatic uveal melanoma. Hepatic cell-surface enzymes, isoenzymes and serum sialic acid levels in early metastatic disease. *Archives of Ophthalmology* **101**, 791–794.

Donoso, L. A., Shields, J. A., Augsburger, J. J., Whitman, J. & Arbizo, V. (1986) Antigenic and cellular heterogeneity of primary uveal malignant melanomas. *Archives of Ophthalmology* **104**, 106–110.

Epstein, G., Jacobson, A. & Levine, R. A. (1981) Tapioca melanoma of the iris arising from a ciliary body melanoma. *Annals of Ophthalmology* **12**, 163–167.

Folberg, R., Verdick, R., Weingeist, T. A. & Montague, P. R. (1986) The gross examination of eyes removed for choroidal and ciliary body melanomas. *Ophthalmology* **93**, 1643–1647.

Font, R. L., Spaulding, A. G. & Zimmerman, L. E. (1968) Diffuse malignant melanoma of the uveal tract: A clinicopathologic report of 54 cases. *Transactions of the American Academy of Ophthalmology and Otolaryngology* **72**, 877–894.

Gonder, J. R., Shields, J. A., Albert, D. M., Augsburger, J. J. & Lavin, P. T. (1982) Uveal melanoma associated with ocular and oculodermal melanocytosis. *Ophthalmology* **89**, 953–960.

Halasa, A. (1970) Malignant melanoma in a case of bilateral nevus of Ota. *Archives of Ophthalmology* **84**, 176–178.

Jensen, O. A. (1976) The 'Knapp–Rønne' type of malignant melanoma of the choroid. *Acta Ophthalmologica* **54**, 41–54.

Juster, R. P. & Char, D. H. (1986) Uveal melanoma: doubling time and mitotic index. *Archives of Ophthalmology* **104**, 174.

Lahav, M. & Gutman, I. (1978) Subretinal pigment cells in malignant melanoma of the choroid. *American Journal of Ophthalmology* **86**, 239–244.

Lambert, S. R., Char, D. H., Howes Jr., E., Crawford, J. B. & Wells, J. (1986) Spontaneous regression of a choroidal melanoma. *Archives of Ophthalmology* **104**, 732–734.

Leonard, B. C., Shields, J. A. & McDonald, P. R. (1975) Malignant melanomas of the uveal tract in children and young adults. *Canadian Journal of Ophthalmology* **10**, 441–449.

McLean, I. W., Foster, W. D., Zimmerman, L. E. & Gamel, J. W. (1983) Modifications of Callender's classification of uveal melanoma at the Armed Forces Institute of Pathology. *American Journal of Ophthalmology* **96**, 502–509.

McLean, I. W., Zimmerman, L. E. & Evans, R. M. (1978) Reappraisal of Callender's spindle A type of malignant melanoma of choroid and ciliary body. *American Journal of Ophthalmology* **86**, 557–564.

Margo, C. E. & McLean, I. W. (1984) Malignant melanoma of the choroid and ciliary body in black patients. *Archives of Ophthalmology* **102**, 77–79.

Michelson, J. B., Felberg, N. T. & Shields, J. A. (1976) Carcinoembryonic antigen. Its role in the evaluation of intraocular malignant tumours. *Archives of Ophthalmology* **94**, 414–416.

Morgan, G. (1973) The history and natural history of malignant melanoma of the uvea. *Transactions of the Ophthalmological Society of the UK* **93**, 71–78.

Noyes, W. D. (1978) Cutaneous melanoma and its relation to melanoma of the uveal tract. *Survey of Ophthalmology* **23**, 143–145.

Pheasant, T. R., Michelson, J. B., Shields, J. A. & Pro, J. M. (1979) Uveal melanoma occurring as fourth primary malignancy: case report. *Annals of Ophthalmology* **11**, 625–627.

Price, M. J., Bell, R. A., Willis, W. E. & Whiteman, D. W. (1981) Tapioca melanoma of the iris: clinicopathological correlation with results of fluorescein angiography. *Canadian Journal of Ophthalmology* **16**, 195–199.

Reese, A. B., Archila, E. A., Jones, I. S. & Cooper, W. C. (1970) Necrosis of malignant melanoma of the choroid. *American Journal of Ophthalmology* **69**, 91–104.

Rodrigues, M. M. & Shields, J. A. (1976) Malignant melanoma of the choroid with balloon cells. A clinicopathologic study of three cases. *Canadian Journal of Ophthalmology* **11**, 208–216.

Samuels, B. (1963) Detachment of the retina in early sarcoma (malignant melanoma) of the choroid. *Archives of Ophthalmology* **69**, 620–627.

Sanke, R. F., Collin, J. R. O., Garner, A. & Packard, R. B. S. (1981) Local recurrence of choroidal malignant melanoma following enucleation. *British Journal of Ophthalmology* **65**, 846–849.

Shields, C. L., Shields, J. A., Yarian, D. L. & Augsburger, J. J. (1987) Intracranial extension of choroidal melanoma via the optic nerve. *British Journal of Ophthalmology* **71**, 172–176.

Shields, J. A. & McDonald, P. R. (1973) Improvements in the diagnosis of posterior uveal melanomas. *Transactions of the American Ophthalmological Society* **71**, 206–209.

Stanford, G. B. & Reese, A. B. (1979) Malignant cells in the blood of eye patients. *Transactions of the American Academy of Ophthalmology and Otolaryngology* **75**, 102–109.

Starr, H. J. & Zimmerman, L. E. (1962) Extrascleral extension and orbital recurrence of malignant melanomas of the choroid and ciliary body. *International Ophthalmology Clinics* **2**, 369–385.

Sunba, M. S. N., Rahi, A. H. S., Garner, A., Alexander, R. A. & Morgan, G. (1980) Tumours of the anterior uvea. III. Oxytalan fibres in the differential diagnosis of leiomyoma and malignant melanoma of the iris. *British Journal of Ophthalmology* **64**, 867–874.

Sunba, M. S. N., Rahi, A. H. S. & Morgan, G. (1980) Tumours of the anterior uvea. I. Metastasizing malignant melanoma of the iris. *Archives of Ophthalmology* **98**, 82–85.

Sunba, M. S. N., Rahi, A. H. S., Morgan, G. & Holborow, E. J. (1980) Lymphoproliferative response as an index of cellular immunity in malignant melanoma of the uvea and its correlation with the histological features of the tumour. *British Journal of Ophthalmology* **64**, 576–590.

Walker, J. P., Weiter, J. J., Albert, D. M., Osborn, E. L. & Weichselbaum, R. R. (1979) Uveal malignant melanoma in three generations of the same family. *American Journal of Ophthalmology* **88**, 723–726.

Wallow, I. H. L. & Tso, M. (1972) Proliferation of the retinal pigmented epithelium over malignant choroidal tumours. *American Journal of Ophthalmology* **73**, 914–926.

Wilhelm, J. L. & Zakov, Z. N. (1982) Choroidal malignant melanoma with liver metastases before enucleation. *Annals of Ophthalmology* **14**, 789–796.

Wolter, J. R. (1983) Orbital extension of choroidal melanoma: within a long posterior ciliary nerve. *Transactions of the American Ophthalmological Society* **81**, 44–59.

Yanoff, M. & Zimmerman, L. E. (1967) Malignant melanoma of the uvea. II. Relationship of uveal naevi to malignant melanomas. *Cancer* **20**, 493–507.

Zakka, K. A., Foos, R. Y. & Sulit, H. (1979) Metastatic tapioca iris melanoma. *British Journal of Ophthalmology* **63**, 744–749.

Prognosis

Albert, D. M. (1978) National Eye Institute — melanoma conference. *American Journal of Ophthalmology* **87**, 422–425.

Davidorff, F. H. & Lang, J. R. (1977) Lymphocytic infiltration in choroidal melanoma and its prognostic significance. *Transactions of the Ophthalmological Society of the UK* **97**, 394–401.

Flocks, M., Gerende, J. H. & Zimmerman, L. E. (1955) The size and shape of malignant melanomas of the choroid and ciliary body in relation to prognosis and histologic characteristics. *Transactions of the American Academy of Ophthalmology and Otolaryngology* **59**, 740–756.

Gamel, J. W. & McLean, I. W. (1984) Modern developments in histopathologic assessment of uveal melanomas. *Ophthalmology* **91**, 679–684.

Hagler, W. S., Jarrett, W. H. & Killian, J. H. (1977) The use of the 32P test in the management of malignant melanoma of the choroid: a five year follow-up study. *Transactions of the American Academy of Ophthalmology and Otolaryngology* **83**, OP 51–60.

Kidd, M. N., Lyness, R. W., Patterson, C. C., Johnston, P. B. & Archer, D. B. (1986) Prognostic factors in malignant melanoma of the choroid: a retrospective survey of cases occurring in Northern Ireland between 1965 and 1980. *Transactions of the Ophthalmological Society of the UK* **105**, 105–121.

McLean, I. W., Foster, W. D. & Zimmerman, L. E. (1977) Prognostic factors in small malignant melanomas of choroid and ciliary body. *Archives of Ophthalmology* **95**, 48–58.

McLean, I. W., Foster, W. D. & Zimmerman, L. E. (1980) Inferred natural history of uveal melanomas. *Investigative Ophthalmology* **19**, 760–770.

Migdal, C. (1983) Effect of method of enucleation on the prognosis of choroidal melanoma. *British Journal of Ophthalmology* **65**, 385–388.

Pach, J. M., Robertson, D. M., Taney, B. S., Martin, J. A., Campbell, R. J. & O'Brien, P. C. (1986) Prognostic factors in choroidal and ciliary body melanomas with extrascleral extension. *American Journal of Ophthalmology* **101**, 325–331.

Paul, E. V., Parnell, B. L. & Fraker, M. (1962) Prognosis of malignant melanoma of the choroid and ciliary body. *International Ophthalmology Clinics* **2**, 387–402.

Rahi, A. H. S. & Agrawal, P. K. (1977) Prognostic parameters in choroidal melanomata. *Transactions of the Ophthalmological Society of the UK* **97**, 368–372.

Shammas, H. F. & Blodi, F. C. (1977) Prognostic factors in choroidal and ciliary body melanomas. *Archives of Ophthalmology* **95**, 63–69.

Wagoner, M. D. & Albert, D. M. (1982) The incidence of metastases from untreated ciliary body and choroidal melanoma. *Archives of Ophthalmology* **100**, 930–940.

Mortality

Greer, C. H., Buckley, C., Buckley, J., Ramsay, R. & La Nauze, J. (1981) An Australian choroidal melanoma survey. Factors affecting survival following enucleation. *Australian Journal of Ophthalmology* **9**, 255–261.

Jensen, O. A. (1982) Malignant melanomas of the human uvea. 25-year follow-up of cases in Denmark, 1943–1952. *Acta Ophthalmologica* **60**, 161–182.

Lang, J. R. (1977) Lost to follow-up. *Archives of Ophthalmology* **95**, 1082.

Packard, R. B. (1980) Pattern of mortality in choroidal malignant melanoma. *British Journal of Ophthalmology* **64**, 565–575.

Seigel, D., Myers, M., Ferris III, F. & Steinhorn, S. C. (1979) Survival rates after enucleation of eyes with malignant melanoma. *American Journal of Ophthalmology* **87**, 761–765.

Thomas, J. V., Green, W. R. & Maumenee, A. E. (1979) Small choroidal melanomas. A long term follow-up study. *Archives of Ophthalmology* **97**, 861–864.

Management

Apple, D. J. & Blodi, F. C. (1980) Pathological observations and clinical approach to uveal melanomas. In *Ocular Pathology Update*, ed. D. H. Nicholson, pp 213–234. Masson, New York.

Burton, T. C. (1976) Iatrogenic breaks in Bruch's membrane in choroidal melanoma. *Transactions of the American Academy of Ophthalmology and Otolaryngology* **81**, OP 841–848.

Damato, E. & Foulds, W. S. (1986) Ciliary body tumours and their management. *Transactions of the Ophthalmological Society of the UK* **105**, 257–264.

Forrest, A. W. (1978) Iridocyclectomy for ciliary body tumours. In *Ocular and Adnexal Tumours*, ed. F. A. Jakobiec, pp 46–60 Aesculapius Publishing Co., Birmingham, Ala.

Fraunfelder, F. T., Boozman III, F. W., Wilson, R. S. & Thomas, A. H. (1977) No-touch technique for intraocular malignant melanomas. *Archives of Ophthalmology* **95**, 1616–1620.

Fraunfelder, F. T. & Wilson, R. S. (1978) A new approach for intraocular malignancy: the 'no-touch' enucleation. In *Ocular and Adnexal Tumours*, ed. F. A. Jakobiec, pp 39–45. Aesculapius Publishing Co., Birmingham, Ala.

Gass, J. D. M. (1980) Changing concepts of natural course and management of uveal melanomas. In *Ocular Pathology Update*, ed. D. H. Nicholson, pp 227–234. Masson, New York.

Hogan, M. J. (1964) Clinical aspects, management and prognosis of melanomas of the uvea and optic nerve. In *Ocular and Adnexal Tumors*, ed. M. Boniuk, pp 203–302. C. V. Mosby Co., St Louis.

Jakobiec, F. A. (1979) A moratorium on enucleation for choroidal melanomas? *American Journal of Ophthalmology* **87**, 842–846.

Kersten, R. C., Anderson, R. L. & Blodi, F. C. (1985) The role of orbital exenteration in choroidal melanoma with extrascleral extension. *Ophthalmology* **92**, 436–443.

Manschot, W. A. & van Peperzeel, H. A. (1980) Choroidal melanoma. Enucleation or observation? A new approach. *Archives of Ophthalmology* **98**, 71–77.

Manschot, W. A. & Van Strik, R. (1987) Is irradiation a justifiable treatment of choroidal melanoma? An analysis of published results. *British Journal of Ophthalmology* **71**, 348–352.

Maumenee, A. E. (1979) An evaluation of enucleation in the management of uveal melanomas. *American Journal of Ophthalmology* **87**, 846–847.

Meyer, E., Navon, D. & Zonis, S. (1987) The role of carcinoembryonic antigen in surveillance of patients with choroidal malignant melanoma: A prospective study. *Annals of Ophthalmology* **19**, 24–25.

Shields, J. A. (1977) Current approaches to the diagnosis and management of choroidal melanomas. *Survey of Ophthalmology* **21**, 443–463.

Zimmerman, L. E. (1979) Discussion of presentations by Dr G. Kara; Drs G. Peyman and M. Raichand; Dr D. M. Albert *et al.*; Dr E. Malbran *et al.*; and Dr L. Joffe *et al. Journal of the American Academy of Ophthalmology* **86**, 1079–1083.

Zimmerman, L. E. (1980) Metastatic disease from uveal melanomas. A review of current concepts concerning future research and prevention. *Transactions of the Ophthalmological Society of the UK* **100**, 34–54.

Zimmerman, L. E. & Mclean, I. W. (1970) An evaluation of enucleation in the management of uveal melanomas. *American Journal of Ophthalmology* **87**, 741–760.

Zimmerman, L. E. & Mclean, I. W. (1979) Metastatic disease from untreated uveal melanomas. *American Journal of Ophthalmology* **88**, 524–534.

Zimmerman, L. E. & Mclean, I. W. (1980) A comparison of progress in the management of retinoblastomas and uveal melanomas. In *Ocular Pathology Update*, ed. D. H. Nicholson, pp 191–212. Masson, New York.

Zimmerman, L. E. & Mclean, I. W. (1984) Do growth and onset of symptoms of uveal melanomas indicate subclinical metastasis. *Ophthalmology* **91**, 685–691.

Zimmerman, L. E., Mclean, I. W. & Foster, W. D. (1978) Does enucleation of the eye containing a malignant melanoma prevent or accelerate the dissemination of tumour cells. *British Journal of Ophthalmology* **62**, 420–425.

Diagnostic problems

Baurmann, H, Schlieter, F. & Bonnin, P. (1978) Irrtumer in der fluoreszangiographischen Diagnostik subretinaler Krankheitsprozesse. *Bucherei der Augenarztes* **73**, 91–96.

Ferry, A. P. (1964) Lesions mistaken for malignant melanomas of the posterior uvea. *Archives of Ophthalmology* **72**, 463–469.

Frazer, D. J. & Front, R. L. (1979) Ocular inflammation and haemorrhage as initial manifestations of uveal malignant melanoma. *Archives of Ophthalmology* **97**, 1311–1314.

Freyler, H. & Egerer, I. (1977) Echography and the histological studies in various eye conditions. *Archives of Ophthalmology* **95**, 1387–1394.

Gass, J. D. M. (1977) Problems in the differential diagnosis of choroidal nevi and malignant melanomas. *Transactions of the American Academy of Ophthalmology and Otolaryngology* **83**, OP 19–48.

Harry, J. (1973) Errors in diagnosis. *Transactions of the Ophthalmological Society of the UK* **93**, 93–103.

Henke, V., Philip, W. & Naumann, G. O. H. (1986) Intraokulare Verknöcherungen bei klinisch unerwarteten malignen Melanomen der Uvea and bei Phthisis Bulbi. *Klinische Monatsblätter für Augenheilkunde* **189**, 243–246.

Michelson, J. B., Stephens, R. F. & Shields, J. A. (1979) Clinical conditions mistaken for metastatic cancer to the choroid. *Annals of Ophthalmology* **11**, 149–153.

Morgan, C. M. & Gragoudas, E. S. (1987) Limited choroidal haemorrhage mistaken for choroidal melanoma. *Ophthalmology* **94**, 41–46.

Pizzuto, D., deLuize, V. & Zimmerman, N. (1986) Choroidal malignant melanoma appearing as acute panophthalmitis. *American Journal of Ophthalmology* **101**, 249–251.

Robertson, D. M. & Campbell, R. J. (1979) Errors in the diagnosis of malignant melanomas of the choroid. *American Journal of Ophthalmology* **87**, 269–275.

Shields, J. A. & Font, R. L. (1972) Melanocytoma of the choroid clinically simulating a malignant melanoma. *Archives of Ophthalmology* **87**, 397–400.

Volcker, H. E. & Naumann, G. O. H. (1976) Klinisch unerwartete maligne Melanome der hinteren Uvea. *Klinische Monatsblätter für Augenheilkunde* **168**, 311–317.

Zimmerman, L. E. (1965) Macular lesions mistaken for malignant melanoma. *Transactions of the American Academy of Ophthalmology and Otolaryngology* **69**, 623–629.

Effects of treatment

Char, D. H. (1986) Radiation therapy for uveal melanomas involving the ciliary body. *Transactions of the Ophthalmological Society of the UK* **105**, 252–256.

Davidorff, F. H., Makley, T. A. & Lang, J. R. (1976) Radiotherapy of malignant melanoma. *Transactions of the American Academy of Ophthalmology and Otolaryngology* **81**, OP849–861.

Duvall, J. & Lucas, D. R. (1981) Argon laser and xenon arc coagulation of malignant choroidal melanomata: histological findings in 6 cases. *British Journal of Ophthalmology* **65**, 464–468.

Hidayat, A. A., LaPiana, F. G., Kramer, K. K., Whitmore, P. V., Wertz, F. D. & Rao, N. A. (1987) The effect of rapid freezing on uveal melanomas. *American Journal of Ophthalmology* **103**, 66–80.

Lee, W. R. (1987) Pseudomelanomas after conservative management of uveal melanomas. *Eye* **1**, 668–675.

MacFaul, P. A. (1977) Local radiotherapy in the treatment of malignant melanoma of the choroid. *Transactions of the Ophthalmological Society of the UK* **97**, 421–427.

MacFaul, P. A. & Morgan, G. (1977) Histopathological changes in malignant melanomas of the choroid after cobalt plaque therapy. *British Journal of Ophthalmology* **61**, 221–228.

Peyman, G. A. & Raichand, M. (1978) Resection of choroidal melanoma. In *Ocular and Adnexal Tumours*, ed. F. A. Jakobiec, pp 61–69. Aesculapius Publishing Co., Birmingham, Ala.

Other primary tumours

Brewitt, H., Huerkamp, B, & Richter, K. (1976) Ein Neurinom der Aderhaut. *Klinische Monatsblätter für Augenheilkunde* **169**, 750–754.

Lister, A. & Morgan, G. (1963) Choroidal haemangio-endothelioma. *British Journal of Ophthalmology* **47**, 215–221.

Smith, P. A., Damato, B. E. & Lyness, R. W. (1987) Anterior uveal neurilemmoma — a rare neoplasm simulating malignant melanoma. *British Journal of Ophthalmology* **71**, 34–40

Secondary tumours

Bloch, R. S. & Gartner, S. (1971) Metastatic carcinoma in eye. *Archives of Ophthalmology* **85**, 673–675.

Ferry, A. P. (1974) The biological behaviour of carcinoma metastatic to the eye and orbit. *Transactions of the American Ophthalmological Society* **71**, 373–425.

Fishman, M. L., Tomaszewski, M. M. & Kuwabara, T. (1976) Malignant melanoma of the skin metastatic to the eye. *Archives of Ophthalmology* **94**, 1309–1311.

Frank, K. W., Sugar, H. S., Sherman, A. L., Beckman, H. & Thomas, S. (1979) Anterior segment metastasis from an ovarian choriocarcinoma. *American Journal of Ophthalmology* **87**, 778–782.

Hutchison, D. S. & Smith, T. R. (1979) Ocular and orbital metastatic carcinoma. *Annals of Ophthalmology* **11**, 869–873.

Nelson, C. C., Hertzberg, B. S. & Klintworth, G. K. (1983) A histopathologic study of 716 unselected eyes in patients with cancer at the time of death. *American Journal of Ophthalmology* **95**, 788–793.

Lymphomata

Michelson, J. B., Michelson, P. E., Bordin, G. M. & Chisari, F. V. (1981) Ocular reticulum cell sarcoma. Presentation as retinal detachment with demonstration of monoclonal immunoglobulin light chains on the vitreous cells. *Archives of Ophthalmology* **99**, 1409–1411.

Nevins, R. C., Frey, W. & Elliott, J. H. (1968) Primary, solitary, intraocular reticulum sarcoma (microgliomatosis). *Transactions of the American Academy of Ophthalmology and Otolaryngology* **72**, 867–876.

Raju, V. K. & Green, W. R. (1982) Reticulum cell sarcoma of the uvea. *Annals of Ophthalmology* **14**, 555–560.

Chapter 9 The lens

DEVELOPMENT

The optic vesicle induces the development of the lens vesicle from surface epithelium. The cells of the posterior wall of the vesicle elongate to form the primary lens fibres and secondary fibres are then laid down in lamellae at the equator. The secondary fibres never become long enough to extend from anterior pole to posterior pole (Fig. 9.1). The junctions between the ends of the fibres at the poles are seen as suture lines. Initially, these are in the form of an erect Y anteriorly and an inverted Y posteriorly, but as more and more layers are added they assume more complex patterns. The fibres lose their nuclei as they mature, but nuclei persist as the 'lens bow' at the equator throughout life (Fig. 9.2). New fibres, albeit at diminishing rate, are generated throughout life. Since the cells cannot be 'desquamated', the lens increases in size slowly throughout life and trebles in weight between birth and the age of 80.

During early development, the lens has a vascular supply fed by the hyaloid artery, the tunica vasculosa lentis, remnants of which may still be seen in the newborn eye.

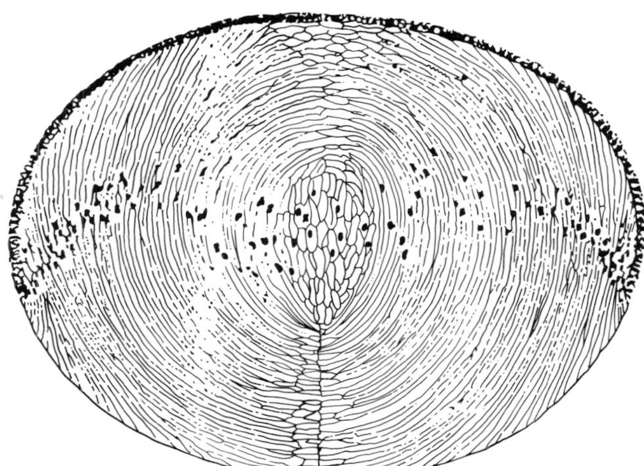

Fig. 9.1 Diagram of lens, in axial section, from a 48 mm human embryo (after Duke-Elder in Bellows, 1975) (×48). The primary lens fibres are compressed at the centre of the lens. They are enclosed by secondary fibres proliferating successively in the equatorial region. An early suture is seen at the junction of the secondary fibres.

NORMAL STRUCTURE

Lens capsule

The capsule is the basement membrane of the epithelium of the lens vesicle. It is thickest anteriorly and thinnest posteriorly. Under the light microscope, it has a hyaline appearance and is strongly PAS-positive. The capsule is freely permeable to water, small ions and protein molecules of 70 000 or less in molecular weight.

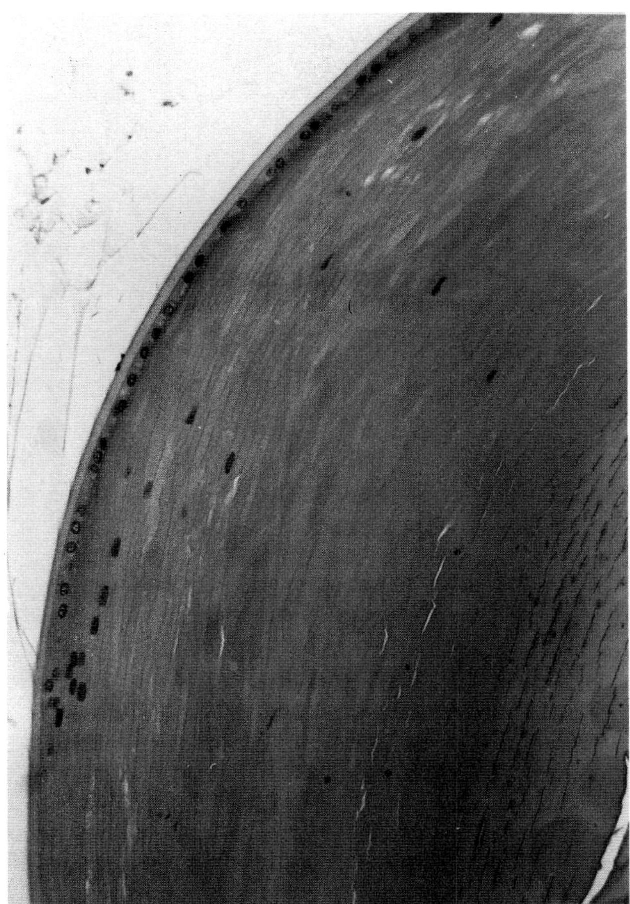

Fig. 9.2 Equator of adult lens to show nuclear bow and epithelium. H & E (×170).

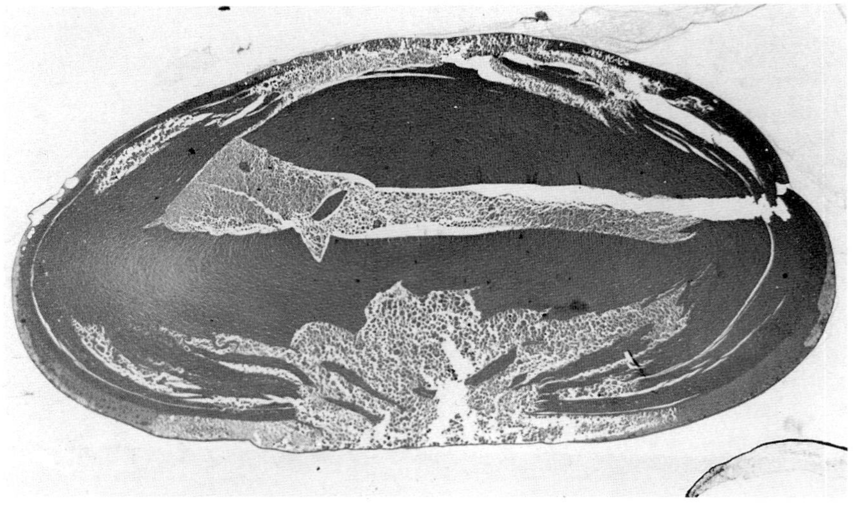

Fig. 9.3 Mature cataract. (a) Low power showing fragmentation of the fibres to form Morgagnian globules.

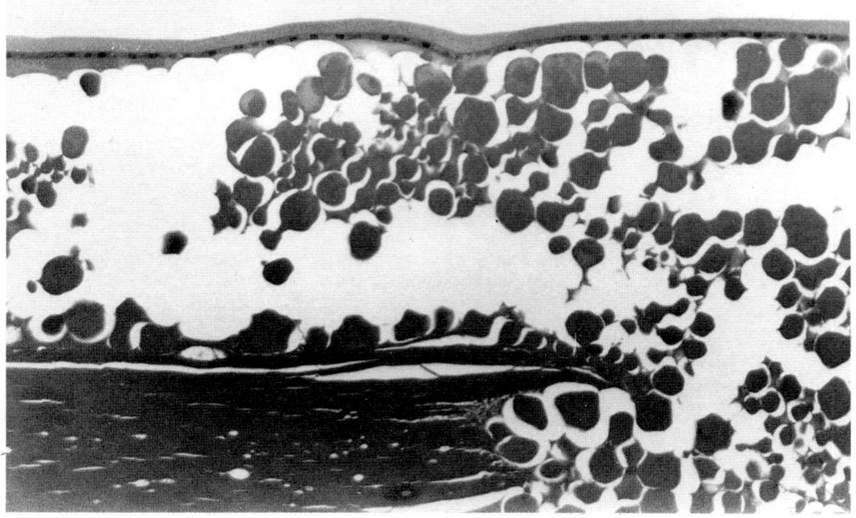

Fig. 9.3 (b) Higher power of anterior capsule showing fragmentation in more detail. Note thinning of capsular epithelium.

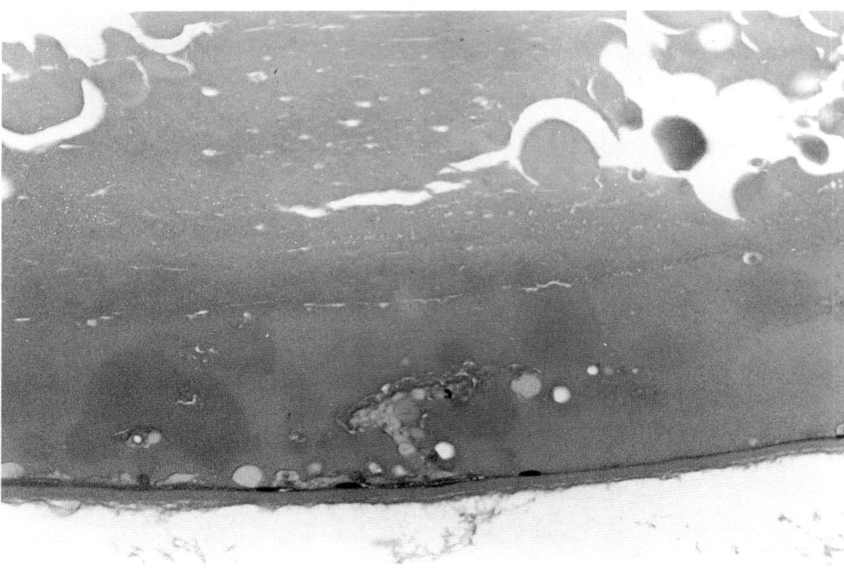

Fig. 9.3 (c) Posterior capsule showing flattened nuclei lying along it.

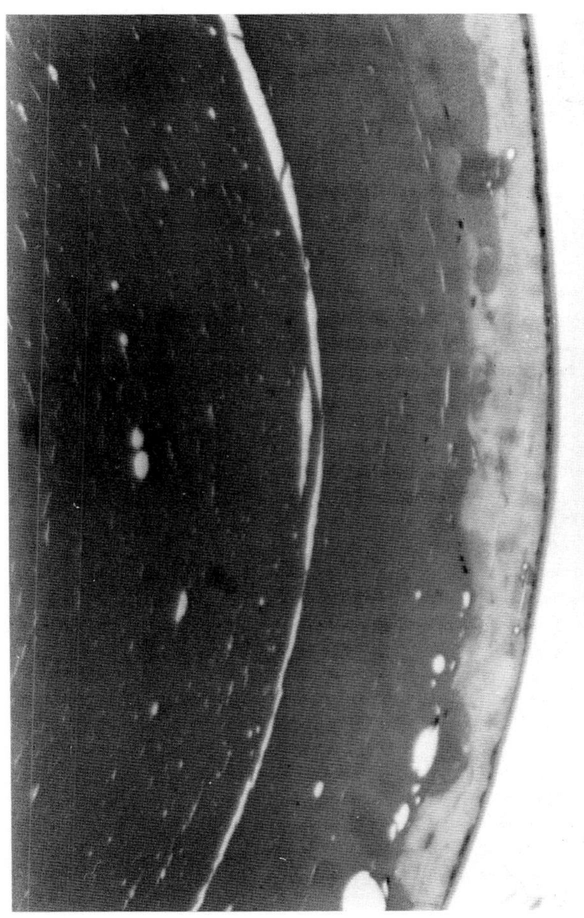

Fig. 9.3 (d) Equator showing absence of lens bow. A thin layer of epithelial nuclei can just be made out. Compare with Fig. 9.2. H & E (×210).

Lens epithelium

The epithelium consists of a single layer of cells located deep to the anterior capsule which appear cubical in sagittal sections and hexagonal in flat preparations. Terminal bar-like structures and interdigitating processes are present between the cells.

Labelling studies have shown that there is continuous slow movement of epithelial cells from a germinal region in the pre-equatorial zone into the lens bow. New fibres are formed in the lens bow throughout life (Fig. 9.2), hence the slow continuous increase in size already mentioned above.

Lens fibres

Lens fibres are hexagonal in cross-section. They are subdivided into cortical, mid-zonal and nuclear fibres. Only the cortical fibres of the lens bow are nucleated. They also contain organelles such as rough endoplasmic reticulum and fine fibrils which disappear in the deeper mid-zonal and nuclear fibres. Desmosomes and terminal bar-like structures are seen between the cortical fibres, but the mid-zone and nuclear fibres show an arrangement which progressively becomes more disorderly, and are joined by interdigitations between the cells. The fibres contain structural protein and the lens crystallins. A thin layer of glycosaminoglycan ground substance is present between them.

The lens is surprisingly malleable as is evident from the deformation which may be observed when it is in contact with a tumour or passes through a corneal perforation.

Lens pigment

The lens contains a yellowish pigment, hydroxykynurenine glucoside, derived from tryptophane which may act as a filter for blue/violet light. The content of this increases with age.

METABOLISM

Hydration of the normal lens is maintained by an active transport mechanism which regulates the balance of sodium and potassium ions. The transport of glucose and amino-acids is also probably linked to this mechanism.

The metabolic turnover of the lens is low. Glucose is the major and probably the only substrate and is metabolised to lactic acid mainly via the Emden–Meyerhof pathway. The oxidation of lactic acid via the tricarboxylic acid cycle occurs almost exclusively in the epithelium.

The lens contains an unusually high concentration of glutathione which can be synthesised and degraded locally. Glutathione is thought to have three functions:

1 Maintenance of the thiol (SH) groups of proteins in a reduced state so that the formation of high molecular weight aggregates of proteins linked by disulphide bonds is prevented. Random arrays of protein aggregates of 50 000 or greater in molecular weight may scatter light and cause opacification.

2 Protection of SH groups involved in the regulation of cation transport and membrane permeability.

3 Protection against oxidative damage by hydrogen peroxide which is normally present in aqueous humour at a very low concentration.

PATHOLOGICAL CHANGES

Cataractous lenses are smaller than normal lenses of comparable age because the development of the cataract is preceded by a cessation of the laying down of new fibres, but imbibition of water may lead to intumescence.

Many different types of cataract are described on

clinical and aetiological grounds, but the variety of pathological changes observed is quite limited, presumably because, apart from spontaneous or traumatic rupture of the capsule, they are the common end-result of various different disturbances in lens metabolism. For practical purposes, therefore, the general pathological responses can best be described in relation to the different components of the lens. They are illustrated in Figs 9.3–9.7.

Capsule

True exfoliation: is classically described in glass-blowers, but examples are rarely encountered in the laboratory. Splitting of the anterior capsule with peeling off of the superfical layer in scrolls is seen.

Pseudo-exfoliation: is not strictly a disease of the lens although deposits occur *inter alia* on the surface of the lens (Chapter 12).

Spontaneous rupture: the capsule may become thin in maturing cataracts and rupture spontaneously. This usually occurs posteriorly where it is normally thinnest.

Traumatic rupture: the capsule may be ruptured by a foreign body penetrating the eye. If the rupture is small, there will be local swelling and opacification, but actual escape of lens fibres may be limited and sealing is possible either by the iris or by local proliferation of the capsular epithelium. A large rupture is followed by rapid swelling and discharge of lens fibres into the anterior chamber. Cortical fibres break rapidly down and usually the debris can be cleared up by macrophages. However, the nucleus may take a long to disintegrate, especially in the elderly. Occasionally lens-induced endophthalmitis may result (Chapter 4).

Epithelium

The epithelium eventually disappears in cataractous lenses. Swollen and vacuolated fibres may be produced (Fig. 9.5a) and the lens bow is lost as germinal activity ceases (Fig. 9.3d). Nucleated cells are seen adjacent to the capsule posterior to the equator (Fig. 9.3c).

Proliferation of the capsular epithelium and subsequent metaplasia of the cells to fibrocyte-like cells which lay down layers of collagen and basement membrane material is common. A dense fibrous plaque (anterior subcapsular cataract) is thus formed which shrinks and causes the overlying capsule to become much folded (Fig. 9.4). In congenital cases, the proliferated fibrous tissue may assume a pyramidal shape (Fig. 9.5b). A similar process may occur under the posterior capsule, but is much less common. Subcapsular fibrosis is seen particularly in secondary cataracts associated with long-standing intraocular disease such as chronic uveitis and old retinal detachments.

Lens fibres

The superficial cortical fibres show swelling and vacuolation. The deeper cortical fibres fragment and clefts appear between them. Lens protein in the form of eosinophilic globules (Morgagnian globules) is released into clefts (Fig. 9.3a & b). The process spreads from the cortex towards the nucleus. The nucleus is slow to liquefy and in a hypermature (Morgagnian) cataract persists after all the cortex has been liquefied (Fig. 9.6). Sometimes imbibition of water occurs during the process of liquefaction so that the lens swells (intumescent cataract). This may result in pupillary block.

Brown discoloration is a conspicuous macroscopic feature and is probably due to the accumulatin of tryptophane degradation products such as hydroxykynurenine glycoside already referred to. The lens may become extremely dense and black (Fig. 9.7a).

A sclerotic nucleus has a dense hyaline appearance which is surprisingly unremarkable in histological sections (Fig. 9.7b). Characteristically it contains calcium oxalate crystals. Birefringent perinuclear retrodots containing calcium oxalate can be observed *in vivo* and *in vitro* in association with cataract in adult lenses, and it

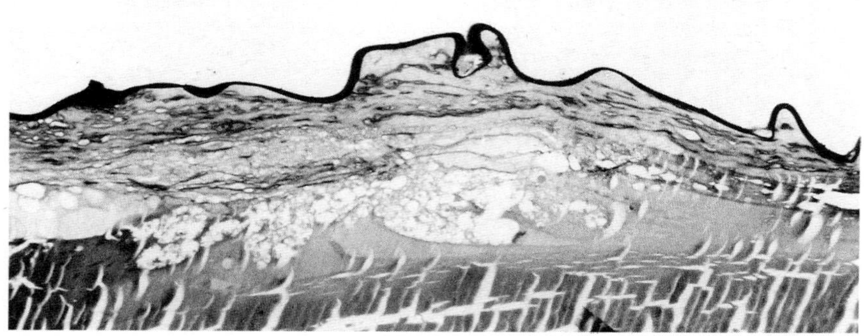

Fig. 9.4 Anterior subcapsular cataract. Fibrous metaplasia of the capsular epithelium to form a layer of collagen beneath the anterior capsule. Layers of PAS-positive material are present in the collagen. PAS/tartrazine (×64).

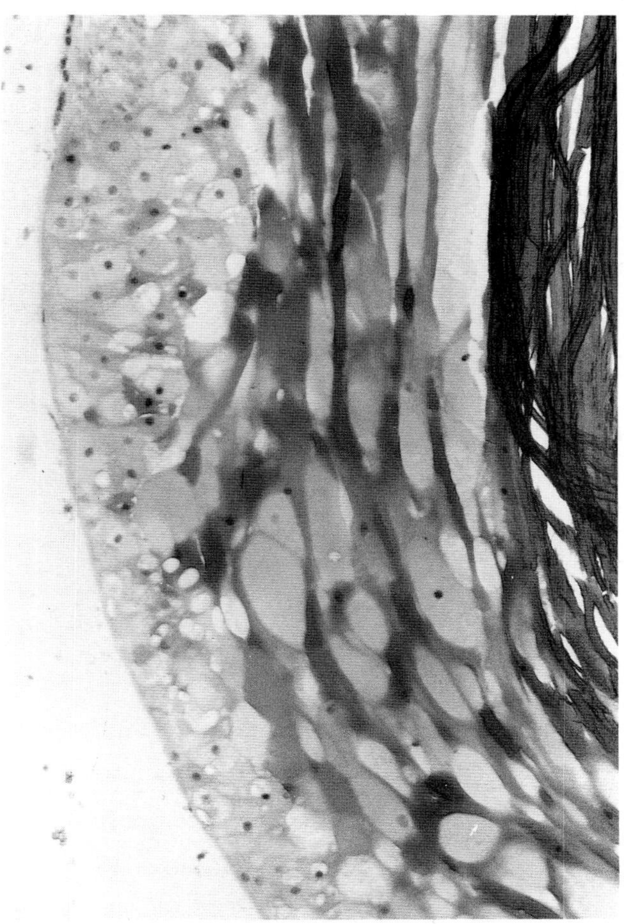

Fig. 9.5 Congenital cataract. (a) Showing production of abnormal fibres at the equator. H & E (×175).

has been suggested that the source is ascorbic acid which probably protects against 'oxidative stress' due to products of photo-oxidation (see below) (Bron & Brown, 1987). Dystrophic calcification is also common in cataracts of long standing.

Ultrastructurally, in senile cataracts the fibres become very dense. Interdigitations and interlocking processes become more numerous and irregular (Fig. 9.7c). In the cortex, globular bodies of varying size and process bodies from degenerating fibres are present in clefts between fibres. In the nucleus, the fibres become tightly packed together.

Complex but regular folding of the fibre membranes has also been observed to produce 'figure of eight' and 'tramline' patterns ultrastructurally as well as lamellar bodies resembling myelin figures.

SENILE CATARACT

The term is applied to cataracts developing in persons aged over 60. The changes are of a non-specific character as described above. Similar cataracts may develop at an earlier age for no apparent reason.

CATARACTA COMPLICATA

Selective opacification of the posterior cortical region occurs in systemic diseases such as myotonia congenita and Turner's syndrome and in ocular diseases such as longstanding uveitis and retinitis pigmentosa or as a complication of steroid therapy or radiation. Such localised cataracts have been known as cataracta complicata. However, they may occur in the absence of other evident disease.

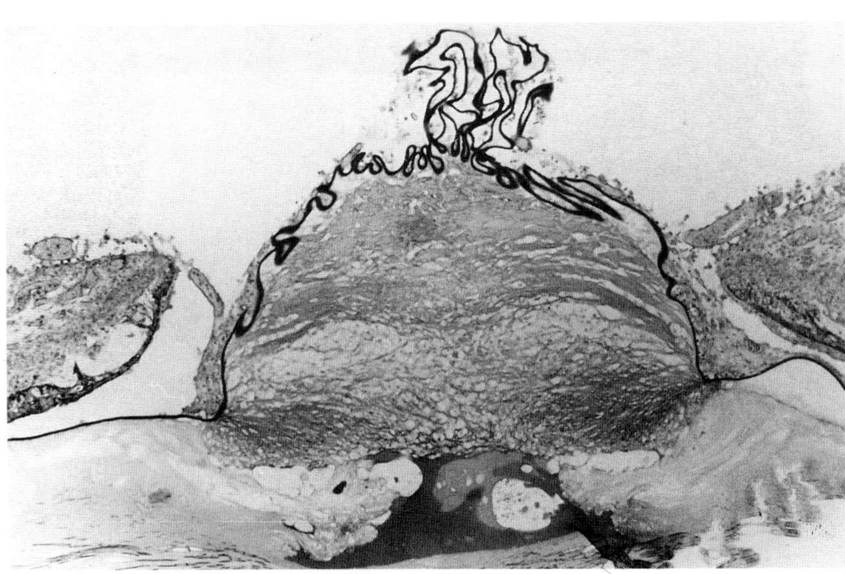

Fig. 9.5 (b) Showing subcapsular fibrosis with complicated folding of the capsule. PAS/tartrazine.

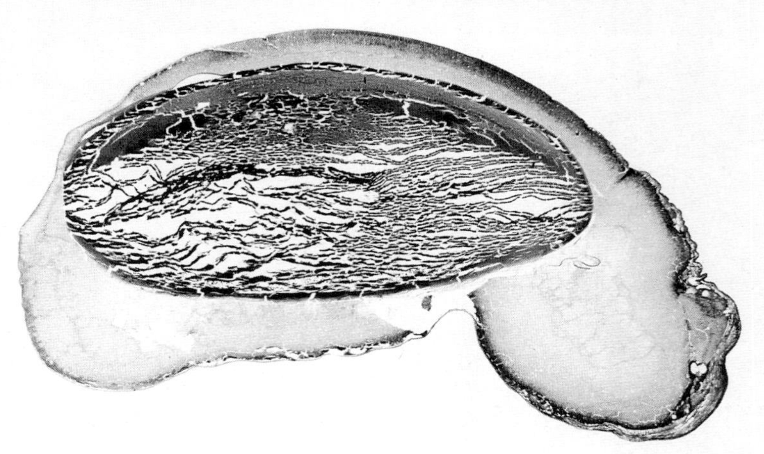

Fig. 9.6 Low power of hypermature cataract. Hard nucleus floating in sac of proteinacous fluid derived from liquefied cortex. H & E.

Observed pathological changes (Eshagian *et al.*, 1981) are liquefactive necrosis and aberrant migration of epithelial cells are of a non-specific character.

CONGENITAL CATARACTS

Anterior polar cataract

The clinical and pathological appearances resemble those of an acquired anterior subcapsular cataract (Fig. 9.5b). No cause is usually discovered, but occasionally the condition is transmitted as an autosomal dominant.

Lenticonus (lentiglobus)

The anterior or posterior surface of the lens has a central conical or hemispherical protuberance over which the capsule is thin, but the epithelium is usually normal.

The condition is usually bilateral. Anterior lenticonus predominantly affects males and may occur in Alport's

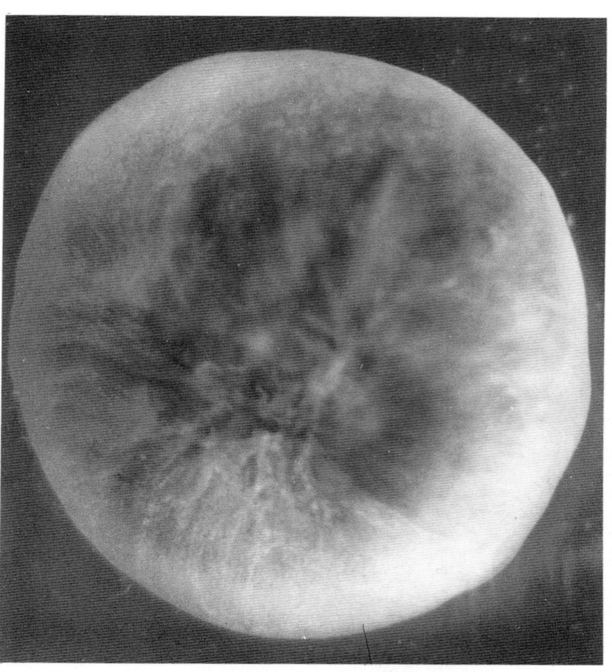

Fig. 9.7 Cataracta nigra. (a) Macroscopic pictures by reflected (left) and transmitted (right) light showing densely opaque lens.

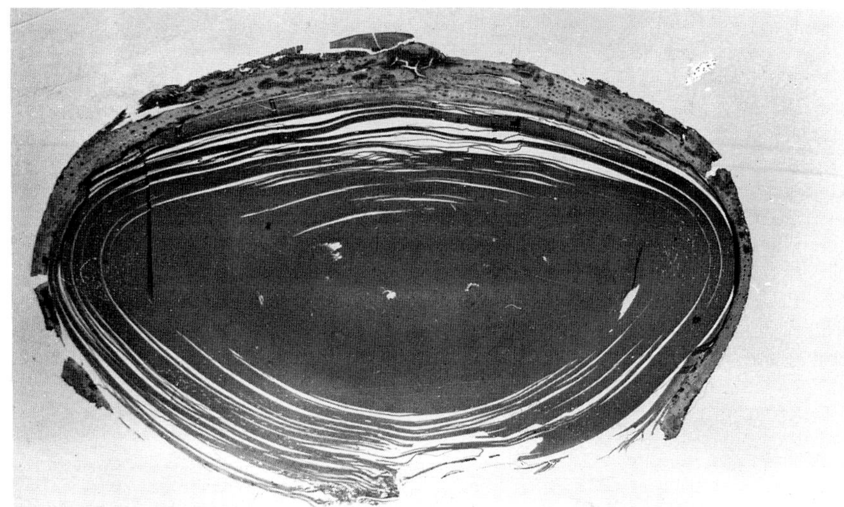

Fig. 9.7 (b) Low power showing hyaline appearance of nucleus. There is some factitious disruption of cortex. H & E.

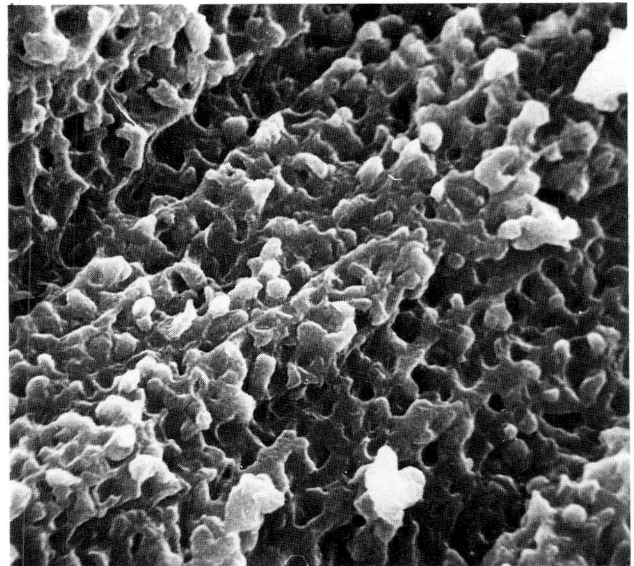

Fig. 9.7 (c) Scanning electron microscopic picture of mid-zonal fibres showing complicated interdigitating processes. (×4800)

syndrome (familial nephritis). Posterior lenticonus affects both sexes, but with a slight female preponderance.

Zonular (lamellar) cataract

Interference with the growth of lens fibres for a limited period may result in a layer of opaque fibres being laid down. These will initially be subcapsular, but, as the lens grows, will become progressively more deeply located in the cortex.

AETIOLOGICAL FACTORS IN CATARACTS

A considerable number of factors (so-called risk factors) have been identified which predispose to the development of cataracts, but, in only one of these (sorbitol pathway in sugar cataracts), has the mechanism been identified. These risk factors include:

1 Sunlight and ultraviolet light.
2 Ionising radiation.
3 Non-ionising radiation (microwave, infrared).
4 Drugs and chemicals (corticosteroids, phenothazines, miotic cholinergics, metals, etc.).
5 Diabetes.
6 Blood pressure.
7 Family history:
  (i) Families with high prevalence.
  (ii) Clear genetic inheritance.
8 Diarrhoea.
9 Malnutrition.
10 Renal failure.

POSSIBLE MECHANISMS OF CATARACT FORMATION

The physical basis of the transparency of the lens is a complex subject beyond the scope of this book. The commonly postulated mechanisms by which it may be disturbed are outlined only briefly.

Sugar cataracts

Fluctuations in blood sugar levels in diabetics often result in refractive changes in the lens. Glucose is converted to sorbitol by aldose reductase, the activity of which is significantly increased in diabetic lenses both in the rat and in man (see Akagi *et al.*, 1987). As this enzyme has a much lower affinity for glucose than hexokinase, most glucose is normally phosphorylated and metabolised via the Emden–Meyerhof pathway. However, if the blood/aqueous glucose is high, the hexokinase pathway is saturated and sorbitol, which does not diffuse readily through membranes, accumulates intracellularly. An osmotic gradient is thus set up which causes hydration of the lens. A high level of glucose in the lens may contribute to this gradient which is accentuated as the blood glucose falls. If the changes are severe enough opacification results.

A similar mechanism accounts for galactose cataracts. Galactose is converted to dulcitol by aldose reductase. However, the affinity of aldose reductase for galactose is greater than for glucose. Increased levels of galactose are thus more rapidly converted to dulcitol. Furthermore, sorbitol dehydrogenase, which converts sorbitol to fructose, is unable to metabolise dulcitol. The hyperosmotic effect of raised galactose levels is thus more severe and occurs more rapidly than that from raised glucose levels.

Sunlight and ultraviolet light

The possible association between high levels of exposure to sunlight and long wavelength ultraviolet light and cataract has been debated over many years.

Tryptophane may be converted to fluorophors. The production of these may involve the transfer of light energy to hypothetical receptors and result in free radical formation. Ultraviolet light can also lead to the formation of hydrogen peroxide and superoxide anions. A combination of these products may result in cataractous changes.

Ionising radiation

The threshold cataractogenic dose in man may be as low as 200 rads. Typically, radiation cataracts initially involve the posterior subcapsular region. The mechanism by which ionising radiation causes cataracts is unknown, though the generation of free radicals is thought to play a role. There is not complete concordance between findings in the experimental animal, but it has long been thought that radiation cataracts result from injury to the epithelial cells of the pre-equatorial germinative zone. This results in failure of the injured cells to form normal fibres and migration of aberrant fibres towards the poles of the lens. It is noteworthy that partial shielding of the lens has a protective effect and apparently facilitates some recovery even in the irradiated area.

Neither the histological changes nor the biochemical changes show specific features not seen in other types of cataract.

Corticosteroids

Prolonged systemic or topical administration of corticosteroids is well known to result in posterior lenticular opacities, though there is considerable individual variation in susceptibility. The opacities seldom cause severe impairment of vision and regression usually follows if treatment is stopped.

The mechanism which results in the formation of the opacities has been the subject of much experimental work and speculation (see Urban & Cotlier, 1987). Glucocorticoids apparently react with specific amino groups of the lens crystallins and induce a conformational change which unveils protein sulphydryl groups. These groups are then able to form disulphide bonds with the result that large light-scattering protein aggregates are formed.

POSSIBLE COMMON PATHWAYS

In conclusion, as already noted, many different pathways may lead to cataract formation, though the precise form the resultant cataract takes may vary. Some of those most commonly postulated have recently been summarised by Harding (1984) in a flowchart (Fig. 9.8).

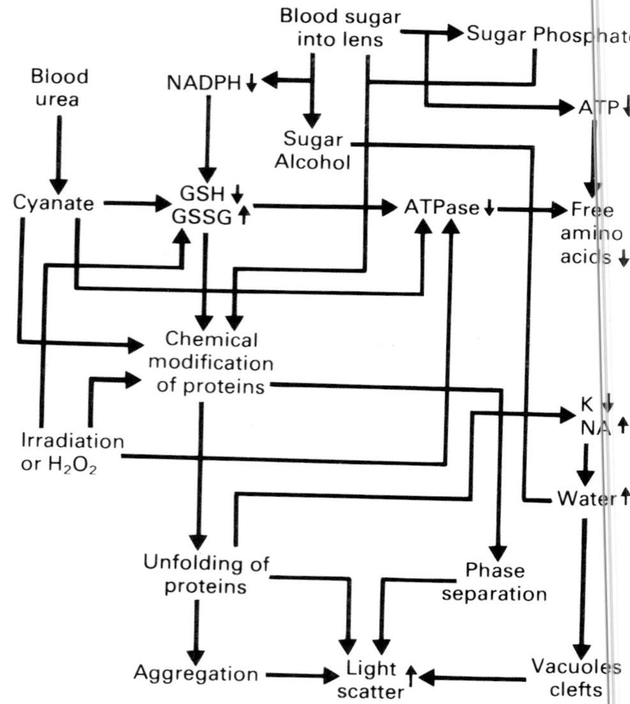

Fig. 9.8 Flow diagram showing possible common pathways in cataract formation. The vertical arrows indicate an increase in activity or content. (After Harding, 1984).

BIBLIOGRAPHY

Akagi, Y, Kador, P. F. & Kinoshita, J. H. (1987) Immunohistochemical localization for aldose reductase in diabetic lenses. *Investigative Ophthalmology and Visual Science* **28**, 163–167.

Bellows, J. G. (1975) *Cataract and Abnormalities of the Lens*. Grune & Stratton, New York.

Bron, A. J. & Brown, N. A. P. (1987) Perinuclear lens retrodots: a role for ascorbate in cataractogenesis. *British Journal of Ophthalmology* **71**, 86–95.

Bron, A. J. & Habgood, J. O. (1976) Morgagnian cataract. *Transactions of the Ophthalmological Society of the UK* **96**, 265–277.

Chylack, L. T. (1984) Mechanisms of senile cataract formation. *Ophthalmology* **91**, 596–602.

Clayton, R. M., Seth, C. J., Phillips, C. I., Bartholomew, R. S. & Reid, J. McK. (1984) Epidemiological and other studies in the assessment of factors contributing to cataractogenesis. In *Human Cataract Formation* (Ciba Foundation Symposium No. 106) eds J. Nugent & J. Whelan, pp 25–40. Pitman, London.

Dilley, K. J., Bron, A. J. & Habgood, J. O. (1976) Anterior and posterior subcapsular cataract in a patient with retinitis pigmentosa: a light-microscopic and ultrastructural study. *Experimental Eye Research* **22**, 155–167.

Dillon, J. & Spector, A. (1980) A comparison of aerobic and anaerobic photolysis of lens protein. *Experimental Eye Research* **31**, 591–599.

Eshagian, J. & Streeten, B. W. (1980) Human posterior subcapsular cataract. An ultrastructural study of the posteriorly migrating cells. *Archives of Ophthalmology* **98**, 134–143.

Eshagian, J., Rafferty, N. S. & Goossens, W. (1981) Human cataracta complicata. *Ophthalmology* **88**, 155–163.

Hanna, C. & O'Brien, J. E. (1961) Cell production and migration in the epithelial layer of the lens. *Archives of Ophthalmology* **66**, 103–107.

Hanna, C. & O'Brien, J. E. (1963) Lens epithelial proliferation and migration in radiation cataracts. *Radiation Research* **19**, 1–11.

Harding, J. J. (1984) General discussion. In *Human Cataract Formation* (Ciba Foundation Symposium No. 106) eds J. Nugent & J. Whelan, p 158. Pitman, London.

Harding, J. J. & Rixon, K. C. (1980) Carbamylation of lens proteins: a possible factor in cataractogenesis in some tropical countries. *Experimental Eye Research* **31**, 567–571.

Iwata, S. & Horiuchi, M. (1980) Studies on experimental cataracts induced by ionophores: *in vitro* effects of Nigericin and Valinomycin on the lenses in mice. *Experimental Eye Research* **31**, 543–541.

Jahn, C. E., Janke, M., Winkowski, H., v. Bergman, K., Leiss, O. & Hockwin, O. (1986) Identification of metabolic risk factors for posterior subcapsular cataract. *Ophthalmic Research* **18**, 112–116.

Kador, P. F. & Kinoshita, J. H. (1984) Diabetic and galactosaemic cataracts. In *Human Cataract Formation* (Ciba Foundation Symposium No. 106) eds J. Nugent & J. Whelan, pp 110–123. Pitman, London.

Littleton, J. T., Durizch, M. L. & Perry, N. (1978) Radiation protection of the lens for patients and users. *Radiology* **129**, 795–798.

Pirie, A., ed. (1962) *Lens Metabolism in Relation to Cataract*. Academic Press, London.

Pirie, A. & Drance, S. M. (1959) Modification of X-ray damage to the lens by partial shielding. *International Journal of Radiation Biology* **1**, 293–304.

Reddy, V. N. & Giblin, F. J. (1984) Metabolism and function of glutathione in the lens. In *Human Cataract Formation* (Ciba Foundation Symposium No. 106) eds J. Nugent & J. Whelan, pp 65–87. Pitman, London.

Richards, R. D., Riley, E. F. & Leinfelder, P. J. (1956) Lens changes following X-irradiation of single and multiple quadrants. *American Journal of Ophthalmology* **42**, 44–50.

Spector, A. (1984) The search for a solution to senile cataracts. *Investigative Ophthalmology and Visual Science* **25**, 130–146.

Urban, R. C. & Cotlier, E. (1987) Cortico-steroid induced cataracts. *Survey of Ophthalmology* **31**, 102–110.

van Heynigen, R. (1976) Experimental studies on cataract. *Investigative Ophthalmology* **15**, 685–679.

von Sallman, L. (1952) Experimental studies on early lens changes after roentgen irradiation. III. Effect of X-radiation on the mitotic activity and nuclear fragmentation of lens epithelium in normal and cysteine-treated rabbits. *Archives of Ophthalmology* **47**, 305–320.

Worgul, B. V., Merriam, G. R., Szechter, A. & Srinivasan, D. (1976) Lens epithelium and radiation cataract. I. Preliminary studies. *Archives of Ophthalmology* **94**, 996–999.

Chapter 10 The retina

NORMAL STRUCTURE

The retina is anatomically part of the brain and, strictly speaking, comprises all those structures derived from the optic vesicle, namely:

1 Pars neuralis.
2 Pars ciliaris.
3 Pars iridica.

In practice, the term 'retina' now effectively means 'pars neuralis retinae'. The retina thus understood is a highly complex arrangment of photoreceptor cells, neurones, glia and blood vessels of which only a brief account can be given here (see Fig. 10.1).

Photoreceptor cells

All photoreceptor cells consist of an outer segment, an inner segment, a cell body and a synaptic expansion. The outer segment, which is a cilium modified to form a photon-trapping device, comprises a continuous membrane folded to form a dense stack of disc-shaped double membranes attached to the inner segment by a thin rootlet. In rods, the arrangement of the membrane stacks is orderly and continuous renewal from the base and phagocytosis by pigmented epithelium at the tip occurs. In cones, the outer segment is shorter and the lamellar arrangement less orderly. Renewal does not occur in the same clearcut manner. The outer segments stain positively by the PAS method and are apparently embedded in a proteoglycan matrix which stains by Hale's colloidal iron method.

The inner segment is the metabolically active 'power house' of the cells which contains mitochondria, a Golgi complex, endoplasmic reticulum and free ribosomes.

The cell body and nucleus of the photoreceptor lie on the vitreous side of the internal limiting membrane and in aggregate form the outer nuclear layer.

The photoreceptor cells terminate in the outer plexiform layer in a synaptic expansion — the rod spherule or cone pedicle. Dendrites from neurones in the inner nuclear layer form synapses with these expansions. Cones receive several dendrites, rods may receive only one. This is precisely the opposite of what had apparently been demonstrated by the Cajal silver staining method. In the foveola, the cones become thinner and their outer segments longer.

Macular yellow pigment

The yellow colour of the macula is due to the xanthophyllic pigment, lutein, which is present in greatest concentration in the inner and outer plexiform layers. It

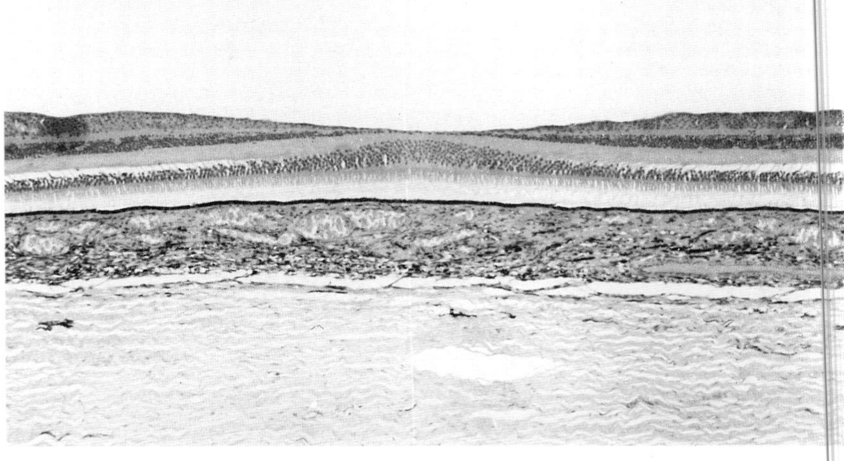

Fig. 10.1. Structure of normal retina (specimen by courtesy of Professor W. R. Lee). (a) Low power view of fovea. ILM = inner limiting membrane, GC = ganglion cells, INL = inner nuclear layer, OF = outer plexfiform layer (Henle's fibre layer), ONL = outer nuclear layer, OLM = outer limiting membrane, PR = photoreceptors, PE = pigmented epithelium. (The choroid appears abnormally thick because the eye was affected by neurofibromatosis.)

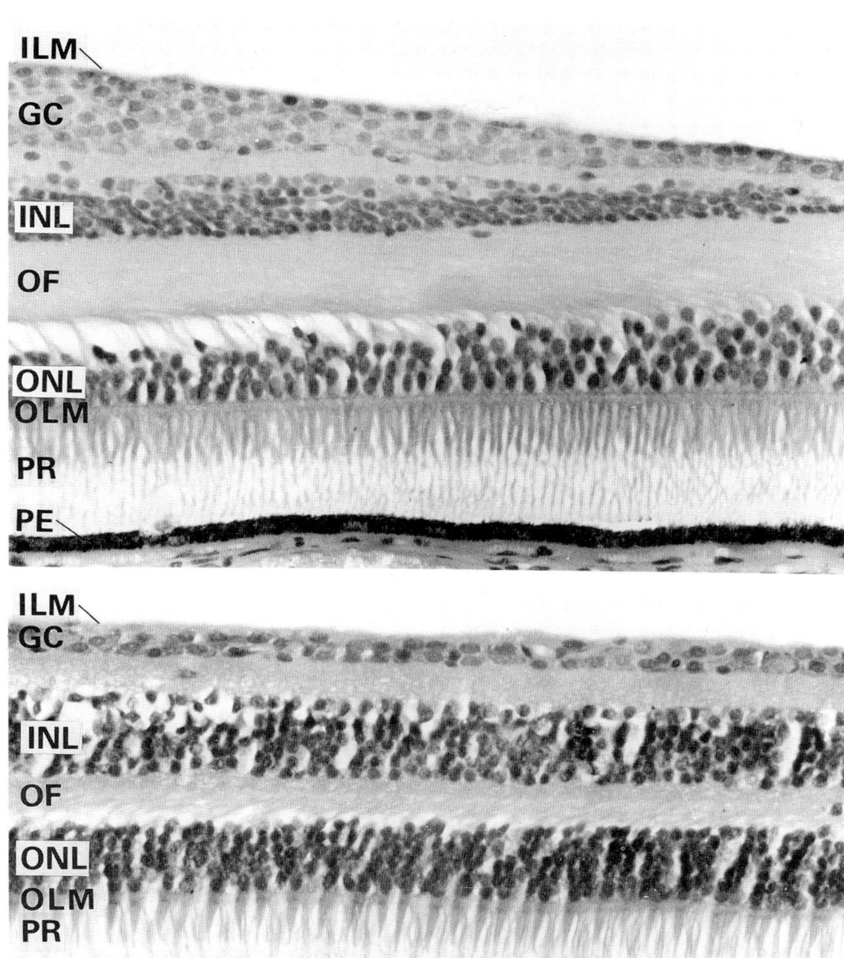

Fig. 10.1 (b) High power to show layers of retina in detail. H & E (×320). The nerve fibres in the outer plexiform layer run almost parallel to the retinal surface. The foveal cones are extremely slender and look morphologically like rods.

Fig. 10.1 (c) Parafoveal retina showing fewer rows of ganglion cells and rods and cones clearly distinguishable. H & E (×320).

Fig. 10.1 (d) (*Below*) SEM of parafoveal rods (R) and cones (C) (×3800).

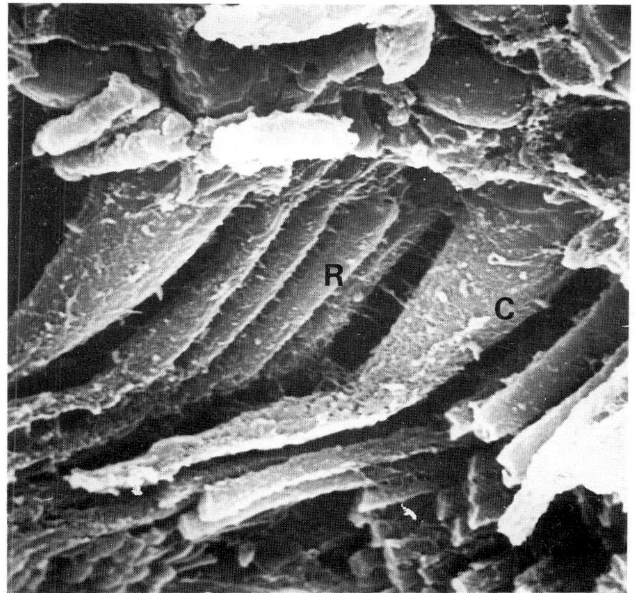

filters out blue light and thus improves chromatic aberration and protects against actinic damage, but a possible role in hereditary or acquired maculopathies has not been established.

Inner nuclear layer

The most numerous cells are the bipolar neurones whose dendrites form synapses in the outer plexiform layer with the photoreceptor cells and in the inner synaptic layer with the ganglion cells. Amacrine cells are large cells with lobulate nuclei which do not have axons, but whose processes make numerous synaptic connections in the inner plexiform layer. The somewhat analogous horizontal cells send processes along the outer border of the inner nuclear layer which enter the synaptic expansions of the photoreceptor cells.

Ganglion cell layer

This layer is composed of large neurones which form a single layer in much of the retina, but in the foveola there are 5–7 rows. The cell bodies contain granular endoplasmic reticulum (Nissl substance). The axons of these cells form the inner fibre layer and eventually run in the optic nerve to the brain. As already mentioned, their dendritic processes form synapses with those of the bipolar cells.

Retinal glia

The principal glial cells of the retina are the Müller fibres. These extend from the inner surface of the retina where their footplates are applied to the internal limiting membrane and to the outer limiting membrane which is formed by terminal bars between the fibres. The nucleus of the cells is located in the inner nuclear layer. Processes extend from the bodies of the cells to envelope the neuronal components of the retina and from the outer limiting membrane to form 'fibre baskets' along the inner segments of the photoreceptors. The body of the cell has a fibrillary structure like a fibrous astrocyte. Smaller astrocytes, mostly fibrous and protoplasmic are found only in the inner layers.

The pigmented epithelium

The pigmented epithelium is a single layer of hexagonal cells derived from the outer layer of the primary optic vesicle. The basal lamina of the cells shows numerous infoldings. From the apex of the cells, microvillous processes extend around the outer segments of the photoreceptors. The cells are linked by terminal bars located towards the apex. The nucleus and mitochondria are located in the base of the cell, while melanin granules are located in the body and apex. The cytoplasm also contains endoplasmic reticulum and free ribosomes.

Pigmented epithelial cells are phagocytic. Phagosomes containing membrane stacks derived from photoreceptor outer segments are often present. Lipofuscin bodies are autofluorescent granules which represent the residual bodies of phagolysosomes involved in the disposal of outer segment material. They correspond to the 'age pigment' found in brain and increase with age.

Melanin granules are synthesised *in utero* and mature in the first decade. They appear to remain more or less static. However, fusion with lysosomes gives rise to melanolysosomes and, in older eyes, complex granules are formed by the fusion of melanolysosomes with lipofuscin granules to form complex melanolipofuscin granules. This suggests that there is a dynamic interrelationship

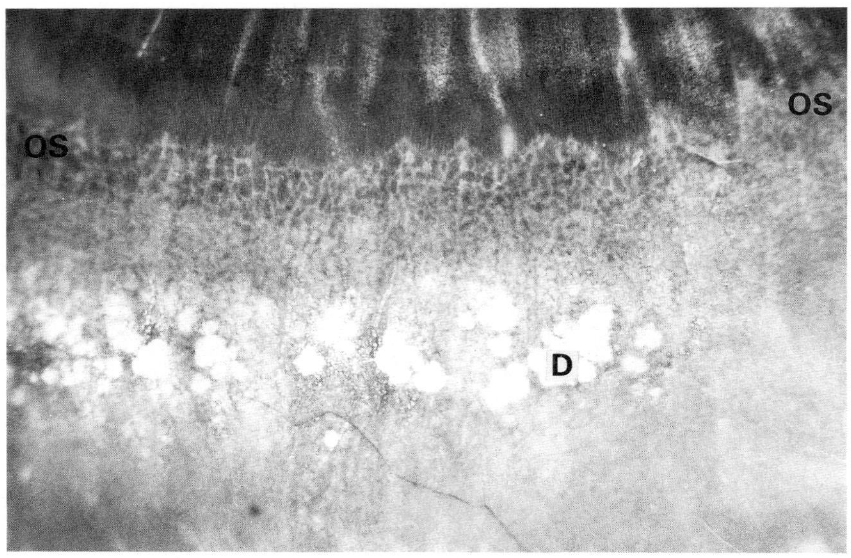

Fig. 10.2 Typical peripheral cystoid degeneration (and drüsen). (a) Macroscopic appearance. OS = ora serrata, D = drüsen.

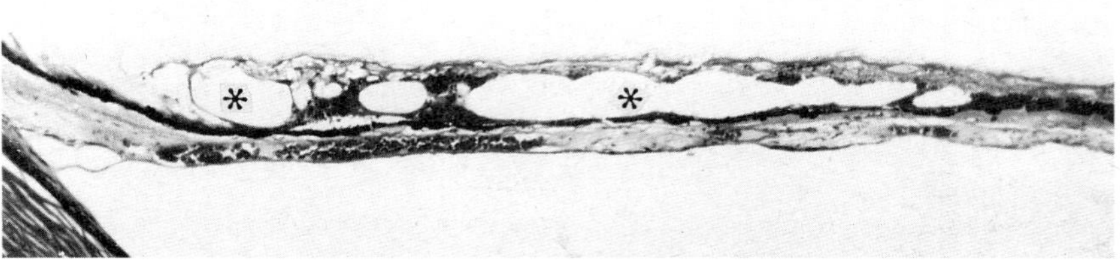

Fig. 10.2 (b) Section through same eye. Cystic spaces affecting central retinal layers indicated by asterisk. H & E (×64).

between the phagolysosomal system and the melanin granules in the pigmented epithelium.

Basement membranes

The inner limiting membrane has a smooth anterior surface and an uneven posterior surface due to irregularities in the footplates of the fibres of Müller to which it is applied. The basement membrane of the pigmented epithelium, the lamina vitrea, forms the inner component of Bruch's membrane.

Limiting membranes

The interweaving neurites of the bipolars and desmosome-like attachments between the synaptic expansions of the photoreceptors form a layer which is sufficiently cohesive to be termed a 'middle limiting membrane'. Similarly the terminal bars between the Müller fibres at the base of the inner segments of the photoreceptors forms an 'outer limiting membrane'. Neither 'membrane' is, of course, a true basement membrane, but they are sufficiently cohesive to limit the passage of exudates and haemorrages for a time.

PART 1: GENERAL DEGENERATIVE DISORDERS

SPONTANEOUS DEGENERATIONS

The degenerations described in this section fall into four categories. The first includes those conditions or circumstances in which the somewhat similar degenerative changes that have been given the descriptive terms 'cystoid' or 'microcystoid' degeneration and 'schisis' may occur. The second and third are the well-established entities of paving or cobble-stone and lattice degenerations and the fourth are those associated with pathological myopia.

Peripheral cystoid degeneration

Two types of peripheral cystoid degeneration are recognised. The typical microcystoid degeneration (Ivanoff–Blessig cysts) affects the peripheral retina of all eyes from early childhood onwards. Reticular cystoid degeneration, which is always seen in association with typical, has been found in nearly 20% of eyes examined post-mortem from adults over the age of 20.

Typical cystoid degeneration

Macroscopically the cysts appear to have rounded margins and are transparent. Microscopically the outer nerve fibre layer is primarily affected (Fig. 10.2). Expanding lacunae, which are usually bridged by columns comprising Müller fibres and compressed neuronal and glial fibres, compress the inner and outer nuclear layers. Coalescence of the lacunae may result in quite substantial cysts and splits. The process is age-related and tends to affect the temporal quadrants most severly.

Reticular cystoid degeneration

Reticular cystoid degeneration usually occurs posterior to a band of confluent typical cystoid degeration and is so called because of the fine surface network and arborising vasculature seen macroscopically. The lateral and posterior margins are bounded by large vessels. Microscopically, the earliest lesion is loss of the nerve fibre layer which is replaced by ramifying lacunae bridged by fibres of Müller. Loss of ganglion cells and considerable separation of the inner limiting membrane and inner nerve fibre layer may occur, but even in severe lesions the process is limited by the latter. Capillaries are seen in relation to the glial pillars and larger vessels remain supported by their fibroglial sheaths. By contrast with the typical form, there is no clear evidence that the lesion extends with increasing age nor does it show a predilection for the temporal quadrants.

Neither type of degeneration appears to predispose to the formation of retinal tears and their pathogenesis is uncertain.

Paving (cobble-stone) degeneration

Macroscopically, groups of yellowish-white spots from 0.1 to 1.5 mm in diameter, sometimes surrounded by a ring of pigment, are seen between the equator and ora serrata. Their incidence increases with age.

Microscopically, there is atrophy of the pigment epithelium and photoreceptors with adhesion of the residual retinal layers to Bruch's membrane. Proliferation of pigment often occurs around the periphery.

The lesions are thought to be due to focal ischaemia, and obliterative changes may be observed in the underlying choriocapillaris. The lesions do not predispose to retinal detachment.

Myopic degenerations

Lacquer cracks are the most important of the degenerative changes affecting the eye with pathological myopia. They represent breaks in the retinal pigment epithelium and Bruch's membrane and may be a source of subretinal neovascularisation or haemorrage.

Fuchs' spot is a dark spot in the macula that may be associated with choroidal haemorrhage. Histopathologically there is a local ingrowth of fibrovascular tissue from the choroid and proliferation of the overlying pigmented epithelium.

Macular haemorrhages occur in myopes in the third and fourth decades. These usually resorb and are thus less serious than Fuchs' spot which is usually progressive.

Lattice degeneration

Lattice degeneration (see Byer, 1979) is of much greater importance than reticular cystoid degeneration because of its association with holes and tears which may give rise to retinal detachment.

Prevalence

In large autopsy series, lattice degeneration has been found in over 10% of cases. In nearly 50% of these the lesion was bilateral. Maximal prevalence is attained by the beginning of the second decade. There is no sexual or racial predilection, though there is an increased incidence to approximately 15% in myopic eyes.

Macroscopic appearance

The lesions, which are oval or elliptical in shape, are usually located between the equator and the ora serrata with their long axis parallel to the latter. The retina adjacent to the vertical meridian superiorly and inferiorly was preferentially involved. The lesions are 0.5–2.0 mm in width and from 1.5 mm upwards in length, sometimes extending around a quadrant. The affected retina is thinned and the overlying vitreous liquefied. The area may be criss-crossed by white vessels or there may be white dots giving the 'snail-track' appearance. At the margins the vitreous is condensed.

Microscopic changes

Loss of neurones occurs from the inner layers and the internal limiting membrane breaks down. In advanced lesions the photoreceptors are also lost and reactive gliosis converts the affected area into a glial plate. Involvement of the pigmented epithelium results in focal depigmentation and reactive hyperplasia with migration of pigment into the lesion, especially along the hyalinised vessels which are invariably present. At the margins of the lesion, the vitreous becomes condensed and there is proliferation of glial filaments forming vitreous bands (Fig. 10.3). Holes or tears may occur.

Pathogenesis

Although there is evidence that genetic factors are involved, no clear mode of inheritance has been established and the pathogenesis of lattice degeneration remains unresolved. It has been attributed to:

1 Vitreous traction.
2 Retinal ischaemia due to local vascular structural abnormalities.
3 Persistence of embryological vascular anastomoses between vitreous and retinal vessels.
4 Local aplasia of the internal limiting membrane, thus locating the primary defect in the Müller fibres.

RETINAL BREAKS (HOLES AND TEARS)

Peripheral breaks

Full thickness breaks in the continuity of the neural retina may be found between the equator and ora serrata in up to about 10% of routine post-mortems on subjects

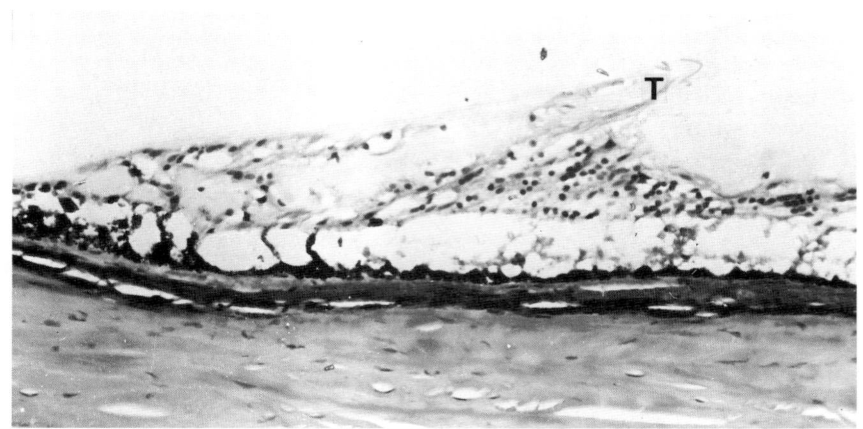

Fig. 10.3 Lattice dystrophy (specimen by courtesy of Dr J. L. S. Smith). There is retinal atrophy with vitreo-glial traction bands (T).

over the age of 20. They may also be observed clinically in the absence of any visual disturbance. They are often associated with lattice degeneration where they appear at the margin of the lesion and are commoner in myopic than emmetropic eyes. Such breaks may be categorised as holes or tears. Holes result from degenerative changes in the retina while tears result from vitreoretinal or zonuloretinal adhesions and traction. The effect of the traction is to raise a flap so that a tear is often horseshoe shaped. The flap is pulled anteriorly towards the vitreous base and may become detached to form an operculum over the break (Plate 4 and Figs 10.4 and 10.5). Holes are a not uncommon incidental post-mortem finding rarely associated with retinal detachment. Most aysmptomatic tears also apparently carry little risk of leading to retinal detachment (see below).

A retinal dialysis is a disinsertion of the retina at the ora serrata. Most such tears result from trauma, but they are seen in the inferotemporal region in childhood.

Macular holes

Macular holes may be full thickness (Fig. 10.6) or lamellar. In the latter the layer of photoreceptors may be partially preserved. Evidence of cystoid macular oedema is usually observed in the retina adjacent to the hole and occasionally actual cysts may be present. Fibroglial proliferation occurs around the margin of the hole on the internal surface of the retina in the majority of cases to form a preretinal membrane, but evidence of vitreous traction is rarely found.

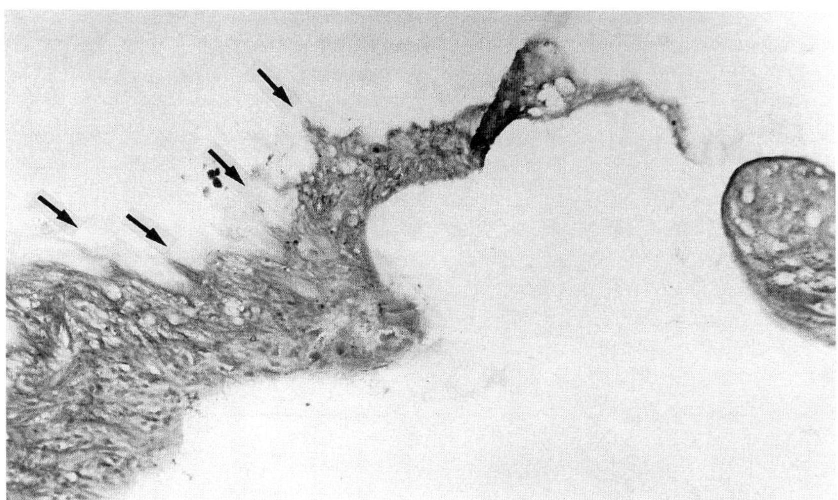

Fig. 10.4 Retinal hole with flap in case of longstanding detachment apparently due to lattice dystrophy. The central margin has a rounded profile while the peripheral margin is raised as a flap and there is evidence of traction (arrows). PAS/tartrazine (×94).

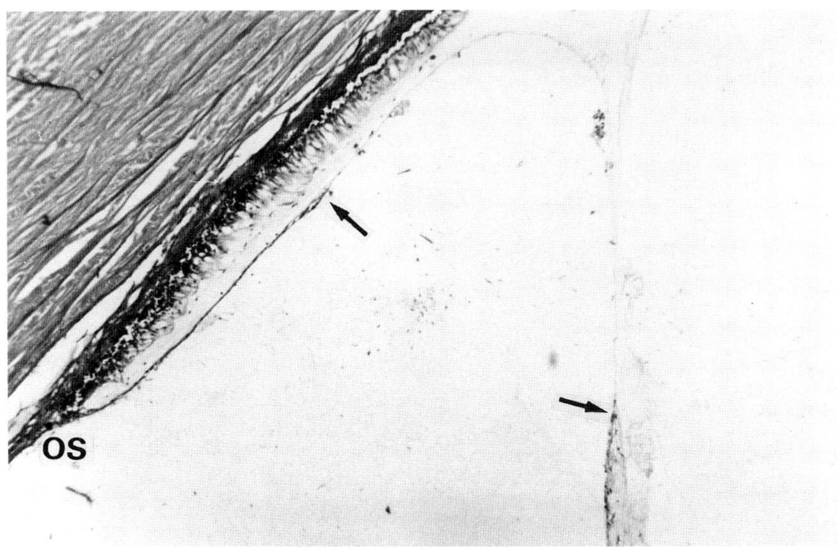

Fig. 10.5 Peripheral retinal break in case of longstanding retinal detachment. Margins of break indicated by arrows. The retina ia greatly thinned and, anterior to the break, reflected forwards. OS = ora serrata. Masson (×64).

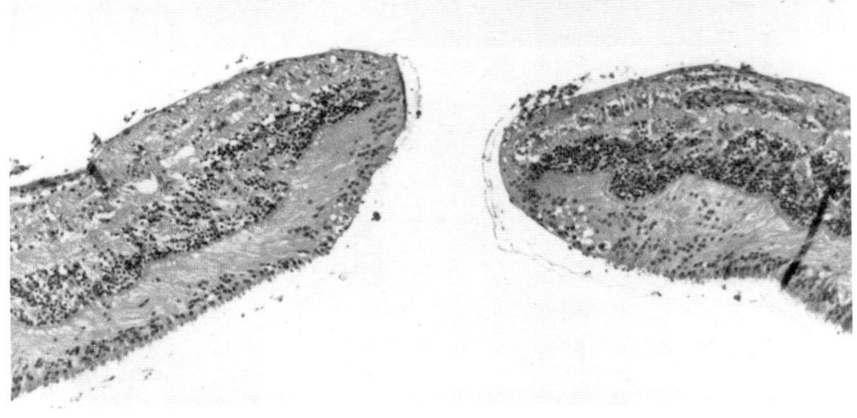

Fig. 10.6 Macular hole. Incidental finding in a large congenitally glaucomatous eye with a desçemetocele. (a) Low power. Note rounded margins of the retina. H & E (×64).

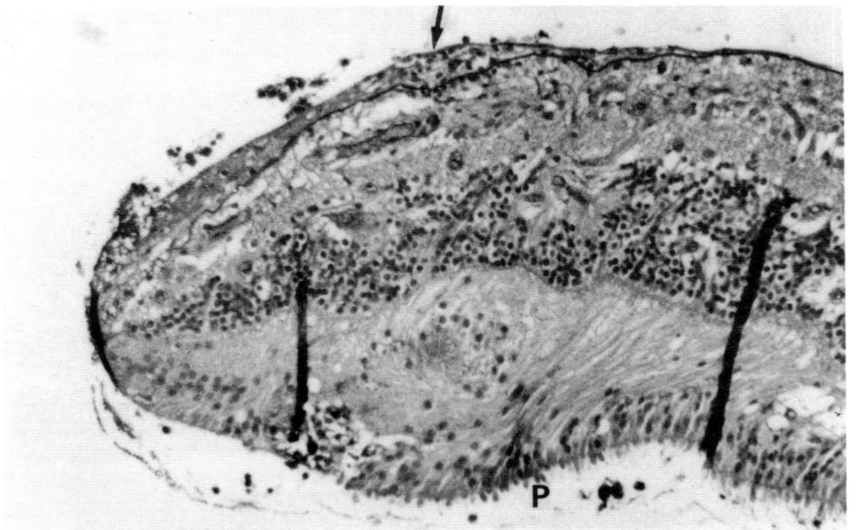

Fig. 10.6 (b) Higher power to show glial proliferation on anterior surface (arrow) and stumpy photoreceptors (P) on posterior surface. PAS/tartrazine (×160).

Pathogenesis

Coalescence of the cystic spaces in cystoid degeneration is probably the commonest cause of macular holes. This accounts for their common association with trauma (see Chapter 18), ocular surgery and diabetes mellitus. Blunt trauma may possibly cause concussive tears which can lead to a macular hole. A few are also apparently related to senile macular degeneration. Preretinal membranes, which may be attached to the margins of the hole, are thought to be a secondary phenomenon.

RETINAL DETACHMENT

Two important factors upon which adhesion of the retina to pigmented epithelium appears to depend are:

1 The proteoglycan ground substance between the outer segments has viscoelastic properties and acts as a cement.

2 Active transport of fluid by the pigmented epithelium maintains a negative pressure and prevents dilution of the proteoglycan.

The term 'retinal detachment' is used with some semantic licence to describe the separation of the neural retina from the pigmented epithelium and concomitant accumulation of fluid in the space thus formed between them which is usually referred to as 'subretinal'.

Detachment of the retina may arise through the operation of three different mechanisms.

Rhegmatogenous detachment

This type of detachment is by definition associated with a retinal break, though the latter may not be easy to identify in globes enucleated with longstanding detachments complicated by intractable secondary glaucoma. Not all the factors which determine whether a break will progress to a retinal detachment are understood (see Foulds, 1987). Those of importance are:

1 *Size:* large breaks are more likely to result in a detachment than small ones.
2 *Shape:* round holes are due to degenerative changes and not to traction and thus rarely give rise to a detachment.
3 *Position with relation to the vitreous base:* the vitreous base is a cortical zone of denser vitreous about 6 mm in width covering the ora serrata with zones of attachment measuring approximately 2 mm and 4 mm to the pars ciliaris retinae and to the peripheral pars neuralis retinae respectively. Breaks within the vitreous base are caused by zonulo-retinal traction and are not subject to vitreous traction. As a result they rarely progress to detachment.
4 *Vitreous degeneration:* liquefaction and posterior detachment of the vitreous result in traction on the margin of the break and seepage of liquefied vitreous between the retina and the pigmented epithelium. The subretinal fluid initially contains little protein, but leakage of larger molecules such as IgA and IgG occurs in a matter of weeks.
5 *Myopia:* retinal detachments are approximately ten times commoner in myopes than in emmetropes. However, it is probable that this merely reflects the greater frequency of breaks in myopic eyes rather than that breaks are more likely to progress to detachment in myopic eyes.

Progression

The rate at which the detachment progresses is very variable. Detachments associated with superiorly situated breaks generally progress rapidly in a matter of hours or days while those from inferiorly located holes may only progress slowly for months. The shape of the detachment is also governed by the position of the hole and helps to locate it clinically.

Exudative detachment

This type of detachment is due to leakage of fluid from vessels, usually as a result of inflammation or neoplasia affecting the uvea. Thus, it is commonly seen in association with malignant melanomata or secondary deposits of carcinoma in the choroid and with retinoblastomata. Other causes are:
1 Coats' disease (see Chapter 10, Part 2).
2 Toxaemia of pregnancy.

The subretinal fluid in exudative detachments has a high protein content.

Tractional detachment

This commonly results from fibrovascular proliferation within the vitreous chamber such as occurs in diabetic retinopathy, retinopathy of prematurity, retinopathy of prematurity and sickle cell haemoglobinopathies. Organisation of vitreous following inflammatory conditions such as vitreous abcess, infestation by *Toxocara* and congenital toxoplasmosis are other causes.

PATHOLOGICAL CHANGES IN RETINAL DETACHMENT

Detachment of the retina is a common artefact in conventionally processed globes and is recognised by the absence of cells or exudate in the subretinal space and the good preservation of the photoreceptors — the tips of which moreover usually have an adherent layer of pigment granules torn from the pigmented epithelium.

Early changes

The opportunity to examine globes with rhematogenous detachments at an early stage rarely arises and much knowledge of early changes is based on animal experiments such as those carried out by Machemer and collaborators (1968a & b, 1975). Similar retinal changes can, however, be observed in eyes enucleated for tumours in which the retina is detached (Fig. 10.7).

Retinal oedema: a diffuse oedema of the inner retinal layers is apparent within a few days. This progresses to the formation of cystoid spaces in the inner nuclear, inner plexiform and ganglion cell layers.

Photoreceptor degeneration: the outer segments become irregular in length and the discs fragmented. Within a short time, pigment-laden macrophages accumulate in increasing numbers around the outer segments and phagocytose the damaged outer segments.

Changes in the pigmented epithelium: pigment granules retract towards the base of the cell and the laminated bodies disappear as phagocytosis of the outer segments ceases. There is evidence of cell divison and some cells are mobilised.

Reversibility of early changes

If re-attachment occurs, the retinal oedema clears, the outer segments rapidly assume a normal appearance and the macrophages are dispersed.

Late changes

Atrophy and gliosis: if the retina remains detached, the photoreceptors undergo progressive atrophy with a variable degree of replacement gliosis.

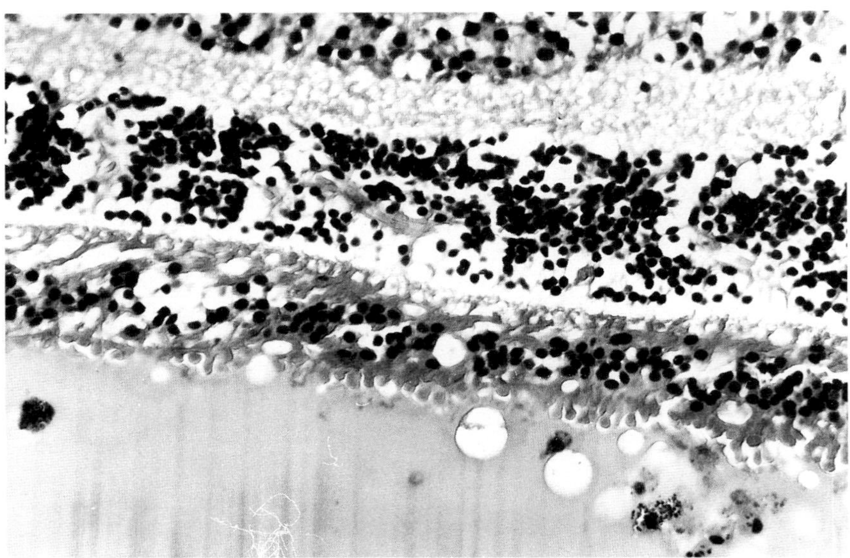

Fig. 10.7 Effects of detachment. Serous detachment due to melanoma of choroid. Note depletion of cells in outer nuclear and stumpy remnants of photoreceptors. The oedema extends into the inner nuclear layer. Several pigment laden cells can be seen in the exudate. H & E (×320).

Pigment proliferation: proliferation of pigmented epithelial cells may occur along the line of attachment of the retina in longstanding cases which have become stabilised. A similar proliferation often occurs at the ora where it is termed Ringschwiele formation (Fig. 10.8).

Cyst formation: thin-walled cysts of variable size are frequently present in longstanding detachments. They usually contain clear fluid. Occasionally they attain a considerable size and haemorrhage may occur into them. Such macrocysts may be misdiagnosed as a tumour.

Epiretinal membranes in rhematogenous detachment

With longstanding detachments, there may be a variable proliferation of fibrocellular membranes on the anterior surface of the retina. Sometimes the proliferation extends to the posterior surfaces of the retina and vitreous. This has been termed massive periretinal proliferation or proliferative vitreopretinopathy. The cells forming these membranes have been identified as:

1 Cells of the pigmented epithelium which migrate through retinal breaks; these may retain their epithelial character or undergo metaplastic transformation to fibroblast-like cells.

2 Fibroblast-like cells not derived from metaplastic pigment epithelium.

3 Astrocytic glia which leave the retina through breaks in the limiting membranes.

4 Myofibroblast-like cells.

5 Macrophages.

The combination of cell types found is variable.

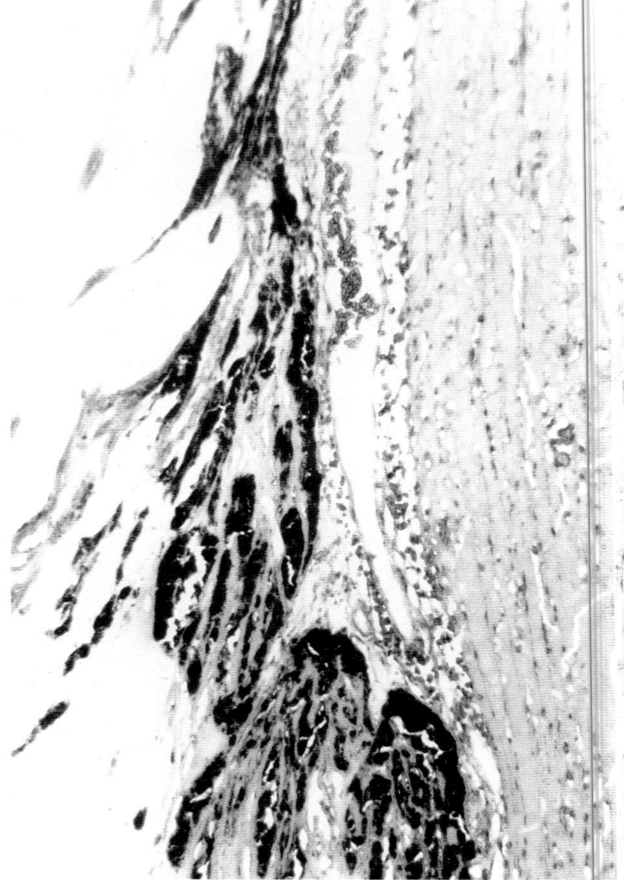

Fig. 10.8 Ringschwiele. Layerwise proliferation of pigmented epithelium at anterior margin of a longstanding post-inflammatory detachment. H & E (×44).

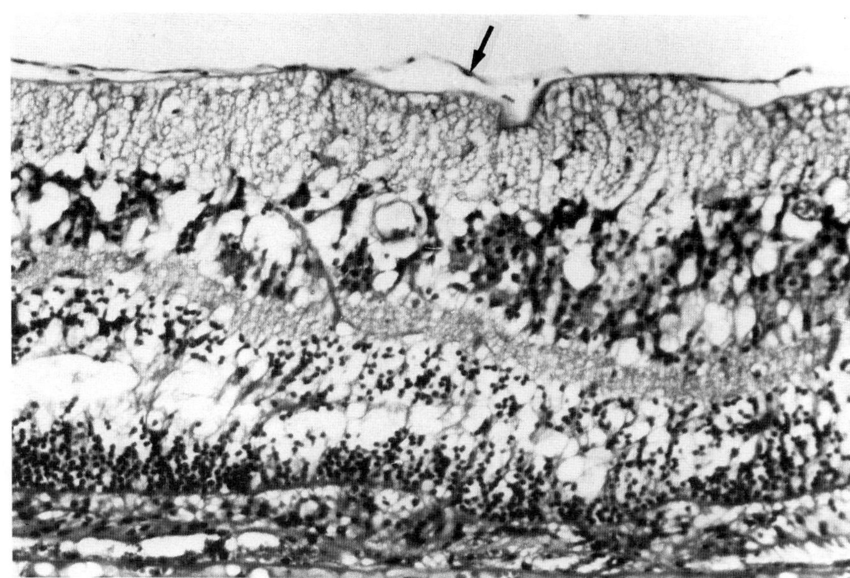

Fig. 10.9 Glial membrane. Delicate membrane on surface of retina (arrow) in a case of longstanding retinal detachment, though the retina appears to have become re-attached in this area. Masson trichrome (×160).

Membrane formation may complicate successfully treated detachments. Contraction of these membranes has serious clinical consequences since it causes puckering of the retinal surface and, eventually, secondary tractional detachment.

Massive periretinal proliferation can be induced in the experimental animal by introducing pigment epithelial cells or fibroblasts into the vitreous. The contractility of epiretinal membranes is thought to depend on the presence of cells containing myofibrils.

Epiretinal membranes in other conditions

Epiretinal membranes have been observed as a complication of a number of other intraocular conditions:

1 Proliferative vascular retinopathies.
2 Intraocular inflammation.
3 Trauma.
4 Vitreous haemorrhage.
5 After retinal photocoagulation.
6 Idiopathic in otherwise normal eyes.

These membranes are commonly glial (Fig. 10.9), but may be fibrocytic. They are usually avascular except when they are related to vascular proliferative retinopathies and do not contain cells derived from the pigmented epithelium.

RETINOSCHISIS

Senile retinoschisis

Posterior extension of peripheral cystoid degeneration may result in a domed tense swelling usually in the infero-temporal region which may be confused with a retinal detachment. The process is often bilaterally symmetrical. The membrane forming the dome is derived from the inner retinal layers and is, therefore, thin. White spots on the surface represent the footplates of the Müller fibres.

Juvenile retinoschisis

Juvenile retinoschisis is a bilateral condition usually encountered in boys as it typically shows a recessive sex-linked mode of inheritance, but may be idiopathic.

By contrast with typical senile retinoschisis, splitting of the retina occurs at the level of the nerve fibre layer so that the internal limiting membrane becomes detached and an expanding cavity filled with thin amorphous proteinaceous material is formed (Fig. 10.10). The anterior wall of the cavity, being composed of internal limiting membrane, is extremely thin, but eventually this becomes reinforced and partially replaced by glial proliferation. The process starts infero-temporally and spreads. As the cavity expands, the vitreous is pushed forwards and sometimes the anterior wall of the cavity forms a retrolenticular membrane.

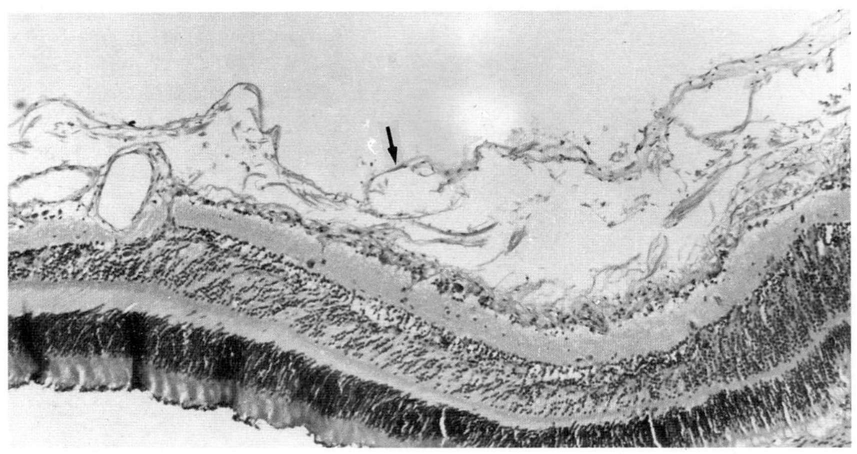

Fig. 10.10 Retinoschisis. The inner limiting membrane of retina (arrow) has become separated. The space appears largely empty apart from strands of glia and nerve fibres. Sporadic case in female aged 12. H & E (×170).

CLASSIFICATION OF INHERITED CHOROIDORETINAL DYSTROPHIES

In the group of disorders to be described below, the photoreceptor cells fail to function adequately usually from an early age and the layer of visual cells undergoes a varying degree of dissolution. The functional failure must ultimately be due to a defect in genetic coding. While it would be convenient and rational to group the disorders according to the cell or cells primarily affected, rods, cones and pigmented epithelium are clearly interdependant to a greater or lesser degree and although a defect in genetic coding might affect them selectively, it is unlikely that the resultant changes would be confined to the cells primarily affected. It may thus in practice be difficult to establish how selective the primary defect actually is. Furthermore, there could, in principle, be a genetically determined failure of the choroidal blood supply which would affect both pigmented epithelium and photoreceptors. Since involutional atrophy of the choriocapillaris may occur in advanced retinal disease, such a primary vascular failure could well be difficult to establish and has not, in fact, been firmly established for any known condition.

Notwithstanding these difficulties, present information permits a tentative classification based on the cell type or types within the visual system which appear to be primarily or, at least, predominantly affected.

DYSTROPHIES PREDOMINANTLY AFFECTING RODS

Retinitis pigmentosa

In a recent symposium (Marmor *et al.*, 1983) it was recommended that the term 'retinitis pigmentosa', though technically incorrect, be used to define 'a set of progressive hereditary disorders that diffusely and primarily affect photoreceptor and pigment epithelial function'. This implies that most cases are hereditary even when no family history can be elicited. Most cases in which there is a family history show an autosomal recessive mode of inheritance, but both X-linked and autosomal dominant modes are also seen. The relative frequency varies in different communities. In general, cases showing autosomal recessive transmission are more severe than those transmitted as an autosomal dominant. In X-linked cases, the disease tends to be severe in males and mild or sometimes asymptomatic in females.

Clinical features

Onset is usually between the ages of 10 and 20 and the disease is slowly progressive. Both eyes are usually affected equally. The early symptoms are of defective vision at night, but vision in daylight is affected later. A characteristic annular scotoma develops, leading to 'tunnel vision'.

Ophthalmoscopically, atrophy of the pigmented epithelium is seen in the post-equatorial fundus followed later by migration of pigment into the retinal along attenuated blood vessels to give the characteristic 'bone corpuscular' or 'spicular' pattern. A glial membrane over the optic disc gives it a waxy appearance.

Numerous variations in the clinical manifestations of retinitis pigmentosa have been described, e.g. retinitis pigmentosa sine pigmento, sectorial, unilateral and inverse variants, and retinitis punctata albescens.

Pathological changes

The pathological changes appear to be similar whatever the pattern of inheritance, although this does influence the rate at which they progress. There is progressive depletion of photoreceptors which starts in the equatorial region and spreads centrally and peripherally.

Most cases have been examined at a late stage of the disease and nearly all the photoreceptors had disappeared except for a few cones in the foveal area (Fig. 10.11a) which were much shorter and stouter than normal. In one comparatively early case of sex-linked retinitis pigmentosa in a male aged 23 (Szamier *et al.*, 1979), the photoreceptors in the fovea were depleted by about 50%. Those remaining were all cones and had severely distorted outer segments. The depletion became progressively more severe through the parafoveal region and, in the zone of 'bone spicule formation', photoreceptors were absent. Anterior to this, however, both rods and cones survived, but had shortened outer segments. A variable amount of neuronal loss and gliosis occurs in the inner retinal layers.

Abnormally large numbers of 'melanolysosomes' were observed in the foveal pigmented epithelium where the photoreceptors were depleted and the number of pigment granules was diminished (Szamier *et al.*, 1979). Similar changes involving both pigmented epithelium and receptors were observed in a female carrier, but they were focal and confined to the mid-periphery of the retina (Szamier & Berson, 1985). Excessive deposition of 'lipofuscin' in the foveal pigmented epithelium with depletion of pigment has also been reported by Kolb and Gouras (1974).

Loss of continuity of the pigmented epithelium occurs and where loss of photoreceptors is complete, proliferation and migration of pigment into the retina is seen and adhesions between retina and Bruch's membrane develop. The migration of pigment often takes place along blood vessels thus giving the spidery pattern of deposition seen macroscopically. The retinal arterioles undergo hyaline sclerosis and, in advanced cases, are seen surrounded by massive aggregations of pigment (Fig. 10.11b). The choriocapillaris may also become atrophic in the late stages.

Widespread deposition of unidentified amorphous

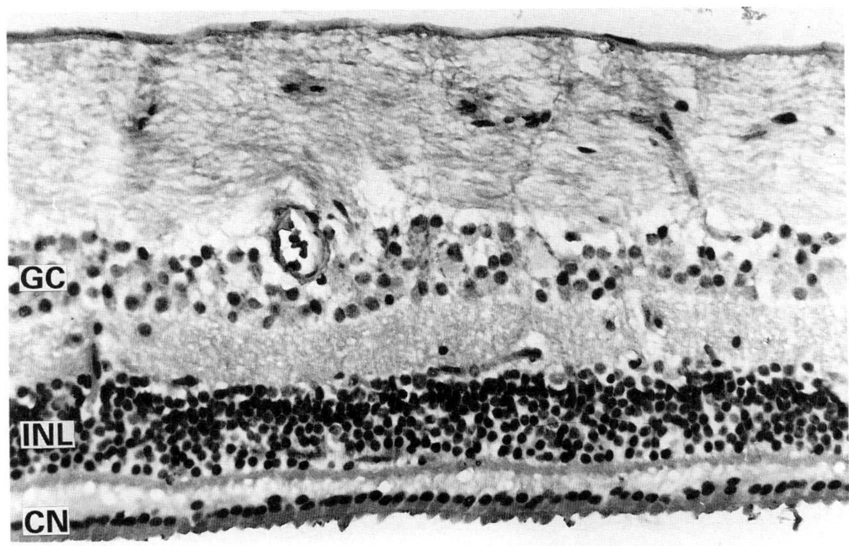

Fig. 10.11 Retinitis pigmentosa. (a) Perifoveal retina. Single residual row of cone nuclei (CN) with stumpy remants of inner segment. H & E (×260). GC = ganglion cells, INL = inner nuclear layer.

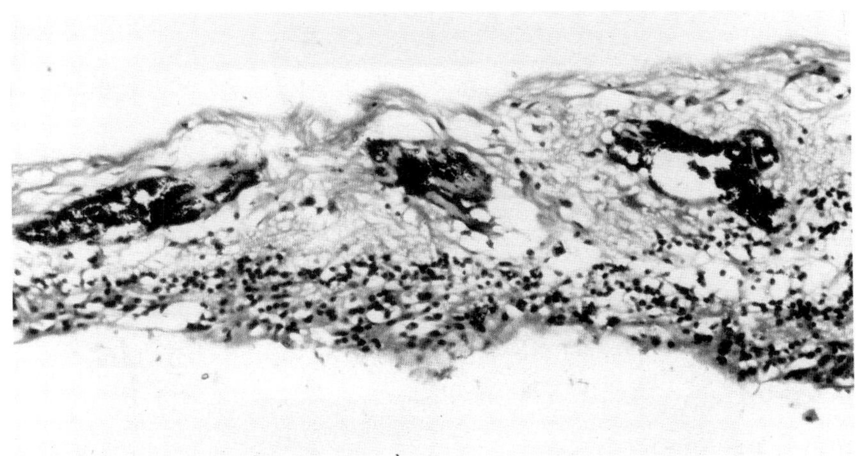

Fig. 10.11 (b) Mid-peripheral retina. Structural disorganisation with masses of pigment around vessels. H & E (×270).

material between the pigmented epithelium and the inner collagenous layer of Bruch's membrane has recently been reported in the eyes of two brothers with dominant retinitis pigmentosa (Duvall *et al.*, 1986).

A fine glial membrane often develops over the optic nerve head. Optic atrophy is not a consistent feature.

Syndromes associated with retinitis pigmentosa

Numerous syndromes have been described in which the eyes show changes resembling retinitis pigmentosa clinically. Of these, the most important are:

Bardet–Biedl (Laurence–Moon) syndrome: this is an autosomal recessive condition in which the principal features are retinal degeneration, mental retardation, obesity, hypogonadism and polydactyly.

Refsum's syndrome: in this autosomal recessive disorder, there is a defect in phytanic acid α-hydroxylase which catalyses the first step in the conversion of phytanic acid to pristanic acid. Phytanic acid, which is formed from phytol (a breakdown product of chlorophyll) accumulates in tissues. In the eye, lipid infiltrates have been observed in sclera, cornea and around the trabecular meshwork and in the sphincter and dilator muscles of the iris, but not in the iris epithelium. The pigmented epithelium of the retina was infiltrated with lipid and showed almost total absence of photoreceptors (Toussaint & Danis, 1971). Other features of the disease include polyneuritis, cerebellar ataxia and cardiac failure.

Bassen–Kornzweig syndrome: the features of this autosomal recessive disease are neuromuscular disorders, acanthocytosis (prickly appearance of erythrocytes in peripheral blood) and absence of β-lipoprotein from the blood due to defective absorption of fats and fatty acids. Pathological changes consistent with advanced retinitis pigmentosa have bee described in the retina.

Cockayne's syndrome: this rare autosomal recessive form of dwarfism is characterised clinically by a 'pepper and salt' retinopathy usually associated with waxy pallor of the optic discs and narrowed retinal vessels. Pathological features include partial depletion of photoreceptors, irregular hypo- and hyperpigmentation of the pigmented epithelium with migration of pigmented cells into the retina. There may be excessive deposition of lipofuscin granules in the peripheral pigmented epithelium. The ganglion cells are depleted and the inner retinal layers and optic nerve undergo atrophy.

Usher's syndrome: in this autosomal recessive condition congenital neurosensory deafness is associated with retinitis pigmentosa.

Kearns–Sayre syndrome: ophthalmoplegia and retinal degeneration occurs in this rare syndrome which has no established pattern of inheritance. Systemic abnormalities include mental retardation and muscular weakness. Death occurs from heart block. The retinal changes are not typical of retinitis pigmentosa. There is loss of photoreceptors and pigmented epithelium at the retinal periphery and around the optic nerve head (McKechnie *et al.*, 1985).

Trauma: contusion of the retina (see Chapter 18) may eventually lead to a histological picture resembling retinitis pigmentosa.

DYSTROPHIES PREDOMINANTLY AFFECTING CONES

Information regarding the pathological changes, especially in the early stages, of the disorders in this group is scanty.

Best's vitelliform foveal dystrophy

1 *Mode of inheritance:* autosomal dominant.
2 *Clinical manifestation:* the typical 'egg-yolk' appearance of the macula is observed soon after birth. This later breaks up and may become invaded by new vessels.
3 *Pathological changes:* in a single relatively early case (Kobrin *et al.*, 1981), there were elevated accumulations of pigmented epithelial cells and diffuse cytoplasmic engorgement with unidentified granular material, probably lipofuscin granules (Weingeist *et al.*, 1982). The photoreceptor outer segments showed atrophic changes in some areas. Free macrophages containing lipofuscin and pigment were present in the subretinal space. Old cases show atrophy of the central retinal pigmented epithelium and choriocapillaris. The disorder may possibly result from accumulation of cone outer segment material in the pigmented epithelium.

Foveomacular vitelliform dystrophy, adult type

A condition resembling Best's vitelliform dystrophy, but with onset in middle life, has recently been recognized. The pathological features of three case studied were also somewhat similar (Gass, 1974; Patrinely *et al.*, 1985)

Stargardt's disease

1 *Mode of inheritance:* autosomal dominant or recessive.
2 *Clinical manifestation:* rapid loss of central vision

occurs over a period of months during the first 15 years of life.

3 *Pathological changes:* there is complete disappearance of the pigmented epithelium and photoreceptors in the macular area. More peripherally, the cells of the pigmented epithelium were crammed with PAS-positive material thought to be abnormal lipofuscin. Posterior to the equator, aggregates of enormously enlarged cells were observed (Eagle *et al.*, 1980).

Dominant macular dystrophy (inherited disciform degeneration)

1 *Mode of inheritance:* autosomal dominant.

2 *Clinical manifestation:* onset is usually in middle life, but may be earlier.

3 *Pathological changes:* Bruch's membrane is primarily affected. Thickening, drüsen formation and ruptures with invasion of vessels deep to the pigmented epithelium have been reported (Ashton & Sorsby, 1951). Thus, the changes closely resemble those seen in senile macular degeneration and angioid streaks.

Dominant drüsen (Doyne's honeycomb choroiditis)

1 *Mode of inheritance:* autosomal dominant.

2 *Clinical manifestations:* onset is usually between 20 and 30 years of age.

3 *Pathological changes:* thickening of Bruch's membrane and drüsen formation predominantly at the posterior pole with overlying degeneration of the outer retina.

CHOROIDAL ATROPHIES AND DYSTROPHIES

Gyrate atrophy of choroid and retina

1 *Mode of inheritance:* autosomal recessive.

2 *Clinical manifestation:* the ophthalmological features of myopia, cataract and chorioretinal atrophy are evident in childhood. The atrophy affects the periphery and mid-periphery. Electroretinographic changes indicative of marked involvement of the rod and cone systems have been demonstrated at an early age.

The patients have a deficiency in ornithine-δ-aminotransferase which leads to hyperornithaemia and ornithinuria. It is not clear how the deficiency is related to the ocular changes.

Choroideraemia

1 *Mode of inheritance:* X-linked.

2 *Clinical manifestation:* males may show pigmentary changes in the first two years of life, but in females the changes occur much later.

3 *Pathological changes:* the outer retinal layers, pigmented epithelium and choriocapillaris show marked atrophy in the mid-peripheral region. The inner retinal layers remain well preserved. A recent study (Cameron *et al.*, 1987) revealed two new features:

(i) Migration of retinal glia through cracks in calcified Bruch's membrane to form Müller footplate-like structures on the choroidal side of Bruch's membrane.

(ii) Deficiency in the basement membrane in uveal capillaries in the anterior choroid and iris with mild atrophic changes in the pigmented epithelium of the iris and dilator muscle. This was interpreted as indicating that there may be a primary vascular factor.

Central areolar choroidal dystrophy (sclerosis)

1 *Mode of inheritance:* autosomal dominant or recessive.

2 *Clinical manifestation:* bilateral loss of central vision occurs at the end of the second decade.

3 *Pathological changes:* a well-demarcated avascular zone has been demonstrated in the choroid between the macula and the optic nerve head. In this zone the choroid is thin and may be fibrotic. The overlying pigmented epithelium is absent and the retina shows loss of photoreceptors. Bruch's membrane remains intact (Ashton, 1953).

GENERAL PERSPECTIVES ON RETINAL DYSTROPHIES

The foregoing is by no means a comprehensive account of inherited retinal or choroidoretinal disorders for some of which no pathological findings are available. It is also clear that histopathological examination has been of limited value in the disorders discussed here because most cases have been examined in the terminal stages of the condition when the important primary features have become obscured by secondary changes. It is not even clear, for example, whether the changes in the pigmented epithelium observed by Szamier *et al.* (1979) are primary or secondary.

This limitation has stimulated an interest in parallel conditions in domestic or laboratory animals in which early morphological and biochemical changes can be studied and correlated with electrophysiological observations. Such findings may lead to a better understanding of related diseases in man.

Retinal dystrophy in the RCS rat

This condition is inherited as an autosomal recessive and becomes manifest a few weeks after birth as the outer rod segments begin to develop. The pigmented epithelium is incapable of phagocytosing the outer segment material which then accumulates between the photoreceptors and the pigmented epithelium. Ultimately, the layer of photoreceptors becomes completely atrophic.

Retinal dystrophy in the mouse

In the mouse a retinal dystrophy, which is also inherited as an autosomal recessive, affects several strains. The condition was originally described as Keeler's 'rodless mice' and is found *inter alia* in C3H mice. By contrast with the rat, the photoreceptors undergo rapid dissolution which begins about 10 days after birth and is complete within 4 weeks (Fig. 10.12). It is now known that the genetic biochemical defect is lack of a light-activated phosphodiesterase in the rod outer segment which catalyses the hydrolysis of cyclic guanosine 3′5′-monophosphate (cGMP).

Retinal dystrophy in the dog

At least four different varieties of progressive retinal atrophy have been described in some 15 different breeds of dog. Of these, a condition affecting the Irish setter appears to correspond to retinal dystrophy in the mouse. Several breeds including the Labrador retriever, Shetland sheepdog and border collie are affected by a pigment epithelial dystrophy which has features in common with that seen in the rat.

Relationship to human disease

It was widely thought that the retinal atrophies and dystrophies in animals were directly comparable with retinitis pigmentosa, but such a simple view is no longer tenable because it has become clear that both retinitis pigmentosa in man and retinal atrophy or dystrophy in animals comprise a spectrum of related conditions in

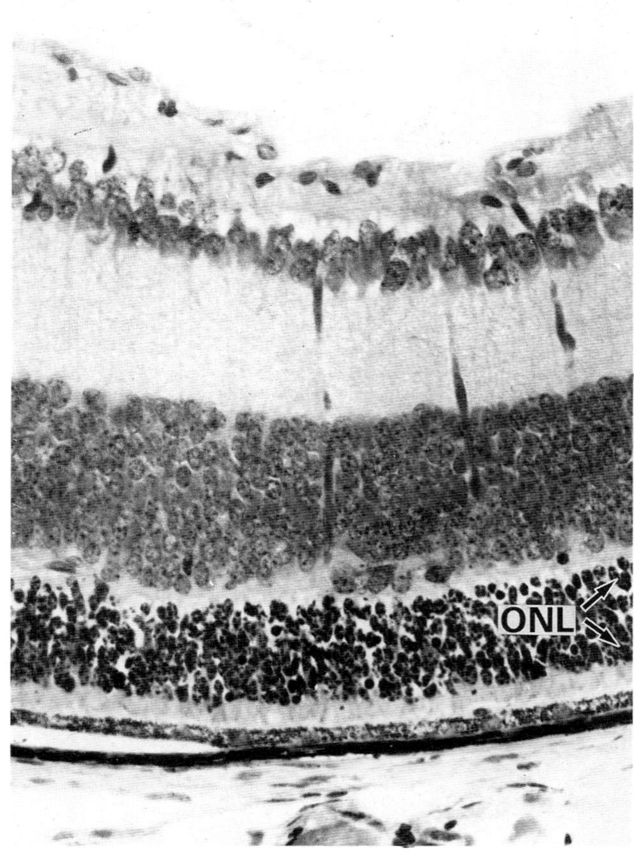

Fig. 10.12 Retinal dystrophy in the C3H mouse. (a) At age 13 days. Outer nuclear (ONL) layer is of normal thickness, although scattered pyknotic nuclei are usually seen. The photoreceptors are as yet very immature.

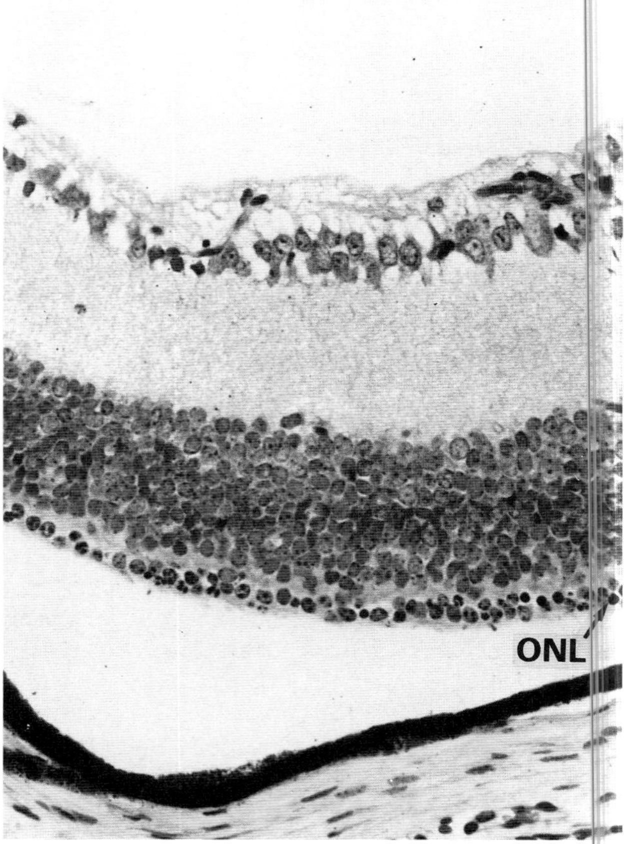

Fig. 10.12 (b) Litter-mate at age 19 days. The outer nuclear layer (ONL) is reduced to one to two rows. Both H & E (×175).

Table 10.1 Classification of blinding disorders by cell type (modified from Lolley, 1983).

Rod preferentially
Retinal dystrophy in the mouse
Progressive retinal atrophy in the dog
Congenital stationary night blindness
Cone preferentially
Hemeralopia in the Alaskan Malamute dog
Stationary cone disorders in man
RPE/rod preferentially
Retinal dystrophy in the rat
Typical retinitis pigmentosa
RPE/cone preferentially
Vitelliform dystrophy
Stargardt's disease
Choroid (endothelium only)
None yet proven
Choroid/receptors/RPE
Choroidal dystrophies
Choroideraemia

which it is highly unlikely that the same pathogenetic mechanism is operative. It also remains uncertain whether, after making allowances for differences in retinal structure which might mask a fundamental similarity in the pathogenetic process in different species, any of the animal conditions has a counterpart in man which is likely to be caused by an identical defect in genetic coding. However, it is possible and conceptually useful to integrate tentatively the animal and human diseases which are primarily involved, according to cell type, into a rational scheme (see Table 10.1).

RETINAL DEGENERATIONS CAUSED BY DRUGS OR TOXIC CHEMICALS

Retinopathy has been associated clinically with a number of drugs of which by far the most important is chloroquine. In the experimental animal, retinal degeneration may be induced by various toxic agents and some of these experimental models have been intensively studied.

Chloroquine retinopathy

Clinical manifestations

The earliest change is a subtle disturbance in macular pigmentation. Later, the macula becomes depigmented and a surrounding ring of increased pigmentation forms. Eventually, the peripheral retina may be affected.

Subepithelial deposition of chloroquine crystals may occur in the cornea.

Relationship to dose

The condition appears to depend on total dosage administered and not on individual idiosyncrasy. Most cases have received a substantial dosage over several years. The dosage required for malaria prophylaxis does not cause the disease, nor does that currently used for the treatment of rheumatoid arthritis. The retinal changes are irreversible, but the corneal crystals gradually disappear following withdrawal of the drug.

Histopathological changes

Extensive loss of the rods and cones and their nuclei is seen, but the fovea is partly spared. Pigmented cells migrate into the remaining inner retinal layers, though not along blood vessels as in retinitis pigmentosa.

Membranous cytoplasmic bodies and clusters of curvilinear tubules have been observed in the retinal ganglion cells. These probably represent altered smooth endoplasmic reticulum and are not a specific effect of chloroquine.

Mode of action

The mechanism for retinal toxicity remains unknown (see Spalton, 1987). Chloroquine binds to melanin and is stored in melanin-containing tissues and also interferes with phagocytosis, but it is not certain that its toxic action on the retina depends on either of these properties. In the experimental animal, the effect of chloroquine administration varies according to the species, but affects primarily the retinal ganglion cells.

Phenothiazine derivatives

Retinal damage simulating retinitis pigmentosa can be produced by a phenothiazine derivative, piperidylethylchlorphenothazine (NP 207). High doses of the closely related thioridazine (Melleril) has also been found to cause retinal damage when used in high doses.

From experimental work on the cat, it is thought that NP 207 activates shedding of the rod outer segments and also disrupts them.

Phenoxyalkanes

Clinically similar blindness was observed during trials of the schistosomicidal agent, 1, 7-di(*p*-dimethylaminophenoxy)heptane. This proved to be one a series of phenoxyalkanes which have been found in the rabbit to produce extensive damage to the visual cells and pigmented epithelium. This is a true retinotoxic effect which can be elicited by quite small doses.

Experimental retinopathies causes by other toxic agents

Interest in these was aroused many years ago when it was found that a therapeutic agent, Septojod, used for treating infections sometimes caused blindness associated with a retinitis pigmentosa-like opthalmoscopic picture. The active agent proved to be sodium iodate. Since then, other agents such as sodium iodoacetate have also been found the affect the retina. To produce retinal damage the agents have to be injected intravenously in nearly lethal doses. Although both agents produce a similar ophthalmoscopic picture, histological studies show that iodate primarily affects the pigmented epithelium while iodoactetate causes necrosis of the visual cells. These agents have proved useful in correlating clinical manifestations of retinal damage with histopathological and biochemical changes and have underlined the fact that ophthalmoscopic changes resembling retinitis pigmentosa can result from unrelated pathological processes.

VITAMIN A DEFICIENCY

It is well known that vitamin A deficiency may lead *inter alia* to night blindness. Degenerative changes have been observed in the photoreceptors of various species. The outer segment is affected first and later there is depletion of the outer nuclear layer. In monkeys, the changes are most severe in the macular and paramacular areas and both rods and cones are affected. Lipid droplets accumulate in the pigmented epithelium.

In rats deprived of vitamin A for several months, degenerative changes appear in the rod outer segments. If the rat is kept alive by supplementing the diet with vitamin A acid, which can substitute for the alcohol for all growth and tissue functions other than its role as a prosthetic group in visual pigments, progressive degeneration of the photoreceptors occurs and eventually the entire visual cell layer disappears apart from perhaps a single row of residual nuclei. An end result closely resembling the inherited dystrophies is thus produced. Somewhat similar degenerative changes can be induced in the rabbit, although, in this species, the pigmented epithelium appears affected and the loss of visual cells is less severe.

RETINAL DAMAGE DUE TO LIGHT

While the retina has evolved to respond to light over an enormous range of levels of irradiance — 9 log units — it may also be damaged by excessive exposure to light within and close to the visible range. Energy is absorbed in the retina by four systems:

1 The visual pigments.
2 Melanin in the pigmented epithelium.
3 Macular pigment.
4 Haemoglobin within blood vessels.

Damage arises as a result of photochemical reactions involving the visual pigments and thermal or thermomechanical effects due to energy being absorbed by the other four systems of which melanin is the most important. Thermal factors may enhance photochemical damage.

Photochemical damage

In the rat and the mouse, prolonged exposure to high levels of fluorescent illumination has been found to cause vesiculation of the rod outer segment discs and increase the rate of shedding of the discs. The visual cell itself may degenerate completely if extensive breakdown of the outer segment occurs from prolonged exposure. The pigmented epithelium is able to phagocytose the outer segment lamellae, but, if exposure is prolonged, it may lose this ability and the lamellar debris accumulates in the subretinal space.

In the monkey and the pigeon, cone outer segments may be damaged by somewhat higher levels of retinal irradiance from fluorescent light sources.

In both the monkey and the rat, a very early change is enlargement of the microvilli of the pigmented epithelium which engulf the separated outer segments.

At present, the main practical implication of these observations is that it is prudent not to overexpose the eyes of under-weight infants undergoing phototherapy for hyperbilirubinaemia.

Exposure to incandescent clinical light sources has also been shown to injure cones and pigmented epithelium in monkeys and may result in cystoid macular oedema. The exposures required are not much greater than those calculated to occur during certain diagnostic and surgical procedures. While light damage is possible but unlikely during such procedures, it is noteworthy that cystoid macular oedema is a common complication of cataract extraction. It must also be borne in mind that injurious effects of light may be attributed to pre-existing disease and thus overlooked.

Thermal damage

Much experimental work has been done on the effects on the retina of narrow beams from high intensity light sources such as lasers or the xenon arc on the experimental animal or on human eyes prior to enucleation for melanomas. Absorption of energy by melanin, haemoglobin or macular pigment results in an intense local increase in temperature sufficient to coagulate tissue proteins. Of these the melanin of the pigmented epithelium is by far the most important. If the energy absorbed is sufficiently great, a micro-explosion may cause additional mechanical damage.

Lesions of moderate severity of similar spot size are similar whether caused by xenon arc or argon laser. The pigmented epithelium rapidly swells up and the melanin content of its cells is released. The photoreceptors overlying the centre of the lesion in the pigmented epithelium undergo coagulative necrosis as shown by loss of cell outlines (Fig. 10.13a & b), increased staining and electron density. At the margin of the lesion, the intensity of the damage shades off to fewer changes such as tubulovesicular degeneration of the outer segments. If the exposure is intense enough, the other retinal layers and the choroid are also affected by heat transfer. The damage becomes progressively less in the inner retina towards the inner limiting membrane. In the choroid under the burn the choriocapillaris may become thrombosed.

Within a few days, macrophages appear and remove the necrotic tissue. The gap in the pigmented epithelium is covered by inward migration of adjacent cells, which may become layered, and Müller's fibres become adherent to the pigmented epithelium where the photoreceptors have been lost (Fig. 10.13c & d).

With the argon laser, damage to the inner retinal layers in the immediate proximity of the macula occurs independently of outer retinal damage even with minimal suprathreshold lesions, as a result of absorption of energy in the foveal pigment. This is of clinical significance because absorption of energy in the inner retina reduces the energy available for the treatment of subretinal lesions and causes unwanted neuroretinal damage.

With minimal suprathreshold lesions from ruby lasers, direct damage to the inner retinal layers does not occur.

The absorption of energy by haemoglobin is much greater with the argon laser than with the ruby laser or xenon arc. Damage to vessel walls and perivascular tissue occurs in argon laser burns, but it has proved difficult to achieve closure of retinal arterioles or venules with a single exposure.

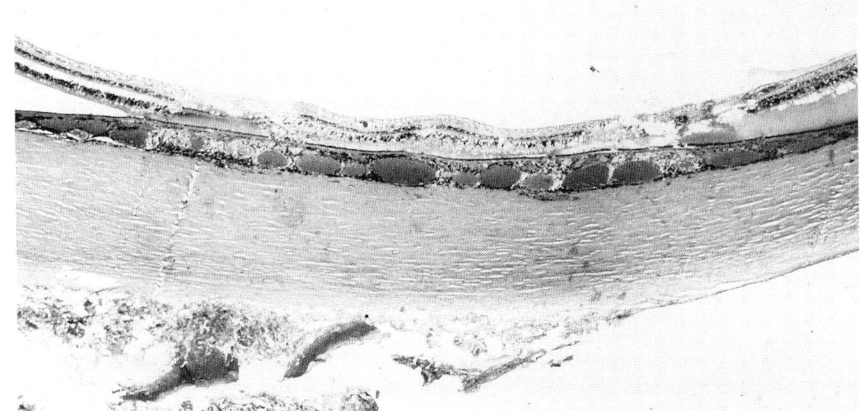

Fig. 10.13 Laser burns. (a) Low power at 24 hours after exposure to show full extent of burn and underlying choroidal swelling. H & E (×20).

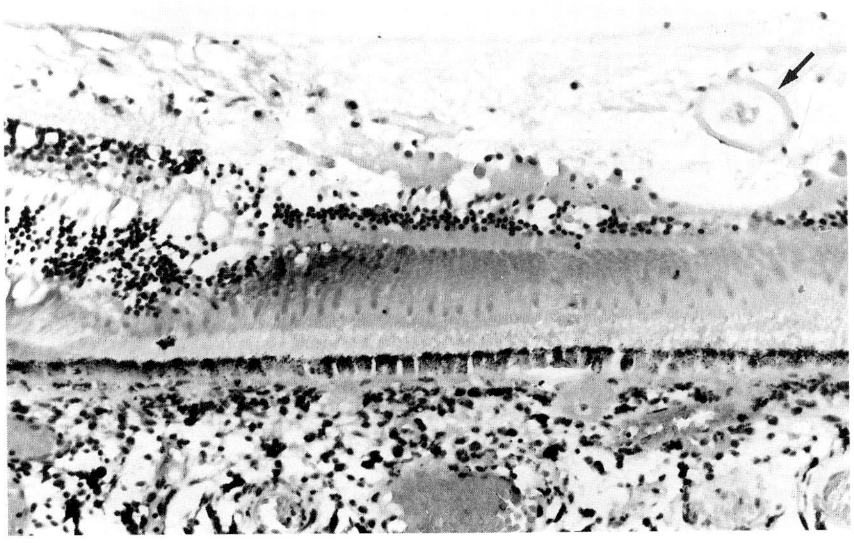

Fig. 10.13 (b) High power of left hand margin of same burn. Note necrosis and peculiar hazy appearance of photoreceptors prior to dissolution. An occluded vessel is indicated (arrow). The pigmented epithelium is swollen and the pigment is in the apical part of the cell. The choroid is infiltrated with lymphocytes. H & E (×160).

Solar burns

Eclipse retinopathy is a well-known clinical entity, but little is known of its pathology.

'Sun-gazing' for an hour has been shown to result in leakage of fluorescein from the choriocapillaris and mild alterations in the capillary endothelium at the fovea. Subtle changes were also noted in the foveal photoreceptors and pigmented epithelium after 48 hours (Tso *et al.*, 1974). It may be noted that thermal burns do not result from looking at the sun unless binoculars or telescopes are used. In such cases, the lesion will be a combination of photic and thermal effects.

EFFECTS OF IONISING RADIATION

The rods are the most radiosensitive component of the retina, and necrosis has been observed in many mammalian species after a single threshold dose of 2000–3000 rads. Since this is above the level used therapeutically in a single treatment, necrosis of the visual cells is not a complication of radiotherapy. Retinal damage may be observed following radiotherapy, usually with total dosage levels exceeding 6000 rads, but results from long-term damage to the retinal vasculature. Narrowing of the retinal vessels and microaneurysms are seen and haemorrhages and exudates appear which may take the form of a circinate retinopathy.

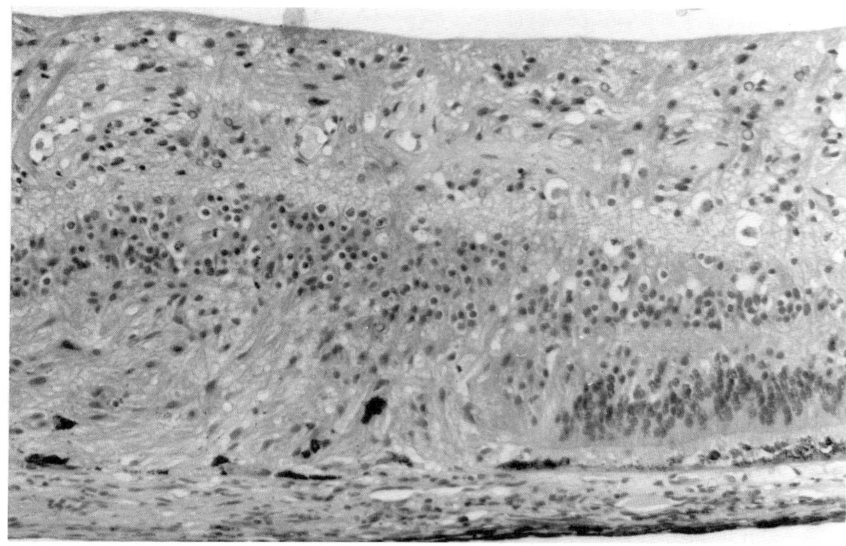

Fig. 10.13 (c) Old burn with destruction and gliosis of outer layers and pigmented epithelium, but partial preservation of inner layers. H & E (×160).

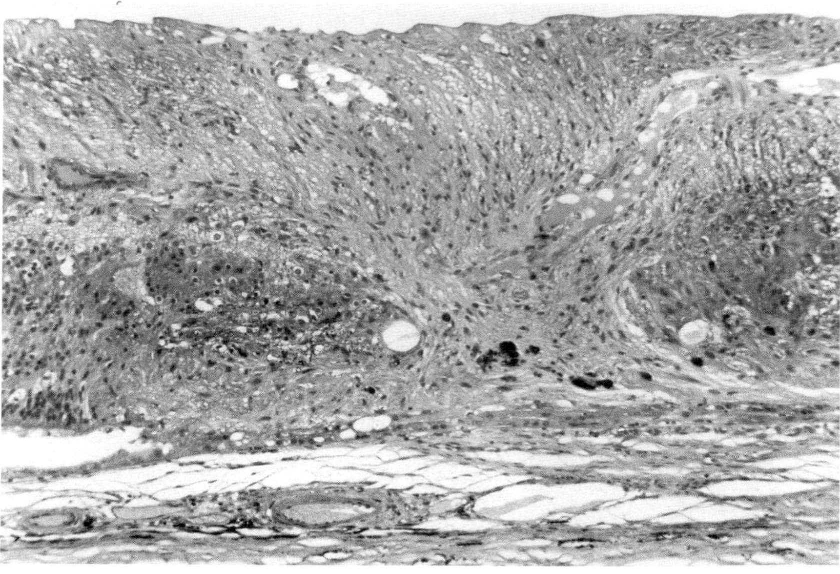

Fig. 10.13 (d) Old burn with destruction and gliosis of all layers. PAS/tartrazine (×94).

DISCIFORM SYNDROMES

This section is devoted principally to a consideration of disciform detachment of the macular neuroepithelium secondary to underlying choroidopathy. The following disciform syndromes will be discussed:
1 Senile macular degeneration.
2 Senile disciform degeneration of the macula.
3 Juvenile disciform degeneration of the macula.
4 Disciform syndromes associated with angioid streaks, choroidal neoplasms, ocular trauma and myopia.

Bruch's membrane

The structure of Bruch's membrane and its relationships with the pigmented epithelium and the choriocapillaris is of crucial importance in understanding the pathology of macular degeneration. Some aspects have already been touched on earlier in the chapter.

The outer and thicker portion of Bruch's membrane is a condensation of collagenous and elastic fibres which forms an inner limiting membrane to the choroidal stroma. The choriocapllaris occupies grooves on the outer aspect of this fibroelastic membrane so that each capillary vessel is separated from its neighbour by a ridge of fibroelastic tissue. These ridges appear in sections as posteriorly directed spurs. Electron microscopy has revealed fenestrations in the inner walls of the capillary vessels where the cytoplasm of the endothelial cell is deficient and the blood in the capillary is thus separated from Bruch's membrane only by a double layer of cell membrane.

The inner or cuticular portion of Bruch's membrane is a very thin layer of basement membrane substance derived from the pigmented epithelium of which it is an integral part, forming complicated folds in the base of the cell. This basement membrane material attaches the pigmented epithelium to the fibroelastic layer of Bruch's membrane. The apices of the pigmented epithelial cells form microvilli which envelope the photoreceptors, but are not firmly attached to them.

As a result of these structural arrangements, fluid trapped between the fibroelastic and cuticular layers of Bruch's membrane forms a blister under the pigmented epithelium. The attachment of the latter to Bruch's membrane round the point of exudation tends to limit the size of the blister and give it a sharp outline. A larger, less well circumscribed lesion will develop if the fluid breaks through the pigmented epithelium into the subretinal space. This is because the loose adhesion of the retina to the pigmented epithelium exercises little restraint on the spread of fluid in the subretinal space.

After intravenous injection of fluorescein, serous fluid confined beneath the retinal pigmented epithelium stains more rapidly and more intensely than fluid in the subretinal space.

Senile macular degeneration

Senile macular degeneration is a common cause of failure of central vision in those over 65 years of age, and is possibly an expression of physiological ageing. Clinically there is pigment stippling and drüsen formation in the macular area first in one eye and then in the other.

Microscopic appearances

1 *Bruch's membrane:* Bruch's membrane is thicker than normal and often granular in appearance. It may be brightly eosinophilic or show variable degrees of basophilia due to calcification. The posteriorly directed intercapillary spurs of Bruch's membrane and the walls of the choriocapillaris are often thickened and hyalinised. These changes may be seen throughout the posterior fundus, but are most obvious beneath the macula and around the optic nerve head.
2 *Retinal pigmented epithelium:* depigmentation, flattening and fragmentation of the pigmented epithelium is a prominent feature and is accompanied by the opposite process of proliferation of some of the pigmented epithelial cells to form small heaps or plaques. Vagrant pigmented epithelial cells are often seen in the retina.
3 *Drüsen:* scattered drüsen are commonly seen in the ageing retina, but increase in size and number with the onset and progress of senile macular degeneration. They appear as hemispherical or placoid deposits of eosinophilic and PAS-positive material beneath the retinal pigmented epithelium (Fig. 10.14a). Although these deposits are known collectively as drüsen or colloid bodies, they are not all alike. Some are homogeneous and glassy while others are finely granular (Fig. 10.14b). The majority of drüsen are probably products of the pigmented epithelium, but the possibility cannot be excluded that proteinous exudates from the choriocapillaris sometimes contribute to their formation.
4 *Basal linear deposit:* one of the earliest changes is the deposition of a finely granular deposit between Bruch's membrane and the pigmented epithelium. This is at first thin and patchy, but gradually forms a continuous layer. The material is eosinophilic and moderately PAS-positive (Fig. 10.15a). Electron microscopy shows the deposit to consist of banded material lying between the linear infoldings of the pigmented epithelium and the basement membrane.
5 *Retina:* the rods and cones are distorted and many are missing so that the external limiting membrane lies against the retinal pigmented epithelium or against Bruch's membrane. The outer nuclear layer of the retina

is replaced by glial cells with large oval or elongated nuclei.

Senile disciform degeneration of the macula

Senile disciform degeneration of the macula is characterised by circumscribed detachment of the macular neuroepithelium due to submacular serous exudation and haemorrhage which is eventually organised to scar tissue. The patients are usually over 60 years of age and in approximately 50% of cases the condition becomes bilateral. Senile disciform degeneration is the result of pathological changes in Bruch's membrane and the choriocapillaris. In its early stages the disciform lesion is characteristically circular in outline and elevated, with flat base on Bruch's membrane and a domed surface in apposition with the rods and cones. In its cicatricial stage the lesion may lose its typical shape and become quite irregular in outline.

Microscopic appearances

1 *Bruch's membrane:* the changes are the same as those already described above under senile macular degeneration. In addition, sclerosis or even obliteration of the choriocapillaris may be evident and small breaks in Bruch's membrane occur. These changes are often difficult to see in sections.

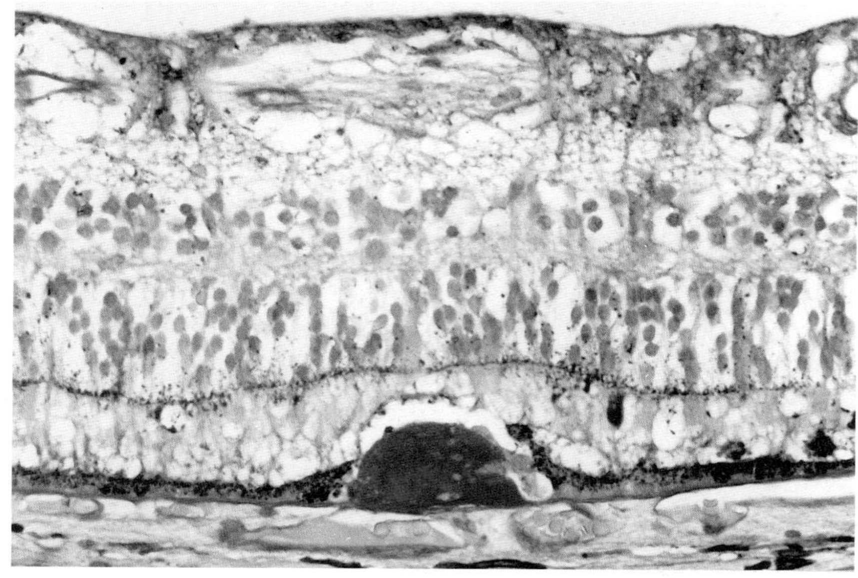

Fig. 10.14 Drüsen. (a) Solitary hemispherical drüse with rupture of pigmented epithelium. PAS/tartrazine (×360).

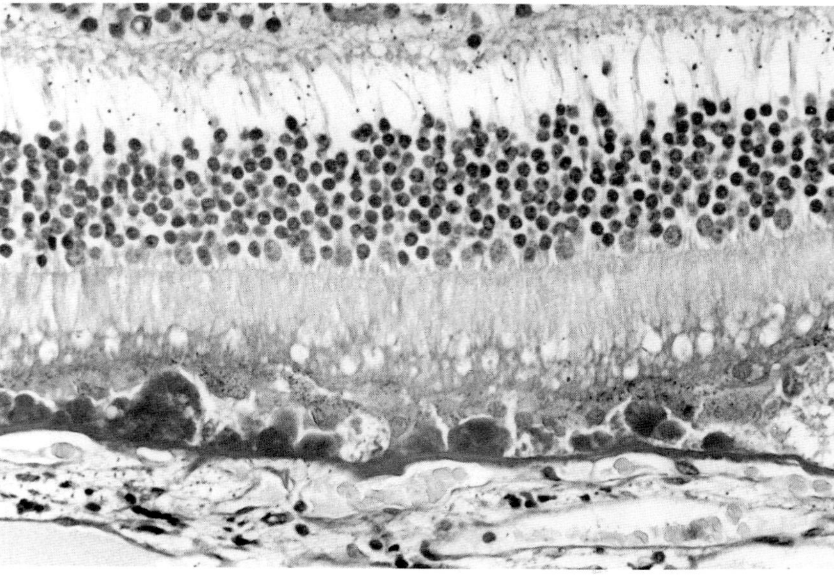

Fig. 10.14 (b) Multiple smaller drüsen with granular debris. PAS/tartrazine (×360).

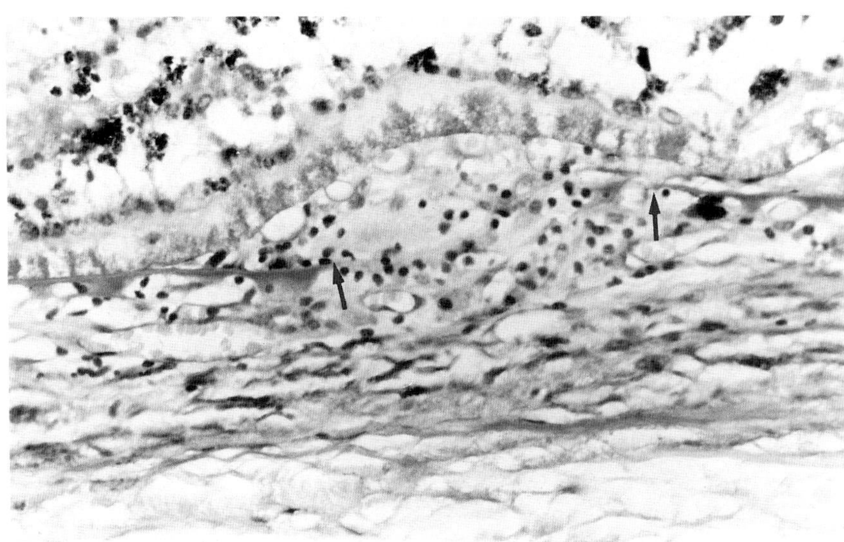

Fig. 10.15 Macular degeneration. (a) Gap in Bruch's membrane (margins indicated by arrows). The gap is bridged by basal linear deposit. PAS/tartrazine (×405).

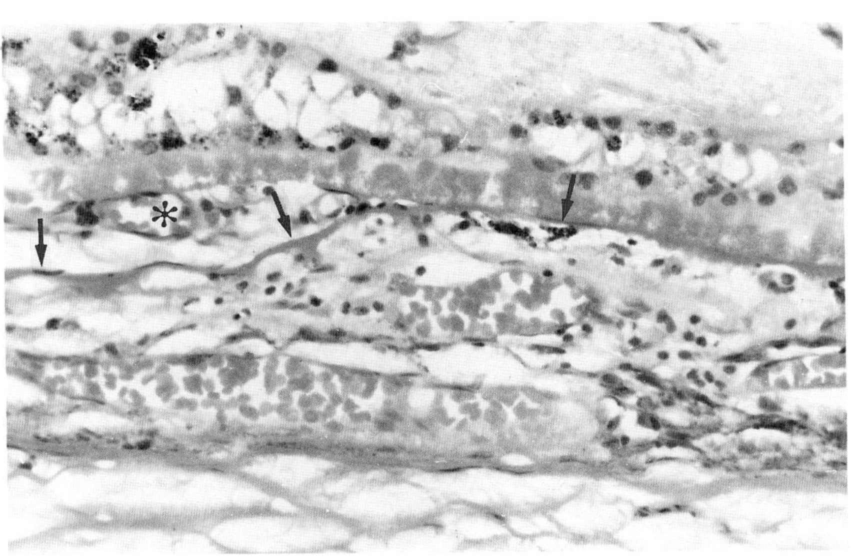

Fig. 10.15 (b) Capillary (asterisk) on retinal side of Bruch's membrane (indicated by arrows). Basal linear deposit is present on Bruch's membrane and is elevated by ingrowing vessel. PAS/tartrazine (×405).

2 *Subretinal-neovascularisation:* new capillary vessels derived from the choroid invade the drüsen on Bruch's membrane and the space between the retinal pigmented epithelium, either through breaks in Bruch's membrane (Fig. 10.15b) or from the margins of the optic nerve head. Capillaries passing through breaks in Bruch's membrane are usually difficult to find and may be missed unless multiple sections are examined.

3 *Exudation and haemorrhage:* serous exudation and haemorrhage stemming from these new vessels and from the choroidal circulation accumulate beneath the retinal pigmented epithelium and may break through into the subretinal space. If the haemorrhage is brisk, the blood may penetrate into the retina and even into the vitreous cavity.

4 *Organisation:* during the ensuing weeks, as a result of breakdown of haemoglobin and release of blood lipids, the submacular haematoma changes colour from dark brown to greyish-white or yellow. These are taken up by macrophages (foam cells) which may migrate into the overlying and surrounding retina. Aggregates of these foam cells may be visible ophthalmoscopically as a macular star, perimacular circinate figures or as irregularly disposed lipid exudates.

Coincident with this degradation of the blood constituents, fibroblasts from the choroid invade the haematoma. At the same time, surviving cells of the retinal pigmented epithelium proliferate and often undergo a curious change into elongated spindly cells. Meanwhile the overlying photoreceptors atrophy. Eventually, a submacular nodule or plaque of fibroglial scar tissue is formed (Fig. 10.16a). This may be seamed by rows of proliferated epithelial cells, many of which have lost their melanin granules. Contraction of the scar tissue distorts the overlying retina.

5 *Secondary haemorrhage and exudation:* further exudates and haemorrhages are a frequent complication in the late stages and sometimes result in large deposits of yellow lipid in the subretinal space and multiple areas of serous detachment (Fig. 10.16b). A picture resembling Coats' disease is thus produced. Massive secondary haemorrhages, which sometimes break through into the vitreous space, may also occur (Fig. 10.17). Such massive haemorrhage have been related to raised blood pressure, anticoagulant therapy and use of salicylates (Baba *et al.*, 1986).

Pathogenesis

The pathogenesis of the drüsen and related basal linear deposit is unknown, but they are generally regarded as manifestations of functional failure of the intracellular digestive system of the pigmented epithelium which results in a build-up of incompletely degraded material within its cells. The maintenance of the photoreceptors is thus compromised and aberrant material (drüsen and linear deposit) deposited on Bruch's membrane (see Eagle, 1984; Havener & Benes, 1986; Young, 1987). The accumulation of this material apparently predisposes to subretinal neovascularisation. The stimulus to capillary growth is unknown, and breaks in Bruch's membrane

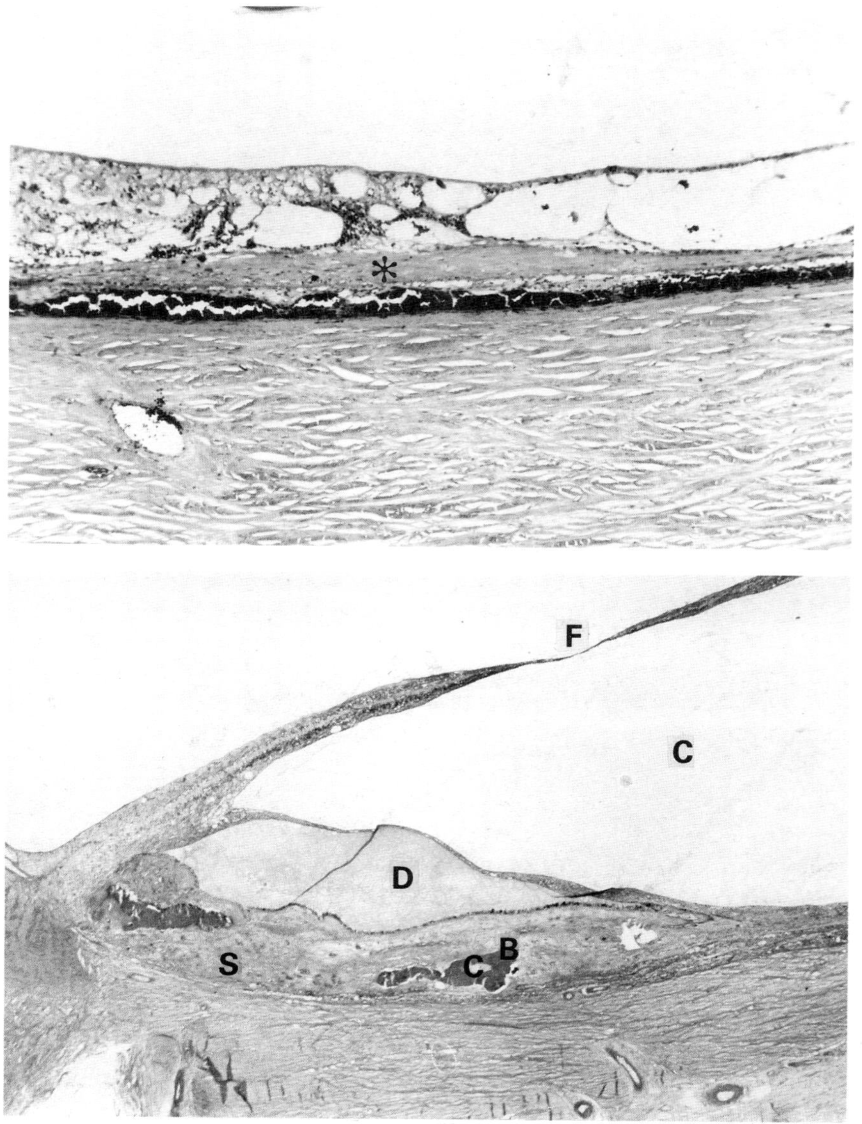

Fig. 10.16 Disciform scars. (a) Simple disciform scar (asterisk) with cystoid degeneration of overlying retina. The dense staining under the scar is due to blood in the choroidal vessels.

Fig. 10.16 (b) More complicated scar (S) with extensive fibrosis in which there has been bone formation (B). There is a giant retinal cyst (C) deep to the fovea (F) and partial detachment of the retina (D) over the scar. H & E (×20).

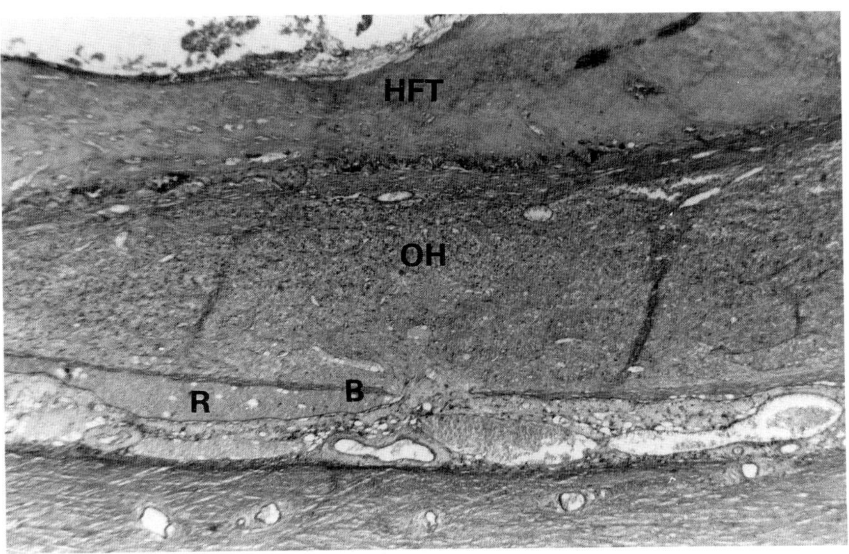

Fig. 10.17 Disciform degeneration with massive successive haemorrhages in a haemophiliac. (a) Low power. Shows a recent haemorrhage (R), a more massive older haemorrhage in process of organisation (OH) and a much older haemorrhage represented by a thick layer of hyaline fibrous tissue (HFT). A gap is present in Bruch's membrane (B) through which choroidal vessels are proliferating into the organising haemorrhage. Note layers created by and dividing successive haemorrhages. PAS/tartrazine (×41).

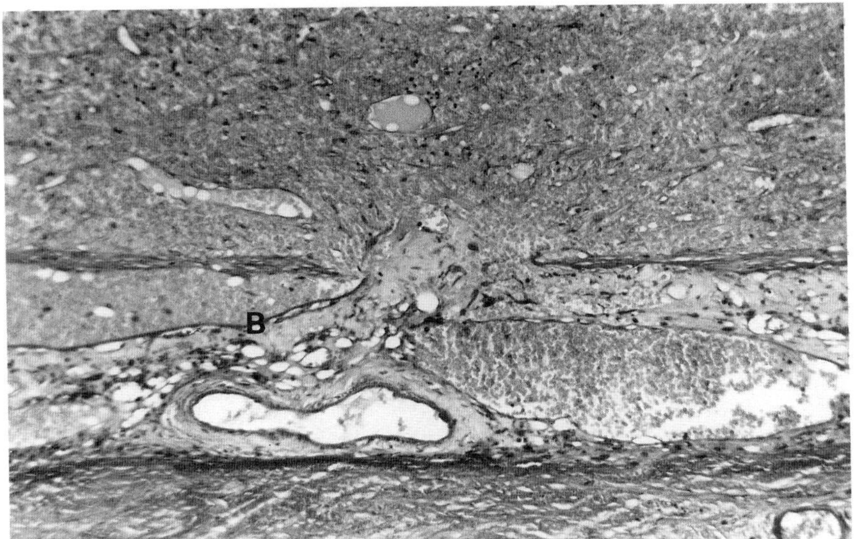

Fig. 10.17 (b) Higher power showing gap in Bruch's membrane in more detail. PAS/tartrazine (×94).

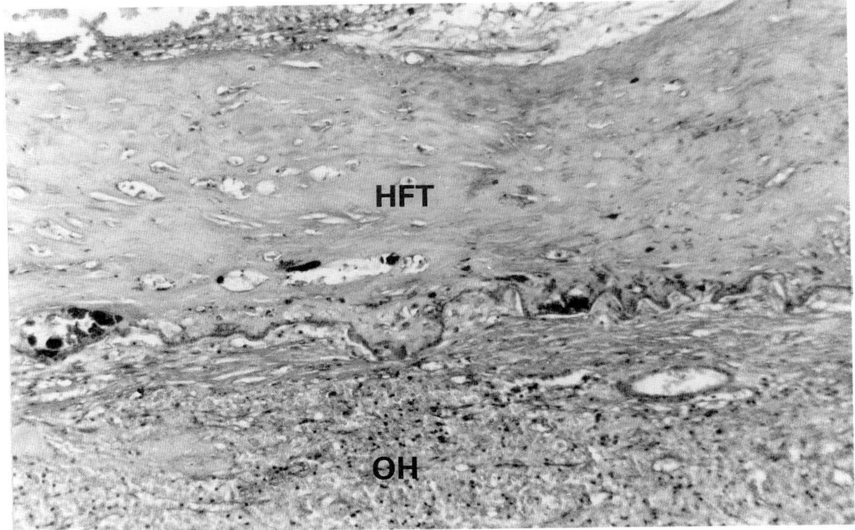

Fig. 10.17 (c) Higher power of boundary zone between organising haemorrhage and hyaline fibrous tissue. Note proliferated pigment and basement membrane-like material. PAS/tartrazine (×94).

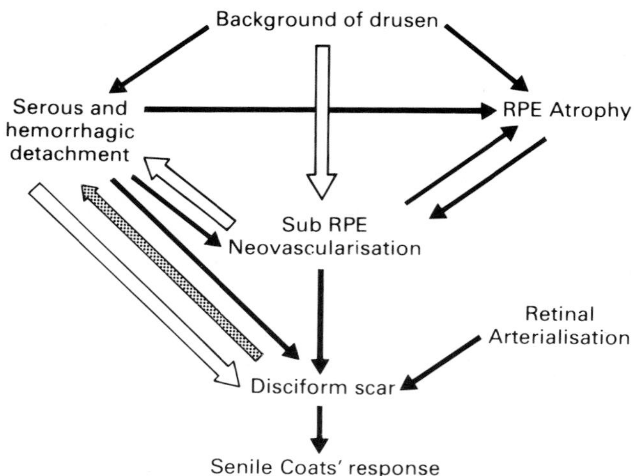

Fig. 10.18 Flow diagram showing relationship between the various forms of macular degeneration. The larger arrows indicate the more common pathways from drüsen to disciform scarring. The smaller arrows indicate other pathways and associated features that may be observed. (Redrawn with permission from Green, 1980.)

may be observed through which no capillaries are seen to pass. The interrelationships of the various stages in the evolution of the lesion are summarised in Fig. 10.18.

In concluding this section, it should be noted that, while involvement of the macular area is usual, the lesion may not be confined to this area.

Juvenile disciform degeneration of the macula

There is a group of middle-aged and young adult patients in otherwise excellent health who suddenly develop haemorrhagic disciform macular detachment in one eye. In 50% of cases the condition becomes bilateral. Often the haemorrhage originates outside the macular area and extends into it. The blood, which may be confined beneath the retinal pigmented epithelium or break through into the subretinal space, is organised to form a submacular scar.

Other disciform syndromes

Disciform lesions sometimes occur in association with the following conditions:

Angioid streaks: angioid streaks are jagged reddish-brown striae radiating from the optic nerve head. They result from breaks in Bruch's membrane along lines of stress. Angioid streaks are always bilateral, often associated with widespread disturbance of the retinal pigmented epithelium and drüsen formation, and sometimes complicated by disciform maculopathy following trauma to the globe.

Angioid streaks are often a manifestation of systemic disease. They are present in 85% of cases of pseudoxanthoma elasticum, in 10–15% of patients with Paget's disease of bone and in 1.5% of cases of sickle cell disease. They have also occasionally been reported in association with many other diseases, but the association may have been coincidental.

Pseudoxanthoma elasticum is a hereditary disorder of elastic tissue in the skin, eyes and blood vessels which is transmitted in an autosomal recessive manner. It is characterised by waxy cutaneous papules in the natural skin folds, angioid streaks in the fundus and evidence of vascular disease and insufficiency such as gastric haemorrhages, intermittent caudication, effort angina, absent peripheral pulses and hypertension.

The pathological basis of pseudoxanthoma elasticum is a degeneration of elastic fibres which swell up, undergo granular disintegration and break up into short curled lengths which usually appear basophilic due to impregnation with calcium phosphate. These changes are best seen in the dermis and in the medial coats of blood vessels. In Bruch's membrane the degeneration is expressed by calcification, basophilia and cracking. In time, fibrovascular tissue from the choroid may grow through the cracks into the space beneath the pigmented epithelium to be followed by serous exudates and haemorrhage and the eventual formation of a submacular scar.

All cases of angioid streaks studied histologically have shown the same changes whatever the associated systemic condition.

Choroidal neoplasm: space occupying lesions of the choroid in the macular area are sometimes complicated by serous exudation and occasionally by haemorrhage which results in detachment of the overlying neuroepithelium. Among such choroidal lesions are naevi, small malignant melanomata, haemangiomata, metastatic carcinomata and leukaemic infiltrations. These choroidal lesions apparently disturb the local microcirculation and induce pathological changes in Bruch's membrane. Neovascular invasion of these drüsen sets the stage for serous or haemorraghic effusions beneath the neuroepithelium.

Ocular trauma: concussional and penetrating injuries of the globe occasionally cause rupture of the choriocapillaris and consequent submacular haemorrhage. Organisation of the haematoma may eventually result in a pigmented disciform scar (see Chapter 18).

Myopic choroidal degeneration: haemorrhagic detachment of the macula occurs as a complication of progressive myopia. The patients are usually middle-aged, high myopes who suffer sudden loss of vision in one eye and are found to have a circular dark spot at the macula with surrounding haemorrhages. It seems that the progressive stretching of the choroid accompanying myopia predisposes to breaks in Bruch's membrane which permit fibrovascular invasion beneath the pigmented epithelium and subsequent haemorrhagic detachment of the macula.

PART 2: VASCULAR DISORDERS

RETINAL BLOOD VESSELS

Arterioles

Like arteries of similar size elsewhere in the body, the central retinal artery consists of an intima (endothelium, subendothelial connective tissue and fenestrated internal elastic lamina), a medial layer of circularly disposed muscle cells and a connective tissue adventitia which is separated by a potential space (corresponding to the Virchow–Robin space of the cerebral vessels) from the pial and astrocytic sheath, which the central vessels carry into the optic nerve where they enter it behind the globe. The arterial lumen is approximately 200 μm in diameter and the ratio of lumen to wall roughly 4:1.

As the central artery passes through the lamina cribrosa, its internal elastic lamina disappears and its muscle coat becomes thin. The intraocular retinal arteries are, in fact, arterioles having endothelium, a thin subendothelial layer, a narrow media composed mainly of collagen fibres together with scanty muscle cells and an inconspicuous adventitia separated by a potential space from the surrounding retinal glia which, in suitable preparations, can be seen to form a definite perivascular sheath. The ratio of lumen to wall is approximately 10:1. The retinal arteries give off short precapillary arterioles which almost immediately break up into capillary nets.

Flat preparations of the retina after partial trypsin digestion have shown that the retinal capillaries ramify extensively in the inner retinal layers and do not form strictly defined strata of vessels at various levels in the retina. In the peripapillary retina, however, there is a distinct layer of capillaries which arise from arterioles near the optic nerve head and pursue a radial and roughly parallel course in the peripapillary nerve fibre layer to which they supply blood. Because these capillaries are long and poor in anastomoses, they may be functionally vulnerable to the effects of raised intraocular tension.

The macula is supplied by branches from the superior and inferior temporal arterioles. They are especially numerous in the perimacular area where they permeate all layers of the inner retina, but diminish progressively towards the central macula and are absent from the fovea.

In the peripheral retina the capillaries are fewer in number than elswhere. Approximately 1 mm behind the ora serrata they loop round to become continuous with the veins.

Blood–ocular barriers

Two main blood–ocular barriers have been proposed: the blood–aqueous barrier which regulates exchanges between the blood and intraocular fluids and the blood–retinal barrier which limits interchange between blood and retina (Fig. 10.19). No convincing blood–vitreous barrier has been demonstrated and diffusion occurs freely between vitreous and posterior chamber or retinal extracellular space.

The blood–aqueous barrier

The blood–aqueous barrier resides in the ciliary body and iris. The capillaries of the sub-epithelial stroma of the ciliary body are fenestrated and freely permeable to plasma proteins and blood-borne tracers of similar size. However, tight junctions between the cells of the non-pigmented ciliary epithelium appear to block the passage of macromolecules such as horseradish peroxidase which can escape from the stromal capillaries.

Iris capillaries are not fenestrated and their endothelial cells are linked by tight junctions. Like retinal capillaries they are impermeable to circulating horseradish peroxidase. However, their tight junctions have been shown to be less stable than those of retinal capillaries.

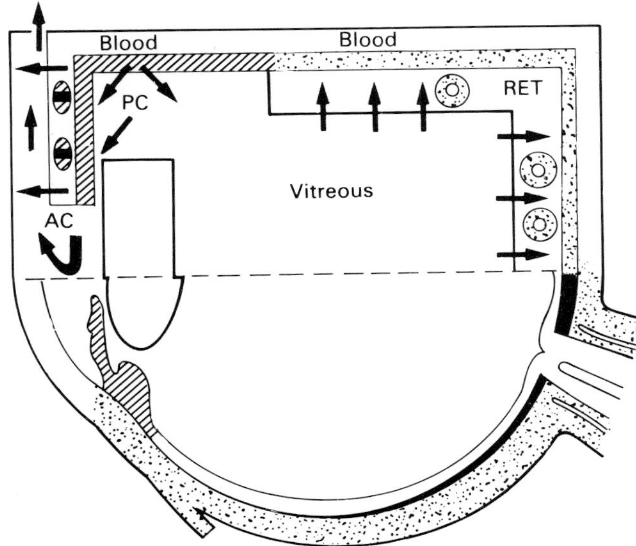

Fig. 10.19 Diagram of the blood–ocular barriers. RET = retina, PC = posterior chamber, AC = anterior chamber. (Redrawn with permission from Cunha-Vaz, 1979.)

The blood–retinal barrier

The blood–retinal barrier is related to blood supply at the level of the retinal capillaries and at the chorioepithelial interface.

Retinal capillaries: these consist of endothelial cells supported on a substantial basement membrane in which are embedded mural cells or pericytes. The endothelial cells are linked together by zonulae occludentes or tight junctions. Outside the basement membrane is a perivascular space which is probably continuous with that which surrounds the central retinal artery and its branches. Surrounding the whole capillary is a dense glial sheath of retinal astrocytes resting on a delicate pial membrane. Retinal capillaries are unresponsive to histamine, and the tight junctions between the endothelial cells appear to block the passage of substances such as trypan blue, thorium dioxide, fluorescein and horseradish peroxidase. The blood–retinal barrier is, therefore, now thought to be at this level rather than in the glial processes which invest the capillaries.

Chorioretinal interface: the capillaries of the choriocapillaris are freely permeable to macromolecules, trypan blue, fluorescein, etc. Bruch's membrane also acts as a diffusion barrier only to molecules of large size. The cells of the pigmented epithelium are, however, joined by zonulae occludentes with similar permeability characteristics to those of the retinal capillary endothelium. Most molecular movements between blood and retina at this level must, therefore, occur transcellularly.

Breakdown of the blood–ocular barriers

Breakdown of the blood–ocular barriers is easily demonstrated clinically by the passage of fluorescein. When the blood–aqueous barrier breaks down, fluorescein leaks into the aqueous and, when the posterior blood–retinal barriers break down, into the retina through the capillary walls and chorioretinal interface. Breakdown of one or other of the barriers is a frequent occurrence in intraocular disease. New vessels and vessels in tumours are permeable to fluorescein.

Venules

The veins in the retina have extremely thin walls and a slightly larger lumen than the corresponding arteries. All that can usually be discerned is endothelium and a fibroelastic wall. At arteriovenous crossings, vein and arteriole share a common adventitia and their walls appear to fuse, a unique circumstance which may well facilitate venous occlusion in arteriolar sclerosis.

The central retinal vein, which is somewhat more robust, has endothelium complete with basement membrane, a media composed of elastic fibres with sparse muscle cells and a thin adventitia. The lumen is approximately the same as that of the central artery, but the ratio of lumen to wall is approximately 10:1.

RETINAL OEDEMA AND EXUDATES

Conditions in which pathological changes occur in the retina which may be grouped under the general heading of oedema are numerous and include diabetic retinopathy, central and branch retinal vein occlusions, hypertensive retinopathy, and trauma, both surgical and accidental.

Cystoid macular oedema

In this condition, cystoid spaces appear in the macula in Henle's layer and are also often widespread in the inner nuclear layer. The spaces usually appear empty and are due initially to imbibition of water by Müller fibres. Later, the cells rupture and the fluid forms pools in Henle's layer (Fig. 10.20). There is some associated necrosis of photoreceptors, but the early stages are reversible.

Disruption of the blood–retinal barrier at the level of the retinal capillaries and pigment epithelium is thought to play an important role in the pathogenesis of cystoid macular oedema.

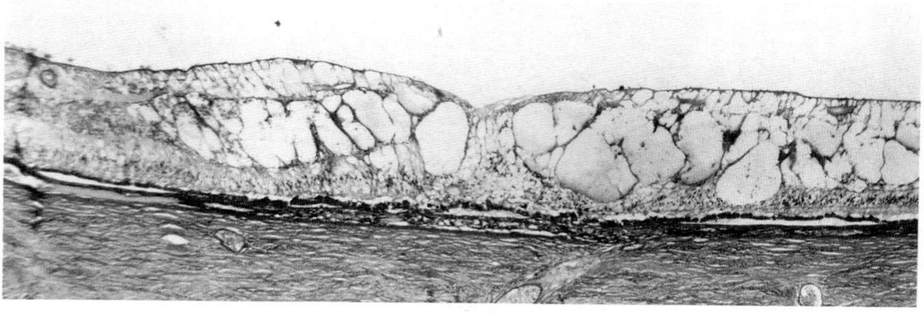

Fig. 10.20 Cystoid macular oedema. The macular area of the retina is virtually destroyed by the massive cystoid accumulations of fluid. In this case a complication of *Pseudomonas endophthalmitis*. PAS/tartrazine (×41).

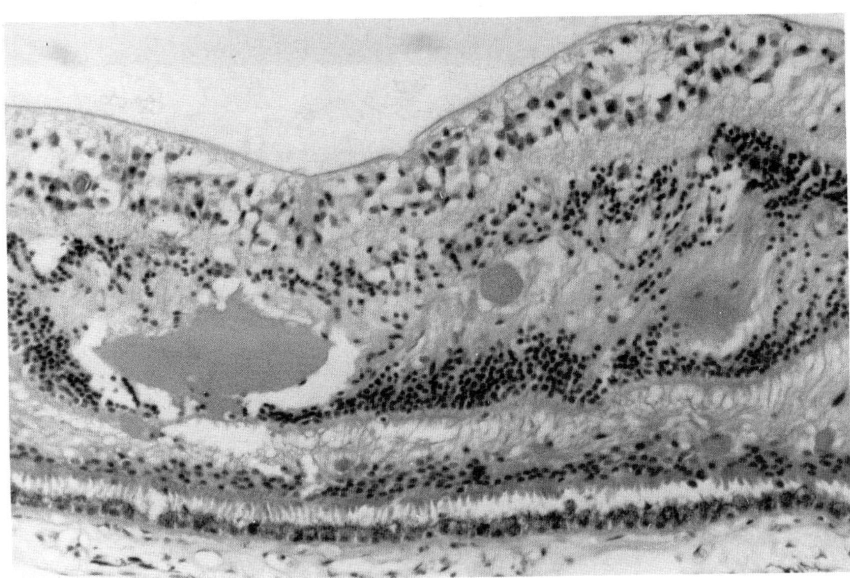

Fig. 10.21 Hard exudates in inner nuclear layer. H & E (×160).

Hard exudates

Hard exudates are seen ophthalmoscopically as glistening yellowish-white exudates between the radial fibres of Henle's layer (macular star) or arranged in an arc or circle around the macula (circinate retinopathy) or aggregated into irregular sheets elsewhere in the fundus.

Microscopically, they appear as pools of exudate in Henle's layer containing proteinaceous material and lipid derived from from blood and necrotic retinal debris (Fig. 10.21). Such deposits attract a macrophagic reaction so that foam cells are seen around them.

Cotton-wool spots

Cotton-wool spots result from arteriolar occlusion and failure of capillary perfusion. They appear as discrete whitish-grey areas often associated with haemorrhages and microaneurysms. They develop in the nerve fibre layer of the optic nerve head or adjacent to it in a variety of conditions in which there is retinal ischaemia.

Microscopically, they consist of swollen axons crammed with mitochondria and other organelles which in cross section resemble giant cells and hence have long been known as cytoid bodies (Fig. 10.22). The axonal swelling occurs on either side of a microinfarct and is due to inhibition of axonal transport in both directions as the nerve fibre passes through the infarct. The margins of the spot perpendicular to the direction of the nerve fibre are thus sharp while the lateral margins are blurred.

INFARCTION OF THE RETINA

Infarction implies necrosis of tissue as the result of obstruction to the arterial inflow or to the venous outflow. Since the central retinal vessels provide virtually the whole of the circulatory pathway serving the inner two-thirds of the retina, obstruction of either the central artery or the central vein has serious effects upon the nerve fibre, ganglion cell and bipolar cell layers.

Occlusion of the central retinal artery

Occlusion of the central retinal artery results in infarction of the inner two-thirds of the retina, reflex constriction of the whole retinal arterial tree and stasis in the retinal capillaries with consequent loss of blood fluid into the tissues. The infarct is ischaemic and haemorrhage is minimal in the absence of concomitant central retinal vein occlusion. The retinal cells undergo cloudy swelling and necrosis, then disintegrate and are phagocytosed by macrophages. Since the debris has a high lipid content these macrophages appear foamy.

In time the oedema is absorbed and the necrotic tissue removed to leave the retina thin and shrunken by the loss of nerve fibres, ganglion cells and bipolar cells. Gliosis is minimal because many of the glial cells are destroyed along with the nerve cells. The optic nerve head shows shallow excavation due to loss of nerve fibres, and there is ascending degeneration of fibres in the optic nerve itself.

Although some circulation is re-established, it is small in volume so that the retinal arteries remain narrow. They may be reduced to white threads like strands of cotton which appear in sections as solid hyaline cords.

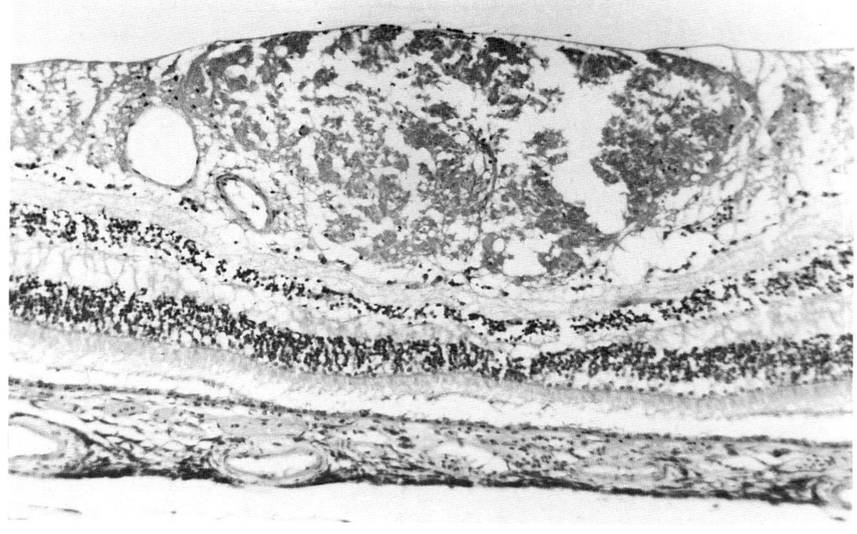

Fig. 10.22 Cotton-wool spot (specimen by courtesy of Dr M. Filipic). (a) Low power showing location in nerve fibre layer. H & E (×64).

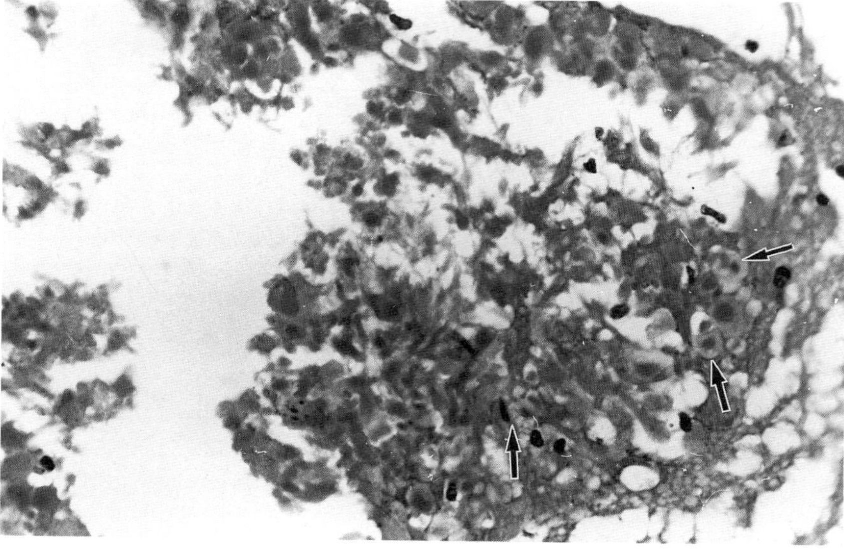

Fig. 10.22 (b) High power showing cytoid bodies (arrows). H & E (×400).

Aetiology

1 *Atherosclerosis of the central retinal artery:* occlusion of the central retinal artery commonly occurs at or in the vicinity of the lamina cribrosa and a frequent cause at this site is atheroma. Atheromatous plaques in the central retinal artery or its immediate branches are seen as subendothelial aggregates of lipid and foam cells which may completely fill the lumen or reduce it to a narrow cleft (Fig. 10.23). Final closure of the vessel may then result from haemorrhage into the plaque or thrombosis on its surface.

Sometimes the occlusion is in the intraneural part of the artery or farther back in the orbit. Serial sections may be required to demonstrate the block and these should be taken transversely since it is difficult to follow the course of the artery in longitudinal sections. Care is required in the interpretation of sections since factitious occlusion is readily produced by clamping the artery during enucleation.

2 *Atherosclerosis of the internal carotid artery:* sudden onset of blindness is common in association with severe atherosclerosis of the internal carotid. Infarction of the retina in such cases is probably due to reduction in the pressure in the central retinal artery in an eye which may already be affected by neovascular glaucoma as a result of ischaemia from the carotid disease. Cerebral infarction is also common in such cases.

3 *Embolism of the central artery:* this not uncommonly occurs as a complication of bacterial endocarditis, myocardial infarction or atherosclerosis of the aortic arch or the innominate and carotid arteries. Small emboli com-

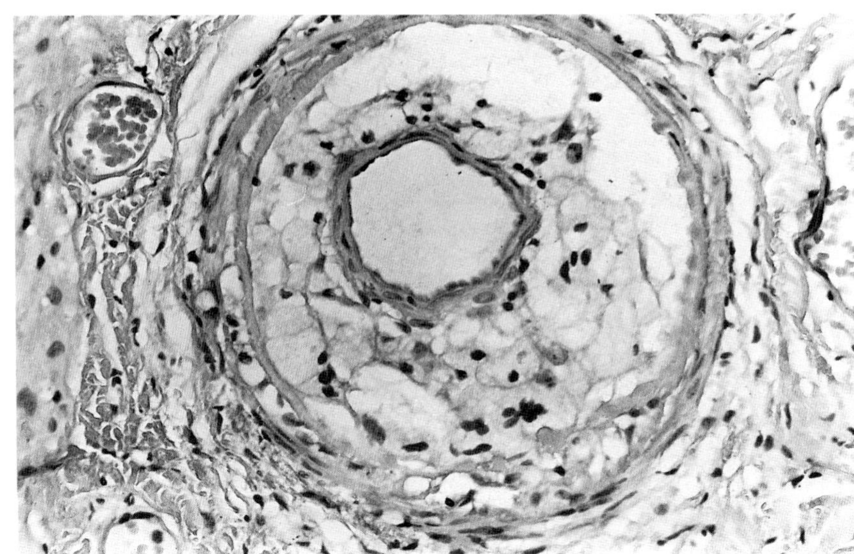

Fig. 10.23 Atheroma of central artery of retina. A massive subintimal accumulation of foam cells has greatly reduced the calibre of the lumen. H & E (×260).

posed of platelets or cholesterol derived from atheromatous plaques in the carotid may occlude branches of the retinal arterioles.

4 *Giant cell arteritis:* approximately 10% of cases.

5 *Occasional causes of occlusion:* these include increased orbital pressure in conditions such as endocrine exophthalmos, retro-ocular haemorrhage or orbital granuloma. Spasm of the retinal arterioles is a cause of transient visual disturbance, but probably does not often cause permanent circulatory impairment in the absence of organic disease such as atherosclerosis.

Complications

The growth of new vessels and subsequent development of neovascular glaucoma (see Chapter 12) has been reported following occlusion of the central retinal artery, but does not occur with the same regularity as following venous occlusions.

Occlusion of the central retinal vein

Occlusion of the central retinal vein occurs most commonly in hypertensive and elderly arteriosclerotic subjects and results in haemorrhagic infarction of the retina with stagnation of the retinal blood flow extending backwards from the veins into the venules, capillaries and arteries.

Haemorrhages in the nerve fibre layer spread in the plane of the fibres and are linear or flame-shaped, while those in the outer retinal layers are retained by Müller's fibres and appear round (dot and blot haemorrhages). Blood may break into the preretinal or subretinal spaces or into the vitreous. Massive oedema and violent effusions of plasma often disrupt the outer plexiform layer and form large spaces filled with sero-fibrinous exudate. Somewhat later, cotton-wool spots and hard exudates appear.

Optico-ciliary venous bypass channels are usually seen and there is new vessel formation in the retina and on its surface, usually from the margins of the optic nerve head. In many cases, new vessels also form on the anterior surface of the iris and lead to the development of neovascular glaucoma which results in a painful blind eye (see Chapter 12). The pathological changes observed in enucleated globes usually, therefore, represent changes due to glaucoma superimposed on those due to the venous occlusion.

In such eyes, the retina shows disorganisation and gliosis. The ganglion cells are absent and there is often substantial depletion of the inner nerve fibre and plexiform layers. Recent hamorrhages into the inner layers and cystoid macular oedema are commonly seen. Branch venules may show recanalised thrombi. The retinal arterioles frequently show marked hyaline mural thickening (Fig. 10.24a) and sometimes an actual occlusion may be found. The arteriolar thickening is not surprising since hypertension is a common predisposing factor, but obliterative change secondary to retinal atrophy may also be involved. Hyalinisation is thought to result from a breakdown in endothelial integrity which allows insudation of plasma into the wall. The insudate gradually loses its affinity for fibrin stains and takes up stains for collagen. Capillary channels may form in the hyalinised walls (Fig. 10.24b) and it has recently been pointed out that proliferation of these new capillaries may extend beyond the vessel wall into the retina and from there through the internal limiting membrane (Manschot & Lee, 1984).

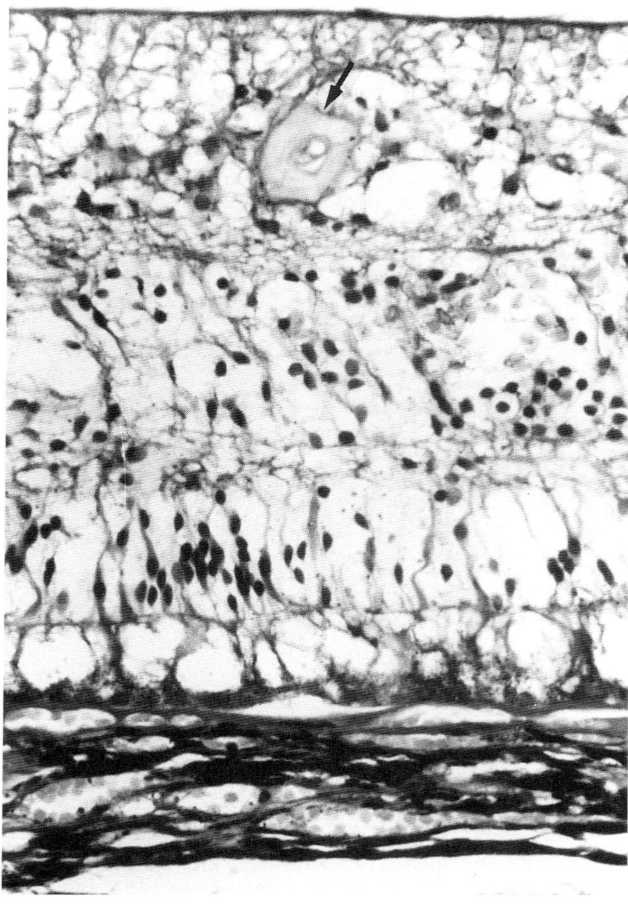

Fig. 10.24 Hyalinised vessels in end-stage neovascular (post-thrombotic) glaucoma complicating hypertension. (a) Vessel with single tiny lumen (arrow). The retina is oedematous. H & E (×340).

Changes in the central vein

To locate the site of occlusion with any certainty it is necessary to cut serial sections through the optic nerve and this cannot be done as a routine procedure. Such special studies have shown that, in the majority of cases, the thrombus is formed just posterior to the lamina cribrosa. The thrombus is initially composed of fibrin, platelets, leucocytes and erythrocytes. Liquefaction occurs following invasion by fibroblasts. This results in the formation of spaces which are lined by proliferating endothelial cells. Channels are thus formed which communicate with the lumen anterior and posterior to the thrombus and may eventually coalesce to form a single channel. Lymphocytic infiltration around the organising thrombus may be a conspicuous feature in the later stages and has led to the belief that endophlebitis is an important predisposing factor.

Lymphocytic infiltration around the central vein is also quite common proximal to the organising thrombus (Fig. 10.25).

Predisposing factors

Many local and systemic factors predispose to occlusion of the central retinal vein.

Local: these fall into three categories:

1 Increased intraocular tension: the central vein is at its narrowest as it emerges from the lamina cribrosa and it is likely that distortion of the latter causes endothelial damage and restriction and turbulence of flow which favour platelet deposition and thrombosis in this part of the vein. Chronic simple glaucoma is the commonest predisposing cause in this category.

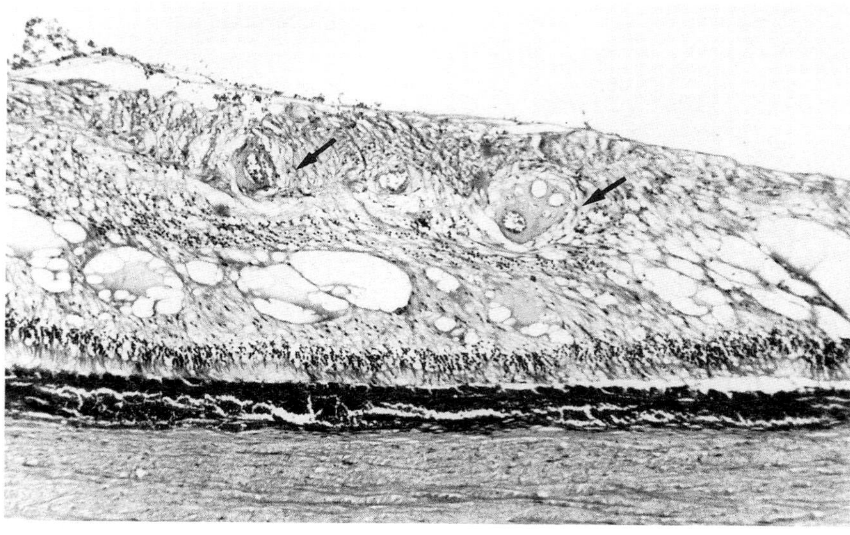

Fig. 10.24 (b) Two hyalised vessels (arrows). One shows what appear to be several channels presumably due to invasion of the wall by new capillaries. The retina shows cystoid oedema. Masson (×94).

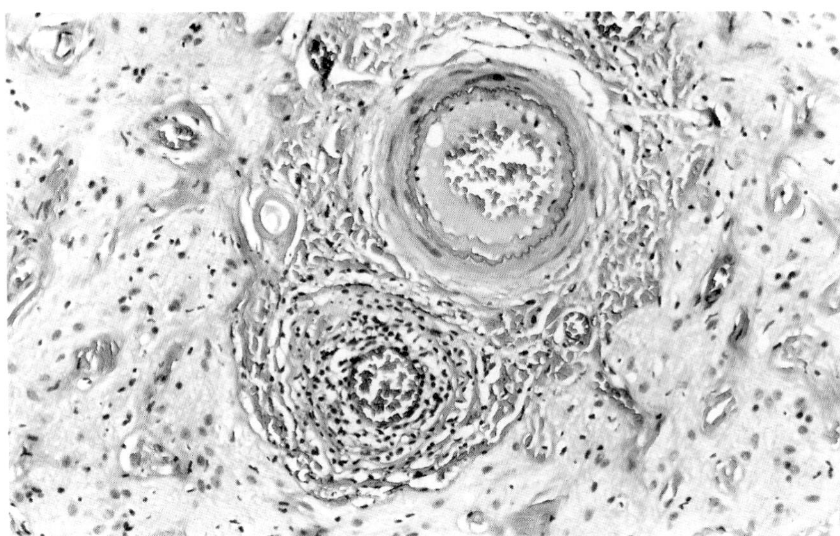

Fig. 10.25 Post-thrombotic glaucoma. Cuffing of collapsed central vein by lymphocytes. H & E (×160).

2 Factors causing mechanical compression of the vein: these include atheromatous plaques in the central retinal artery, papilloedema and large drüsen of the nerve head.
3 Local endophlebitis such as may occur in Behçet's disease or Eales' disease.

Systemic: these comprise cardiovascular disease and changes in the blood.
1 Cardiovascular disease: the most important systemic factors are arteriosclerosis and hypertension. Arterial disease may, indeed, play a primary role in producing the typical clinical picture of occlusion of the central retinal vein (Paton *et al.*, 1964).

In the experimental animal, occlusion of both central vein and artery as they enter the optic nerve in the orbit was necessary to produce retinal haemorrhages and oedema (Hayreh, 1965, 1971). In his view, the retinal haemorrhages, which occurred only with combined arterial and venous occlusion, are attributable to capillary ischaemia. However, obstructing the central retinal vein alone within the nerve head does produce a necrotic hamorrhagic retinopathy (Fujino *et al.*, 1969).

In an attempt to resolve the relative importance of arterial and venous factors, the clinical findings were compared in patients with and without cilio-retinal arteries who had suffered an occlusion of the central vein (McLeod, 1975). The territory supplied by the cilio-retinal artery is independent of the central retinal artery, but shares a common venous drainage through the central vein. It might, therefore, be expected that this territory would be spared after occlusion of the central vein if the hypothesis that concomitant occlusion of the central artery and resulting hypoxia was necessary to produce the typical clinical picture of occlusion of the central vein was correct. However, haemorrhages were observed in this territory as elsewhere. Though this did not deny the importance of hypoxia, it emphasised the importance of intraluminal pressure changes as opposed to perfusion changes in the causation of haemorrhage and oedema after venous occlusion.
2 Changes in the blood: occlusion of the central vein has been reported in association with various disorders of the blood including leukaemia and polycythaemia and systemic conditions affecting blood coagulability such as macroglobulinaemia and haemodialysis.

It has recently been found (Trope *et al.*, 1983) that, in longstanding cases of venous occlusion complicated by capillary non-perfusion of new vessels, blood viscosity is increased and the platelet count is lower than in cases without these complications, but it is not clear whether these changes are of causal significance.

Venous stasis retinopathy

Cases of occlusion of the central retinal vein without significant hypoxia due to arterial disease have been termed 'venous stasis retinopathy'. Such cases tend to occur in younger age groups, probably as a result of endophlebitis, and have a better prognosis (Hayreh, 1977).

Occlusion of branch veins

Occlusion of branch veins usually occurs at arteriovenous crossings and is often seen in hypertensives with arteriolar sclerosis. This is presumably because kinking of the vein causes local turbulence. Predisposing factors other than hypertension are the same as those associated with occlusion of the central vein. The superior temporal quadrant is most commonly affected because there are more arteriovenous crossings in this quadrant than in any other.

Occlusion is followed by intraretinal haemorrhage mainly in the nerve fibre layers and capillary collaterals develop within a few days. Local ischaemia is not essential for the development of local venous infarction since experimental occlusion by laser photocoagulation of branch veins readily reproduces the clinical picture. However, the persistent oedema and preretinal neovascularization which sometimes complicate the clinical condition were not seen in the experimental model (Hamilton *et al.*, 1979).

Pathological changes: investigation of the experimental material (Hockley *et al.*, 1979) showed that circulating peroxidase leaked through capillaries within a few hours of the occlusion before there was any morphological evidence of endothelial damage. Degenerative changes were observed in the endothelium and pericytes after 6 hours and were accompanied by focal thrombosis and haemorrhage into the retina. After 7 days, the oedema and haemorrhage gradually resolved and the affected capillaries became permanently closed by entry of processes of proliferating glial cells through breaks in the basement membrane.

In pathological material, the occlusion site can be demonstrated by serial sectioning, usually as a multichannel vessel adjacent to a sclerotic arteriole. Intravitreal or intra-retinal neovascularisation and cystoid macular oedema may be seen in some cases (Frangieh *et al.*, 1982).

Complications: the most important are:

1 Chronic macular oedema.

2 Neovascularization with consequent vitreous haemorrhage from posteriorly located new vessels (Fig. 10.26a) and neovascular glaucoma from those located on the anterior surface of the iris (Fig. 10.26b). These result in anterior peripheral synechiae which are responsible for post-thrombotic glaucoma (see Chapter 12).

HYPERTENSIVE RETINOPATHY

Hypertensive retinopathy is the expression in the retina of vascular changes going on all over the body as a result of raised blood pressure from any cause. The retinal vasculature has considerable autoregulatory capacity which enables it to maintain an appropriate physiological milieu in the face of wide fluctuations in blood pressure. Pathological changes in the vessels occurring as a result of sustained hypertension are of two types:

1 Structural breakdown when the vessel wall can no longer withstand the internal pressure.

2 Structural alterations which enable the sustained rise in intravascular pressure to be contained. Some of these changes appear to represent an acceleration and intensification of the normal ageing process.

The type of change which will predominate is governed by the period over which the rise in blood pressure occurs and the age of the subject. Most cases of hypertension are of the so-called essential type in which there is a breakdown in the complicated homeostatic mechanisms which regulate blood pressure. Essential hypertension manifests itself in two forms often called benign and malignant which may be regarded as phases of the same process.

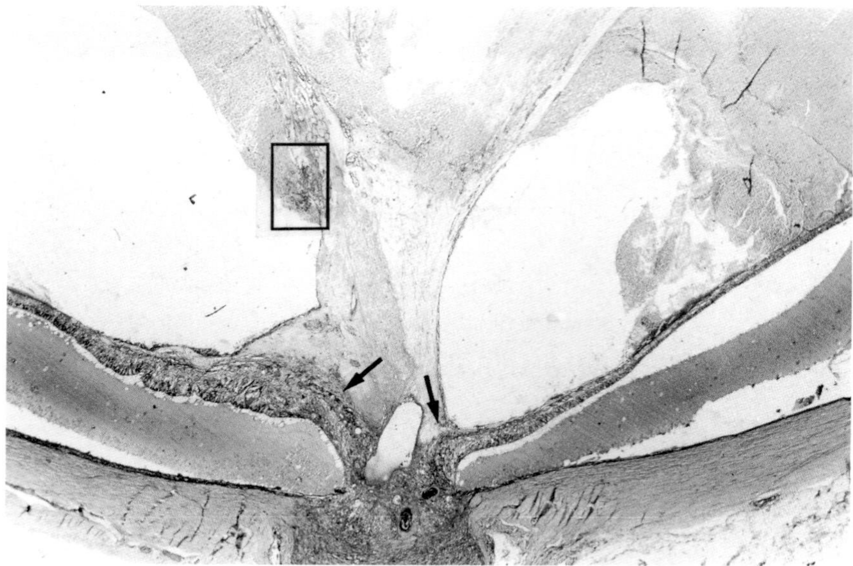

Fig. 10.26 Neovascularisation in post-thrombotic glaucoma. (a) Around optic nerve head. Fibrovascular tissue (arrows) proliferating from margins of optic nerve head along anterior surface of retina and into vitreous which has retracted forwards. PAS/tartrazine.

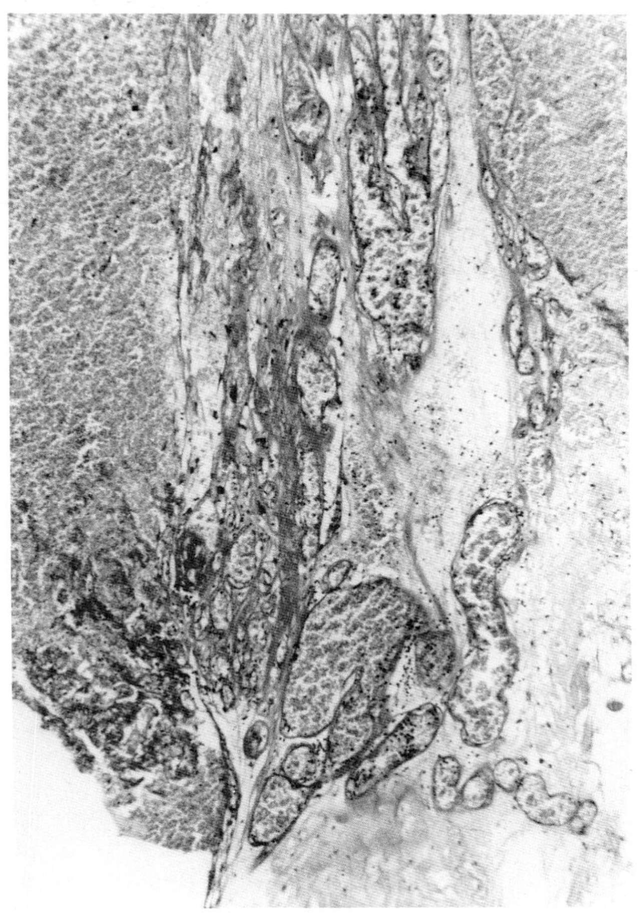

Fig. 10.26 (b) Detail of blood vessels in area in box. PAS/tartrazine (×71).

Benign phase

In the benign phase of hypertension, blood pressure rises gradually over a more prolonged period and compensatory structural changes result. The arterioles are at first constricted, and eventually their walls become thickened and hyalinised as muscle cells are replaced by collagen. The lumen may be greatly reduced in calibre. Thickening and increased density of the arteriolar wall is responsible for the diffusion of the arteriolar wall light reflex and nicking at arteriovenous crossings where the sclerotic arteriole obscures and compresses the underlying vein. In more advanced cases, the sclerotic vessels assume an appearance of copper or silver wire due to progressive screening of the blood column from view. This type of arteriolosclerosis resembles normal ageing seen, for example, in the splenic arterioles in normotensive subjects and may represent an acceleration of the ageing process.

A degree of vascular sclerosis appears to offer limited protection against the effects of malignant hypertension. Thus, the effects of malignant hypertension are less severe in older subjects or in patients who have been in a benign phase for some time. Atheroscleosis is also well known to be accelerated in hypertensives.

Retinal macroaneurysms are seen in elderly hypertensives with generalised arteriosclerosis and often elevated serum cholesterol and triglyceride levels. These arise in one or both eyes on major retinal arterioles within the first three orders of bifurcation from the optic nerve head. They may be single or multiple, sometimes pulsate and commonly give rise to intraretinal haemor-

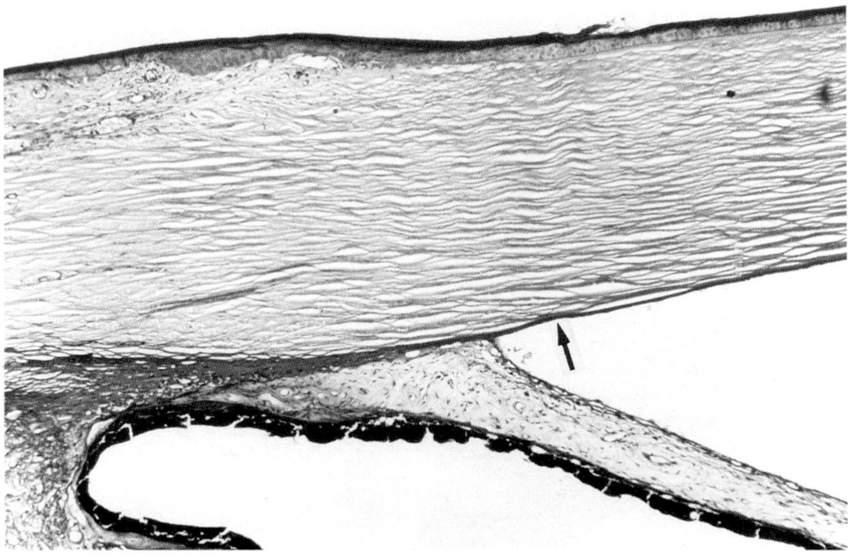

Fig. 10.26 (c) On anterior surface of iris with occlusion of angle by anterior peripheral synechiae. Arrow indicates Desçemet's membrane. PAS/tartrazine (×64).

rhage, oedema and exudates. During fluorescein angiography the aneurysms fill immediately and may leak.

It should also be noted that hypertensive changes similar to those found in the kidney affect the choroidal vasculature.

Accelerated (malignant) phase

Rapid sustained rise in blood pressure results in widespread arteriolar damage. The early ultrastructural changes have been studied in the experimental animal. Initially, there is focal spasm of the precapillary arterioles. This is thought eventually to result in damage to the smooth muscle cells in the wall, which undergo necrosis, so that dilatation occurs. Damage to the endothelium results and plasma seeps into the vessel wall. Secondary reduction in lumen may occur as a result of this influx. At the level of light microscopy, the arteriolar damage is seen as fibrinoid necrosis. There is focal replacement of the arteriolar wall by smudgy, brightly eosinophilic material.

Capillary closure occurs in relation to the arterioles affected by fibrinoid necrosis and capillary microaneurysms may also be seen. In addition, cotton-wool spots and hard exudates appear.

Characteristic linear haemorrhages result from blood escaping through the damaged vessel walls tracking along the nerve fibres.

DIABETIC RETINOPATHY

Although the pathological changes in the retinal vasculature which characterise diabetic retinopathy have been known and elegantly demonstrated for many years, their pathogenesis remains largely speculative.

Changes affect the arterioles, capillaries and veins. They include hyaline arteriolosclerosis, thickening of the capillary basement membrane, degeneration of pericytes, capillary closure, microaneurysm formation and increased tortuosity of the veins. Such changes form the pathological basis of what is known clinically as 'background retinopathy'. Later, the disease may enter a more serious phase in which the growth of new vessels occurs on the surface of the retina. Haemorrhage from these poses a threat to vision.

Hyaline arteriosclerosis

The walls of the arterioles become greatly thickened by hyaline material which, although it usually stains for collagen, is probably the consequence of insudation of plasma components. There is a resulting diminution in luminal diameter.

Basement membrane thickening

Increase in the amount of basement membrane substance is characteristic of diabetic capillaries in many areas of the body including the retina and kidney and is apparently mainly due to the deposition of glycoprotein, though osmiophilic material and cell debris may also be present. The significance of this striking feature of diabetic angiopathy is unknown.

Pericyte loss

An unsolved riddle is the widespread degeneration and disappearance of the retinal capillary pericytes. Although these cells form a substantial part of the capillary wall and are thought to be concerned with the maintenance of capillary tone, their function is not known for certain and the significance of the loss is thus difficult to assess.

Capillary closure

Another characteristic feature of diabetic retinopathy is the presence of small areas of closed or non-functioning capillaries which are quite devoid of cells and consist of tubes of basement membrane substance. Running through these areas are distended capillaries showing endothelial proliferation.

It is debatable whether these so-called shunt vessels are a factor in causing closure of the capillary bed or develop only because the capillary bed has already shut down. The arteriolar narrowing and occlusion is probably an important prerequisite for this type of capillary closure.

Microaneurysms

Although characteristic of diabetic retinopathy, retinal microaneurysms also occur in other diseases such as central venous occlusion and hypertension and in conditions where there is hyperviscosity of the blood such as macroglobulinaemia and myelomatosis. Aneurysms are not as a rule found in diabetic capillaries elswhere in the body. They first appear as minute red dots at the posterior pole and gradually increase in number until eventually they may involve the whole retina. Their excessive permeability makes them the source of serous and lipid exudates and haemorrhages mainly in the outer synaptic layer. These, together with cotton-wool spots at the margins of microinfarcts in the nerve fibre layer and cystoid macular oedema contribute to the clinical picture of diabetic retinopathy.

Microaneurysms may be identified in histological sections where they protrude into the outer plexiform

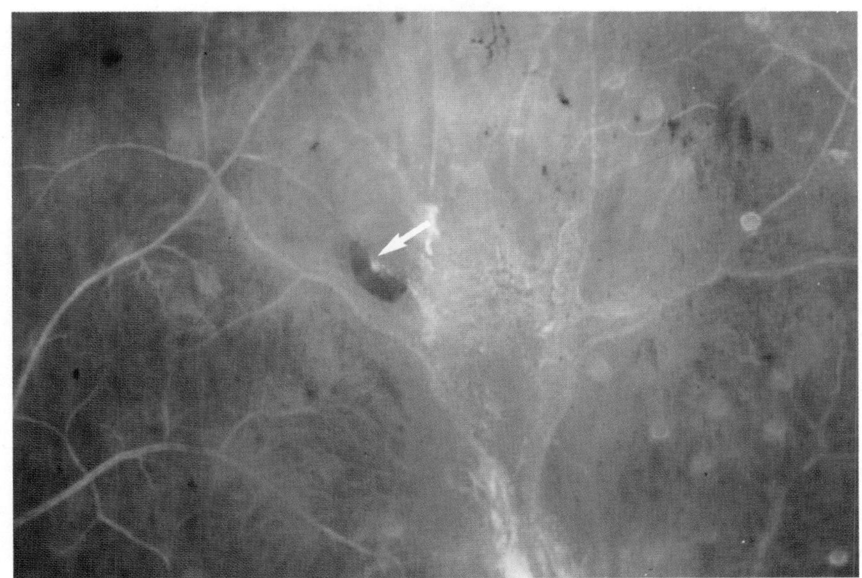

Plate 4 Retinal hole in case of longstanding retinal detachment apparently due to lattice dystrophy. The upper (peripheral) part of the hole (arrow) has a hazy appearance and is raised as a flap (see Fig. 10.4 for the microscopic appearance).

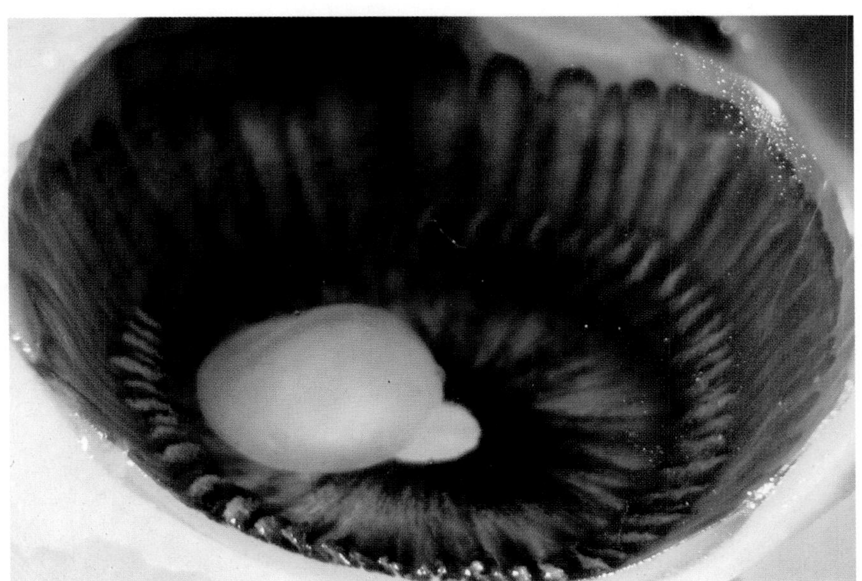

Plate 5 Marfan's syndrome. Macroscopic picture showing subluxated lens, which is small, opaque and rounded.

layer (Fig. 10.27), but are best demonstrated in flat trypsin digested preparations of the retina which have been injected with indian ink or stained by the PAS method to show up the vasculature. Such preparations show that clusters of microaneurysms are frequently found near areas of capillary closure.

The pathogenesis of capillary microaneurysms remains debatable. Digest preparations suggest that they arise as thin-walled capillary out-pouchings rather than by fusion of the walls of a dilated U-shaped capillary loop. Whether this occurs as a result of weakening of the capillary wall by loss of pericytes remains uncertain. In time the wall of the aneurysm becomes greatly thickened. Stagnation of blood and thrombosis may occur in the lumen. The clustering of aneurysms around areas of capillary closure has led to the suggestion that they are abortive attempts at new vessel formation in hypoxic areas.

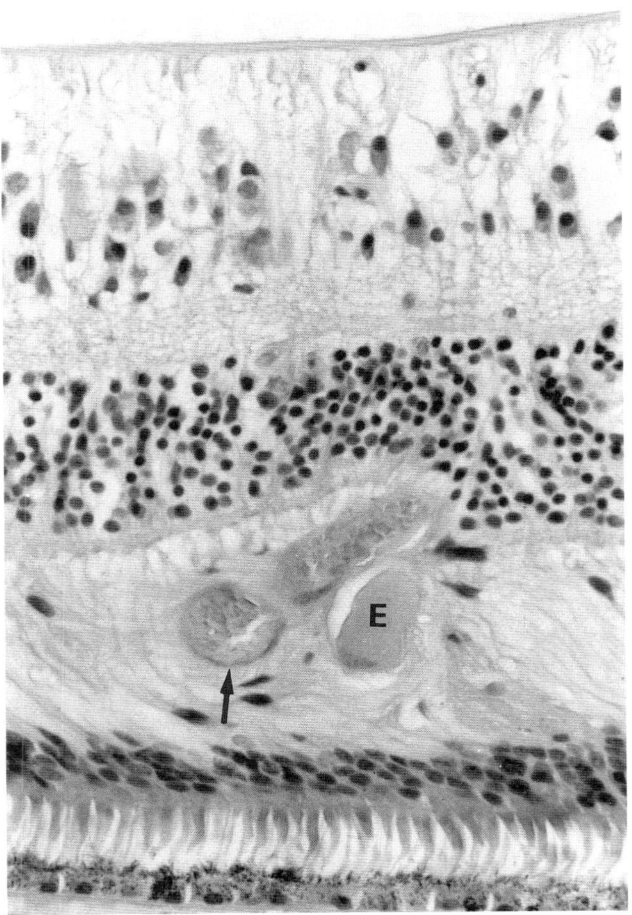

Fig. 10.27 Diabetic retinopathy. Microaneurysm in outer plexiform layer (arrow) with small adjacent exudate (E) presumably due to leakage. H & E (×350).

Venous changes

The veins become increasingly beaded, tortuous and dilated. Occasionally dilated loops appear to be drawn through the inner limiting membrane by vitreous strands and may thus become a potential source of vitreous haemorrhage.

Diabetic iridopathy

Although not obviously related to vascular changes it is convenient to mention in this context that a characteristic feature of diabetes is vacuolation of the pigmented epithelium of the iris due to accumulation of glycogen in the epithelial cells.

NEOVASCULARISATION

A serious complication of diabetic retinopathy is the proliferation of new capillaries on the retinal surface. This predisposes to preretinal haemorrhage, vitreoretinal adhesions and retinal detachment. Such proliferative retinopathy has a poor prognosis for vision. It may be seen, usually in a less florid form, in other conditions. Its occurrence after occlusion of the central retinal vein or a major branch has already been described.

The new capillaries, which are derived from the venous side of the retinal circulation particularly around the nerve head, extend at first along the inner retinal surface. Later, some of them grow into the vitreous body or into the retrovitreal space if, as often happens, the vitreous has retracted. Capillaries which have attached themselves to the posterior face of the retracting vitreous are liable to rupture and bleed. The mesenchyme from which the proliferating vessels are derived is also the source of fibroblasts so that the vessels become enveloped in connective tissue which, when it contracts, tends to detach the retina. Retinal neovascularisation may be accompanied by the growth of new vessels on the iris leading to peripheral anterior adhesions and secondary angle closure glaucoma (Chapter 12).

Effect of photocoagulation

The efficacy of panretinal photocoagulation in retarding the progress of proliferative diabetic retinopathy appears beyond doubt. The treatment is not directed primarily at the new vessels, but at the surrounding presumptively ischaemic retina. Possible mechanisms by which the hypoxia may be alleviated and the stimulus to new vessel formation abolished are:

1 Destruction of the photoreceptors, which have a high consumption of oxygen makes the oxygen supplied by the choriocapillaris available to the hypoxic inner layers.

2 Increased oxygen tension in the inner layers might constrict the retinal vessels feeding the new vessels.
3 Decreased capacity of surviving retinal tissue to synthesise angiogenic factor.

Angiogenic factors

It is now over 40 years since the existence in the retina of a factor associated with its metabolism capable of initiating capillary growth was postulated and the mode of new vessel formation during development related to that which occurs in certain retinal diseases. In particular, diseases such as diabetic retinopathy which call for the accession of new vessels to insufficiently vascularised situations (Michaelson, 1948). Angiogenic factors have now been isolated from normal retina of several species. They have a low molecular weight, but, as they have not yet been characterised, it is not clear whether they are identical in all species. Similar angiogenic factors have been isolated from many neoplasms. That from the Walker 256 carcinoma cross-reacts antigenically with angiogenic factors isolated from bovine retina. In normal retina, the effect of the angiogenic factor must clearly be suppressed and there is evidence that the vitreous contains an anti-angiogenic factor.

Other angiogenic agents

Other agents that may be capable of inducing neovascularisation in the retina include lactic acid and inflammatory cells. Activated lymphocytes and macrophages release prostaglandins. Prostaglandins are also released when platelets aggregate. Since prostaglandins of the E series have been shown experimentally to stimulate vascular growth in the cornea, they must be considered as possible mediators through which growth of new vessels in the retina is stimulated.

PERIPHERAL RETINAL NEOVASCULARISATION

Localised areas of capillary non-perfusion may develop under certain conditions because retinal and choroidal blood flow is less at the periphery than at the posterior pole. The resultant retinal ischaemia stimulates the growth of new vessels.

Sickle cell haemoglobinopathies

The commonest cause of peripheral neovascularisation is sickle cell desease in which the so-called sea fans develop, usually at the temporal periphery. It is probable that the slow transit time at the periphery allows sickling to occur with resultant arteriolar plugging.

Hyperviscosity syndrome

Grossly elevated white blood cell counts, especially in chronic myeloid leukaemia can result in hyperviscosity of the blood. In the peripheral retina, this may result in capillary non-perfusion, perivenous sheathing and microaneurysm formation. Fan-like tufts have also been observed at the margins of non-perfused areas of retina.

RETINOPATHY OF PREMATURITY (RETROLENTAL FIBROPLASIA)

In 1942, Terry described a conditon which he believed was due mainly to persistence of the hyaloid artery and tunica vasculosa lentis and overgrowth of embryonic connective tissue behind the lens. The key pathogenetic role of oxygen was not recognised until the widespread use of oxygen therapy for the treatment of respiratory distress in premature infants apparently resulted in an outbreak of epidemic proportions in the fifties.

Experimental work in various species has shown that exposure of the immature retina to high ambient concentrations of oxygen results in vaso-obliteration. When the animal is subsequently returned to air, vasoproliferation in the form of capillary budding occurs.

A similar process has been observed in the human infant both *in vivo* and in pathological specimens. During development, proliferating mesenchymal spindle-cells migrate from the optic nerve head in the nerve fibre layer towards the retinal periphery. Differentiation of the spindle-cells into the retinal blood vessels follows as a peripherally migrating wave.

It appears that, under conditions of high oxygen tension, arterioles and venules are not affected, but capillary closure occurs and migration of the spindle-cells is inhibited. Anterior to the wave front of vascular differentiation the spindle-cells proliferate. At the wave front itself endothelial proliferation occurs to form a knot of capillary channels (Fig. 10.28a) which have been shown by fluorescein angiography to be arteriovenous shunts. Subsequently, dilated tortuous new vessels may proliferate on the surface of the retina posterior to the shunt (Fig. 10.28b). Partial or complete regression occurs if the avascular retina posterior to the shunt is revascularised by proliferation of capillaries from the shunt. If this fails to occur, the vascular abnormalities persist and further proliferation, exudation and haemorrhage lead to the avascular retina becoming detached and organised into a retrolental cicatrising mass.

With a view to introducing descriptive uniformity the disease has recently been categorised into stages by an international committee (Garner, 1984).

While prematurity and hyperoxia are important factors, occasional cases occur in full-term infants and in

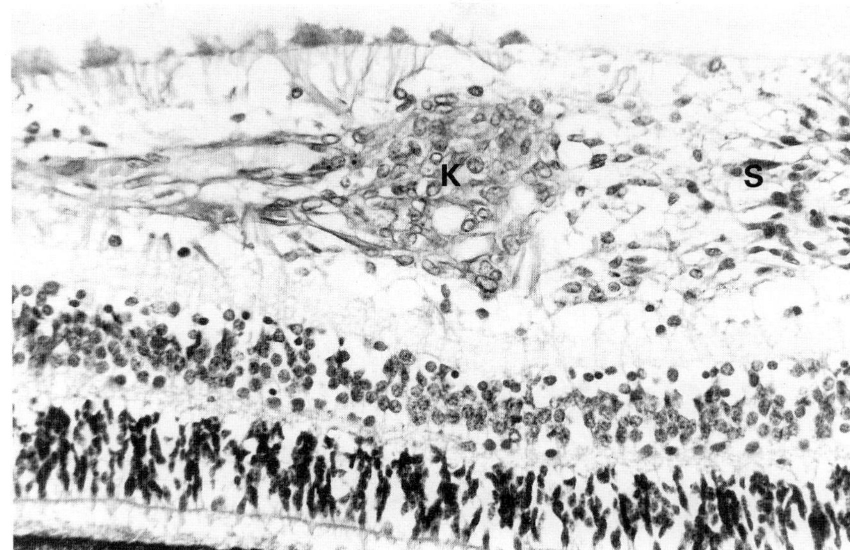

Fig. 10.28 Retinopathy of prematurity. (a) Capillary knot (K) in nerve fibre layer with adjacent spindle cells (S) orientated parallel to retinal surface. PAS/tartrazine (×260).

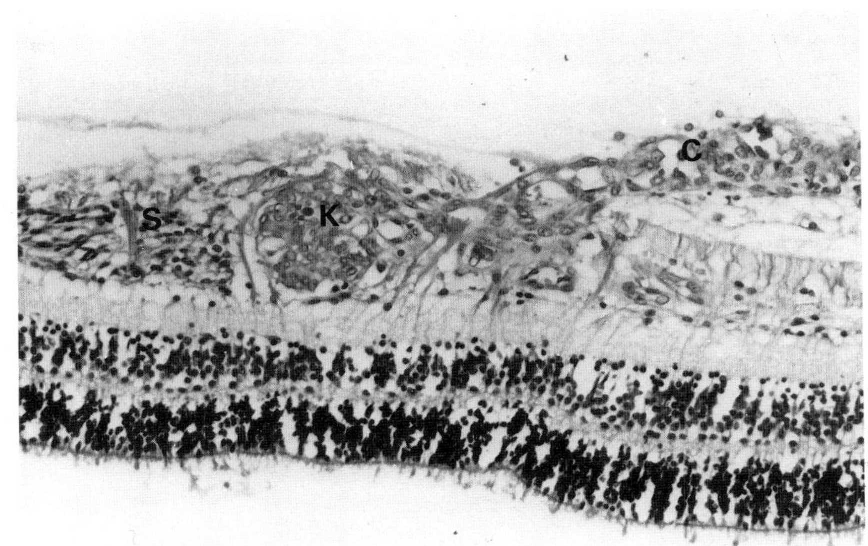

Fig. 10.28 (b) Capillary knot (K) within nerve fibre layer from which capillaries (C) are seen proliferating onto the anterior retinal surface. Spindle cells (S) can also be seen adjacent to proliferating capillaries. Masson trichrome (×160).

infants who have never been exposed to oxygen therapy. Large doses of vitamin E protect pre-term infants exposed to continuous oxygen therapy against the development of retinopathy of prematurity. It has been suggested that, under hyperoxic conditions, a population of spindle cells is generated which is not primed for endothelial differentiation and that large doses of vitamin E inhibits this (Kretzer *et al.* 1982).

COATS' DISEASE

In 1908, George Coats wrote his classical paper describing three forms of 'haemorrhagic retinitis' in which there was massive exudation. These comprised:

1 Cases without gross retinal vascular disease.
2 Cases with gross retinal vascular disease.
3 A peculiar group characterised by the formation of large arteriovenous communications.

The cases in the third group are now considered to be identical with von Hippel's disease while the first two are termed Coats' disease, Types 1 and 2 respectively.

Clinical features

The disease commonly affects males under the age of 21, is unilateral and non-familial. There is usually no related systemic disorder and no early anterior segment disease.

The principal ocular findings are:

1 *Exudative mass:* a yellowish or greyish-white raised mass of woolly or flocculent exudate is present between the retina and the choroid usually near the posterior pole. Glittering spots suggestive of cholesterol crystals

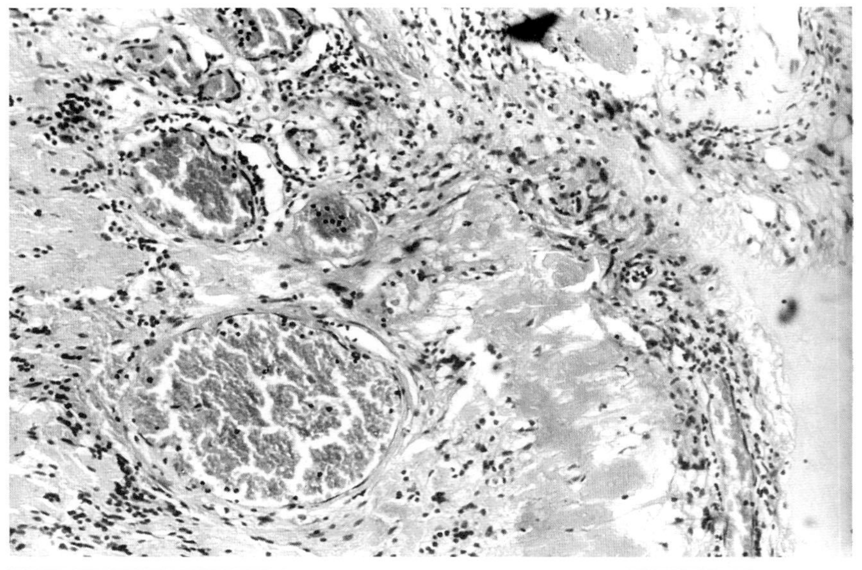

Fig. 10.29 Coats' disease. (a) Peripheral telangiectasia. The thin-walled blood vessel on the left measured approximately 200 μm in diameter. Exudate is seen streaming away towards the subretinal space below.

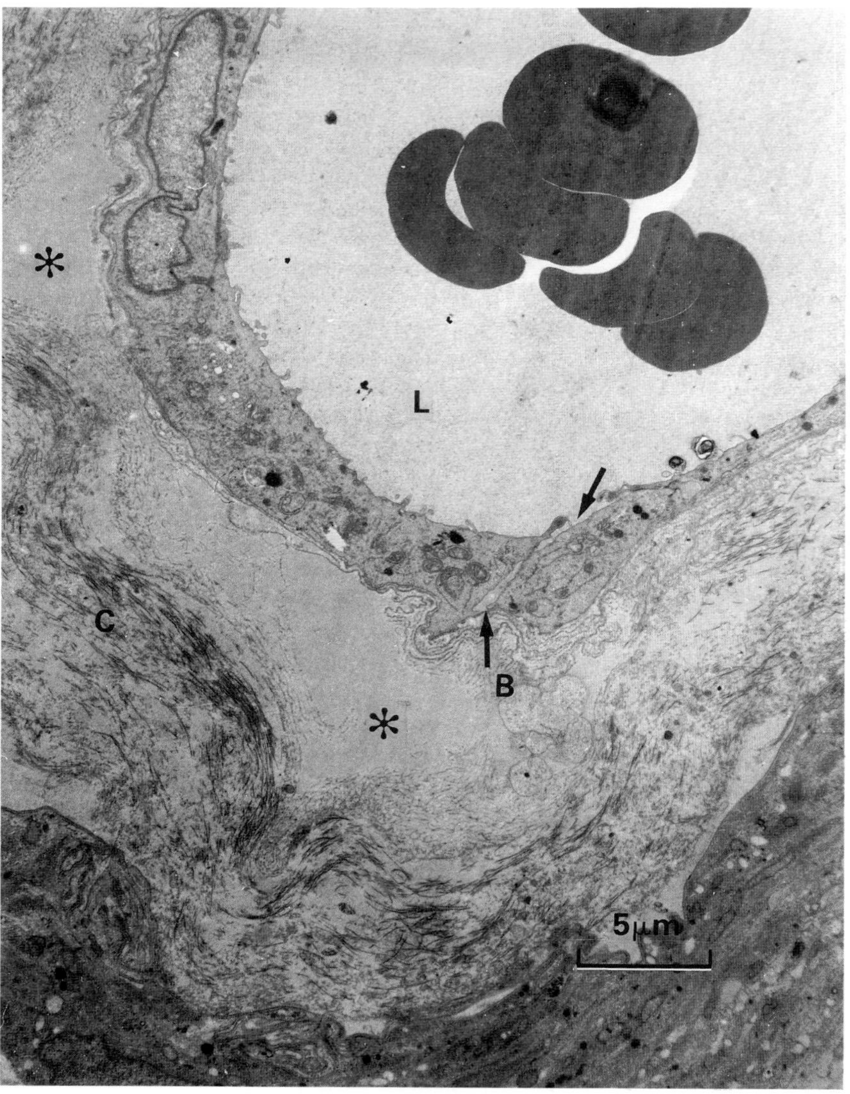

Fig. 10.29 (b) Electron micrograph of capillary showing insudation of plasma of plasma beneath endothelium. * = plasma, L = lumen, B = basement membrane material, C = collagen. Junction between endothelial cells indicated by arrows.

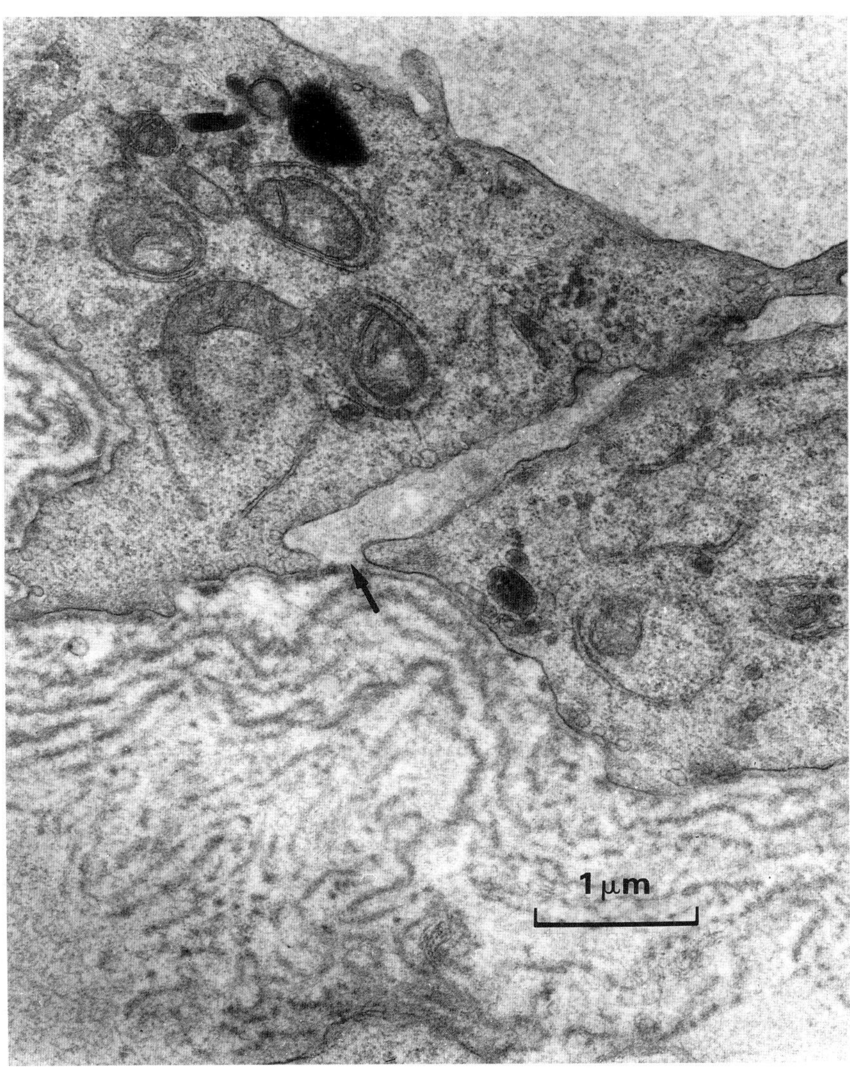

Fig. 10.29 (c) Detail of gap between endothelial cells (arrow). (Fig. 10.29b & c reproduced with permission from McGettrick & Loeffler 1987.)

are characteristically present in the mass and sometimes in the healthy fundus as well. This is often accompanied by retinal haemorrhages.

2 *Retinal detachment:* there is commonly detachment of the retina in some part of the fundus and the detached retina appears thick and rigid as if there was something solid beneath it.

3 *Retinal vascular disease:* in Type 1 cases the retinal vessels appear normal. In Type 2 cases they show beading, tortuosity, looping and sheathing.

Pathological features

Most cases that come to enucleation have been diagnosed clinically as possible retinoblastoma.

Macroscopically there is partial or complete detachment of the retina with a proteinaceous subretinal exudate containing shimmering crystals of cholesterol.

Microscopically the retina is usually disorganised and shows cystic degeneration and secondary gliosis. Serous exudates and haemorrhages are seen in the deeper layers. Massive infiltration with foamy macrophages is characteristic. Some doubt exists as to whether the macrophages are derived primarily from the pigmented epithelium, or incoming monocytes from the blood. Glial cells are also capable of ingesting lipid.

In many cases, careful search will reveal clusters of capillaries and groups of large, thin-walled vessels in the inner retinal layers (Fig. 10.29a). Some of these are 300 μm or more in diameter, i.e. larger than the central retinal vein in the optic nerve. Other vessels may exhibit gross mural thickening which has been shown by electron microscopy to be the result of insudated lipid, plasma and fibrin together with abundant basement membrane-like material and cellular debris. In early lesions, the endothelium remained intact, though showing cytoplasmic vacuolation. In advanced lesions, however, it disappeared. More recent work (McGettrick & Loeffler, 1987) has suggested that the leakage of plasma into the vessel wall occurs through gaps between the endothelial cells (Fig. 10.29b & c). Fenestrations were also found in endothelial cells lining a hyalinised vessel. Cuffing of vessels by lymphocytes may also be seen.

In the subretinal space there is organising haemorrhage with many foamy macrophages and cholesterol clefts around which may be found giant cells. Sometimes a fibroglial cholesterol granuloma may form.

Although light lymphocytic infiltration of the choroid may be present, evidence of inflammation in any part of the eye is usually lacking.

While the pathological picture is quite characteristic, ocular changes in other conditions such as the 'battered baby syndrome' may simulate Coats' disease in that features such as cholesterol crystals and lipoidal macrophages in serosanguineous exudates may be observed.

Pathogenesis

Retinal haemorrhage

Coats believed that the condition he described was the result of haemorrhage from the retinal capillaries into the outer layers of the retina and subretinal space, followed by breakdown and organisation of the clot. In Type 2 cases with gross vascular abnormalities this seemed a reasonable hypothesis, but could not easily account for Type 1 cases in which vascular changes are absent or minimal.

Retinal telangiectasis

In 1956, Reese described the condition of retinal telangiectasis (Leber's multiple retinal aneurysms) which he believed could be a precursor of Coats' disease. Retinal telangiectasis is usually uniocular and occurs in both children and adults. Its characteristic lesion is a single circumscribed slightly elevated area anywhere in the fundus, over which dilated blood vessels appear as numerous sharply outlined red globules.

Usually, the telangiectases remain symptomless, but in a minority of cases substantial haemorrhage occurs and courses through the external layers of the retina into the subretinal space inducing a dark bullous detachment. Subsequently the blood breaks down and organises. Reese considered that the term Coats' disease should be restricted to cases of this type. However, this is not what Coats described although it may well represent a phase of the disease which he had no opportunity to observe.

Breakdown of the blood–retinal barrier

Tripathi and Ashton (1971) interpreted their electron microscopic findings as indicating that an abnormality in endothelial permeability occurs early in Coats' disease, that is a structural or functional breakdown in the blood–retina barrier. Insudation of plasma into the walls of small vessels and loss of endothelial lining would render them weak and porous and thus allow telangectatic dilatation, exudation and haemorrhage to occur. On this interpretation, Type 1 may be regarded as an early stage of Type 2 disease. The recent work by McGettrick and Loeffler (1987) has indicated the probable nature and location of the initial structural breakdown.

Inflammation

The possibility of inflammation as an aetiological factor in some cases was reviewed by Woods and Duke (1963a & b) who found that four adults with classical signs of the disease all had histories of uveitis. All four patients also had hypercholestrinaemia. On the basis of these and other findings, they concluded that the essential pathological feature of Coats' disease in adults was the deposition of cholesterol in the outer retina and subretinal space. They postulated that this deposition was triggered by uveal inflammation in the presence of hypercholestrinaemia and was mediated by a tissue factor, probably an acid mucopolysaccharide. The hypothesis is not applicable to juvenile Coats' disease in which there is rarely a history of uveitis and in which plasma lipid values are within normal limits.

BIBLIOGRAPHY

Part 1. General degenerative disorders

General structure and function

Anderson, D. H., Fisher, S. K., Erickson, P. A. & Tabor, G. A. (1980) Rod and cone disc shedding in the rhesus monkey retina: a quantitative study. *Experimental Eye Research* **30**, 559–574.

Besharse, J. C. & Hollyfield, J. G. (1979) Turnover of mouse photoreceptor outer segments in constant light and darkness. *Investigative Ophthalmology and Visual Science* **18**, 1019–1024.

Cohen, A. I. (1961a) Electron microscopic observations of the internal limiting membrane and optic fibre layer of the retina of the rhesus monkey (*M. mulatto*). *American Journal of Anatomy* **108**, 179–198.

Cohen, A. I. (1961b) The fine structure of the extrafoveal receptors of the rhesus monkey. *Experimental Eye Research* **1**, 128–136.

Dowling, J. E. & Boycott, B. B. (1966) Organization of the primate retina: electron microscopy. *Proceedings of the Royal Society B* **166**, 80–111.

Duvall, J. (1987) Structure, function and pathological responses of pigment epithelium. A review. *Seminars in Ophthalmology* **2**, 130–140.

Feeney, L. (1978) Lipofuscin and melanin of human retinal pigment epithelium. *Investigative Ophthalmology and Visual Science* **17**, 583–600.

Fine, B. S. (1961) Limiting membranes of the sensory retina and pigment epithelium. *Archives of Ophthalmology* **66**, 847–860.

Fine, B. S. (1963) Ganglion cells in the human retina. *Archives of Ophthalmology* **69**, 83–96.

Fine, B. S. & Zimmerman, L. E. (1962) Müller's cells and the 'middle limiting membrane' of the human retina. *Investigative Ophthalmology* **1**, 304–326.

Fine, B. S. & Zimmerman, L. E. (1963) Observations on the rod and cone layer of the human retina. *Investigative Ophthalmology* **2**, 446–459.

Foos, R. Y. (1972) Posterior vitreous detachment. *Transactions of the American Academy of Ophthalmology and Otolaryngology* **76**, 480–496.

LaVail, M. M. (1983) Outer segment disc shedding and phagocytosis in the outer retina. *Transactions of the Ophthalmological Society of the UK* **103**, 397–404.

Michaelson, I. C. (1980) *Textbook of the Fundus of the Eye*, 3rd edn. Churchill Livingstone, Edinburgh.

Noell, W. K., (1958) Differentiation, metabolic organization, and viability of the visual cell. *Archives of Ophthalmology* **60**, 702–733.

Nussbaum, J. J., Pruett, R. C. & Delori, F. C. (1981) Macular pigment. The first 200 years. *Retina* **1**, 296–310.

Young, R. W. (1976) Visual cells and the concept of renewal. *Investigative Ophthalmology* **15**, 700–725.

Zinn, K. M. & Marmor, M. F., eds (1979) *The Retinal Pigment Epithelium*. Harvard University Press, Cambridge, Massachusetts.

Spontaneous degenerations

Byer, N. E. (1979) Lattice degeneration of the retina. *Survey of Ophthalmology* **23**, 213–248.

Foos, R. Y. & Feman, S. S. (1970) Reticular cystoid degeneration of the peripheral retina. *American Journal of Ophthalmology* **69**, 392–403.

Foos, R. Y. & Simons, K. B. (1984) Vitreous in lattice degeneration of the retina. *Ophthalmology* **91**, 452–457.

O'Malley, P. F., Allen, R. A., Straatsma, B. R. & O'Malley, C. C. (1965) Paving stone degeneration of the retina. *Archives of Ophthalmology* **73**, 169–172.

Rabb, M. F., Garoon, I. & La Franco, F. P. (1981) Myopic macular degeneration. *International Ophthalmology Clinics* **21**, 51–69.

Straatsma, B. R., Zeegen, P. D., Foos, R. Y., Feman, S. S. & Shabo, A. L. (1974) Lattice degeneration of the retina. *Transactions of the American Academy of Ophthalmology and Otolaryngology* **78**, OP 87–113.

Retinal breaks (holes and tears)

Aaberg, T. M. (1970) Macular holes: a review. *Survey of Ophthalmology* **15**, 139–162.

Byer, N. E. (1974) Prognosis of asymptomatic retinal breaks. *Archives of Ophthalmology* **92**, 208–215.

Foos, R. Y. & Allen, R. A. (1967) Retinal tears and lesser lesions of the peripheral retina in autopsy eyes. *American Journal of Ophthalmology* **64**, 643–655.

Frangieh, G. T., Green, W. R. & Engel, H. M. (1981) A histopathologic study of macular cysts and holes. *Retina* **1**, 311–336.

Lincoff, H. & Gieser, R. (1971) Finding the retinal hole. *Archives of Ophthalmology* **85**, 565–569.

Sigelman, J. (1980) Vitreous base classification of retinal tears: clinical application. *Survey of Ophthalmology* **25**, 59–74.

Retinal detachment

Chaine, G., Sebag, J. & Coscas, G. (1983) The induction of retinal detachment. *Transactions of the Ophthalmological Society of the UK* **103**, 480–485.

Foulds, W. S. (1987) Is your vitreous really necessary? The role of the vitreous in the eye with particular reference to retinal detachment and the mode of action of vitreous substitutes. *Eye* **1**, 641–664.

Kroll, A. J. & Machemer, R. (1968) Experimental retinal detachment in the owl monkey. *American Journal of Ophthalmology* **66**, 410–427.

Laqua, H. & Machemer, R. (1975) Glial cell proliferation in retinal detachment (massive periretinal proliferation). *American Journal of Ophthalmology* **80**, 602–618.

Machemer, R. (1968a) Experimental retinal detachment in the owl monkey. II. Histology of retinal and pigment epithelium. *American Journal of Ophthalmology* **66**, 396–410.

Machemer, R. (1968b) Experimental retinal detachment in the owl monkey. IV. The reattached retina. *American Journal of Opthalmology* **66**, 1075–1091.

Machemer, R. (1975) Clinico-pathological correlation in massive periretinal proliferation. *American Journal of Ophthalmology* **80**, 913–929.

Machemer, R. & Laqua, H. (1975) Pigment epithelium proliferation in retinal detachment (massive periretinal proliferation). *American Journal of Ophthalmology* **80**, 1–23.

Machemer, R. & Norton, E. W. D. (1968) Experimental retinal detachment in the owl monkey. I. Methods of production and clinical picture. *American Journal of Ophthalmology* **66**, 338–396.

Epiretinal membranes

Clarkson, J. G., Green, W. R. & Massof, D. (1977) A histopathologic review of 168 cases of preretinal membrane. *American Journal of Ophthalmology* **84**, 1–17.

Haefliger, E. A. & Daicker, B. (1979) Netzhautfaltelung und epiretinale Membranen bei haemorrhagischem Sekundarglaukom. *Klinische Monatsblätter für Augenheilkunde* **174**, 548–556.

Hamilton, C. W., Chandler, D., Klintworth, G. K. & Machemer, R. (1982) A transmission and scanning electron microscopic study of surgically excised preretinal membrane proliferations in diabetes mellitus. *American Journal of Ophthalmology* **94**, 473–488.

Hiscott, P. S., Grierson, I. & McLeod, D. (1984) Retinal pigment epithelial cells in epiretinal membranes: an immunohistochemical study. *British Journal of Ophthalmology* **68**, 708–715.

Hiscott, P. S., Grierson, I., Trombetta, C. J., Rahi, A. H. S., Marshall, J. & McLeod, D. (1984) Retinal and epiretinal glia — an immunohistochemical study. *British Journal of Ophthalmology* **68**, 698–707.

Kampik, A., Kenyon, K. R., Michels, R. G., Green, W. R. & de la Cruz, Z. C. (1981) Epiretinal and vitreous membranes. Comparative study of 56 cases. *Archives of Ophthalmology* **99**, 1445–1454.

Radtke, N. D., Tano, Y., Chandler, D. & Machemer, R. (1981) Simulation of massive periretinal proliferation by autotransplantation of retinal pigment epithelial cells in rabbits. *American Journal of Ophthalmology* **91**, 76–87.

Retinoschisis

Manschot, W. A. (1972) Pathology of hereditary juvenile retinoschisis. *Archives of Ophthalmology* **88**, 131–138.

Yanoff, M., Rahn, E. K. & Zimmerman, L. E. (1968) Histopathology of juvenile retinoschisis. *Archives of Ophthalmology* **79**, 49–53.

Inherited choroidoretinal dystrophies

Ashton, N. (1953) Central areolar choroidal sclerosis. A histopathological study. *British Journal of Ophthalmology* **37**, 140–147.

Ashton, N. & Sorsby, A. (1951) Fundus dystrophy with unusual features. *British Journal of Ophthalmology* **35**, 751–764.

Barnett, K. C. & Curtis, R. (1983) Retinal degenerations in the dog and the cat as models for retinitis pigmentosa. *Transactions of the Ophthalmological Society of the UK* **103**, 448–452.

Cameron, J. D., Fine, B. S. & Shapiro, I. (1987) Histopathologic observations in choroideraemia with emphasis on vascular changes of the uveal tract. *Ophthalmology* **94**, 187–196.

Duvall, J., McKechnie, N.M., Lee, W. R., Rothery, S. & Marshall, J. (1986) Extensive subretinal pigment deposit in two brothers suffering from dominant retinitis pigmentosa. *Graefe's Archive for Clinical and Experimental Ophthalmology* **224**, 299–309.

Eagle Jr., R. C., Lucier, A. C., Bernadino Jr., V. B. & Yanoff, M. Y. (1980) Retinal pigment epithelial abnormalities in fundus flavimaculatus. A light and electron microscopic study. *Ophthalmology* **87**, 1189–1200.

Ferry, A. P., Llovera, I. & Shaffer, D. M. (1972) Central areoloar choroidal dystrophy. *Archives of Ophthalmology* **88**, 39–43.

Francois, J. (1982) Metabolic tapetoretinal degenerations. *Survey of Ophthalmology* **26**, 293–333.

Gartner, S. & Henkind, P. (1982) Pathology of retinitis pigmentosa. *Ophthalmology* **89**, 1425–1432.

Gass, J. D. M. (1974) A clinicopathologic study of a peculiar foveomacular dystrophy. *Transactions of the American Ophthalmic Society* **72**, 139–156.

Herron, W. L., Riegel, B. W. & Rubin, M. L. (1969) Retinal dystrophy in the rat — a pigment epithelial disease. *Investigative Ophthalmology* **8**, 595–604.

Kaiser-Kupfer, M. I., Ludwig, I. H., de Monasterio, F. M., Valle, D. & Krieger, I. (1985) Gyrate atrophy of the choroid and retina. Early findings. *Ophthalmology* **92**, 394–401.

Kobrin, J. L., Apple, D. J. & Hart, W. B. (1981) Vitelliform dystrophy. *International Ophthalmology Clinics* **21**, 167–184.

Kolb, H & Gouras, P. (1974) Electron microscopic observations of human retinitis pigmentosa. *Investigative Ophthalmology* **13**, 487–498.

Krill, A. E. & Archer, D. B. (1971) Classification of choroidal atrophies. *American Journal of Ophthalmology* **72**, 562–585.

Levin, P. S., Green, W. R., Victor, D. I. & Maclean, A. (1983) Histopathology of the eye in Cockayne's syndrome. *Archives of Ophthalmology* **101**, 1093–1097.

Lolley, R.N. (1983) Cell dysfunction in inherited blindness. *Transactions of the Ophthalmological Society of the UK* **103**, 438–443.

Lucas, D. R. (1956) Retinitis pigmentosa: pathological findings in two cases. *British Journal of Ophthalmology* **40**, 14–23.

McCulloch, C. (1950) The pathologic findings in two cases of choroideraemia. *Transactions of the American Academy of Ophthalmology and Otolaryngology* **56**, 565–572.

McCulloch, C. (1969) Choroideraemia: a clinical and pathologic review. *Transactions of the American Ophthalmological Society* **67**, 145–191.

McKechnie, N. M., King, M. & Lee, W. R. (1985) Retinal pathology in the Kearns–Sayre syndrome. *British Journal of Ophthalmology* **69**, 63–75.

McMarland, C. B. (1955) Heredodegeneration of the macula lutea. *Archives of Ophthalmology* **53**, 224–228.

Marmor, M. F., Aguire, G., Arden, G., Berson, E., Birch, D. G., Boughman, J. A., Carr, R., Chatrian, G. E., Del Monte, M., Dowling, J., Enoch, J., Fishman, G. A., Fulton, A. B., Garcia, C. A., Gouras, P., Heckenlively, J., Hu, D., Lewis, R. A., Niemeyer, G., Parker, J. A., Perlman, I., Ripps, H., Sandberg, M. A., Siegel, I., Weleber, R. G., Wolf, M. L., Wu, L. & Young, R. S. L. (1983) Retinitis pigmentosa. A symposium on terminology and methods of examination. *Ophthalmology* **90**, 126–131.

Meyer, K. T., Heckenlively, J. R., Spitznas, M. & Foos, R. Y. (1982) Dominant retinitis pigmentosa. A clinicopathologic correlation. *Ophthalmology* **89**, 1414–1424.

Mizuno, K. & Nishida, S. (1967) Electron microscopic studies of human retinitis pigmentosa. 1. Two cases of advanced retinitis pigmentosa. *American Journal of Ophthalmology* **63**, 791–803.

Mullen, R. J. & LaVail, M. M. (1976) Inherited retinal dystrophy: primary defect in pigment epithelium determined with experimental rat chimeras. *Science* **194**, 799–801.

Patrinely, J. R., Lewis, R. A. & Font, R. L. (1985) Foveomacular vitelliform dystrophy, adult type. A clinicopathologic study including electron microscopic observations. *Ophthalmology* **92**, 1712–1718.

Rafuse, E. F. & McCulloch, C. (1968) Choroideremia. A pathological report. *Canadian Journal of Ophthalmology* **3**, 347–352.

Ross, C. F., Crome, L. & Mackenzie, D. Y. (1956) The Laurence–Moon–Biedl syndrome. *Journal of Pathology and Bacteriology* **62**, 161–172.

Szamier, R. B. (1981) Ultrastructure of the preretinal membrane in retinitis pigmentosa. *Investigative Ophthalomology and Visual Science* **21**, 227–236.

Szamier, R. B. & Berson, E. L. (1985) Retinal histopathology of a carrier of X-chromosome-linked retinitis pigmentosa. *Ophthalmology* **92**, 271–278.

Szamier, R. B., Berson, E. L., Klein, R. & Meyers, S. (1979) Sex-linked retinitis pigmentosa: ultrastructure of photoreceptors and pigment epithelium. *Investigative Ophthalmology and Visual Science* **18**, 145–160.

Toussaint, D. & Danis, P. (1971) An ocular pathologic study of Refsum's syndrome. *American Journal of Ophthalmology* **72**, 342–347.

Verhoeff, F. H. (1931) Microscopic observations in a case of retinitis pigmentosa. *Archives of Ophthalmology* **5**, 392–407.

Sallmann, L., von Gelderman, A. A. & Laster, L. (1969) Ocular histopathologic changes in A-β-lipoproteinaemia (Bassen–Kornzweig syndrome). *Documenta Ophthalmologica* **26**, 451–460.

Weingeist, T. A., Kobrin, J. L. & Watzke, R. C. (1982) Histopathology of Best's macular dystrophy. *Archives of Ophthalmology* **100**, 1108–1121.

Degenerations caused by drugs and chemicals

Bernstein, H. & Ginsberg, J. (1964) The ocular pathology of chloroquine toxicity. *Archives of Ophthalmology* **71**, 238–245.

Editorial (1962) Retinal damage from drugs. *British Medical Journal* **i**, 929.

Editorial (1967) Delayed chloroquine sensitivity. *British Medical Journal* **i**, 254.

Gregory, M. H., Rutty, D. A. & Wood, R. D. (1970) Differences in the retinotoxic action of chloroquine and phenothiazine derivatives. *Journal of Pathology* **102**, 139–150.

Jones, C. J. P. & Jayson, M. I. V. (1984) Chloroquine: its effect on leucocyte auto- and heterophagocytosis. *Annals of Rheumatic Diseases* **43**, 205–212.

Newhouse, J. P. & Lucas, D. R. (1959) Effects of parenteral iodoactetate and other thiol reagents on the rabbit retina. Relation of histological to biochemical lesions. *British Journal of Ophthalmology* **43**, 528–539.

Ramsey, M. S. & Fine, B. S. (1972) Chloroquine toxicity in the human eye. Histopathologic observations by electron microscopy. *American Journal of Ophthalmology* **73**, 229–235.

Sorsby, A. & Nakajima, A. (1958) Experimental degeneration of the retina. IV. Diaminodiphenoxyalkanes as inducing agents. *British Journal of Ophthalmology* **42**, 563–571.

Spalton, D. J. (1987) Chloroquine and the eye. *The British Journal of Clinical Practice* **41**, suppl. **52**, 50–55.

Wetterholm, D. H. & Winter, F. C. (1964) Histopathology of chloroquine retinal toxicity. *Archives of Ophthalmology* **71**, 82–87.

Vitamin A deficiency

Carter-Dawson, L., Kuwabara, T., O'Brien, P. J. & Bieri, J. G. (1979) Structural and biochemical changes in Vitamin A-deficient rat retinas. *Investigative Ophthalmology and Visual Science* **18**, 437–446.

Retinal damage due to light

Apple, D. J., Goldberg, M. F. & Wyhinny, G. (1973) Histopathology and ultrastructure of the argon laser lesion in human retinal and choroidal vasculature. *American Journal of Ophthalmology* **75**, 593–609.

Dobson, V. (1976) Phototherapy and retinal damage. *Investigative Ophthalmology* **15**, 595–598.

Ham, W. T., Ruffolo Jr., J. J., Mueller, H. A. & Guerry III, D. (1980) The nature of retinal radiation damage: dependence on wavelength, power level and exposure time. *Vision Research* **20**, 1105–1111.

Lanum, J. (1978) The damaging effects of light on the retina. Empirical findings, theoretical and practical implications. *Survey of Ophthalmology* **22**, 221–249.

McKechnie, N. M. & Ghafour, I. M. (1982) Potential retinal light damage from the use of therapeutic instruments. *Transactions of the Ophthalmological Society of the UK* **102**, 140–145.

Marshall, J. (1984) Light damage and the practice of ophthalmology. In *Intraocular Lens Implantation*, eds E. S. Rosen, W. M. Haining & E. J. Arnott, pp 182–207. Mosby, St Louis.

Marshall, J., Hamilton, A. M. & Bird, A. C. (1975) Histopathology of ruby and argon laser lesions in monkey and human retina. A comparative study. *British Journal of Ophthalmology* **59**, 610–630.

Tso, M. O. M., Fine, B. S. & Zimmerman, L. E. (1972) Photic maculopathy produced by the indirect ophthalmoscope. 1. Clinical and histopathologic study. *American Journal of Ophthalmology* **73**, 686–699.

Tso, M. O. M., Wallow, I. H. L. & Elgin, S. (1977) Experimental photocoagulation of the human retina. I. Correlation of physical, clinical, and pathologic data. *Archives of Ophthalmology* **95**, 1035–1040.

Wallow, I. H. L., Tso, M. O. M. & Elgin, S. (1977) Experimental photocoagulation of the human retina. II. Electron microscopic study. *Archives of Ophthalmology* **95**, 1041–1050.

Effects of ionising radiation

Bagan, S. M. & Hollenhorst, R. W. (1979) Radiation retinopathy after irradiation of intracranial lesions. *American Journal of Ophthalmology* **88**, 694–697.

Bedford, M. A., Bedotto, C. & McFaul, P. A. (1970) Radiation retinopathy after the application of a cobalt plaque. *British Journal of Ophthalmology* **54**, 505–509.

Chee, P. H. Y. (1968) Radiation retinopathy. *American Journal of Ophthalmology* **66**, 860–865.

Cibis, P. A. & Brown, D. V. L. (1955) Retinal changes following ionising radiation. *American Journal of Ophthalmology* **40**, 84–88.

Lucas, D. R. (1961) The effect of X-radiation on the mouse retina at different stages of development. *International Journal of Radiation Biology* **3**, 105–124.

Disorders of Bruch's membrane and the disciform syndromes

Baba, F. E., Jarrett II, W. H., Harbin, T. S., Fine, S. L., Michels, R. G., Schachat, A. P. & Green, W. R. (1986) Massive haemorrhage complicating age-related macular degeneration. *Ophthalmology* **93**, 1581–1592.

Clarkson, J. G. & Altman, R. D. (1982) Angioid streaks. *Survey of Ophthalmology* **26**, 235–246.

Eagle Jr., R. C. (1984) Mechanisms of maculopathy. *Ophthalmology* **91**, 613–625.

Farkas, T. G., Sylvester, V. & Archer, D. B. (1971) The ultrastructure of drüsen. *American Journal of Ophthalmology* **71**, 1196–1205.

Farkas, T. G., Sylvester, V., Archer, D. B. & Altona, M. (1971) The histochemistry of drüsen. *American Journal of Ophthalmology* **71**, 1206–1215.

Garner, A. (1975) Pathology of macular degeneration in the elderly. *Transactions of the Ophthalmological Society of the UK* **95**, 54–61.

Gass, J. D. M. (1967) Pathogenesis of disciform detachment of the neuroepithelium. *American Journal of Ophthalmology* **63**, 573/1–711/139.

Green, W. R. (1980) Clinicopathologic studies of senile macular degeneration. In *Ocular Pathology Update*, ed. D. H. Nicholson, pp 115–144. Masson, New York.

Gregor, Z., Bird, A. C. & Chisholm, I. H. (1977) Senile disciform macular degeneration in the second eye. *British Journal of Ophthalmology* **61**, 141–147.

Havener, W. H. & Benes, S. C. (1986) Posterior decompensation syndrome: macular failure versus senile macular degeneration. *Annals of Ophthalmology* **18**, 271–272.

Hogan, M. J. (1972) The role of the retinal pigment epithelium in macular disease. *Transactions of the American Academy of Ophthalmology and Otolaryngology* **76**, 64–80.

Klien, B. A. (1964) Some aspects of the classification and differential diagnosis of senile macular degeneration. *American Journal of Ophthalmology* **58**, 927–939.

Maumenee, A. E. (1967) Further advances in the study of the macula. *Archives of Ophthalmology* **78**, 151–165.

Sarks, S. H. (1973) New vessel formation beneath the retinal pigmented epithelium in senile eyes. *British Journal of Ophthalmology* **57**, 951–965.

Sarks, S. H. (1976) Ageing and degeneration in the macular region: a clinico-pathological study. *British Journal of Ophthalmology* **60**, 324–341.

Sarks, S. H. (1980) Drüsen and their relationship to senile macular degeneration. *Australian Journal of Ophthalmology* **8**, 117–130.

Young, R. W. (1987) Pathophysiology of age-related macular degeneration. *Survey of Ophthalmology* **37**, 291–306.

Part 2. Vascular disorders

General

Ashton, N. (1957) Retinal vascularisation in health and disease. *American Journal of Ophthalmology* **44**, 7–17.

Michaelson, I. C. (1948) The mode of development of the vascular system of the retina, with some observations on its significance for certain retinal diseases. *Transactions of the Ophthalmological Society of the UK* **68**, 137–180.

Michaelson, I. C. & Campbell, A. C. P. (1940) The anatomy of the finer retinal vessels. *Transactions of the Ophthalmological Society of the UK* **60**, 71–112.

Toussaint, D., Kuwabara, T. & Cogan, D. G. (1961) Retinal vascular patterns. Part II. Human retinal vessels studied in three dimensions. *Archives of Ophthalmology* **65**, 575–581.

Blood–ocular barriers

Ashton, N. (1965) The blood–retinal barrier and vaso-glial relationships in retinal disease. *Transactions of the Opthalmological Society of the UK* **85**, 199–229.

Cunha-Vaz, J. G. (1966) Studies on the permeability of the blood–retinal barrier. II. Breakdown of the blood–retinal barrier by injury. *British Journal of Ophthalmology* **50**, 454–462.

Cunha-Vaz, J. (1979) The blood–ocular barriers. *Survey of Ophthalmology* **23**, 279–296.

Cunha-Vaz, J. G., Shakib, M. & Ashton, N. (1966) Studies on the permeability of the blood–retinal barrier. I. On the existence, development, and site of a blood–retinal barrier. *British Journal of Ophthalmology* **50**, 441–453.

Cotton-wool spots, retinal oedema and exudates

Fine, B. S. & Brucker, A. J. (1981) Macular edema & cystoid macular edema. *American Journal of Ophthalmology* **92**, 466–481.

Irvine, R. A. (1976) Cystoid maculopathy. *Survey of Ophthalmology* **21**, 1–17.

McLeod, D. (1981) Reappraisal of the cotton-wool spot. *Journal of the Royal Society of Medicine* **74**, 682–686.

McLeod, D., Marshall, J., Kohner, E. M. & Bird, A. C. (1977) The role of axoplasmic transport in the pathogenesis of retinal cotton-wool spots. *British Journal of Opthalmology* **61**, 177–191.

Shakib, M. & Ashton, N. (1966) Focal retinal ischaemia. *British Journal of Ophthalmology* **50**, 325–389.

Tso, M. O. M. (1982) Pathology of cystoid macular oedema. *Ophthalmology* **89**, 902–914.

Vascular occlusions

Appen, R. E., Wray, S. H. & Cogan, D.G. (1975) Central retinal artery occlusion. *American Journal of Ophthalmology* **79**, 374–381.

Archer, D. B., Ernest, J. T. & Maguire, C. J. F. (1976) Experimental branch retinal vein obstruction. In *Vision and Circulation*, ed. J. S. Cant. Kimpton, London.

Dahrling II, B.E. (1965) The histopathology of early central retinal artery occlusion. *Archives of Ophthalmology* **73**, 506–510.

Dryden, R. M. (1965) Central retinal vein occlusions and chronic simple glaucoma. *Archives of Ophthalmology* **73**, 659–663.

Fujino, T., Curtin, V. T. & Norton, E. W. D. (1969) Experimental central retinal vein occlusion. *Archives of Ophthalmology* **81**, 395–406.

Frangieh, G. T., Green, W. R., Barraquer-Somers, E. & Finkelstein, D. (1982) Histopathologic study of nine branch retinal vein occlusions. *Archives of Ophthalmology* **100**, 1132–1140.

Green, W. R., Chan, C. C., Hutchins, G. M. & Terry, J. M. (1981) Central retinal vein occlusion: a prospective histopathologic study of 29 eyes in 28 cases. *Retina* **1**, 27–55.

Hamilton, D. M., Kohner, E. M., Rosen, D., Bird, A. C. & Dollery, C. T. (1979) Experimental retinal branch vein occlusion in monkeys. I. Clinical appearances. *British Journal of Ophthalmology* **63**, 377–387.

Hayreh, S. S. (1965) Occlusion of the central retinal vessels. *British Journal of Ophthalmology* **49**, 626–645.

Hayreh, S. S. (1971) Pathogenesis of occlusion of central retinal vessels. *American Journal of Ophthalmology* **72**, 998–1011.

Hayreh, S. S. (1977) Central retinal vein occlusion. *Transactions of the American Academy of Ophthalmology and Otolaryngology* **83**, OP 379–391.

Hockley, D.J., Tripathi, R. C. & Ashton, N. (1979) Experimental retinal branch vein occlusion. III. Histopathological and electron microscopical studies. *British Journal of Ophthalmology* **63**, 393–411.

McLeod, D. (1975) Cilio-retinal arterial circulation in central vein occlusion. *British Journal of Ophthalmology* **59**, 486–492.

Orth, D. H. & Patz, A. (1978) Retinal branch vein occlusion. *Survey of Ophthalmology* **22**, 357–376.

Paton, A., Rubinstein, S. & Smith, V. H. (1964) Arterial insufficiency in retinal venous occlusion. *Transactions of the Ophthalmological Society of the UK* **84**, 559–586.

Perraut, L. E. & Zimmerman, L. E. (1959) The occurrence of glaucoma following occlusion of the central retinal artery. *Archives of Ophthalmology* **61**, 845–865.

Rosen, D. A., Marshall, J., Kohner, E. M., Hamilton, A. M. & Dollery, C. T. (1979) Experimental retinal branch vein occlusion in rhesus monkeys. II. Retinal blood flow studies. *British Journal of Ophthalmology* **63**, 388–392.

Stern, W. H. & Archer, D. B. (1981) Retinal vascular occlusion. *Annual Review of Medicine* **32**, 101–106.

Trope, G. E., Lowe, G. D. O., McArdle, B. M., Forbes, C. D., Prentice, C. M. & Foulds, W. S. (1983) Abnormal blood viscosity and haemostasis in long-standing retinal vein occlusion. *British Journal of Ophthalmology* **67**, 137–142.

Wolter, J. R. (1972) Double embolism of the central retinal artery and one long posterior ciliary artery followed by secondary hamorrhagic glaucoma. *American Journal of Ophthalmology* **73**, 651–657.

Wolter, J. R. & Phillips, R. L. (1959) Secondary glaucoma following occlusion of the central retinal artery. *American Journal of Ophthalmology* **47**, 335–340.

Zimmerman, L. E. (1965) Embolism of central retinal artery secondary to myocardial infarction with mural thrombosis. *Archives of Ophthalmology* **73**, 822–826.

Hypertensive retinopathy

Asdourian, G. K., Goldberg, M. F., Jampol, L. & Rabb, M. (1977) Retinal macroaneurysms. *Archives of Ophthalmology* **95**, 624–628.

Ashton, N. (1972) The eye in malignant hypertension. *Transactions of the American Academy of Ophthalmology and Otolaryngology* **76**, 17–40.

Tso, M. O. M. & Jampol, L. M. (1982) Pathophysiology of hypertensive retinopathy. *Ophthalmology* **89**, 1132–1145.

Diabetic retinopathy

Ashton, N. (1961) Neovascularisation in ocular disease. *Transactions of the Ophthalmological Society of the UK* **81**, 145–161.

Ashton, N. (1974) Vascular basement membrane changes in diabetic retinopathy. *British Journal of Ophthalmology* **58**, 344–366.

Bresnick, G. H., Davis, M. D., Myers, F. L. & De Venecia, G. (1977) Clinicopathologic correlations in diabetic retinopathy II. Clinical and histologic appearances of retinal capillary microaneurysms. *Archives of Ophthalmology* **95**, 1215–1220.

De Venecia, G., Davis, M. & Engerman, R. (1976) Clinicopathologic correlations in diabetic retinopathy. I. Histology and fluorescein angiography of microaneurysms. *Archives of Ophthalmology* **94**, 1766–1773.

Garner, A. (1970) Pathology of diabetic retinopathy. *British Medical Bulletin* **26**, 137–142.

Hersh, P. S., Green, W. R. & Tomas, J. V. Tractional venous loops in diabetic retinopathy. *American Journal of Ophthalmology* **92**, 661–671.

Kincaid, M. C., Green, W. R., Fine, S. L., Ferris, F. L. & Patz, A. (1983) An ocular clinicopathologic study of six patients from the diabetic retinopathy study. *Retina* **3**, 218–238.

Yanoff, M. (1969) Ocular pathology of diabetes mellitus. *American Journal of Ophthalmology* **67**, 21–38.

Neovascularisation

Ashton, N. (1961) Neovascularisation in ocular disease. *Transactions of the Ophthalmological Society of the UK* **81**, 145–161.

Hayreh, S. S. (1982) Ocular neovascularization with retinal vascular occlusion II. Occurrence of in central and branch retinal artery occlusion. *Archives of Ophthalmology* **100**, 1585–1596.

Jampol, L. M. & Goldbaum, M. H. (1980) Peripheral proliferative retinopathies. *Survey of Ophthalmology* **25**, 1–14.

Manschot, W. A. & Lee, W. R. (1984) Retinal neovascularisation arising from hyalinised blood vessels. *Graefe's Archive for Clinical and Experimental Ophthalmology* **222**, 63–70.

Patz, A. (1982a) Clinical and experimental studies on retinal neovascularization. *American Journal of Ophthalmology* **94**, 715–743.

Preis, I., Langer, R., Brem, H. & Folkman, J. (1977) Inhibition of neovascularization by an extract derived from vitreous. *American Journal of Ophthalmology* **84**, 323–327.

Angiogenic factors

Ben Ezra, D. (1978) Neovasculogenic ability of prostaglandins, growth factors and synthetic chemotactants. *American Journal of Ophthalmology* **86**, 455–461.

Kissun, R. D., Hill, C. R., Garner, A., Kumar, S. & Weiss, J. B. (1982) A low molecular weight angiogenic factor in cat retina. *British Journal of Ophthalmology* **66**, 165–169.

Retinopathy of prematurity

Ashton, N. (1954) Pathological basis of retrolental fibroplasia. *British Journal of Ophthalmology* **38**, 385–396.

Ashton, N. (1970) Some aspects of the comparative pathology of oxygen toxicity in the retina. *Ophthalmologica* **160**, 54–71.

Ashton, N., Ward, B. & Serpell, G. (1954) Effect of oxygen on developing retinal vessels with particular reference to the problem of retrolental fibroplasia. *British Journal of Ophthalmology* **38**, 397–432.

Flynn, J. T., O'Grady, G. E, Herrera, J. & Kushner, B. J. (1977) Retrolental fibroplasia: I. Clinical observations. *Archives of Ophthalmology* **95**, 217–223.

Garner, A. (1984) An international classification of retinopathy of prematurity prepared by an international committee. *British Journal of Ophthalmology* **68**, 690–697.

Kretzer, F. L., Hittner, H. M., Johnson, A. T., Mehta, R. S. & Godio, L. B. (1982) Vitamin E and retrolental fibroplasia: ultrastructural support of clinical efficacy. *Annals of the New York Academy of Sciences* **393**, 145–164.

Kushner, B. J., Essner, D., Cohen, I. J. & Flynn, J. T. (1977) Retrolental fibroplasia. II. Pathologic correlation. *Archives of Ophthalmology* **95**, 29–38.

Naiman, J., Green, W. R. & Patz, A. (1979) Retrolental fibroplasia in hypoxic newborn. *American Journal of Ophthalmology* **88**, 55–58.

Patz, A. (1969) Retrolental fibrolasia. *Survey of Ophthalmology* **14**, 1–29.

Patz, A. (1982b) Retrolental fibroplasia (retinopathy of prematurity). *American Journal of Ophthalmology* **94**, 552–554.

Patz, A. (1983) Current therapy of retrolental fibroplasia. *Ophthalmology* **90**, 425–427.

Patz, A. (1984) Retinal neovascularisation: early contributions of Professor Michaelson and recent observations. *British Journal of Ophthalmology* **68**, 42–46.

Silverman, W. A. (1980) *Retrolental Fibroplasia: A Modern Parable*. Grune & Stratton, New York.

Terry, T. L. (1942) Extreme prematurity and fibroblastic overgrowth of persistent vascular sheath behind the crystalline lens. I. Preliminary report. *American Journal of Ophthalmology* **25**, 203–204.

CHAPTER 10

Coats' disease

Coats, G. (1907–1908) Forms of retinal disease with massive exudation. *Royal London Ophthalmic Hospital Reports* **17**, 440–525.

Chang, M., McLean, I. W. & Merritt, J. C. (1984) Coats' disease: a study of 62 histologically confirmed cases. *Journal of Pediatric Ophthalmology and Strabismus* **21**, 163–168.

Henkind, P. & Morgan, G. (1966) Peripheral retinal angioma with exudative retinopathy in adults (Coats' lesion). *British Journal of Ophthalmology* **50**, 2–11.

McGettrick, P. M. & Loeffler, K. U. (1987) Bilateral Coats' disease in an infant (A clinical, angiographic, light and electron microscopic study). *Eye* **1**, 136–145.

Manschot, W. A. & de Bruijn, W. C. (1967) Coats' disease: definition and pathogenesis. *British Journal of Ophthamology* **31**, 145–157.

Mushin, A. & Morgan, G. (1971) Ocular injury in the battered baby syndrome. *British Journal of Ophthalmology* **55**, 343–347.

Reese, A. B. (1956) Telangiectasis of the retina and Coats' disease. *American Journal of Ophthalmology* **42**, 1–8.

Tripathi, R. & Ashton, N. (1971) Electron microscopical study of Coats' disease. *British Journal of Ophthalmology* **55**, 289–301.

Woods, A. C. & Duke, J. R. (1963a) Coats' disease. I. Review of literature, diagnostic criteria, clinical findings and plasma lipid studies. *British Journal of Ophthalmology* **47**, 385–412.

Woods, A. C. & Duke J. R. (1963b) Coats' disease. II. Studies on the identity of the lipids concerned and probable role of mucopolysaccharides in its pathogenesis. *British Journal of Opthalmology* **47**, 413–434.

Chapter 11 Tumours of neuroepithelium

RETINOBLASTOMA

Retinoblastoma is a malignant neoplasm composed of embryonic neuronal cells. Although it is the commonest intraocular tumour of infancy and childhood, it is by no means common. Its frequency is approximately one in every 15 000 to 20 000 live births and it constitutes about 3% of childhood malignancies. An increase in the number of reported cases has occurred in recent years mainly as a result of reduced mortality of those bearing the retinoblastoma gene.

Boys and girls are affected in about equal numbers except that the rare diffuse infiltrating type almost always occurs in boys. Retinoblastomata are bilateral in 25–30% of cases and such neoplasms are unconnected, independent foci of growth, often asynchronous in appearance and unequal in size. Retinoblastomata may commence in foetal life and so be present at birth. In most patients the neoplasm is discovered before the age of 3 years and first presentation after the age of 6 years is rare. Again the diffuse infiltrating type is exceptional since the majority have presented in boys between 6 and 11 years of age. Most retinoblastomata reported as occurring in adults seem to have been growths arising from the pars ciliaris retinae.

Inheritance

In describing retinoblastomata it is customary to differentiate between familial and sporadic cases or between bilateral and unilateral tumours, but the fundamental distinction is between genetic and non-genetic retinoblastomata.

Genetic retinoblastoma

A genetic retinoblastoma is the result of a germinal mutation in the antecedents of the afflicted child, the antecedents being either a family member in some previous generation or one of the child's parents. The mutation gives rise to an autosomal dominant gene with incomplete penetrance estimated at approximately 80%.

1 *Past germinal mutation in a previous generation:* in this case there will be evidence of inheritance in the family in an autosomal dominant manner (familial retinoblastoma). In such pedigrees, a generation is sometimes skipped, transmission then being through an unaffected, but carrier parent with retinoblastomatous near relatives. Familial retinoblastomata, most of which are bilateral, account for 6–8% of new cases seen.

2 *New germinal mutation in a parent:* retinoblastomata occurring as a result of new parental mutations appear sporadically in previously healthy families. They make up a minority of sporadically occurring retinoblastomata and are more often bilateral than unilateral. Of all retinoblastoma cases, 25–30% are bilateral and genetic, while 10–20% are unilateral and genetic. Survivors of genetic retinoblastomata will transmit the disease to 40–45% of their offspring.

Non-genetic retinoblastoma

A non-genetic retinoblastoma is the result of a somatic mutation in the retina of the affected child. There is no way of distinguishing them either clinically or pathologically from sporadically occurring unilateral genetic retinoblastomata.

Chromosomal abnormalities

Most patients with retinoblastomata have normal karyotypes, but about 20% of patients with partial deletion of the long arm of chromosome 13 (13q-syndrome) develop retinoblastoma. In most of these cases the retinoblastomata were bilateral and some of the children were mentally retarded. The locus at which the retinoblastoma mutation occurs has been confirmed by linkage studies of the esterase D gene locus in hereditary families to be at 13q14. The normal allele at this locus probably regulates differentiation and in its absence uncontrolled proliferation occurs. Two steps are thought to be necessary to induce the malignancy. The first occurs in a single somatic retinal cell (non-hereditary) or on the germ-line (hereditary). In both hereditary and non-hereditary tumours, the second step is a somatic event in the cell that becomes malignant.

An association between retinoblastoma and Down's syndrome (trisomy 21 and XXX trisomy 21) has also occasionally been noted.

Gross appearance

Most retinoblastomata arise in the fundal retina and multiple foci of growth may be evident macroscopically. When the enucleated globe is opened, the neoplasm is often found to be more extensive than the ophthalmoscopic findings had suggested.

In formalin-fixed eyes, the neoplastic tissue is pinkish-white or cream coloured, compact or fluffy and often nodular on its free surfaces (Fig. 11.1). The cut surface of the growth is rarely homogeneous, but shows yellowish-white areas of necrosis, dead-white calcium flecks and pink to brown areas of haemorrhage. Often a very fine honeycomb pattern can be seen where grey perivascular mantles of surviving cells are enclosed by white necrotic tissue. This appearance is pathognomonic of retinoblastoma. The growth may be predominantly posterior to the retina so that the retina is detached (exophytum type, see Fig. 11.1a) or anterior (endophytum type, see Fig. 11.1b). The former is commoner.

Small clumps of cells of retinoblastomata readily adhere to cutting implements even after fixation, it is, therefore, advisable to cut the optic nerve stump before cutting the globe to avoid any risk of transfer. Invasion of the optic nerve can usually be detected macroscopically if present.

Microscopic appearances

Retinoblastomata are intensely cellular neoplasms with a minimum of supportive stroma (Fig. 11.2). Blood vessels are quite numerous and usually well formed, but the blood supply seems to be inadequate to the demands of the neoplastic tissue so that patchy necrosis is often widespread, leaving multilayered perivascular mantles of surviving cells (Fig. 11.3). The necrotic cells tend to remain *in situ* and rarely excite any marked inflammatory reaction and it may be for this reason that retinoblastomatous eyes so often remain relatively white and uninflamed. The necrotic areas readily calcify, however, forming gritty flecks which can be seen clinically and demonstrated radiologically. This is an important diagnostic sign since intraocular calcification in childrens' eyes is uncommon in any other condition. At the ultra-

Fig. 11.1 Macroscopic appearances of retinoblastoma. (a) Exophytum type (child aged 5 months). The mouth of the funnel of detached retina (R) is seen in contact with the lens which is displaced forwards. Note the opaque flecks of calcification on the cut surface of the tumour.

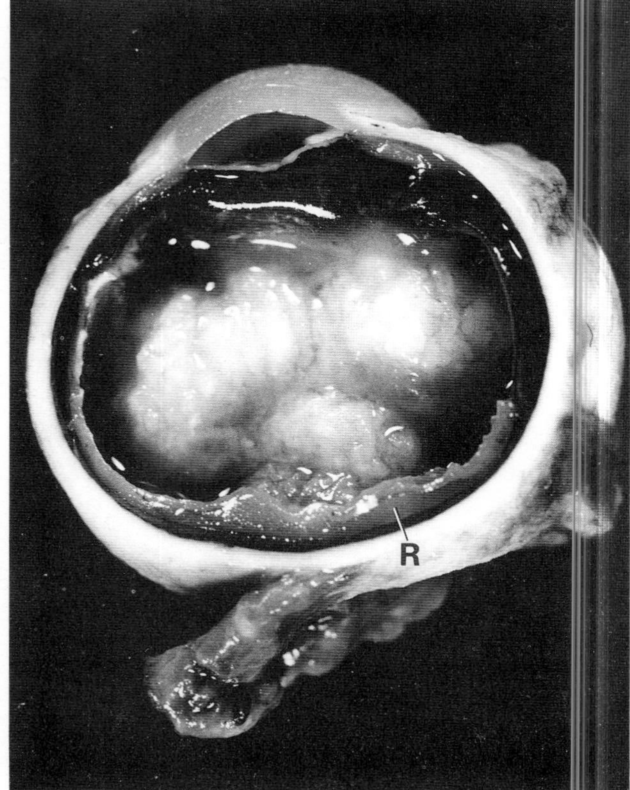

Fig. 11.1 (b) Endophytum type (child aged 3 years 11 months). The tumour occupied the nasal half of the globe and the temporal aspect of the tumour is illustrated. Growth has been forwards into the vitreous and the anterior part of the tumour is in contact with the lens. The retina (R) is seen posteriorly and is not detached.

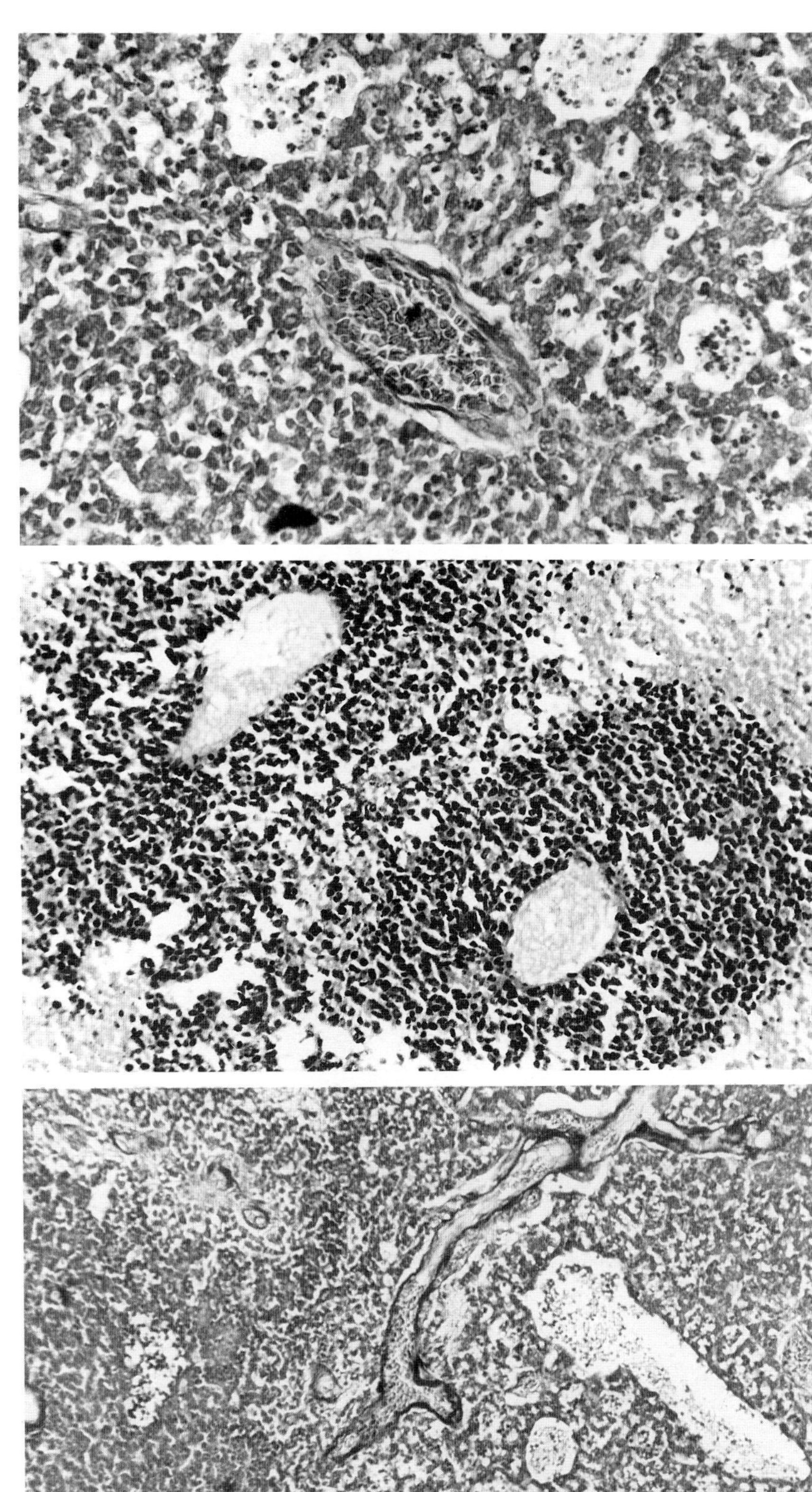

Fig. 11.2 Undifferentiated retinoblastoma surrounding a blood vessel. Nuclear fragments are seen throughout the field as dark spots. In addition, three lacunae filled with cellular debris have formed.

Fig. 11.3 Mantles of cells around blood vessels. H & E (×260).

Fig. 11.4 Basophilic deposit of complexed DNA on a blood vessel.

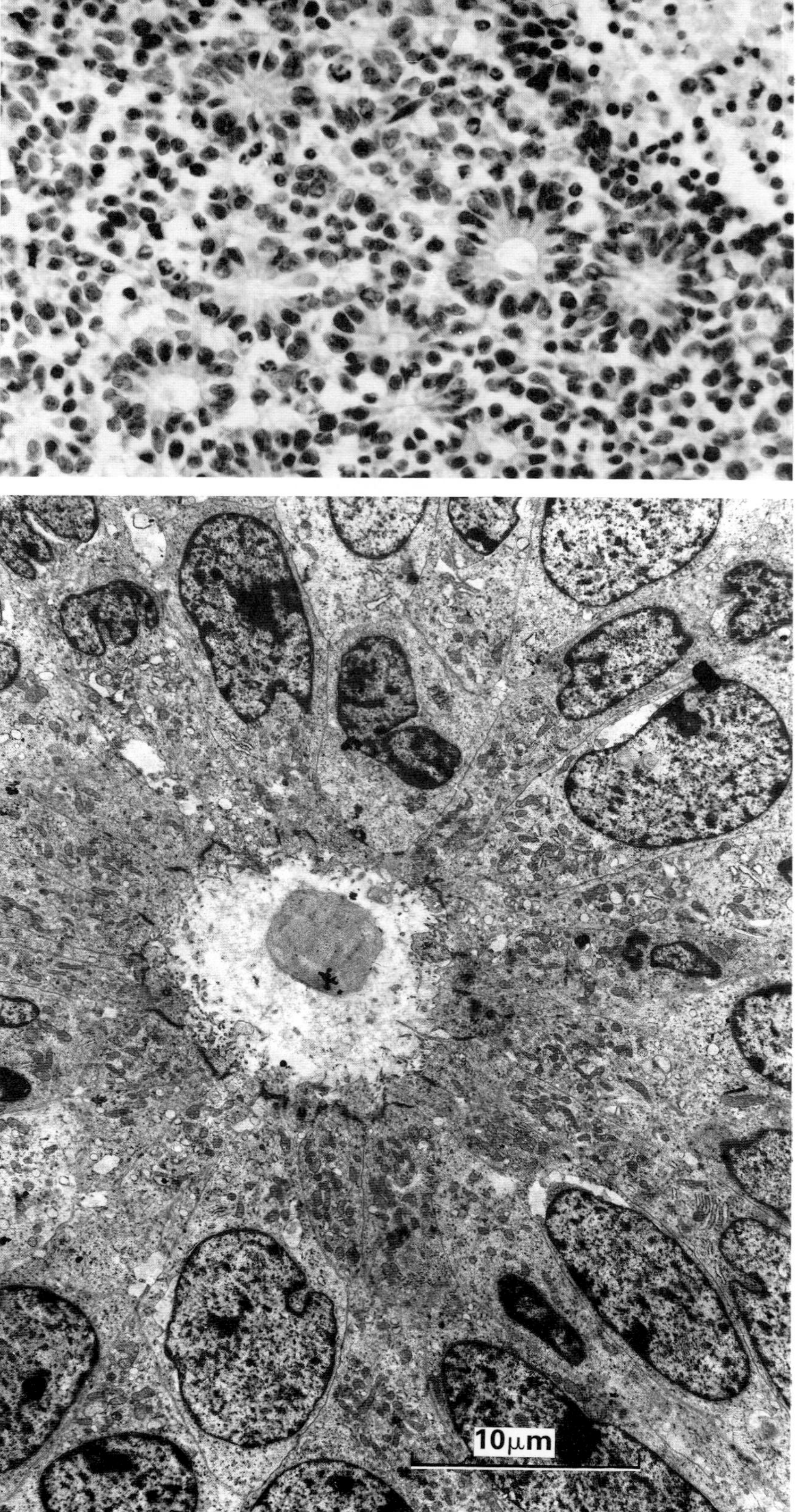

Fig. 11.5 Flexner–Wintersteiner rosette. (a) Light microscopic appearance in H & E section. Small cells with generally hyperchromatic nuclei are arranged radially around a central space demarcated by a limiting membrane. (×405).

Fig. 11.5 (b) Low power electron micrograph of a rosette. (×4310).

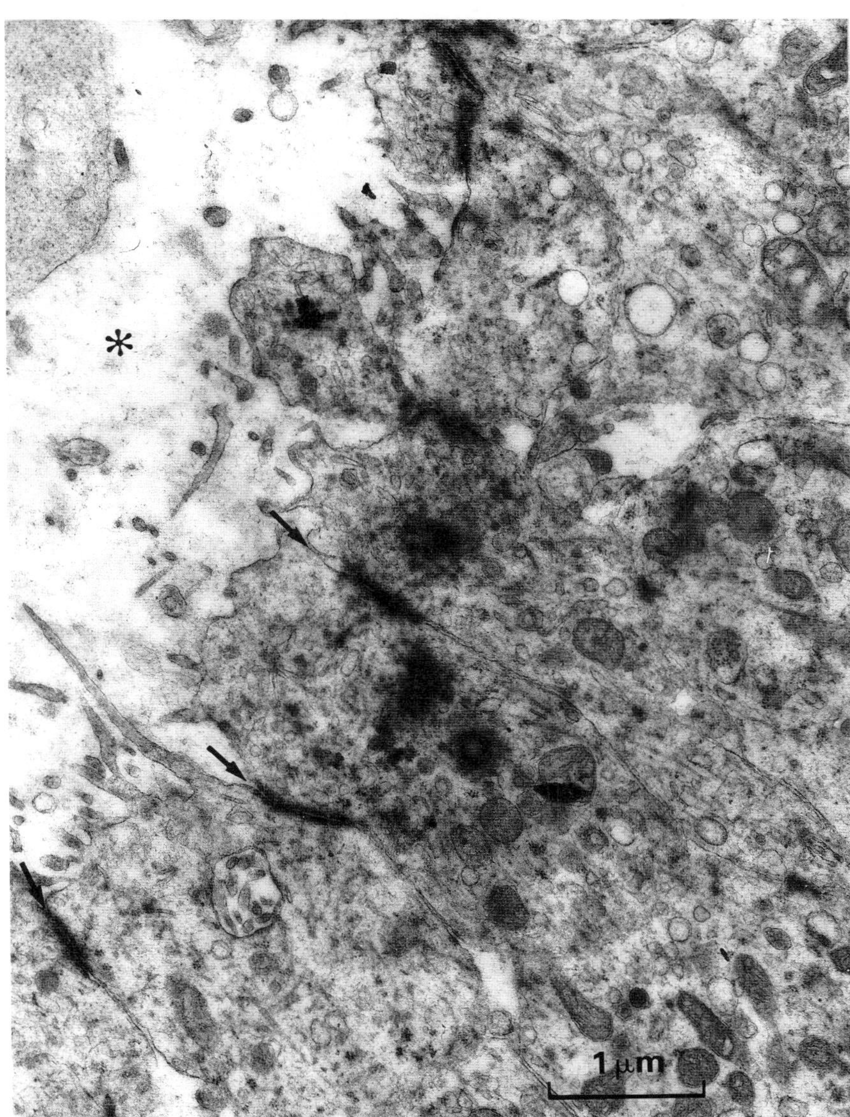

Fig. 11.5 (c) Higher power of cells around central space (asterisk) showing terminal bars (arrows). Fine filaments can be seen projecting from the apices of the cells, but photoreceptor-like structures are lacking. (×21 180).

structural level, needle-like calcium deposits form within the mitochondrial membranes following disruption of the plasmalemma (Lin & Tso, 1983).

In tumours showing extensive necrosis, dense, strongly basophilic accumulations of calcium–DNA complexes are sometimes evident as free globules or encrustations on the blood vessels (Fig. 11.4).

Most retinoblastomata exhibit both undifferentiated and rosetted types of growth, the former always predominating. A small minority of retinoblastomata show, in addition, areas of photoreceptor differentiation, but as a rule these areas form only a small part of the whole tumour.

Undifferentiated growth: the densely packed neoplastic cells are devoid of special arrangement (Fig. 11.2). They have round, oval, elongated or polygonal nuclei with deeply staining punctate chromatin, but usually no nucleoli. Deep infolding of the nuclear membrane is often seen under the electron micrscope. Nuclear fragmentation is widespread and mitotic figures are numerous. By light microscopy, the cytoplasm is scanty and poorly demarcated, but carrot shaped cytoplasmic rudiments may occasionally be seen.

As already described, the undifferentiated cells readily undergo necrosis both spontaneously and after radiotherapy.

Rosetted growth (Fig. 11.5a): a rosetted pattern forms part of many retinoblastomata. Rosettes are small formations of 15–40 tapering, elongated cells arranged radially about a round or oval central cavity 10–60 μm or more in diameter. This central cavity may contain a few neoplastic cells, but never contains blood vessels. The lumen of the Flexner–Wintersteiner rosette, which is so characteristic of the retinoblastoma, is demarcated by a limiting membrane is made up of terminal bars and is analogous to the outer limiting membrane of the retina (11.5b & c). The rosetted cells sometimes exhibit fine processes trailing out from their peripheral ends. Rosettes are rather constant in size and almost always circular or oval in outline. Larger, elongated or horseshoe forms are, however, occasionally seen.

Rosettes are regarded as evidence of partial differentiation towards photoreceptors. There is some evidence that the younger a retinoblastoma is, as judged by the age of the patient and the duration of the disease, the more rosettes it contains. Heavily rosetted growths are somewhat less lethal than those principally composed of undifferentiated cells.

Photoreceptor differentiation: more advanced differentiation of tumour cells to form photoreceptor elements occurs in a minority of retinoblastomata. Under low magnification, areas with photoreceptor differentiation are pale and eosinophilic compared with the densely basophilic areas of undifferentiated growth. This is because the differentiated cells have smaller, less hyperchromatic nuclei and more cytoplasm and are separated by more intercellular matrix. These cells form eosinophilic cytoplasmic processes 15–20 μm in length projecting through a fenetrated membrane often in clusters like the petals of a flower or a formal fleur-de-lys (fleurettes) (Fig. 11.6).

The absence of any evidence of Müller cell formation helps to confirm the belief that retinoblastomata are neuronal neoplasms. In areas showing photoreceptor differentiation, mitotic figures are rare, necrosis is absent and calcium deposition, if present, is small in amount.

Other features which may be seen under the electron microscope are plentiful cilia and appendages (Fig. 11.7) which, in common with photoreceptors, have nine double tubules with no central pair. Annulate lamellae (cytomembranes resembling the nuclear envelope) are also commonly seen and numerous dense core secretory granules have been observed. Immunohistochemical staining for retinal S-antigen is positive, especially in differentiated cells and in cells forming Flexner–Wintersteiner rosettes.

There is evidence that cells showing photoreceptor differentiation are more radioresistant than undifferentiated retinoblastoma cells. This accords with the rule that radiosensitivity of cells varies inversely with their degree of differentation. Following radiotherapy, surviving tumour nodules composed of cells showing photoreceptor differentiation, either alone or mixed with glial tissue, have a grey 'fish-flesh' appearance through the ophthalmoscope.

Neuronal differentiation: neurone-specific enolase is a specific marker for cells of neuronal, neuroendocrine and neurotactile origin which can be identified by immunohistochemical staining. As would be expected, many cells in a retinoblastoma react for neurone-specific enolase. Some cells giving a strong cytoplasmic reaction may show no evidence of photoreceptor differentiation. It is possible that these are differentiating along other neuronal lines.

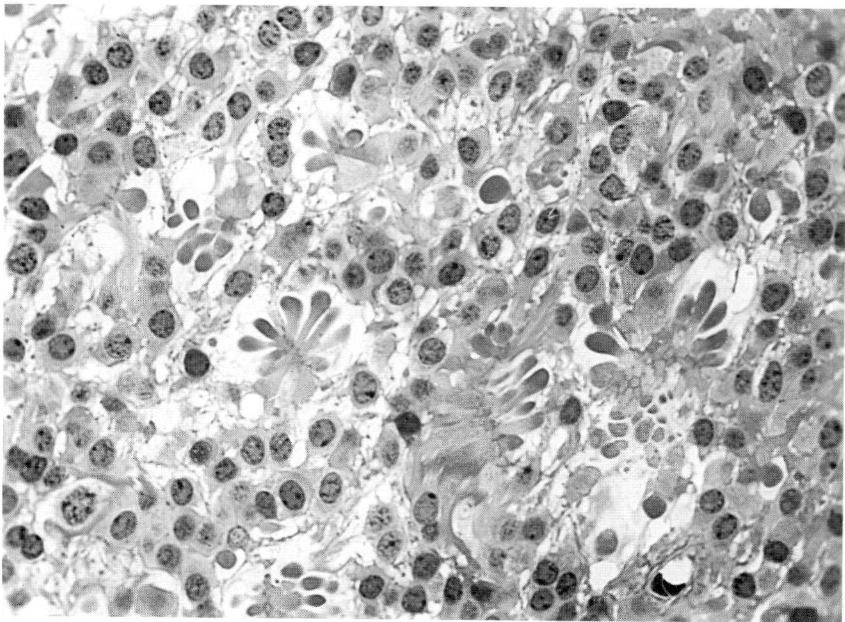

Fig. 11.6 Fleurettes. Photoreceptor elements are seen as club-ended processes related to a fenestrated membrane. The cells from which they originate are out of focus. 1 μ Epon section stained by paraphenylene diamine. (×550). (Reproduced with permission from Tso *et al.*, 1970a.)

Fig. 11.7 (*Opposite*) Electron micrograph showing cell containing a centriole (C) and possible neurosecretory granules (arrows). (×9010).

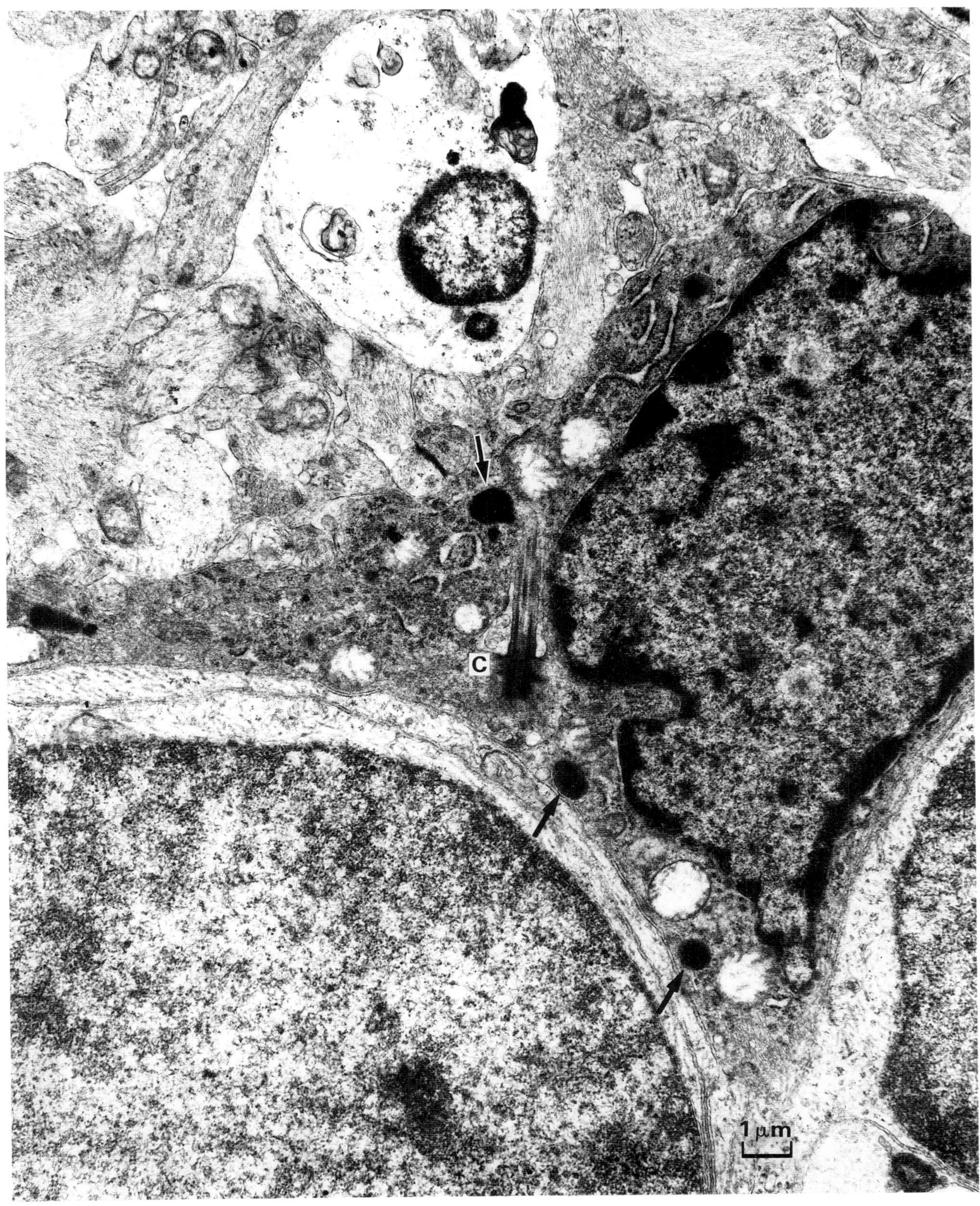
C
1 μm

Astrocytic differentiation: glial cells are regularly observed in retinoblastomata and cells can also be demonstrated that react with antibodies to glial fibrillary acidic protein. While these are probably mainly reactive rather than neoplastic astrocytes, it is possible that the tumour cells can occasionally develop along glial lines.

Types and growth

Retinoblastomata are classified into three main types according to the mode of growth they exhibit:

Exophytum type: in this, the commonest type, the main mass of growth is directed outwards with progressive retinal detachment (Figs 11.1a & 11.8a). Tumour seeding occurs via the subretinal fluid to the outer layers of other parts of the retina and on to the pigmented epithelium. The detached retina may be pressed forwards behind the lens and thus obscure a clear ophthalmoscopic view of the actual tumour.

Endophytum type: growth is directed mainly into the vitreous, the retina remaining undetached (Figs 11.1b & 11.8b). Groups of neoplastic cells migrate through the vitreous to other parts of the retina and even to the anterior segment (Fig. 11.9). Seedling tumours may thus be established on the ciliary body, iris and corneal endothelium and a sediment of malignant cells be deposited in the filtration angle inferiorly. Ophthalmoscopically, the neoplastic tissue in the retina and and anterior segment can be viewed directly. Some retinoblastomata grow simultaneously outwards into the subretinal space and inwards into the vitreous thus exhibiting features of both types of growth.

In either type, as the neoplasm grows larger, it infiltrates and replaces the retina (Fig. 11.10) and incorporates the secondary implants. Degeneration and atrophy of the intraocular structures ensues. The increasing volume of the intraocular mass may lead to glaucoma, expansion of the globe, thinning of the corneoscleral envelope and the formation of staphylomata. Later the lens may become cataractous, its capsule ruptured and its fibres absorbed (Fig. 11.11a). Eventually by seeding and infiltration, the neoplasm may invade all the ocular layers and cavities and perforate the globe (Fig. 11.11b). Endophthalmitis or panophthalmitis may occasionally supervene, extensively destroying the growth and quite obscuring its clinical presentation.

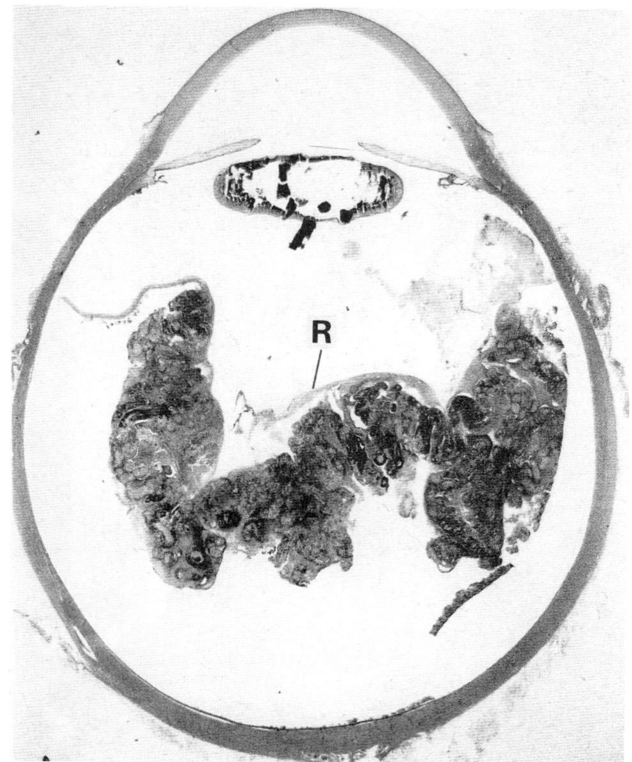

Fig. 11.8 Types of retinoblastoma. (a) Exophytum type. The tumour is posterior to the retina.

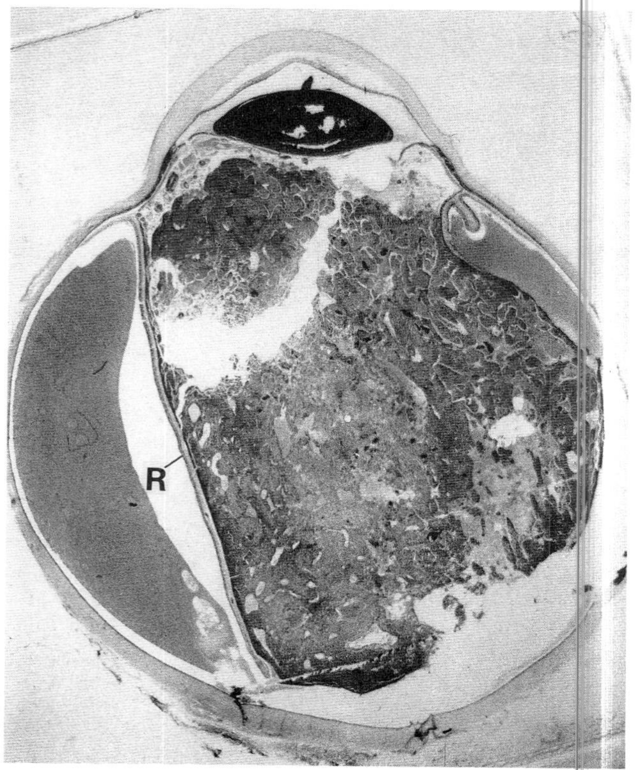

Fig. 11.8 (b) Endophytum type. The tumour is anterior to the retina and in apposition with the lens. R = retina.

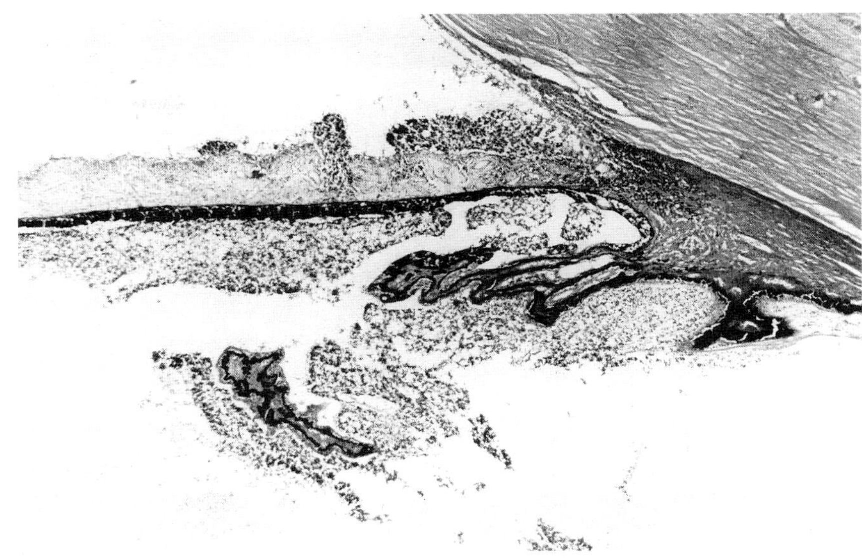

Fig. 11.9 Spread in anterior segment. Necrotic seedlings on ciliary processes, both surfaces of iris and in chamber angle.

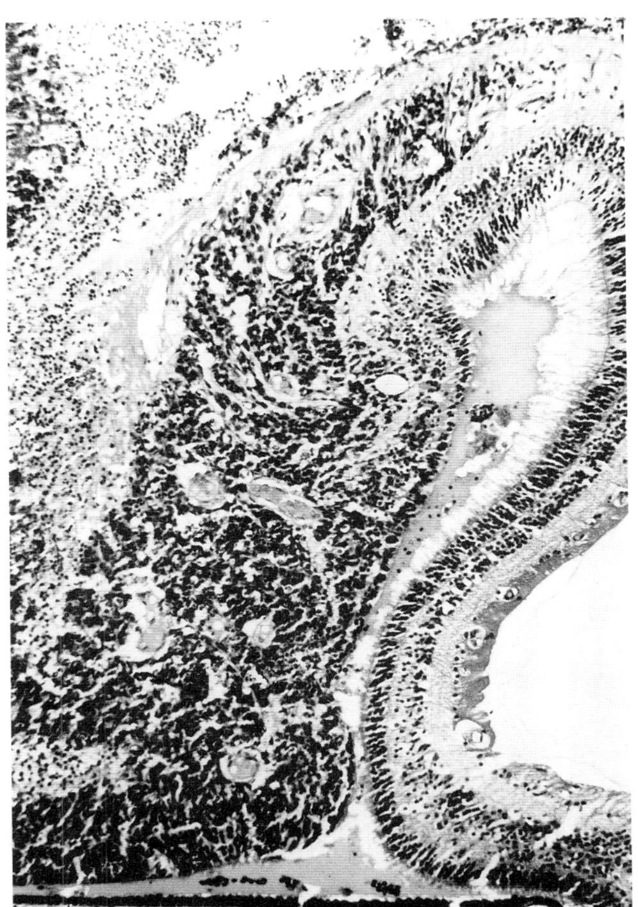

Fig. 11.10 Retinal infiltration at margin of a retinoblastoma. H & E (×105).

Diffuse infiltrating type: this rare variant most commonly originates in the peripheral retina which is replaced, but only slightly thickened, by typical retinoblastomatous cells. Mitotic activity, rosette formation and necrosis is not, however, marked. No macroscopic tumour mass is formed and retinal detachment is slight or absent, but there is a constant discharge of malignant cells into the aqueous. In the course of time, neoplastic cells replace the ciliary epithelium, infiltrate the ciliary body, uveoscleral meshwork and iris, and may invade the fundal retina and extend into the optic nerve if the eye is retained long enough. The majority of reported cases have occurred in boys between the age of 6 and 11 years who presented with an apparent uveitis with hypopyon or an apparent hypopyon with raised intraocular tension. Examination of aspirated aqueous revealed clumps of malignant cells but neither organisms nor polymorphonuclear leucocytes. In most of the recorded cases, the eye was enucleated before extraocular extension had occurred.

Spread and metastasis

1 The commonest route by which retinoblastomata escape from the globe is along the optic nerve (Fig. 11.12) and the consequent intracranial extension is a common, if not the commonest, cause of death, often by hydrocephalus. Growth along the nerve proceeds by destroying and replacing the nerve tracts and may even reach the chiasma. Where adequate diagnostic facilities are available it is now rare to find, at operation, extension along the nerve as far back as the point at which the central retinal vessels enter and leave (approximately 10 mm from the globe). This is a danger point since it allows

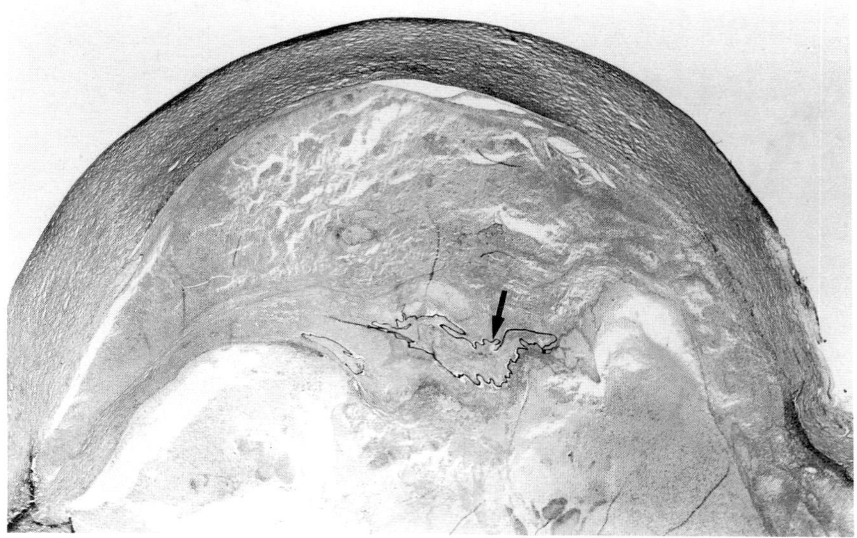

Fig. 11.11 A neglected retinoblastoma in child aged 3. (a) Anterior chamber showing remnants of lens capsule (arrow) in necrotic tumour. PAS/tartrazine.

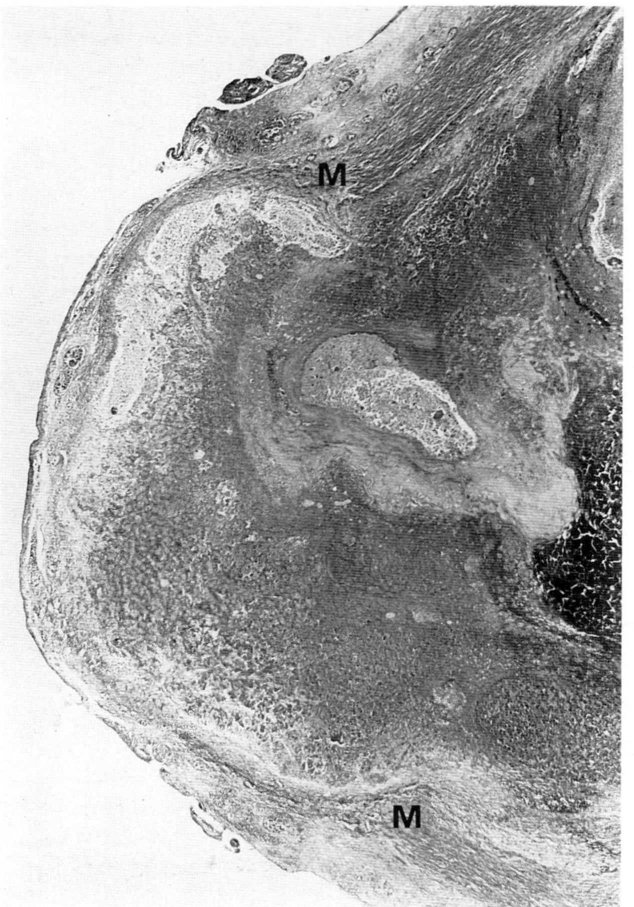

Fig. 11.11 (b) Section at level where limbal rupture had occurred and necrotic tumour is prolapsing through sclera. M = margins of scleral rupture. H & E.

access to the subarachnoid space. However, growth may enter the subarachnoid space before reaching the 10 mm point or, very occasionally, without invading the nerve at all. Once in the subarachnoid space, the neoplasm is rapidly disseminated to the leptomeninges, ventricles, brain and spinal cord and even into the opposite orbit, but is restrained from extension into the calvarium and vertebrae by the dura mater.

2 A somewhat less frequent route of extraocular extension is round the margin of Bruch's membrane at the nerve head into the choroid and thence, either into the orbit along the scleral emissary channels or into the bloodstream via the choroidal vessels. Choroidal invasion (Fig. 11.13) and extrascleral extension occur more frequently with undifferentiated tumours exhibiting few or no rosettes. Evidence of choroidal invasion is a poor prognostic sign, probably because it is a prelude to blood-borne dissemination.

3 Once in the orbit the neoplasms may invade the orbital bones and those of the face or skull (and even extend into the paranasal sinuses, nose and mouth) thence to metastasise by lymphatic channels to cervical, mediastinal and more distant lymph nodes.

4 Blood-borne metastases from the ocular or orbital growth are most frequently to bones, e.g. skull, ribs, humerus and less often to viscera and muscles. The lungs are usually spared. Haematogenous metastases are very often found at autopsy. Extraocular extensions, orbital recurrences and metastatic growths rarely exhibit any rosette formation.

Prognosis

Treatment by irradiation is an alternative to enucleation of the eye. The probable response can be judged by

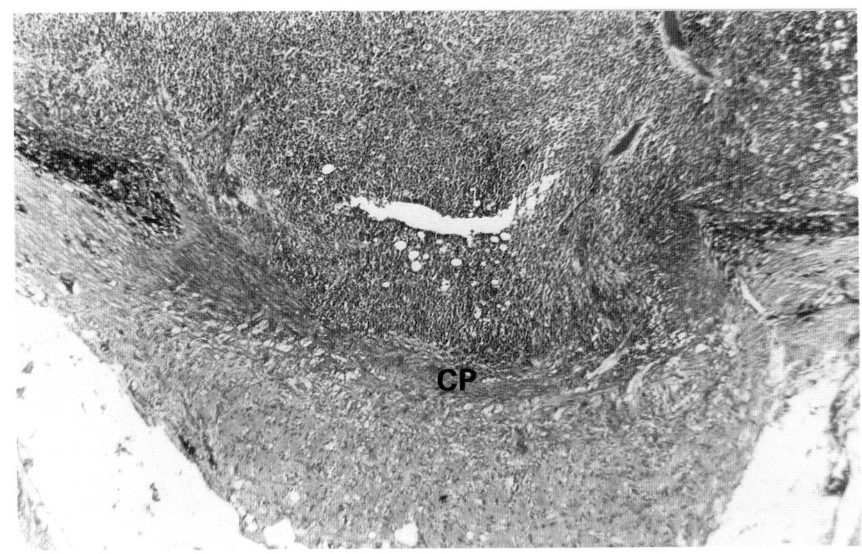

Fig. 11.12 Invasion of optic nerve. (a) Low power showing tumour occupying nerve head and causing some bowing of cribriform plate (CP). Masson trichrome (×41).

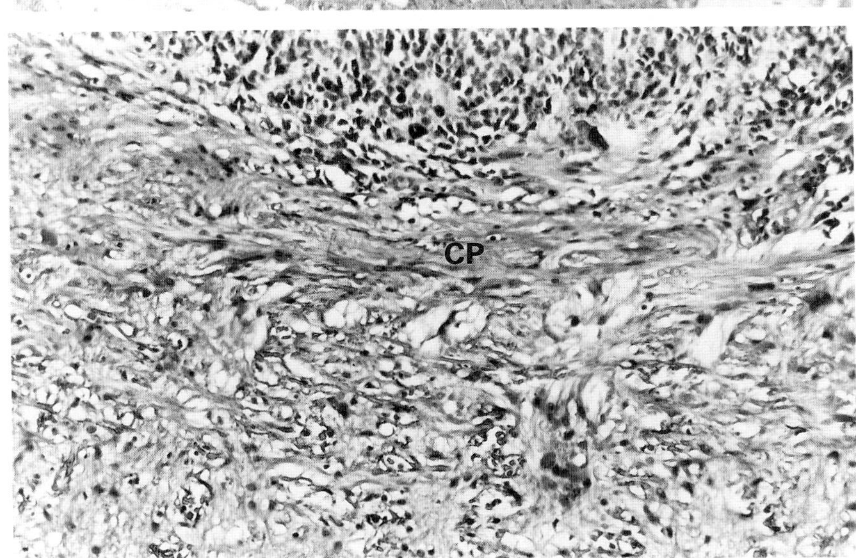

Fig. 11.12 (b) Higher power showing tumour just beginning to enter post-cribriform part of nerve.

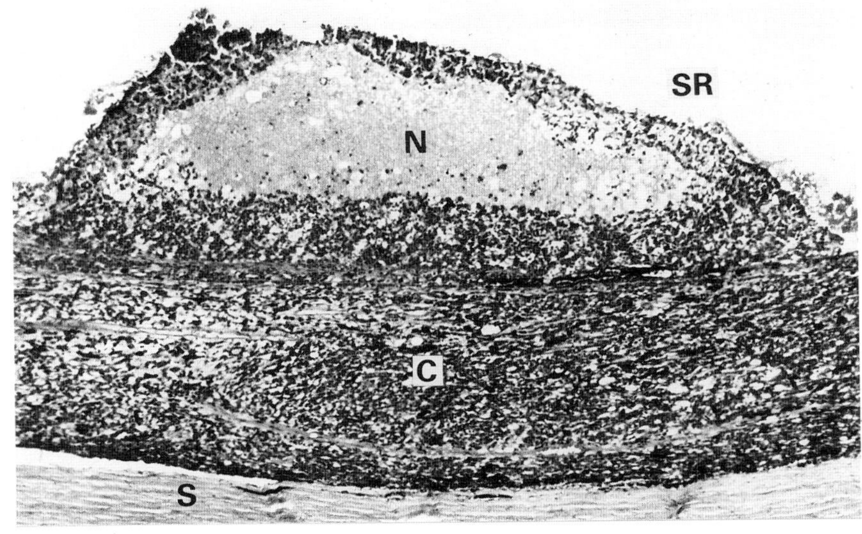

Fig. 11.13 Choroidal invasion. Retinoblastoma infiltrating full thickness of choroid (C). A necrotic seedling (N) is present in overlying subretinal space (SR). S = sclera. H & E (×64).

classifying the tumours into groups according to their size, number and location in the eye (Reese, 1976).

When enucleation is done, as much optic nerve as possible should be removed with the globe and examined histologically to establish:

1 If the nerve is free of growth and there is no evidence of orbital extension, risk of recurrence is not great and prognosis will largely depend on the probability of a second neoplasm developing in the other eye. This probability is much higher when there is an inherited liability to the disease. If a second neoplasm does appear, the prognosis still remains quite favourable provided the growth is promptly and totally eradicated. Estimates of cure by enucleation alone, in cases without evidence of extraocular extension vary from 50–90% of cases. Early diagnosis and prompt enucleation naturally increases the prospect of cure.

2 If the optic nerve is infiltrated, i.e. the growth has extended through the *lamina cribrosa*, the outlook is much worse. A fatal outcome is to be expected in approximately 50% of such cases. If the growth has extended to the point of exit of the central vessels from the nerve, the mortality rate rises to approximately 65%.

3 If neoplastic infiltration extends to the cut end of the optic nerve the line of excision has passed through malignant tissue. Recurrence is then almost certain and the prognosis is grave. Recurrence, which usually occurs within 6 months of enucleation, is most commonly in the orbit, but occasionally within the cranium or even at some distant metastatic site.

Spontaneous regression and arrest

Since 1952, spontaneously regressed retinoblastomata have been reported in some 85 eyes (Aaby *et al.*, 1983). Such cases fall into two categories:

1 *In phthisical globes:* a number of phthisical globes mostly from close relatives of retinoblastoma cases have been found to contain calcified remnants of tumour. Necrosis of the tumour probably occurs for vascular reasons and results in subsequent shrinkage of the globe. The necrosis may be incomplete so that islands of viable cells persist. A 'regressed' retinoblastoma in a phthisical globe may be associated with a 'viable' tumour in the other eye.

2 *In functional globes:* calcified lesions have been observed, usually in the eyes of parents of retinoblastoma cases, which are sufficiently characteristic clinically to justify a diagnosis of 'regressed' retinoblastoma. A few such cases have been examined histologically. They are usually flattish tumours composed of 'benign-looking' cells exhibiting photoreceptor differentiation. They show no mitotic or invasive activity. It is not at present clear whether they represent 'regressed' or 'arrested' tumours.

Various names have been proposed for tumours falling within this category: 'retinoma' (Gallie *et al.*, 1982); 'retinoblastoma group 0' (Aaby *et al.*, 1983); 'retinocytoma' (Margot *et al.*, 1983). Whatever their status, for the purposes of genetic counselling, they carry the same risk as retinoblastomata.

Differential diagnosis

The rather anachronistic term 'pseudoglioma' is still sometimes used for lesions which simulate retinoblastoma in their clinical presentation. These conditions may be classified into four groups:

1 Vascular malformations of the retina, e.g. Coats' disease (Chapter 10, Part 2) and angiomatosis retinae (Chapter 15).

2 Endophthalmitis. Intraocular inflammation leading to retinal detachment or granuloma formation due to metastatic bacteria or fungi, *Toxocara canis*, *Toxoplasma gondii* (Chapter 2).

3 Retrolental connective tissue (persistent hyperplastic primary vitreous) (Chapter 17).

4 Miscellaneous conditions.

A useful differential point worth remembering is that the retinoblastomatous eye is, more often than not, white and of normal size or slightly larger for the age with a normal to deep anterior chamber.

Trilateral retinoblastoma

Retinoblastoma occasionally occurs in association with intracranial tumours, particularly of the pineal. Pinealoblastomata closely resemble retinoblastomata histologically and it has been shown that some cases react positively for retinal S-antigen (Donoso *et al.*, 1987).

Second malignancies in retinoblastoma survivors

Patients with bilateral retinoblastoma have a 15–20% chance of developing a second non-ocular malignancy. Second malignancies are much rarer in unilateral cases. The time interval extends from 1 to 42 years. Three groups can be recognised:

1 Tumours arising in cases treated by radiotherapy in the field of irradiation. This group constitutes 70% of the cases and by far the commonest tumour is an osteogenic sarcoma (see Chapter 14).

2 Tumours arising in cases treated by radiotherapy outside the field of irradiation. Most of these were osteogenic sarcomata of the lower extremities.

3 Tumours arising in cases treated by enucleation alone. These comprised three out of 22 cases. They consisted of a rhabdomyosarcoma, a malignant melanoma and an osteogenic sarcoma.

4 In a few cases, no clear distinction could be made between a late metastasis of the retinoblastoma and a second primary tumour.

The prognosis for cases developing second malignancies was poor. Eighty five per cent died of them (see Abramson *et al.* 1975; 1979; 1980).

TUMOURS OF THE PARS CILIARIS RETINAE

Tumours of the ciliary epithelium are too rare to warrant more than brief consideration here. Most arise from the non-pigmented epithelium. They are divisible into the two following groups:

1 Embryonal tumours, medulloepitheliomata, which are believed to develop from ciliary epithelium that is still immature. They are almost always detected in childhood.

2 Acquired tumours and tumour-like lesions. These arise from fully differentiated ciliary epithelium and typically appear in adults.

Medulloepitheliomata

1 Benign medulloepitheliomata vary from tiny excrescences on the ciliary surface to large masses which have replaced most of the anterior segment of the globe and induced cataract, glaucoma and retinal detachment. Sometimes there is an associated defect of the neuroepithelial layers which allows the tumour to spread into the uvea. Occasionally the growth spreads as a flat white sheet over the pars plana, ciliary processes, zonular fibres, iris and posterior corneal surface.

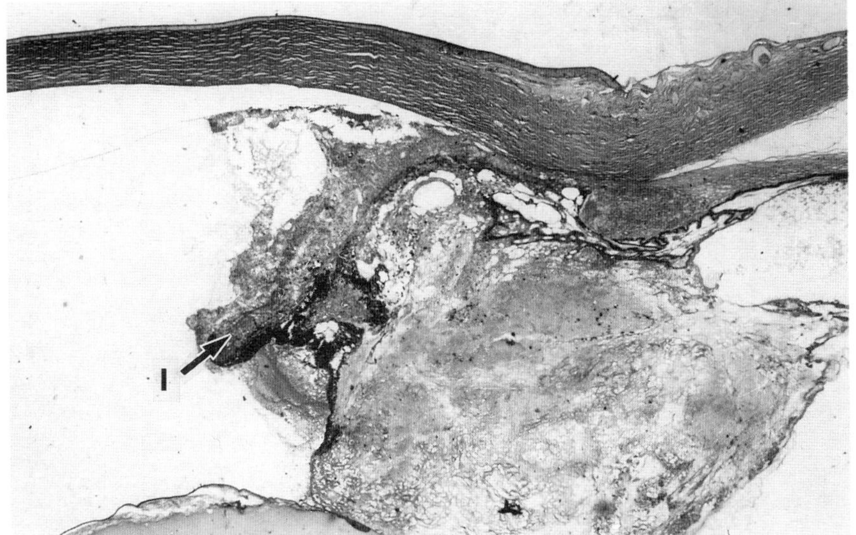

Fig. 11.14 Malignant medulloepithelioma. (a) Low power showing large mass of largely necrotic tumour arising from ciliary body and spreading into anterior chamber through iris (I).

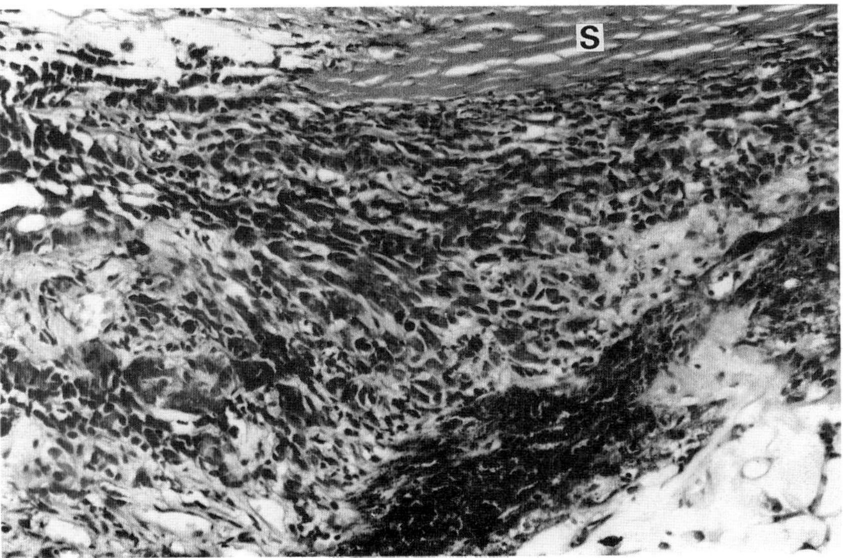

Fig. 11.14 (b) Higher power of tumour in region of trabecular meshwork (S = sclera). Note pleomorphic and hyperchromatic character of tumour cells. H & E (×190).

Typically, much of the tumour consists of multilayered membranes and cords of medullary epithelium which often bear a striking resemblance to embryonic retina and ciliary epithelium. From one surface of the neoplastic cords and membranes, protoplasmic extensions of the cells project into the slightly fibrillary myxoid stroma of the tumour. This stroma is rich in hyaluronic acid and its relationship to the tumour cells is reminscent of the relationship of the vitreous to the ciliary epithelium and retina in the embryonic eye. A definite limiting membrane corresponding to the external limiting membrane is often visible on the opposite surface of the neoplastic membranes. No glycosaminoglycan is demonstrable along this surface.

2 Malignant medulloepitheliomata are more aggressive and infiltrate the ciliary body, iris, sclera and cornea (Fig. 11.14). If the eye is retained long enough, they may penetrate the sclera, invade the orbit and brain and metastasise by the bloodstream. Microscopically the growth retains the characteristic tendency of medulloepithelioma to form cellular membranes and cords, but the consituent cells are larger and more mitotically active. In addition, there are areas of densely packed hyperchromatic cells resembling retinoblastomatous tissue. Although these cells do not usually undergo the necrosis and calcification characteristic of retinoblastoma, rosettes resembling Flexner–Wintersteiner rosettes may be formed.

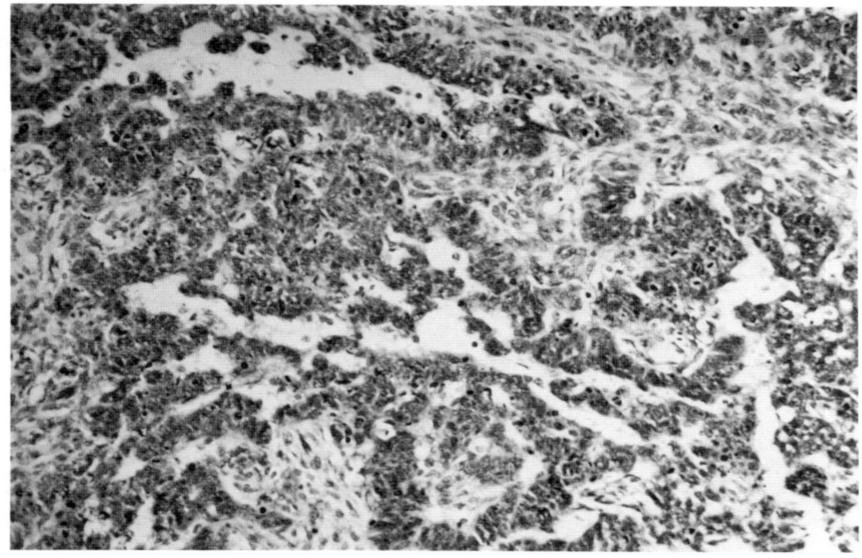

Fig. 11.15 Teratoid medulloepithelioma. (a) Epithelial component showing disorderly growth with a tendency to form crude tubular structures. H & E (×165).

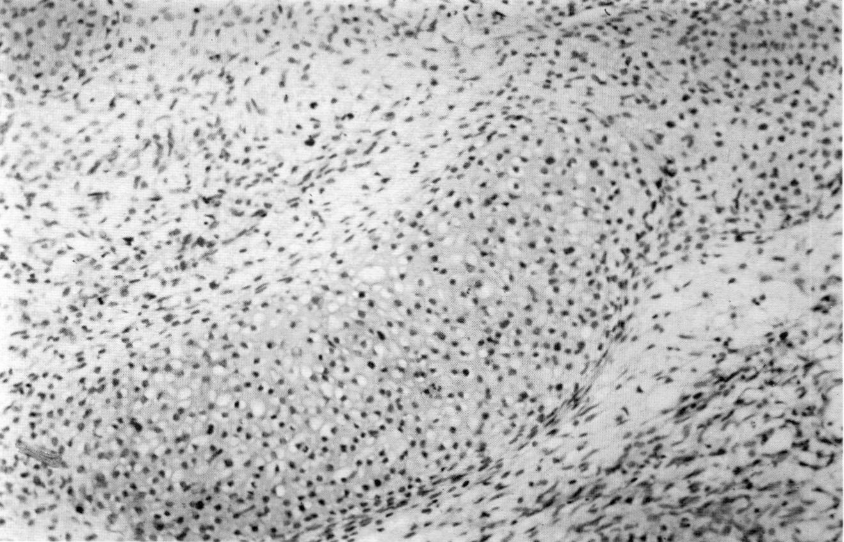

Fig. 11.15 (b) Heterotopic component of embryonic cartilage. H & E (×165). (Specimen by courtesy of Professor A. C. P. Campbell.)

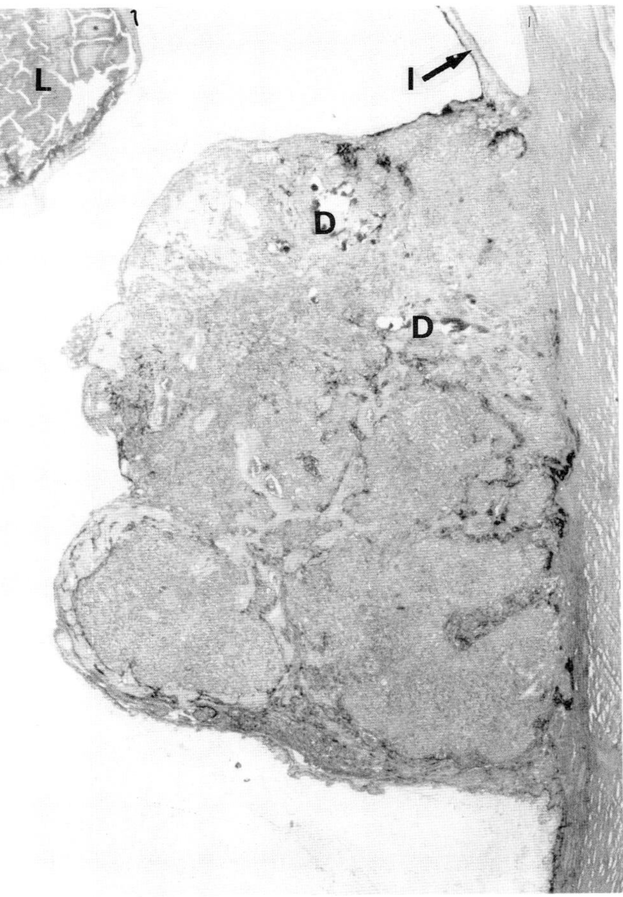

Fig. 11.16 Large ciliary nodule which was an incidental finding in a case of longstanding glaucoma. The case exemplifies the difficulty of distinguishing between hyperplasia and neoplasia in some ciliary lesions. (a) Low power. D = calcified drüsen which have tended to break out during sectioning, L = lens, I = iris. H & E (×21).

3 Teratoid medulloepithelioma is the name proposed for a group of medulloepitheliomata which, in addition to the sheets and cords of neuroepithelial cells common to all medulloepitheliomata, exhibit differentiation into brain tissue or contain elements such as cartilage and striated muscle not normally present in human eyes (Fig. 11.15). Benign and malignant variants are recognised by the same criteria which are applicable to the more simply constituted medulloepitheliomata.

The term diktyoma, widely used for the three types of neoplasm described above, refers to the net-like pattern of interlacing cords of cells seen in the majority of medulloepitheliomata.

Acquired tumours and tumour-like lesions

1 Fuchs' adenoma is a nodular hyperplasia of the ciliary epithelium occurring in adult eyes as a manifestation of ageing. The nodule, which is small and symptomless, is really an ampulla filled by strands of unpigmented ciliary epithelium and an eosinophilic secretion of the cells which is rich in hyaluronic acid.

2 Reactive hyperplasia typically occurs in response to low grade inflammation. There may be a history of past injury to the eye. The lesion, which is often ovoid in shape, may grow large enough to become visible ophthalmoscopically and press upon the lens causing cataract. Distinction between these formations and true adenomata is sometimes difficult, but evidence of injury and inflammation , the production of abundant basement membrane substance by the epithelial cells and the participation of both the unpigmented and pigmented epithelium indicate hyperplasia rather than adenoma (Fig. 11.16).

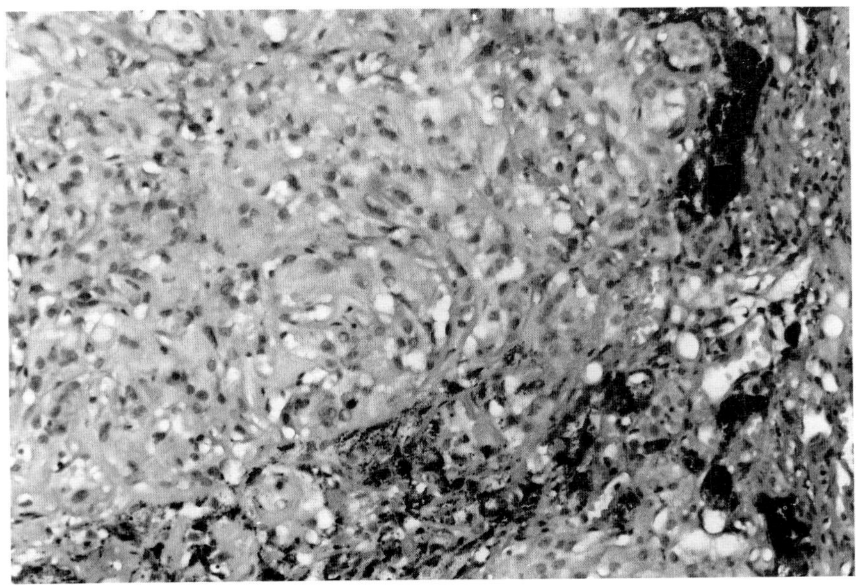

Fig. 11.16 (b) Showing disorderly proliferation of large poorly defined non-pigmented cells and rather fewer pigmented cells. H & E (×165).

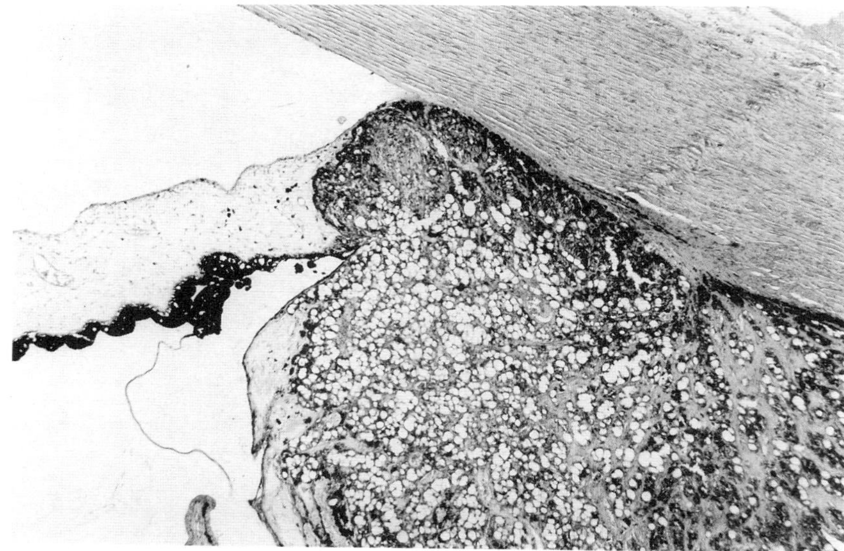

Fig. 11.17 Pigmented ciliary adenoma. (a) Low power showing tumour invading iris root and trabecular meshwork. The extensive vacuolation gives the tumour a laciform appearance.

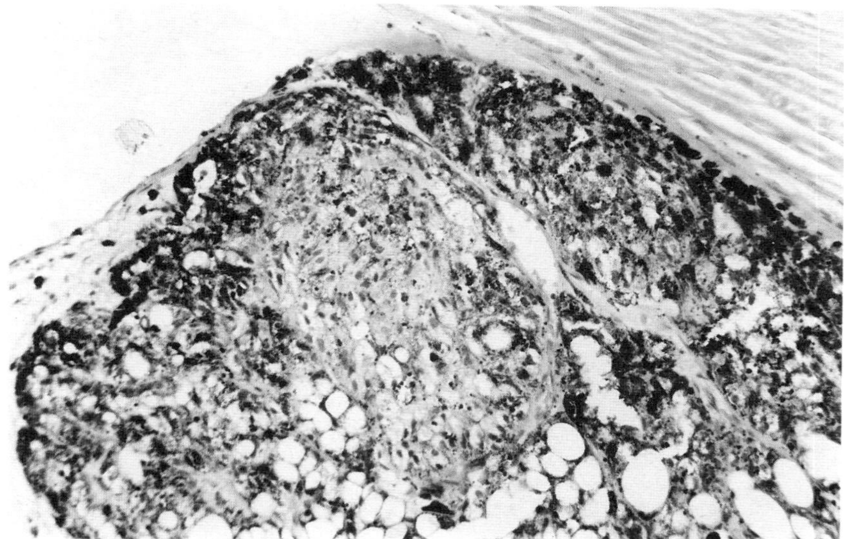

Fig. 11.17 (b) Showing melanin-laden cells and prominent vacuolation. H & E (×160).

3 Adenomata (benign epitheliomata) almost always occur in adults. Deterioration of vision and the presence of an enlarging mass arising from the ciliary body are the commonest presenting manifestations.

Microscopically, adenomata are composed of cuboidal and columnar cells in solid masses, membranes, tubules and papillae, but there are no formations resembling embryonic ciliary epithelium or retina. Pigmented and unpigmented variants occur. Stroma is usually minimal in amount and sometimes contains hyaluronic acid. The pigmented variety may show a characteristic vacuolated structure (Fig. 11.17). Though the vacuoles give the apppearance of being intracellular, electron microscopy has shown them to be intercellular (Streeten & McGraw, 1972).

4 Adenocarcinomata (or malignant epitheliomata) are very rare neoplasms of the ciliary epithelium in adults (Fig. 11.18) which occasionally show anaplasia, marked mitotic activity and invasiveness. Most are only locally invasive and metastasis beyond the globe is almost unknown.

BIBLIOGRAPHY

Retinoblastoma

General

Boniuk, M., ed. (1964) *Ocular and Adnexal Tumours*, Section II. C. V. Mosby Co., St Louis,

Jakobiec, F. A., ed. (1978) *Ocular and Adnexal Tumours*, Section II. Aesculapius Publishing Co., Birmingham, Ala.

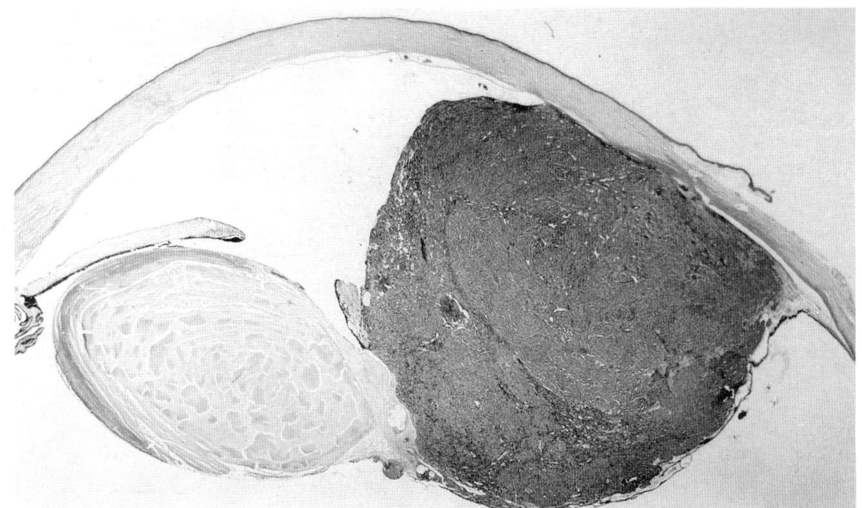

Fig. 11.18 Ciliary adenocarcinoma which had been present for 6 years in a female of 58. H & E (×160). (a) Low power showing how tumour expanded iris, displaced lens and occupied part of the anterior chamber. The growth remains relatively well circumscribed.

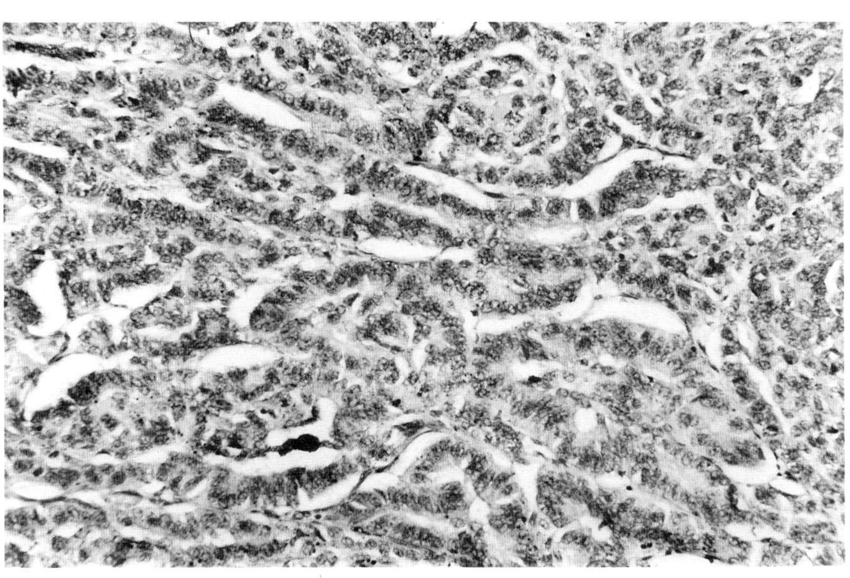

Fig. 11.18 (b) Higher power showing adenocarcinomatous appearance of the tumour. H & E (×160). (Specimen by courtesy of Dr M. Filipic.)

Lennox, E. L., Draper, G. J. & Sanders, B.M. (1975) Retinoblastoma: a study of natural history and prognosis of 268 cases. *British Medical Journal* **3**, 731–734.

Reese, A. B. (1976) *Tumours of the Eye*, 3rd Edn, pp 89–132. Harper & Row, New York.

Smith, J. L. S. & Bedford, M. A. (1974) In *Recent Results in Cancer Research*, eds H. B. Marsden & J. K. Steward, vol. 13. Springer-Verlag, Berlin.

Genetic aspects

Abramson, D. H. (1983) Retinoma, retinocytoma, and the retinoblastoma gene. *Archives of Ophthalmology* **101**, 1517–1518.

Gallie, B. L. & Phillips, R. A. (1984) Retinoblastoma: a model of oncogenesis. *Ophthalmology* **91**, 666–672.

Microscopical, histochemical and immunochemical topics

Donoso, L. A., Rorke, L. B., Shields, J. A., Augsburger, J. J., Browstein, S. & Lahoud, S. (1987) S-antigen immunoreactivity in trilateral retinoblastoma. *American Journal of Ophthalmology* **103**, 57–62.

Lin, C. C. L. & Tso, M. O. M. (1983) An electron microscopic study of calcification of retinoblastoma. *American Journal of Ophthalmology* **96**, 765–774.

Messmer, E. P., Font, R. L., Kirkpatrick, J. B. & Hoepping, W. (1985) Immunohistochemical demonstration of neuronal and astrocytic differentiation in retinoblastoma. *Ophthalmology* **92**, 167–173.

Mullaney, J. (1969) Retinoblastomas with DNA precipitation. *Archives of Ophthalmology* **82**, 454–456.

Perentes, E., Herbort, C. P., Rubenstein, L. J., Herman, M. M., Uffer, S., Donoso, L. A. & Collins, V. P. (1987) Immunohistochemical characterization of human retinoblastomas *in situ* with multiple markers. *American Journal of Ophthalmology* **103**, 647–658.

Radnot, M. (1975) Synaptic lamellae in retinoblastoma. *American Journal of Ophthalmology* **79**, 393–404.

Rodrigues, M. M., Wilson, M. E., Wiggert, B., Krishna, G. & Chader, G. J. (1986) Retinoblastoma. A clinical, immunohistochemical and electron microscopic case report. *Ophthalmology* **93**, 1010–1015.

Rootman, J., Hofbauer, J., Ellsworth, R. M. & Kitchen, D. (1976) Invasion of the optic nerve by retinoblastoma: a clinicopathological study. *Canadian Journal of Ophthalmology* **11**, 106–114.

Sang, D. N. & Albert, D. M. (1982) Retinoblastoma: clinical and histopathologic features. *Human Pathology* **13**, 133–147.

Stowe, III, G. C., Zakov, Z. N., Albert, D. M., Smith, T. R., Sang, D. N. & Craft, J. L. (1979) Vascular basophilia in ocular and orbital tumours. *Investigative Ophthalmology and Visual Science* **18**, 1068–1075.

Tso, M. O. M., Zimmerman, L. E. & Fine, B. S. (1970a) The nature of retinoblastoma. I. photoreceptor differentiation: a clinical and histopathologic study. *American Journal of Ophthalmology* **69**, 339–348.

Tso, M. O. M., Zimmerman, L. E. & Fine, B. S. (1970b) The nature of retinoblastoma. II. photoreceptor differentiation: an electron microscopic study. *American Journal of Opthalmology* **69**, 350–359.

Tso, M. O. M., Zimmerman, L. E. Fine, B. S. & Ellsworth, R. M. (1970c) A cause of radioresistance in retinoblastoma: photoreceptor differentiation. *Transactions of the American Academy of Ophthalmology and Otolaryngology* **74**, 959–989.

Spontaneous arrest or regression

Aaby, A. A., Price, R. L. & Zakov, Z. N. (1983) Spontaneously regressing retinoblastomas, retinoma, or retinoblastoma group 0. *American Journal of Ophthalmology* **96**, 315–320.

Andersen, S. R. & Jensen, O. A. (1974) Retinoblastoma with necrosis of central retinal artery and vein and partial spontaneous regression. *Acta Ophthalmologica* **52**, 183–193.

Boniuk, M. & Zimmerman, L. E. (1962) Spontaneous regression of retinoblastoma. *International Ophthalmology Clinics* **2**, 525–542.

Gallie, B. L., Phillips, R. A., Ellsworth, R. M. & Abramson, D. H. (1982) Significance of retinoma and phthisi bulbi for retinoblastoma. *Ophthalmology* **89**, 1392–1399.

Khodadoust, A. A., Rootzitalab, H. M. & Green, W. R. (1977) Spontaneous regression of retinoblastoma. *Survey of Ophthalmology* **21**, 467–478.

Margot, C., Hidayat, A., Kopelman, J. & Zimmerman, L. E. (1983) Retinocytoma. A benign variant of retinoblastoma. *Archives of Ophthalmology* **101**, 1519–1531.

Sanborn, G. E., Augsburger, J. J. & Shields, J. A. (1981) Spontaneous regression of bilateral retinoblastoma. *British Journal of Ophthalmology* **66**, 685–690.

Smith, J. L. S. (1974) Histology and spontaneous regression of retinoblastoma. *Transactions of the Ophthalmological Societies of the UK* **94**, 953–967.

Steward, J. K., Smith, J. L. S. & Arnold, E. L. (1956) Spontaneous regression of retinoblastoma. *British Journal of Ophthalmology* **40**, 449–461.

Second malignancies

Abramson, D. H., Ellsworth, R. M. & Kitchin, D. F. (1980) Osteogenic sarcoma of the humerus after cobalt plaque treatment for retinoblastoma. *American Journal of Ophthalmology* **90**, 374–376.

Abramson, D. H., Ellsworth, R. M. & Zimmerman, L. E. (1975) Nonocular cancer in retinoblastoma survivors. *Transactions of the American Academy of Ophthalmology and Otolaryngology* **81**, OP 454–457.

Abramson, D. H., Ronner, H. J. & Ellsworth, R. M. (1979) Second tumours in nonirradiated bilateral retinoblastoma. *American Journal of Ophthalmology* **87**, 624–627.

Tumours of the pars ciliaris retinae

Andersen, S. R. (1962) Medulloepithelioma of the retina. *International Ophthalmology Clinics* **2**, 483–506.

Brownstein, S., Barsoum-Homsy, M., Conway, V. H., Sales, S. & Condon, G. (1984) Nonteratoid medulloepithelioma of the ciliary body. *Ophthalmology,* **91**, 1118–1122.

Shields, J. A., Augsburger, J. J., Wallar, P. H. & Shah, H. G. (1983) Adenoma of the nonpigmented epithelium of the ciliary body. *Ophthalmology* **90**, 1528–1530.

Streeten, B. W. & McGraw, J. L. (1972) Tumour of the ciliary pigment epithelium. *American Journal of Ophthalmology* **74**, 420–429.

Zimmerman, L. E. (1970) The remarkable polymorphism of tumours of the ciliary epithelium. *Transactions of the Australian College of Ophthalmologists* **2**, 114–125.

Zimmerman, L. E. (1971) Verhoeff's 'Teratoneuroma': a critical reappraisal in the light of new observations and current concepts of embryonic tumours. *Transactions of the American Ophthalmological Society* **69**, 210–236.

Chapter 12 Glaucoma

THE AQUEOUS OUTFLOW PATHWAY

Drainage of aqueous takes place through two pathways:
1 The major 'conventional' pathway is through the trabecular meshwork into the canal of Schlemm.
2 The accessory drainage routes include uveoscleral drainage, transcorneal flux and diffusion along iris vessels and through the vitreous. These do not make a significant contribution to aqeous outflow.

The trabecular meshwork is wedge shaped in profile. The tip of the wedge is continuous with Desçemet's membrane and the base straddles the scleral spur which divides it into the corneoscleral and uveal portions (Fig. 12.1).

The trabeculae are flattened perforated sheets composed of collagen and elastic fibres coated with a basal lamina and covered by a layer of flattened endothelial cells which are capable of phagocytosing debris such as melanin granules and of migrating. Hydrophilic glycosaminoglycans (mucopolysaccharides) are present in the intertrabecular spaces of corneoscleral portion of the meshwork and are a potential cause of obstruction to outflow.

Schlemm's canal encircles the globe between the meshwork and the cornea. The trabecular wall of the canal is lined by spindly cells in which giant vacuoles may be present. Various types of particle, including red blood cells, are readily taken up in these vacuoles after introduction into the anterior chamber and it is thought they may play a significant role in the passage of aqueous across the endothelial barrier of Schlemm's canal. No permanent direct channels apparently exist between Schlemm's canal and the trabecular meshwork, but the giant vacuoles appear to undergo a cycle and occasionally a cell may be found with a vacuole opening both into the meshwork and the canal.

DEFINITION AND CLASSIFICATION OF GLAUCOMA

The term 'glaucoma' comprises a wide variety of disorders in which, as a result of obstruction to aqueous drainage from the anterior chamber, intraocular tension is raised to a level sufficient to damage various component tissues of the eye, especially the retina and optic nerve. The pathological changes thus fall into two categories:
1 Changes resulting directly in obstruction to the outflow of aqueous which are unique to each type of glaucoma.
2 Changes in component tissues of the eye which are similar whatever the cause of the glaucoma.

In many eyes with longstanding glaucoma which are

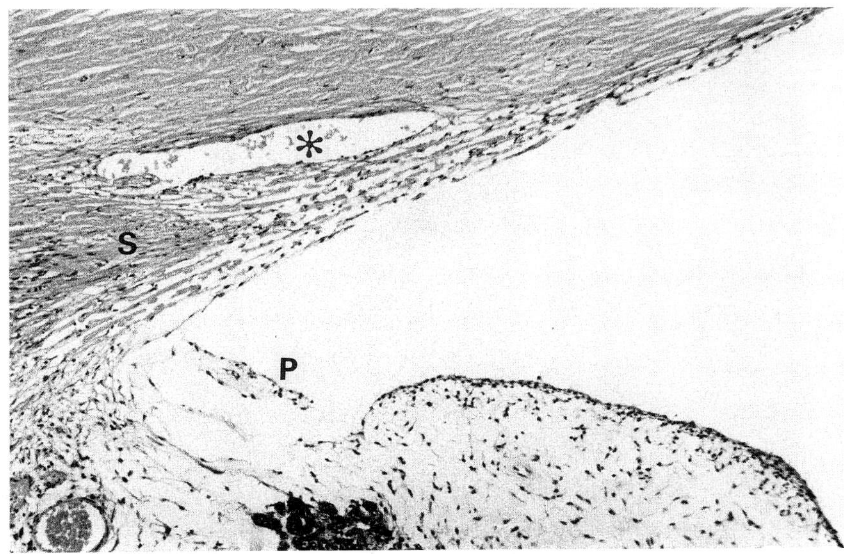

Fig. 12.1 Normal appearance of drainage angle and trabecular meshwork. Asterisk is in the canal of Schlemm. S = scleral spur, P = strand of pectinate ligament. H & E (×94).

removed because they have become blind and painful, the secondary changes dominate the pathological picture and it may be difficult to identify the primary pathology.

Glaucoma is conveniently classified according to the nature of the process resulting in obstruction to aqueous outflow:

1 Primary angle closure glaucoma.
2 Primary open angle glaucoma.
3 Congenital glaucoma.
4 Secondary glaucoma:
   (i) Closed angle.
   (ii) Open angle.
   (iii) Pupillary block.
   (iv) Due to intraocular tumours.

Primary angle closure glaucoma

Eyes predisposed to angle closure glaucoma characteristically have a shallow anterior chamber and narrow filtration angle. These result from a combination of several anatomical factors:

1 The lens is axially thicker and more anteriorly placed than normal.
2 The corneal diameter is small.
3 The angle is asymmetric, being narrower superiorly.
4 The axial length of the scleral envelope is shorter than normal.

In such eyes, contact between lens and iris tends to be excessive and may result in pupillary block. Aqueous backup behind the iris will then tend to push it forwards and so close the already narrow angle. Progressive growth of the lens with increasing age or swelling of a cataractous lens increases the likelihood of angle closure. Another possible operative factor is misdirection of aqueous posteriorly into the vitreous cavity pushing the lens forwards.

During the attack, the filtration angle is closed by contact between the swollen peripheral iris and the inner face of the trabecular meshwork. In the early stages this is reversible, but, after repeated attacks, irido-trabecular adhesions close the angle permanently, the trabecular meshwork becomes fibrotic and Schlemm's canal is compressed and eventually obliterated (Fig. 12.2).

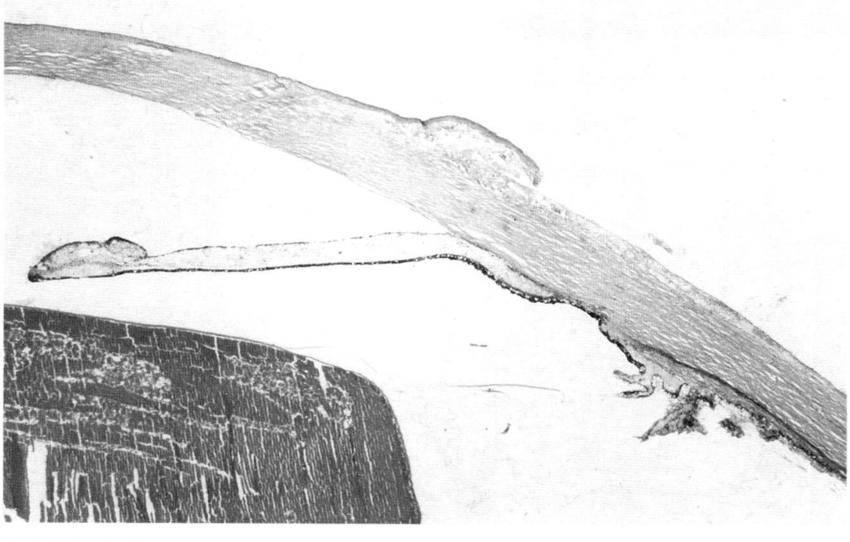

Fig. 12.2 Angle-closure glaucoma. (a) Anterior segment. Root of iris covers trabecular meshwork and no canal of Schlemm is seen. The iris and ciliary body are atrophic. H & E (×20).

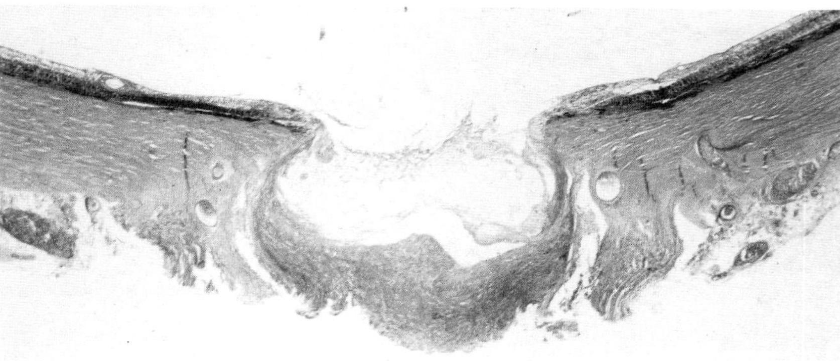

Fig. 12.2 (b) Posterior segment to show associated cupping of optic nerve head. H & E (×20).

Primary open angle glaucoma (chronic simple glaucoma)

This type of glaucoma is bilateral, although the onset is not necessarily synchronous in the two eyes. Onset is normally in middle age or later. The condition has a familial incidence and the patients' relatives have a higher raised intraocular tension and respond positively to steroids or to the 'water-drinking test' more frequently than the general population.

Simple glaucoma is characterised by an increased resistance to aqueous outflow, but the primary pathological changes responsible for the increase remain to be identified. This is because much of the material available for study is unsatisfactory. Trabeculectomy specimens sample only a tiny sector of the outflow apparatus and often inevitably show changes due to trauma. Eyes obtained at post-mortem have usually been affected for many years, while those enucleated for intractable pain may have superimposed neovascular changes. The changes observed in routine H & E sections are unimpressive (Fig. 12.3). With more refined methods, the changes observed in the outflow apparatus include:

1 Thickening of the trabecular cores with degeneration of regular collagen and elastic fibrils and increased deposition of 'curly' collagen.

2 Deposition of what appear to be 'plaques' of amorphous material in the extracellular spaces. Some of these plaques are actually sheaths of elastic-like tissue around the trabeculae.

3 Compaction of the uveal meshwork, hyalinization and atrophy of the adjacent ciliary muscle and atrophy of the root of the iris leading to an exaggerated scleral spur.

4 Narrowing of Schlemm's canal.

5 Depletion of the endothelial cell population of the trabecular meshwork.

The structural changes may be the result of the sustained raised intraocular tension rather than the cause. Similar, but usually less marked changes are seen in ageing eyes.

The possibility that depletion of the trabecular cell population might be of primary importance has attracted recent interest. It is likely that these cells, like those of the corneal endothelium, have little, if any, capacity to replace loss from any cause. Chronic simple glaucoma could thus be regarded as a congenital deficit in these cells which is not manifest until depletion through age reaches a critical level (Alvarado *et al.*, 1984; see also Grierson, 1987).

Congenital glaucoma

There are two main categories of congenital glaucoma:

1 Primary (infantile) glaucoma.

2 Secondary.

Primary congenital glaucoma

Congenital glaucoma is usually inherited as an autosomal recessive and affects boys more often than girls. In 70% of cases, both eyes are affected.

Incomplete separation of iris and trabecular tissue produces the microscopic appearance of anterior insertion of the iris on the trabecular meshwork. The angle recess and ciliary processes are displaced anteriorly and the longitudinal fibres of the ciliary muscle insert directly onto the trabeculae instead of the scleral spur which is poorly developed. The appearance thus closely resembles that of a normal infantile angle (Fig. 12.4).

The presence of a mesodermal membrane (Barkan's membrane) or congenital absence of Schlemm's canal

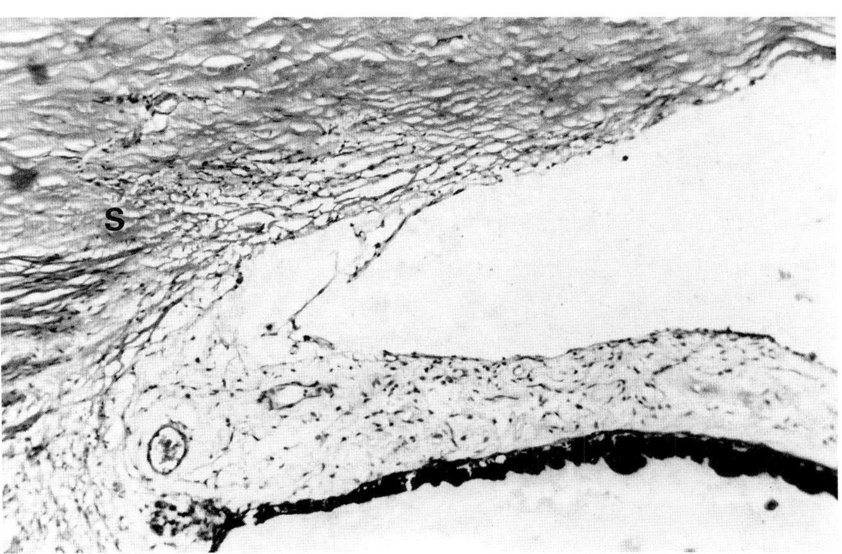

Fig. 12.3 Chronic simple glaucoma. The drainage angle is open. The trabeculae appear somewhat irregular at the magnification and no canal of Schlemm is present. S = scleral spur. H & E (×41).

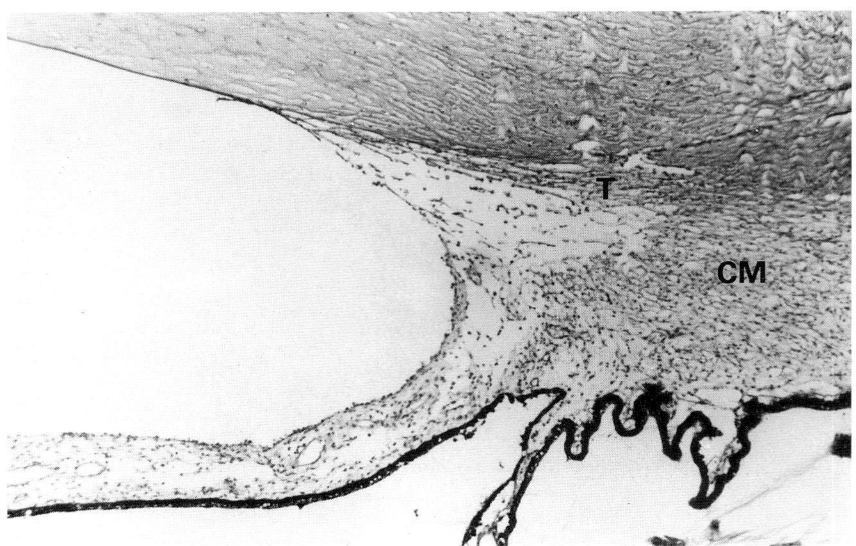

Fig. 12.4 Congenital glaucoma. Infant aged 8 days with probable Kniest's dysplasia which has 'bulging eyes'. There is no scleral spur and the scleral trabeculae (T) appear to insert into ciliary muscle (CM). Note how far forwards the circumferential fibres of the ciliary muscle appear to be situated. PAS/tartrazine (×63).

have not been established as regular causes of congenital glaucoma.

Secondary congenital glaucoma

Secondary congenital glaucoma may occur:
1 As a result of rubella in pregnancy.
2 As a complication of neurofibromatosis, the Sturge–Weber syndrome (Chapter 15), aniridia, retrolental fibroplasia, persistent hyperplastic primary vitreous and dysgenesis involving the anterior segment of the globe such as occurs in Rieger's and Peter's anomalies (Chapter 17).

Secondary glaucoma

Mechanical obstruction to aqueous outflow occurs as a complication of many intraocular inflammatory, traumatic, vascular and neoplastic conditions. Secondary glaucoma is, therefore, commonly unilateral.

Secondary angle closure glaucoma

Synechiae

Secondary glaucoma due to the formation of adhesions between the iris root and the trabecular meshwork may complicate any condition in which inflammatory exudate or blood, even in small amounts, organises in angles already narrowed or closed by such conditions as post-operative or post-traumatic flattening of the anterior chamber, oedematous or inflammatory swelling of the iris or ciliary body or the pressure of a posterior intraocular tumour. Peripheral adhesions may also develop as a result of delayed post-operative reformation of the anterior chamber due to iris prolapse, incarceration of the lens capsule or fistularisation.

In iritis, annular adhesions sometimes form between the iris and the lens, obstructing the flow of aqueous from the posterior chamber. The iris is ballooned forwards by aqueous trapped behind it (iris bombé) and the consequent apposition with the trabecular meshwork leads to the formation of adhesions which permanently block the angle (Fig. 12.5). Iris bombé is also often seen in eyes with old retinal detachments in which there is commonly low-grade inflammation in the anterior segment.

Neovascularisation of the iris

Neovascularisation of the iris with occlusion of the angle by fibrovascular adhesions causes intractable glaucoma which results in a painful blind eye. Such eyes frequently require enucleation. Neovascular glaucoma is indeed one of the most common reasons for therapeutic enucleation.

The proliferation of new vessels on the iris is invariably secondary to numerous other ocular or systemic diseases of which the most important are:
1 Occlusion of central retinal vein.
2 Diabetes mellitus.
3 Glaucoma, especially primary open angle.
4 Uveitis.
5 Trauma.
6 Tumours, especially retinoblastoma.

Thrombotic glaucoma: most eyes enucleated with 'end-stage' neovascular glaucoma are the late result of thrombotic occlusion of the central retinal vein; hence the term 'thrombotic' or, more strictly, 'post-thrombotic'

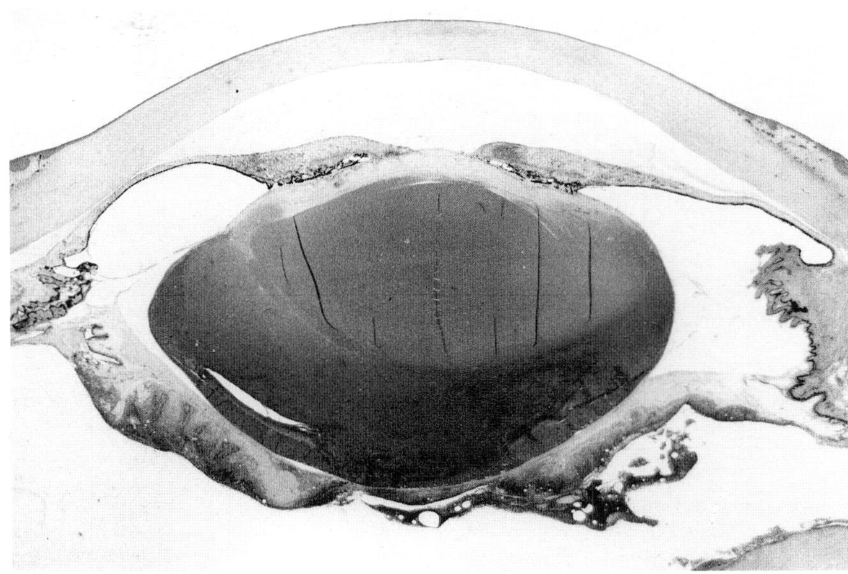

Fig. 12.5 Iris bombé. The pupillary border of the iris is tightly bound to the anterior surface of the lens. The pale area is hyaline fibrous tissue deep to the lens capsule anteriorly. Detached retina is adherent to the posterior surface of the lens. H & E.

glaucoma. Both diabetes and raised intraocular tension also increase the incidence of thrombotic occlusion of the central vein. Following the venons occlusion, about 20% of cases show evidence of raised intraocular tension and neovascularisation of the iris within 3 months (see Chapter 10, Part 2).

Growth of the new vessels on the iris begins separately at the pupil and at the periphery by endothelial budding from capillaries or venules in the iris. As growth progresses, the two areas coalesce and fibrous tissue including a myofibroblastic component is laid down. This eventually contracts to cause ectropion of the pupil. Sometimes new vessels extend across the pupil and form pupillary membranes. At the periphery, an extension of Desçemet's membrane may be laid down over the false angle and fibrovascular layer on the anterior surface of the iris (see Fig. 10.26b).

The precise pathogenetic mechanism has not been established. In many of the conditions in which neovascularisation occurs, retinal circulation is impaired and a widely held theory is that hypoxic retina releases an angiogenic factor which diffuses forwards to stimulate the growth of new vessels on the iris (Chapter 10, Part 2).

The iridocorneal endothelial (ICE) syndrome

This term has been used to embrace the iris naevus syndrome, Chandler's syndrome and essential iris atrophy. The syndrome affects predominantly young to middle-aged females and is a cause of unilateral glaucoma.

The common pathological features are anterior synechiae and extension of the corneal endothelium over the filtration angle and anterior surface of the iris to form an endothelial membrane. In Chandler's syndrome, corneal oedema is prominent due to dystrophic changes in the corneal endothelium and small anterior peripheral synechiae form in the angles. In essential iris atrophy, focal peripheral anterior synechiae appear early and atrophic holes result in the iris both at the site of the synechiae and in the contra-lateral mid-peripheral iris. In the iris naevus syndrome, a diffuse naevus covers the anterior surface of the iris. This is associated with anterior peripheral synechiae and eversion of the pupillary border.

Earlier reports that some endothelial cells might acquire epithelial characteristics as in posterior polymorphous dystrophy have not been confirmed (Rodrigues *et al.*, 1986).

The acronyms ICE and NUDE (iris *N*odules, *U*nilateral glaucoma and extension of *D*esçemet's membrane and the corneal *E*ndothelium) have been proposed for the syndrome (Eagle *et al.*, 1979; Spencer, 1979).

Secondary open angle glaucoma

Secondary glaucoma without the formation of anterior peripheral adhesions is less common than angle closure glaucoma. It may be due to blockage of the drainage channels by particulate matter or cells, or to structural changes in the outflow apparatus itself.

The pseudoexfoliation syndrome

The pseudoexfoliation syndrome is a disease of unknown pathogenesis which is often bilateral and frequently associated with open angle glaucoma or cataracts or both.

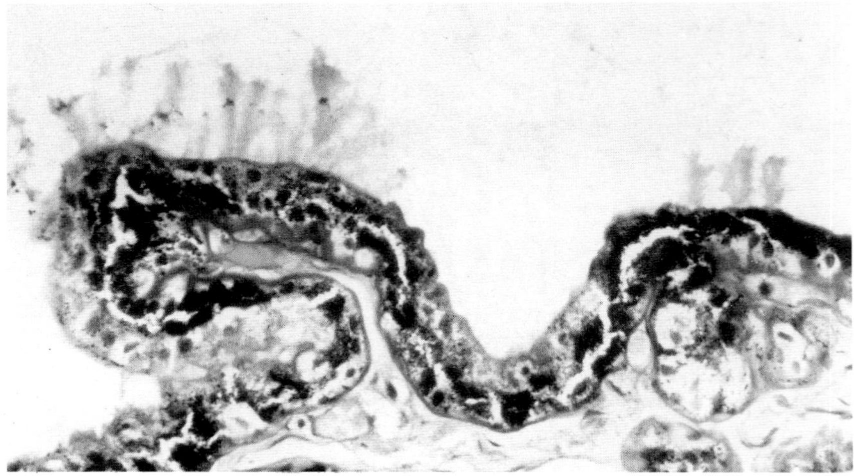

Fig. 12.6 Pseudoexfoliation. (a) Light microscopy showing tufts of the pseudoexfoliative material on ciliary processes. PAS/tartrazine (×320).

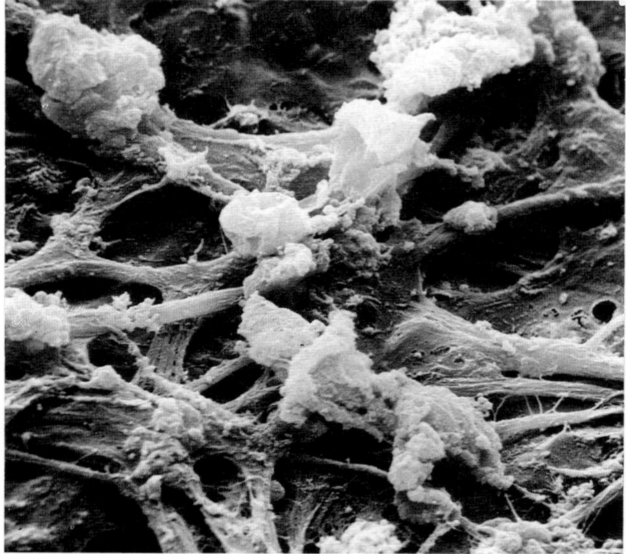

Fig. 12.6 (b) Scanning electron micrograph of material on trabecular meshwork. (×950). (Photograph by courtesy of Professor G. W. Crock.)

While originally thought to be relatively uncommon outside Scandinavia, more recent surveys have shown it to have a world-wide distribution and to affect all races. The disease is commoner in men than in women and its incidence increases with age.

Clinically, characteristic deposits of grey, fluffy, 'dandruff-like' material are seen on the anterior lens surface in an area corresponding to the smallest pupillary diameter and in a peripheral pre-equatorial band.

Microscopically, the deposits appear as finely granular, faintly eosinophilic, weakly PAS-positive tufts which are widely distributed on the anterior and posterior surfaces of the lens, the suspensory ligaments, the ciliary processes (Fig. 12.6a) and the anterior face of the vitreous. By electron microscopy they may also be demonstrated in the trabecular meshwork (Fig. 12.6b) and in pits on the anterior surface of the iris.

Ultrastructurally, the material has a fibrillary structure resembling amyloid, but does not give a positive reaction with Congo red. The fibres are 35–40 nm in width and show major cross-banding at 50 nm.

Histochemical and other evidence indicates than the material is a gel of proteoglycans, but its source remains obscure.

Glaucoma occurs in about 50% of patients affected with the pseudoexfoliation syndrome (glaucoma capsulare) and it seems probable that deposits in the trabecular meshwork are the cause, or, at least, an important contributory factor. It must also be noted that, due to an unexplained degeneration of the iris pigment epithelium, there are often heavy deposits of melanin in the filtration angle. The pigment granules are found within the trabecular meshwork and in macrophages lodged therein.

Phacolytic glaucoma

Phacolytic glaucoma is due to sudden blockage of aqueous outflow either by particulate lens matter released from a hypermature cataractous lens or by macrophages engorged with such material. There is, however, no allergic reaction to the lens matter. Phagocytosis of lens matter may also occur without causing glaucoma, but is then presumably a slower more gradual process.

Clinical features: persons over 70 years of age are commonly affected and the onset of the glaucoma is sudden and unilateral. The angle is open. There is an aqueous flare due to liquid lens protein and sometimes lens floccules and crystals may be seen in the anterior chamber, but neither keratic precipitates nor adhesions are formed. Removal of lens substance often gives prompt relief and some restoration of vision.

Microscopic appearances: these are conveniently segregated into five components:

1 The lens cortex is broken down into eosinophilic globules and liquefied. The nucleus is small and may be fissured. The lens substance may escape through ruptures in the capsule or exude through microscopic holes to appear in the anterior chamber as a weakly eosinophilic, finely granular precipitate. Capsular ruptures are usually posterior, but in about 20% of cases no rupture is found. In contrast to lens-induced endophthalmitis (Chapter 4), there is no invasion of the lens by polymorphs, and macrophages do not become adherent to the capsule.

2 Numerous large globular macrophages with abundant, finely granular cytoplasm are found around the lens and related anterior segment structures and may be observed crowding the filtration angle, intertrabecular spaces and even Schlemm's canal (Fig. 12.7a & b). Owing to an unexplained degeneration of the iris pigmented epithelium, there are often heavy deposits of melanin in the filtration angle, the pigment granules being found both within the trabecular meshwork and in macrophages lodged therein.

3 There is no inflammatory infiltration of the uvea and adhesions are not formed. The aqueous does not contain fibrinogen and does not, therefore, clot. The macrophages do not adhere to one another or to the cornea so that keratic precipitates are not formed.

4 Similar eosinophilic macrophages may be found on the retina and optic nerve head. In most cases, cupping of the nerve head is slight, presumably because the eye has been removed for acute glaucoma before this can develop.

5 In 25% of eyes enucleated for phacolytic glaucoma,

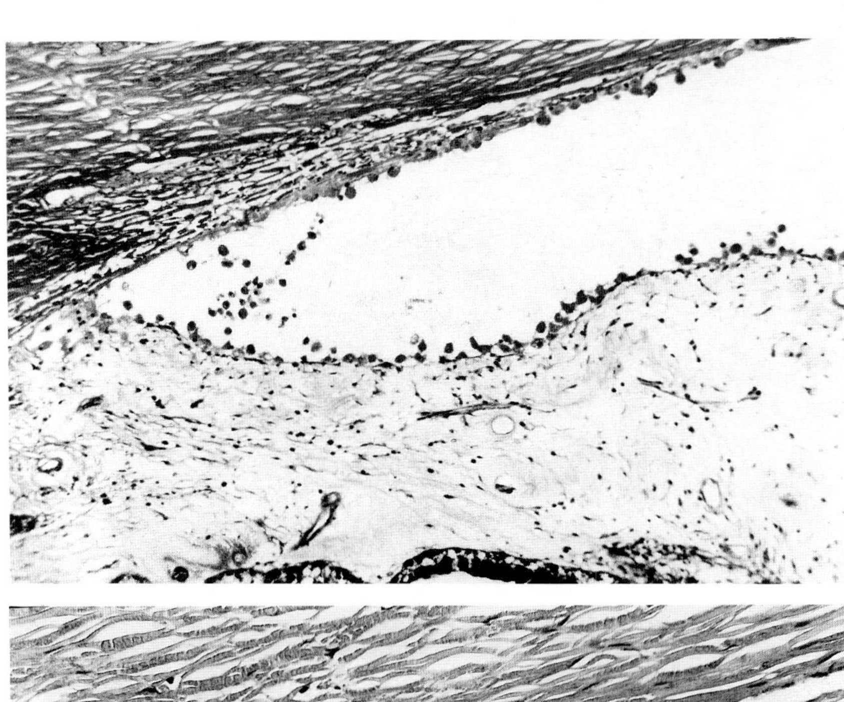

Fig. 12.7 Phacolytic glaucoma. (a) Angle showing macrophages lying free and on surface of iris and trabecular meshwork. H & E (×95).

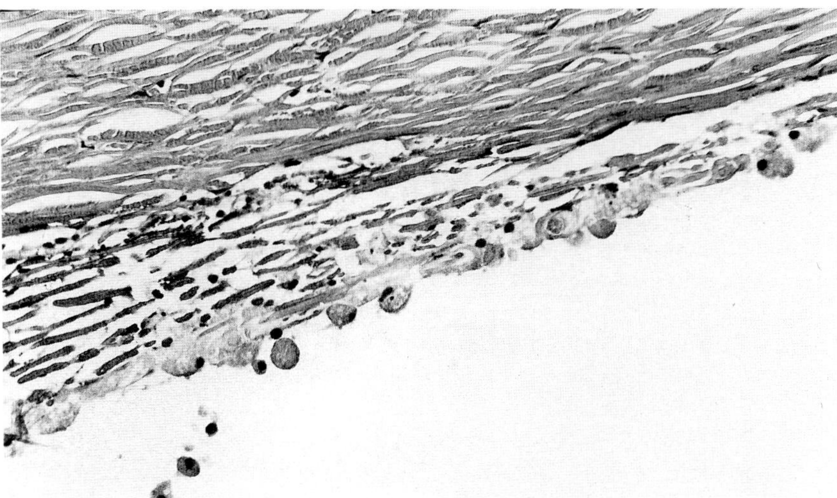

Fig. 12.7 (b) Detail of meshwork showing some insinuation of the macophages into the superficial pores. H & E (×260).

there is histological evidence of post-contusive angle cleavage, an injury known to be followed eventually by glaucoma (Smith & Zimmerman, 1965). In such cases, the lens-laden macrophages may simply precipitate the onset of glaucoma by completing blockage of an already partially incompetent outflow apparatus.

Finally, it may be noted that changes observed in eyes enucleated for phacolytic glaucoma may be minimal because most of the macrophages have left the anterior chamber by the time the eye is enucleated. Moreover, if the plane of section through the eye is horizontal, the residual macrophages may not be seen because they are concentrated in the drainage angle inferiorly.

Pigmentary dispersion syndrome

While deposition of pigment on the posterior aspect of the cornea and in the filtration angle may be observed as a degenerative phenomenon in senile or diseased globes (Fig. 12.8), the pigmentary dispersion syndrome typically affects males between the ages of 20 and 45. The affected eyes are myopic and have a deep anterior chamber. Clinically, transillumination defects due to atrophy of the pigmented epithelium are seen in the mid-peripheral iris. Heavy deposits of pigment are observed on the posterior aspect of the cornea in the form of the Krükenberg spindle and in the trabecular meshwork between the trabeculae and within the endothelial cells. About half of the cases develop glaucoma, but it is not clear whether this can be explained on the basis of simple mechanical obstruction of the outflow pathways or whether these are already functionally inadequate, and pigment deposition exacerbates the inadequacy.

Corticosteroid glaucoma

Information is scanty on the pathological basis of corticosteroid glaucoma. Substantial deposits of fibrillar material never seen in normal or glaucomatous eyes were demonstrated in the trabecular meshwork in two cases (Rohen *et al.*, 1973).

Membrane formation

Open angle glaucoma is occasionally due to the trabecular meshwork becoming covered by corneal epithelium invading the anterior chamber after operations or injuries which involve the cornea or limbus. In addition, after traumatic inflammation or iridocyclitis, a hyaline membrane may be laid down over the filtration angle and along the iris surface by proliferating corneal or trabecular endothelium. In some instances, the glaucoma is really of secondary angle closure type since the epithelium or membrane covers an angle already closed by adhesions occasioned by trauma or inflammation.

Traumatic cleavage of the chamber angle

In a small proportion of cases, contusion of the globe causes tears through the anterior ciliary muscles, rupture of the iris root and even disinsertion of the ciliary muscles from the scleral spur. As a result the iris root and ciliary processes are displaced backwards, the anterior chamber is laterally deepened and the filtration angle becomes deeper than normal. In the succeeding months or years the traumatised tissues atrophy and may disappear while the drainage of aqueous is gradually im-

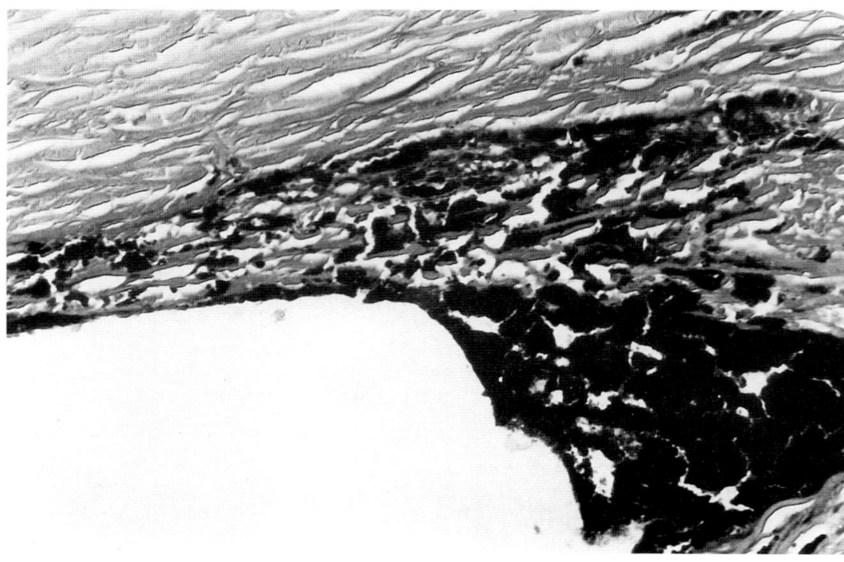

Fig. 12.8 Heavy deposit of pigment in angle and trabecular mesh-work. H & E (×320).

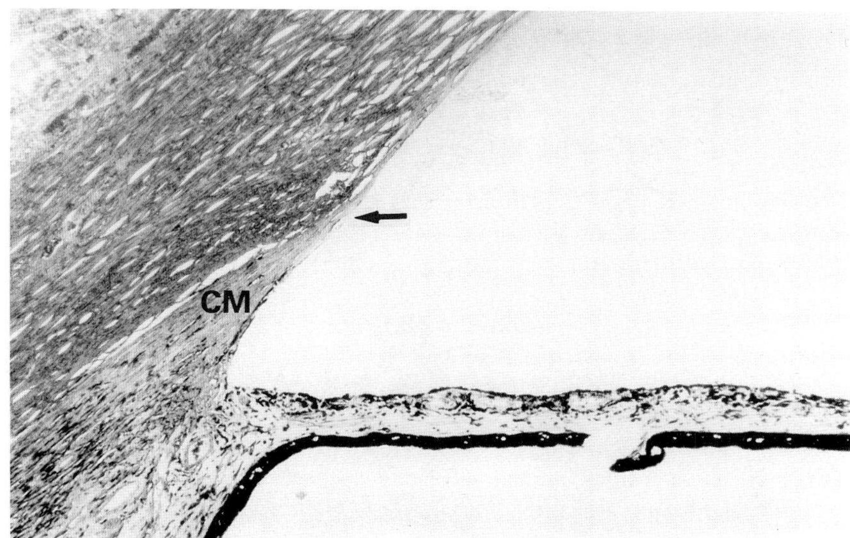

Fig. 12.9 Post-contusion angle deformity. Note the abnormally anterior location of the scleral spur with relation to the recessed angle. The trabecular meshwork can barely be identified and there is no canal of Sclemm. Masson trichrome (×160).

paired resulting eventually in glaucoma of insidious onset. Histological sections show a recessed and scarred open angle together with compaction of the trabecular meshwork which may be covered by an extension of the corneal endothelium and Desçemet's membrane as described below (Fig. 12.9).

Histological evidence of traumatic angle cleavage is seen in the majority of eyes with posterior dislocation of the lens, and the association with phacolytic glaucoma has already been noted.

Haemolytic glaucoma

Occasional cases of vitreous haemorrhage are complicated by glaucoma. The mechanism is thought to be obstruction of the trabecular meshwork by haemorrhagic debris and macrophages.

Siderosis

Late secondary open angle glaucoma sometimes complicates retained iron foreign bodies probably because deposition of iron salts in the trabecular meshwork leads to degeneration and sclerosis of the fibres.

Displacements of lens and vitreous

Dislocation or subluxation of the lens

Raised intraocular tension frequently complicates dislocation or subluxation of the lens whether this is due to developmental defects of the zonule as in Marfan's syndrome (Chapter 17) or weakening of the zonular fibres by stretching, inflammation or degeneration.

Anterior dislocation: in Marfan's syndrome, displacement is usually forwards, but incomplete so that the lens blocks the pupil. Dilatation of the pupil relieves the tension, a paradox also found in congenital spherophakia when the rounded, bulging anterior face of the lens obstructs aqueous outflow.

Trauma may displace the lens completely into the anterior chamber. In this position it blocks the pupil from the front so that continued aqueous secretion pushes the iris against the trabecular meshwork.

Posterior dislocation: glaucoma may also result from posterior dislocation of the lens, but its onset is often delayed for years. In many instances the cause is not the dislocation itself, but traumatic cleavage of the angle due to the contusive injury which displaced the lens.

Intumescence of the lens

Swelling of the lens during development of a cataract or as the result of a small capsular opening due to surgical or other trauma pushes the anterior part of the ciliary body and root of iris forwards. Concomitant oedema of the ciliary processes, probably due to circulatory embarrassment, displaces the lens itself forwards with resulting blockage of the pupil.

Pupillary blockage by vitreous

In aphakic eyes, synechiae may form between the pupil and anterior face of the vitreous. Aqueous then pools in the posterior chamber detaching the vitreous anteriorly or tracks behind a posteriorly detached vitreous to push it forwards into the pupil.

Intraocular tumours

Extensive invasion of of the aqueous drainage channels in the angle by neoplasms involving the iris root or ciliary body causes secondary glaucoma. Such neoplasms are:

1 Diffuse naevus.
2 Malignant melanoma (particularly ring melanoma of the iris root, see Chapter 8).
3 Juvenile xanthogranuloma.
4 Leukaemic deposits.

Melanomalytic glaucoma is due to obstruction of the outflow pathways by macrophages laden with pigment and necrotic debris derived from necrosis of anteriorly located melanomas.

Large, posteriorly located neoplasms associated with a massive serous retinal detachment may displace the lens–iris diaphragm forwards. This leads to adhesions between lens and iris, iris bombé and secondary peripheral anterior adhesions.

As already mentioned above, neovascularisation of the iris with consequent secondary glaucoma may occur in association with intraocular melanomata and retinoblastomata, particularly the latter. Such tumours possibly release tumour angiogenic factor.

THE HISTOLOGICAL SIGNS OF RAISED TENSION

Cornea

Intercellular and intracellular epithelial oedema are characteristic of glaucoma probably because of damage to the corneal endothelium by the raised intraocular tension. The epithelial cells appear bloated and stain weakly. Clear vesicles develop between the cells and in time watery bullae form between the epithelium and Bowman's membrane. A delicate connective tissue begins to spread from the periphery between Bowman's membrane and the epithelium (degenerative pannus). Eventually, this connective tissue segregates islands of epithelium and erodes through Bowman's membrane into the superficial stroma (Chapter 5). A thick fibrovascular layer containing numerous discrete hyaline granules may spread over most of the cornea.

Endothelial damage is also the probable cause of persistant stromal oedema following severe attacks of angle closure oedema which remain unrelieved for 24 hours or more.

Corneoscleral envelope

The adult corneoscleral envelope is resistant to stretching and rarely exhibits more than a moderate degree of thinning and expansion. Sustained high pressure causes ectasias (staphylomas) at points of weakness such as the equatorial exits of the vortex veins, limbal scars and the ciliary sclera in cyclitis. At the margins of such local ectasias, the sclera appears to taper off quite sharply.

In infants, the ocular coats are much more stretchable so that in the course of congenital glaucoma or secondary glaucoma in early life the globe may become enormously expanded in all directions (buphthalmos). During the process:

1 The anterior chamber becomes deep.
2 Desçemet's membrane ruptures allowing aqueous to enter the corneal stroma.
3 The zonule degenerates with consequent subluxation of the lens.
4 The uvea and retina are markedly stretched.

Lens

In acute glaucoma, focal accumulations of necrotic debris occur in the superficial cortex deep to areas of local damage to the capsular epithelium (glaukomflecken).

Uveal tract

Acute congestion of the iris root in severe glaucoma may so damage the blood supply to the iris that it undergoes segmental ischaemic necrosis. The iris stroma becomes rarified and the sphincter and dilator muscles atrophy while the iris pigment epithelium disintegrates releasing its pigment granules which are deposited on the lens and cornea and in the trabecular meshwork.

In chronic glaucoma, the ciliary muscles undergo progressive ischaemic atrophy and appear flat and fibrotic. The ciliary processes shrink and become fibrosed and hyalinised.

The choroid resists the effects of the pressure longer than other ocular structures, but in longstanding glaucoma appears attenuated, compressed and fibrotic.

Optic nerve

It has been noted (Chapter 13) that swelling of the optic nerve head may occur in acute glaucoma. In chronic glaucoma, the nerve fibres atrophy and the lamina cribrosa shows a variable degree of ectasia as exemplified in the case of angle closure glaucoma (Fig. 12.2b). Sometimes there is glial proliferation in the floor of the resulting cup. These changes are accompanied by thickening of the pial septa and replacement of the lost axons by proliferated astrocytes (Fig. 12.10a & b).

Occasionally, the disappearance of the axons is accompanied by degeneration of the glial cells so that the interseptal spaces of the anterior orbital part of the nerve

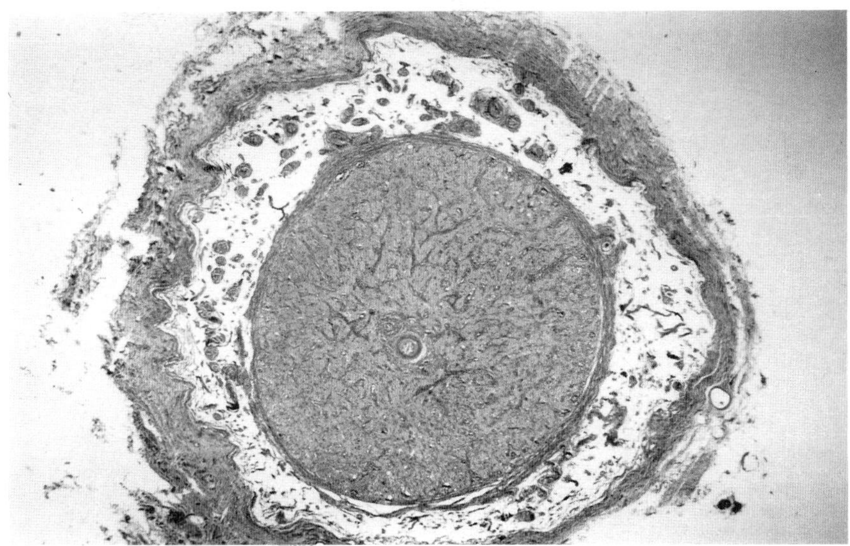

Fig. 12.10 Typical glaucomatous atrophy of optic nerve. (a) Low power showing wrinkling of dural sheath and wide pial space. H & E (×20).

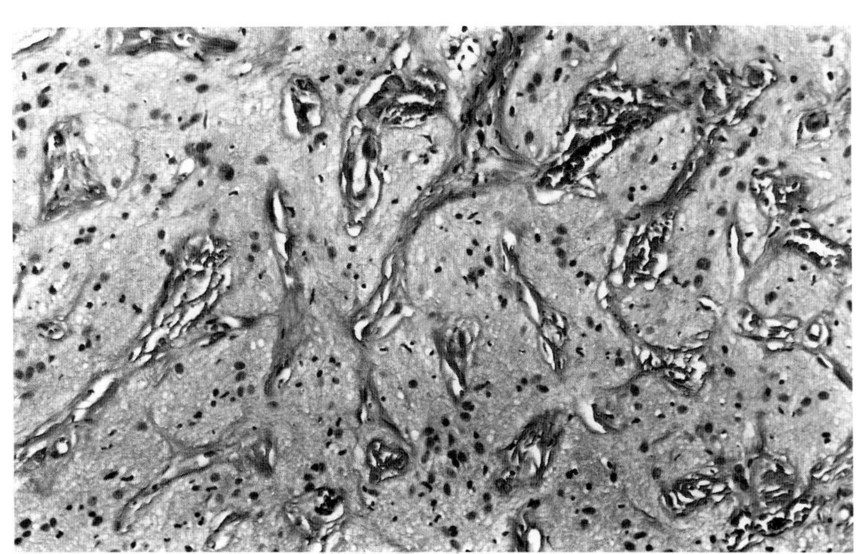

Fig. 12.10 (b) Higher power to show thickened fibrous septa with nerve fibres completely replaced by glial tissue. H & E (×160).

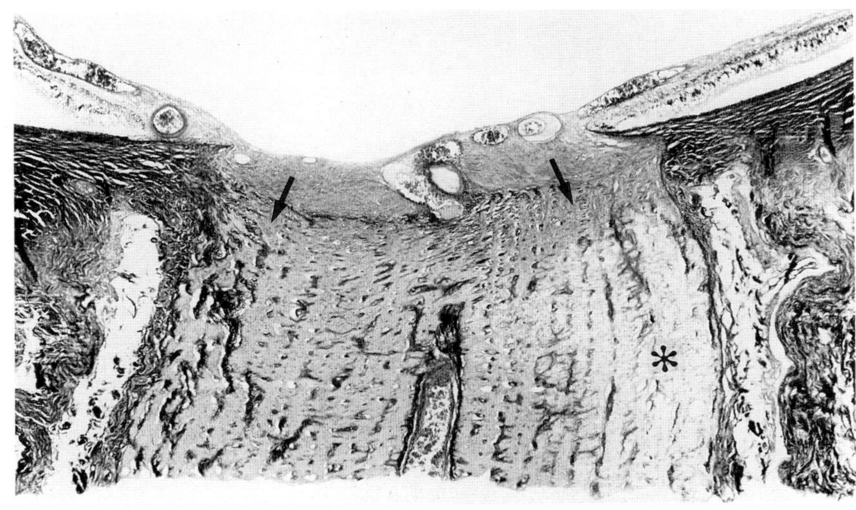

Fig. 12.11 Schnabel's type of cavernous atrophy. (a) Longitudinal section showing slight outward bowing of the lamina cribrosa (arrows). There does not appear to be much cupping but there is a layer glia anterior to the lamina. The cavernous atrophy (asterisk) affects the post-laminar part of the nerve. Masson trichrome.

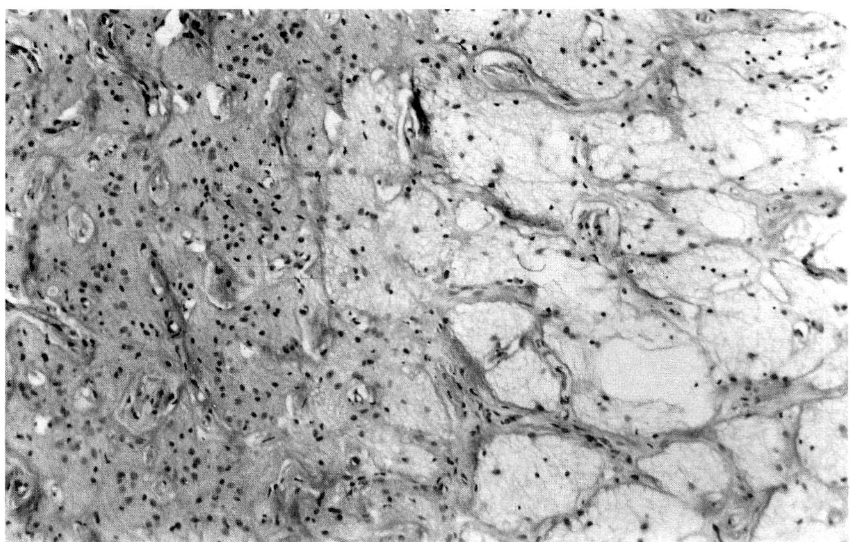

Fig. 12.11 (b) Transverse section of post-laminar portion of nerve showing adjacent areas of 'normal' and 'cavernous' atrophy. H & E (×94).

appear empty — cavernous (Schnabel's) atrophy (Fig. 12.11a & b). Staining by Alcian blue shows that the spaces contain hyaluronic acid which is thought to be derived from the vitreous. This type of damage can affect both pre- and post-laminar portions of the optic nerve and is thought to be a form of ischaemic infarction typically seen in acute glaucoma (Chapter 13).

The precise pathogenesis of the damage to the optic nerve in glaucoma is not clear at present. A widely accepted hypothesis is that the circulation of the nerve head is impaired by raised intraocular pressure and ischaemia destroys the axons and astroglia. However, distortion of the lamina cribrosa precedes visual loss and axonal damage could result from direct compression or compromise of the laminar capillaries. Moreover, a direct effect of pressure on axons and astroglia cannot be ruled out.

Retina

The loss of nerve fibres in the optic nerve is accompanied by loss of ganglion cells from the retina. This is most obvious in the fovea where the ganglion cells are most numerous (Fig. 12.12).

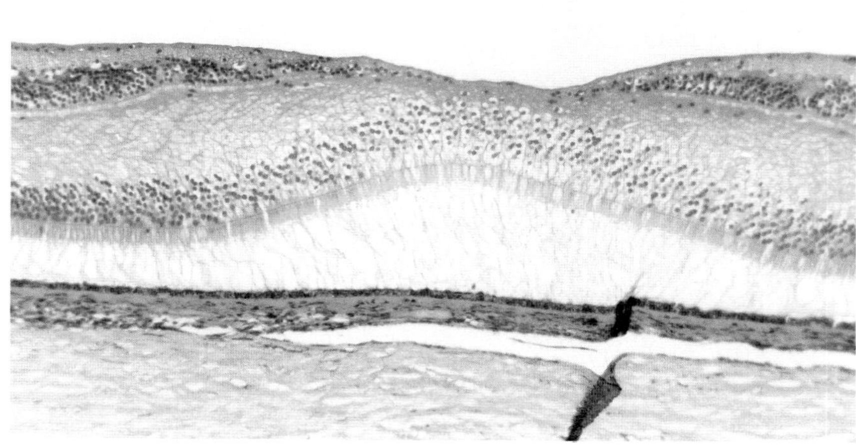

Fig. 12.12 Fovea in glaucoma showing complete loss of ganglion cells (cf. Fig. 10.1). H & E (×41).

BIBLIOGRAPHY

Structure and function

Anderson, D. R. (1977) The vascular supply of the optic disc. In *Scientific Foundations of Ophthalmology*, eds E. S. Perkins & D. W. Hill, pp 18–26. Heinemann, London.

McMenamin, P. G., Lee, W. R. & Aitken, D. A. N. (1986) Age-related changes in the human outflow apparatus. *Ophthalmology* **93**, 194–209.

Tripathi, R. C. (1971) Mechanism of aqueous outflow across the trabecular wall of Schlemm's canal. *Experimental Eye Research* **11**, 116–121.

Tripathi, R. C. (1977) The aqueous outflow pathways in vertebrate eyes. In *Scientific Foundations of Ophthalmology*, eds E. S. Perkins & D. W. Hill, pp 1–7. Heinemann, London.

General

Anderson, D. R. (1972) Pathology of the glaucomas. *British Journal of Ophthalmology* **56**, 146–157.

Open angle glaucoma

Alvarado, J., Murphy, C. & Juster, R. (1984) Trabecular meshwork cellularity in primary open-angle and non-glaucomatous normals. *Ophthalmology* **91**, 564–579.

Alvarado, J. A., Yun, A. J. & Murphy, C. G. (1986) Juxtacanalicular tissue in primary open angle glaucoma and in non-glaucomatous individuals. *Archives of Ophthalmology* **104**, 1517–1528.

Ashton, N. (1958) Discussion on the trabecular structure in relation to the problem of glaucoma. *Proceedings of the Royal Society of Medicine* **52**, 69–72.

Fine, B. S. (1964) Observations on the drainage angle in man and rhesus monkey: a concept of the pathogenesis of chronic simple glaucoma. *Investigative Ophthalmology* **3**, 609–646.

Fine, B. S., Yanoff, M. & Stone, R. A. (1981) A clinicopathologic study of four cases of primary open-angle glaucoma compared to normal eyes. *American Journal of Ophthalmology* **91**, 88–105.

Fink, A. I., Felix, M. D. & Fletcher, R. C. (1978) The anatomic basis for glaucoma. *Annals of Ophthalmology* **10**, 397–411.

Grierson, I. (1987) What is open angle glaucoma? *Eye* **1**, 15–28.

Rohen, J. W. (1970) The morphologic organization of the chamber angle in normal and glaucomatous eyes. *Advances in Ophthalmology* **22**, 80–96.

Rohen, J. W. (1978) Chamber angle in glaucoma. In *Conceptions of a Disease*, eds K. Heilmann & K. T. Richardson, pp 26–43. W. B. Saunders, Philadelphia.

Rohen, J. W. (1983) Why is intraocular pressure elevated in chronic simple glaucoma? Anatomical considerations. *Ophthalmology* **90**, 758–765.

Segawa, K. (1977) Electron microscopic changes of the trabecular tissue in primary open-angle glaucoma. *Annals of Ophthalmology* **9**, 1429–1430.

Tripathi R. C. (1972) Aqueous outflow in normal and glaucomatous eyes. *British Journal of Ophthalmology* **56**, 157–174.

Angle closure glaucoma

Phillips, C. I. (1972) Aetiology of angle-closure glaucoma. *British Journal of Ophthalmology* **56**, 248–253.

Wilensky, J. T. (1977) Current concepts in primary angle-closure glaucoma. *Annals of Ophthalmology* **9**, 963–972.

Congenital glaucoma

DeLuise, V. P. & Anderson, D. R. (1983) Primary infantile glaucoma (congenital glaucoma). *Survey of Ophthalmology* **28**, 1–19.

Kwitko, M. L. (1973) *Glaucoma in Infants and Children*. Appleton-Century-Crofts, New York.

ICE syndrome

Campbell, D. G., Shields, M. B. & Smith, T. R. (1978) The corneal endothelium and the spectrum of essential iris atrophy. *American Journal of Ophthalmology* **86**, 317–323.

Eagle, R. C., Jr., Font, R. L., Yanoff, M. & Fine, B. S. (1979) Proliferative endotheliopathy with iris abnormalities. The iridocorneal syndrome. *Archives of Ophthalmology* **97**, 2104–2111.

Rodrigues, M. M., Stulting, R. D. & Waring III, G. O. (1986) Clinical, electron microscopic and immunohistochemical study of the corneal endothelium and Desçemet's membrane in the iridocorneal endothelial syndrome. *American Journal of Ophthalmology* **101**, 16–27.

Scheie, H. G., Yanoff, M. & Kellog, W. T. (1976) Essential iris atrophy. *Archives of Ophthalmology* **94**, 1315–1320.

Shields, M. B. (1979) Progressive essential iris atrophy, Chandler's syndrome, and the uris naevus (Cogan–Reese) syndrome: a spectrum of disease. *Survey of Ophthalmology* **24**, 3–20.

Shields, M. B., Campbell, D. G. & Simmons, R. J. (1978) The essential iris atrophies. *American Journal of Ophthalmology* **85**, 749–759.

Spencer, W. H. (1979) Proliferating terminology and the NUDE syndrome. *Archives of Ophthalmology* **97**, 2103.

Pseudoexfoliation syndrome

Aasved, H. (1979) Prevalence of fibrillopathia epitheliocapsularis (pseudoexfoliation) and capsular glaucoma. *Transactions of the Ophthalmological Society of the UK* **99**, 293–301.

Aasved, H. (1979) Relationship of intraocular pressure and fibrillopathia epitheliocapsularis. *Transactions of the Opthalmological Society of the UK* **99**, 310–311.

Dark, A. J., Streeten, B. W. & Cornwall, C. C. (1977) Pseudoexfoliative disease of the lens: a study in electron microscopy and histochemistry. *British Journal of Ophthalmology* **61**, 462–472.

Davanger, M. (1978) A note on the pseudoexfoliation fibrils. *Acta Ophthalmologica* **56**, 114–120.

Davanger, M. (1978) On the molecular composition and physicochemical properties of pseudo-exfoliation material. *Acta Ophthalmologica* **56**, 621–633.

Dickson, D. H. & Ramsey, M. S. (1979) Fibrillopathia epitheliocapsularis. Review of the nature and origin of pseudoexfoliative deposits. *Transactions of the Ophthalmological Society of the UK* **99**, 284–292.

Mizuno, K., Hara, Ishiguro, S & Takei, Y. (1980) Acid phosphatase in eyes with pseudoexfoliation. *American Journal of Ophthalmology* **89**, 482–489.

Roth, M. & Epstein, D. L. (1980) Exfoliation syndrome. *American Journal of Ophthalmology* **89**, 477–480.

Smith, R. (1979) Nature of glaucoma in the pseudoexfoliation syndrome. *Transactions of the Ophthalmological Society of the UK* **99**, 308–309.

Taylor, H.R. (1979) Pseudoexfoliation, an environmental disease? *Transactions of the Ophthalmological Society of the UK* **99**, 302–307.

Other secondary glaucomata

Epstein, D. L. (1979) Pigment dispersion and glaucoma. *Annals of Ophthalmology* **11**, 917–918.

Fenton, R. H. & Zimmerman, L. E. (1963) Haemolytic glaucoma. *Archives of Ophthalmology* **70**, 236–239.

Fine, B. S., Yanoff, M. & Scheie, H. G. (1974) Pigmentary glaucoma, a histologic study. *Transactions of the American Academy of Ophthalmology and Otolaryngology* **78**, 314–325.

Flocks, M., Litturin, C. S. & Zimmerman, L. E. (1955) Phacolytic glaucoma. *Archives of Ophthalmology* **54**, 37–45.

Francois, J. (1977) Corticosteroid glaucoma. *Annals of Ophthalmology* **9**, 1075–1080.

Iwamoto, T., Witmer, R. & Landolt, E. (1971) Light and electron microscopy in absolute glaucoma with pigment dispersion phenomena and contusion angle deformity. *American Journal of Ophthalmology* **72(2)**, 420–434.

Jay, B. (1972) Glaucoma associated with sudden displacement of the lens. *British Journal of Ophthamology* **56**, 258–262.

Kupfer, C., Kuwabara, T. & Kaiser-Kupfer, M. (1975) The histopathology of pigment dispersion syndrome with glaucoma. *American Journal of Ophthalmology* **80**, 857–862.

Richardson, T. M., Hutchinson, B. T. & Grant, W. M. (1977) The outflow tract in pigmentary glaucoma. A light and electron microscope study. *Archives of Ophthalmology* **95**, 1015–1025.

Rohen, J. W. Linner, E. & Witmer, R. (1973) Electron microscopic studies of the trabecular meshwork in two cases of corticosteroid glaucoma. *Experimental Eye Research* **17**, 19–31.

Shaffer, R. N. (1954) The role of vitreous detachment in aphakic and malignant glaucoma. *Transactions of the American Academy of Ophthalmology and Otolaryngology* **58**, suppl., 217–231.

Smith, M. E. & Zimmerman, L. E. (1965) Contusive angle recession in phacolytic glaucoma. *Archives of Ophthalmology* **74**, 799–804.

Optic nerve damage

Emery, J. M., Landis, D. & Paton, D., Boniuk, M. & Craig, J. M. (1974). Lamina cribrosa in normal and glaucomatous eyes. *Transactions of the American Academy of Ophthalmology and Otolaryngology* **78**, 290–297.

Hayreh, S. S. (1972) Optic disc changes in glaucoma. *British Journal of Ophthalmology* **56**, 175–185.

Hayreh, S. S. (1978) Structure and blood supply of the optic nerve. In *Glaucoma. Conceptions of a Disease*, eds K. Heilmann & K. T. Richardson, pp 78–103. W. B. Saunders, Philadelphia.

Maumenee, A. E. (1983) Causes of optic nerve damage in glaucoma. *Ophthalmology* **90**, 741–702.

Minckler, D. S. & Spaeth, G. L. (1981) Optic nerve damage in glaucoma. *Survey of Ophthalmology* **26**, 128–148.

Quigley, H. A. (1987) Reappraisal of the mechanisms of glaucomatous optic nerve damage. *Eye* **1**, 318–322.

Quigley, H. A., Hohman, R. M., Addicks, E.M., Massoff, R. W. & Green, W. R. (1983) Morphologic changes in the lamina cribrosa correlated with neural loss in open-angle glaucoma. *American Journal of Ophthalmology* **95**, 673–691.

Yablonski, M. E. (1979) An analysis of the 'vascular hypothesis' concerning optic disc pathology in glaucoma. *Annals of Ophthalmology* **11**, 67–69.

Yablonski, M. E. (1979) An analysis of the 'mechanical hypothesis' of glaucomatous optic disc cupping. *Annals of Ophthalmology* **11**, 427–428.

Other

Gartner, S. & Henkind, P. (1978) Neovascularization of the iris (rubeosis iridis). *Survey of Ophthalmology* **22**, 291–312.

John, T., Sassani, J. W. & Eagle, R. C., Jr. (1983) The myofibroblastic component of rubeosis iridis. *Ophthalmology* **90**, 721–728.

Chapter 13 Optic nerve

NORMAL STRUCTURE AND FUNCTION

As an introduction to the disorders of the optic nerve some important structural and functional considerations are summarised below.

Optic nerve head

The optic nerve head comprises the surface layer of nerve fibres, the pre-laminar region and the lamina cribosa region.

The surface nerve fibre layer

In this anterior layer, compact nerve fibres converge from all parts of the retina and bend posteriorly towards the brain. The layer is separated from the vitreous by the internal limiting membrane.

The pre-laminar region

In this region the nerve fibres become segregated into bundles by glial septa in which there is a capillary network.

The lamina cribrosa region

The lamina cribrosa itself is a lamellar structure composed of collagen bundles with a variable content of elastic tissue alternating with glial sheets. It is continuous peripherally with the sclera and centrally with the adventitial sheath of the central artery and vein. The nerve fibres pass through numerous rounded or oval apertures of varying size and are separated from the connective tissue by a glial membrane.

Anterior orbital part of optic nerve

In this part the nerve fibres are myelinated. The nerve itself becomes much thicker and is enclosed in a sheath of dura and pia arachnoid. The nerve fibres are separated into bundles by connective tissue septa containing blood vessels from which they are, however, separated by an astroglial layer.

Blood supply

A continuous capillary network is present from the optic nerve head and adjacent retina to the anterior orbital part of the optic nerve. The network is fed mainly by branches of the short posterior ciliary arteries and circle of Zinn, but, in the anterior nerve fibre layer, branches are received from the retinal arterioles. The network is separate from the choroidal capillary network and the capillaries have pericytes and non-fenestrated endothelial cells with tight junctions as elsewhere in the CNS. They do not leak fluorescein. In the anterior orbital part of the optic nerve there is both a centripetal supply from the pial vessels and a centrifugal supply from the central retinal artery.

Axoplasmic transport

The cytoplasmic constituents of neurones are in a constant state of flow which may be defined by direction, rate and constituents carried. There are at least three components.

1 *The orthograde rapid component:* is probably concerned with synaptic transmission. It moves at the rate of 200–1000 mm/day. Metabolites synthesised in the perikaryon are delivered, probably via the microtubular system in the axoplasm, to the nerve terminals.

2 *The orthograde slow component:* is probably concerned with growth and maintenance. It moves at the rate of 0.5–3.0 mm/day. Up to 80% of the proteins moving in an orthograde direction may be carried in this component. Mitochondria move at the same rate, although they exhibit a back and forth motion.

3 *The retrograde component:* is concerned with feedback. It moves at the rate of only 50 mm/day and transports acetylcholinesterase, nerve growth factor and lysosomal enzymes. Axoplasmic transport in the optic nerve head may be affected by:

(i) Changes in intraocular pressure.
(ii) Changes intracranial pressure.
(iii) Circulatory disturbances.

PAPILLOEDEMA

Though originally defined as a non-inflammatory swelling of the optic nerve head due to raised intracranial pressure, it is well recognised that an essentially similar swelling may also result from sudden increases or decreases in intraocular tension. It has been established experimentally that, whatever the cause of the papilloedema, axoplasmic transport is slowed down and both fast and slow components accumulate in the region of the cribriform plate. This disturbance in axoplasmic transport may thus represent a final common pathway. Histologically, the swelling of the nerve head is seen to displace the layers of the retina away from its margins and the nuclear layers appear 'stepped' (Fig. 13.1).

Electron microscopy has shown that the increase in tissue volume is almost entirely due to swelling of the nerve fibres.

Degeneration of the nerve fibres may occur, and, if the condition is protracted, atrophy and gliosis are likely to ensue.

ATROPHY, NEURITIS AND NEUROPATHY

Few terms give rise to greater confusion than the above when used in relation to the optic nerve. This is largely because they are widely used clinically for conditions seldom seen under the microscope.

Myelinated nerve tracts within the CNS such as the optic nerve undergo two types of degeneration:

1 Wallerian-type degeneration in which both myelin sheaths and axons are affected and function is lost.

2 Demyelination in which the myelin sheath degenerates, but the axons survive and continue to conduct impulses at a lower than normal rate and may eventually recover partially or completely if the myelin sheath is restored.

If the destructive process is rapid, a phagocytic reaction by the microglia is provoked and there is replacement gliosis. If the degeneration progresses slowly, the replacement gliosis procedes in an orderly fashion preserving the general architecture. The nerve is greatly reduced in size and the dural sheath tends to become convoluted (Fig. 13.2).

OPTIC ATROPHY

Atrophy is the end result of the degenerative process. The clinical appearance of the disc and pathological changes in the nerve are governed by the nature and cause of the process and the glial response it provokes. Based on these considerations, four types of atrophy can be described:

1 Descending atrophy follows lesions in the CNS proximal to the optic nerve. It is characterised by an absence of gliosis or fibrosis in the nerve head. The lamina cribrosa is covered only by a layer of residual glia after atrophy of the nerve fibres and the disc appears unduly white. The atrophy seen in tabes dorsalis, often misleadingly referred to as 'primary atrophy', is typical, but other lesions within the CNS such as hydrocephalus, tumours and transection of the optic nerve give rise to a similar picture.

2 Ascending atrophy is much commoner and follows disease processes affecting the retinal ganglion cells within the globe such as glaucoma (Chapter 12), retinal infarction, chorioretinitis, etc. If there is swelling of the nerve head, fibroglial proliferation will occur in it so that the disc does not have the 'clean' white appearance described above.

3 Secondary atrophy may follow pathological processes occurring within the optic nerve itself. These include various types of neuritis and neuropathy considered below. Clearly, however, there is, as for example in the

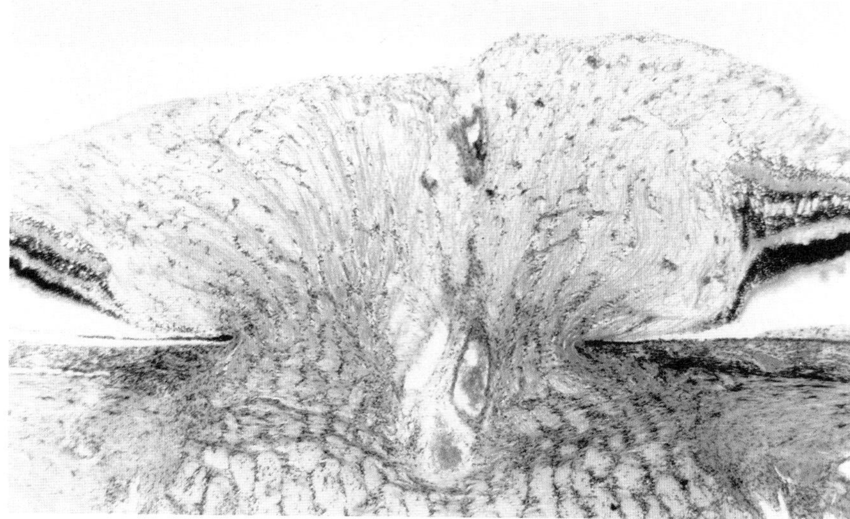

Fig. 13.1 Papilloedema due to an intracranial tumour. Note swelling of nerve head and outward displacement of retina.

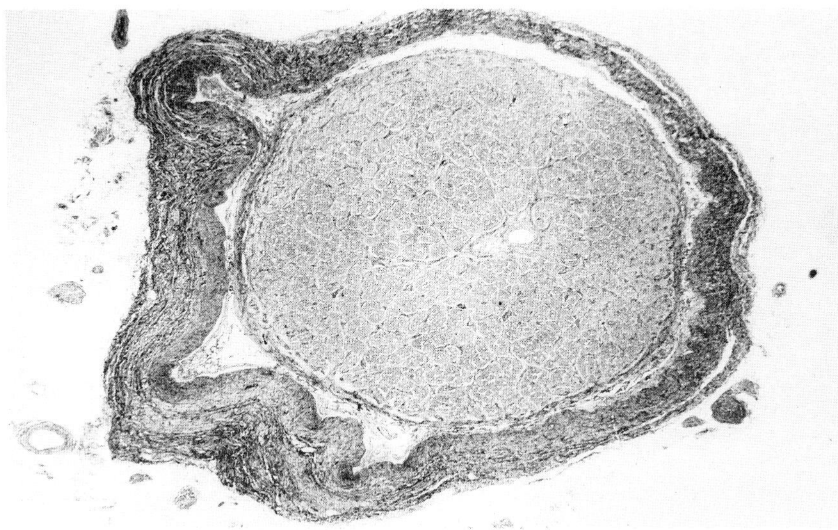

Fig. 13.2 Optic atrophy. Optic nerves removed post-mortem from an unusual case of indirect atrophy. (a) Normal nerve. Masson trichrome (×25).

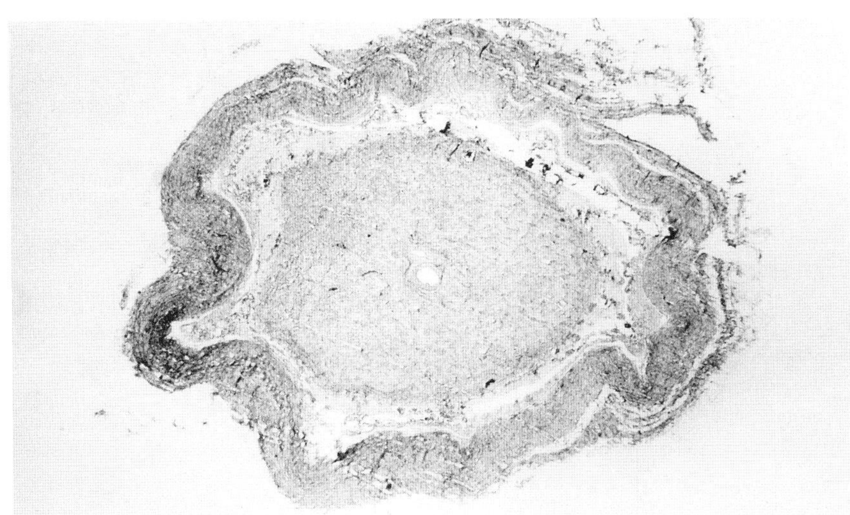

Fig. 13.2 (b) Atrophied nerve showing great reduction in cross-sectional diameter. Masson trichrome (×20).

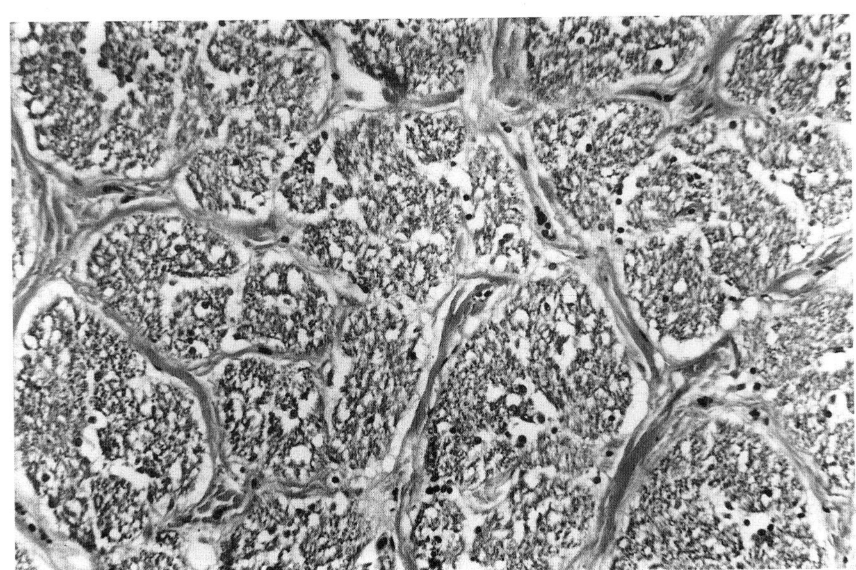

Fig. 13.2 (c) Normal nerve. Masson trichrome (×210).

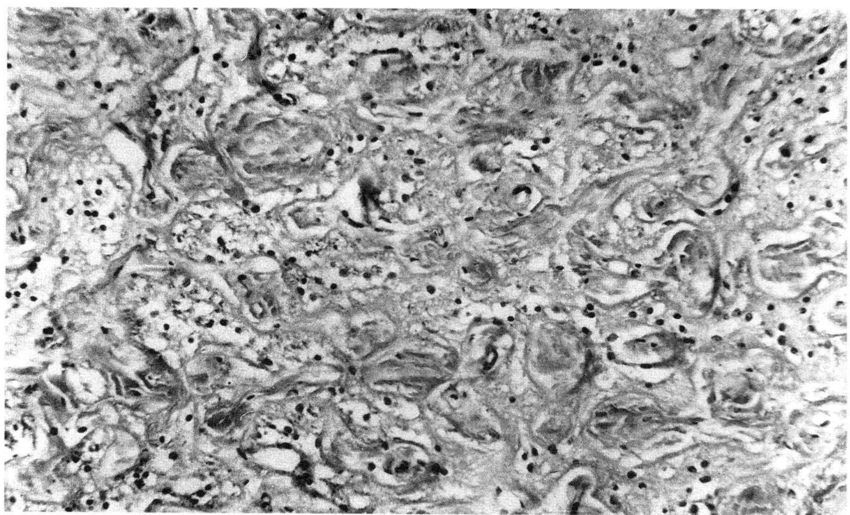

Fig. 13.2 (d) Atrophied nerve. The nerve fibre bundles have disappeared leaving erratically arranged collagenous septa interspersed with microglia. Masson trichrome (×160).

case of papilloedema, some overlap between this category and the other two which are also 'secondary atrophies'. There may or may not be fibroglial proliferation on the nerve head so that the clinical appearances are variable.

So-called indirect atrophy follows an injury to the head or orbit which does not involve the optic nerve directly, but results in contusion or tearing of the optic nerve or chiasma or haemorrhage into the arachnoid. Rarely, indirect optic atrophy follows an apparently trivial external injury (Fig. 13.2).

4 Hereditary atrophies occur as three principal types:

(i) infantile hereditary optic atrophy which shows two forms: (a) recessive form — characterised by onset soon after birth and subsequent severe visual loss; and (b) dominant form — characterised by slow decrease in vision throughout life.

(ii) Behr's disease which is transmitted as an autosomal recessive. Visual loss is not total and remains static after the second or third decade. A variety of neurological disturbances are associated, such as cerebellar ataxia, spasticity and pyramidal tract abnormalities.

(iii) Leber's optic atrophy which affects men and usually shows an X-linked recessive mode of inheritance. Onset occurs in the second or third decade with sudden rapid loss of central vision. Some slow recovery of vision may occur and there may be mild neurological disturbances.

Microscopic changes: in the few cases that have been studied, the changes were similar in dominant optic atrophy and Leber's disease. There was atrophy and degeneration of the retinal ganglion cells with demyelination of the nerve fibres in the optic nerve and in the chiasma. The papillomacular bundle was most severely affected. Degenerative changes were also present in the lateral geniculate body.

OPTIC NEURITIS

Microbial

The optic nerve may become involved by spread of inflammatory processes:

1 In the globe: examples include toxoplasmic retinochoroiditis and infective endophthalmitis, especially fungal.

2 In the skull: acute bacterial, tuberculous, syphilitic and fungal meningitis may all spread along the dural sheath of the optic nerve and into the optic nerve itself via the pial septa thus affecting peripheral part of the nerve most severely.

3 In the orbit: orbital cellulitis due to sinusitis is the usual cause.

Encephalitic

Visual failure occasionally complicates encephalitis following viral infections and vaccination, but little is known of the pathological changes in the optic nerves.

Degenerative 'optic neuritis'

The term 'optic neuritis' is commonly applied clinically to a condition which is not strictly inflammatory, but degenerative. The essential pathological process is demyelination and the commonest identifiable cause is multiple sclerosis (Fig. 13.3). Visual failure is indeed a common presenting symptom in multiple sclerosis. Estimates vary widely (0–85%) as to how many cases presenting clinically with 'optic neuritis' actually progess to multiple sclerosis. The changes in the nerve consist of local loss of myelin sheaths and oligodendroglia. After phagocytosis of the myelin and axonal debris there as

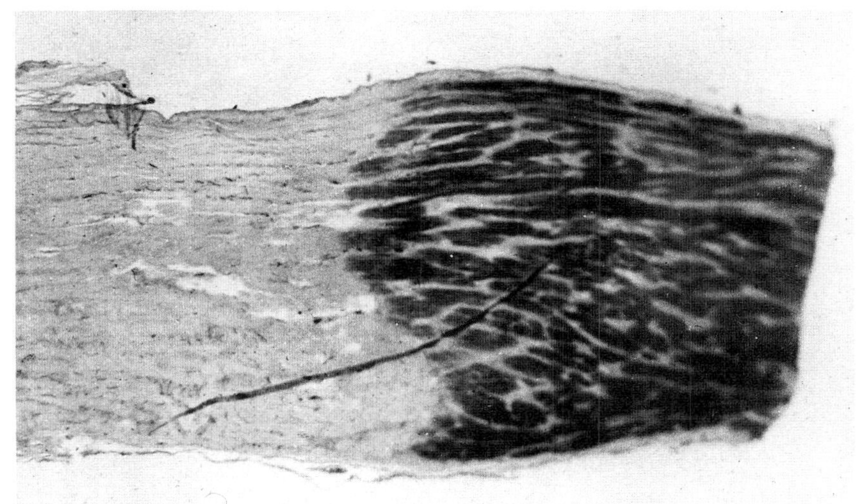

Fig. 13.3 Demyelination of optic nerve in multiple sclerosis shown by Weigert–Pal staining. Note abrupt boundary between normal area and affected area. (Photograph by courtesy of Professor P. O. Yates.)

astrocytic proliferation and a local plaque is formed. Small vessels may show lymphocytic cuffing, especially in older plaques. The causative mechanism remains unknown.

Devic's disease (neuromyelitis optica), which is thought to be an acute form of multiple sclerosis, is characterised by necrotising lesions in the optic nerve, optic chiasma, optic tract and spinal cord.

ISCHAEMIC OPTIC NEUROPATHY

Ischaemic optic neuropathy commonly affects the elderly and presents as acute visual failure in one or both eyes. Most cases are caused either by arteriosclerosis or cranial arteritis involving the ciliary vessels supplying the anterior portion of the optic nerve, but they may also result from embolism of these vessels.

Microscopically, there is initially a well demarcated liquefaction necrosis of the pre- or retrolaminar part of the optic nerve which provokes a lymphocytic and astrocytic reaction (Fig. 13.4a). In the early stages the appearances may resemble those seen in the cavernous atrophy which occasionally occurs in acute glaucoma (Chapter 12) and deposition of acid mucopolysaccharide (glycosaminoglycan) presumably of vitreal origin has been reported (Hinzpeter & Naumann, 1976). Ascending and descending degeneration of the nerve fibres directed towards the retina and optic chiasm respectively follow and the affected part of the nerve eventually becomes fibrotic.

Giant cell arteritis

Because giant cell arteritis is such an important cause of

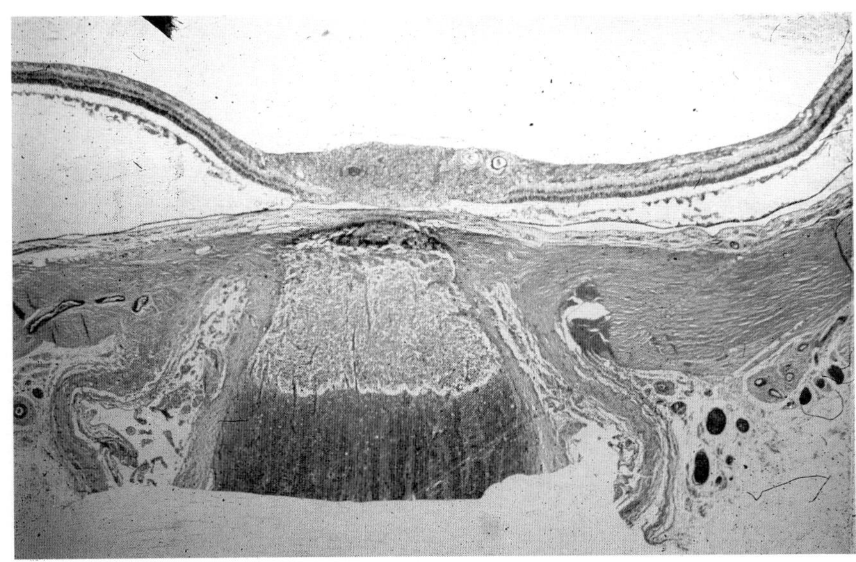

Fig. 13.4 Cranial arteritis. (a) Retrolaminar infarction of the optic nerve. (Reproduced with permission from Cullen & Coleiro, 1976).

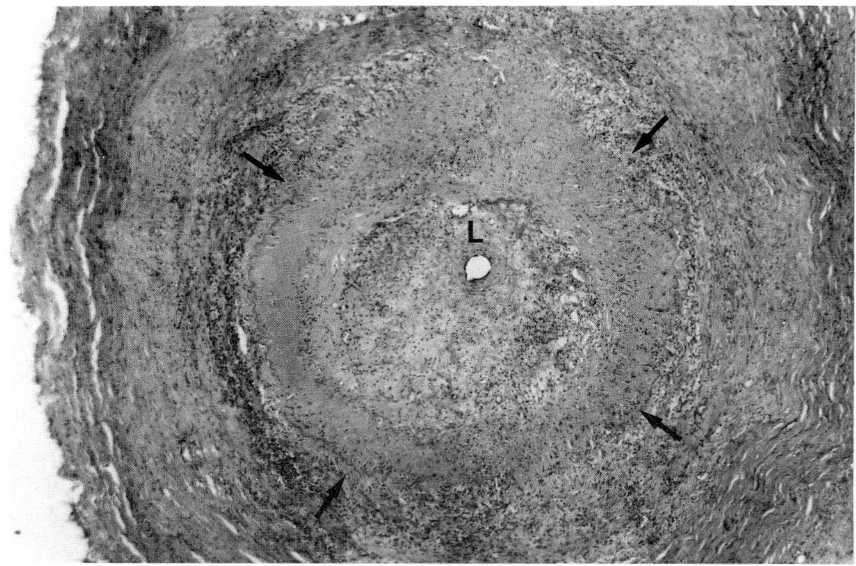

Fig. 13.4 (b) An affected temporal artery. The vascular lumen (L) is much reduced by a massive chronic inflammatory infiltrate. Much of the internal elastic lamina has been destroyed, but segments where it survives are indicated by arrows. H & E.

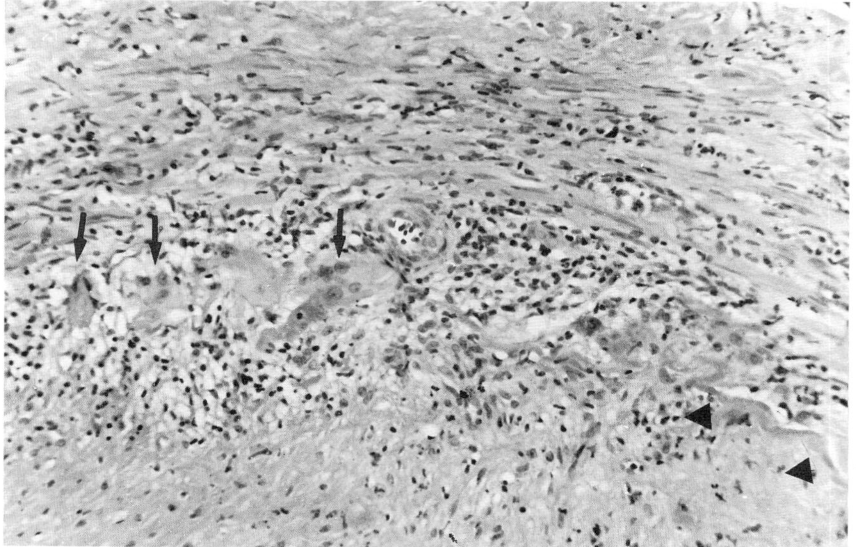

Fig. 13.4 (c) Higher power of area indicated by circle showing giant cells (arrows) in a cellular inflammatory infiltrate related to surviving remnants of elastic lamina (arrowheads). H & E (×160).

ischaemic optic neuropathy it is convenient to consider the disease in more detail at this point. It is a chronic granulomatous inflammation of unknown aetiology involving arteries in many different parts of the the body including the aorta and coronary and renal arteries, but having a predilection for those of carotid distribution. Both sexes are equally susceptible and the patients are usually over 60 years of age.

Most patients suffer from headache due to involvement of the cranial arteries while many also have anorexia, loss of weight and low-grade fever. Pain on chewing is a common and diagnostically useful symptom which may, however, be wrongly attributed to arthritis of the mandibular joint. The temporal arteries are often thick, nodlar, pulseless and tender and on biopsy display characteristic histological features.

Ocular complications

Ocular involvement occurs in nearly 50% of patients. Sometimes ocular symptoms and signs precede other evidence of disease while a few patients go blind without having suffered any appreciable headache or constitutional disturbance.

The ocular symptoms range from diplopia, sixth and third nerve palsies and visual defects, through episodes of transient visual loss to permanent blindness in one or both eyes, sometimes of sudden onset. Ophthalmoscopically there is usually slight to moderate pallid oedematous swelling of the disc which may progress to optic atrophy. Sometimes there is more generalised oedema of the retina at the posterior pole accompanied by attenuated vessels, small haemorrhages and cotton-wool spots while, in a minority of cases, the fundus presents the characteristic appearance of ischaemic infarction with milky oedema of the retina in the macular area and a cherry-red foveal spot (Chapter 10, Part 2). These symptoms and signs are the result of progressive occlusion of the ophthalmic artery and its branches causing ischaemia of the retina, the optic nerve and the extra-ocular muscles. the commonest cause of blindness in giant cell arteritis is ischaemia of the optic nerve. It is often impossible to determine clinically the site or sites of arterial occlusion but pathological studies have shown them to be in the ophthalmic and posterior ciliary arteries and in the orbital extent of the central retinal artery. The intraneural extent of the central retinal artery is only rarely involved in the arteritic process while the choroidal arteries seem to be completely exempt.

Microscopic appearances

In the characteristic granulomatous phase of the disease (Fig. 13.4b) the wall of the artery is thickened by an inflammatory infiltrate consisting of histiocytes and lymphocytes, a variable number of foreign bodies and Langhan's type giant cells and occasional neutrophils and eosinophils. This reaction appears to be directed against the medial muscle cells and the internal elastic lamina. Ultrastructural studies have shown phagocytosis of degenerated smooth muscle cell basement membrane by macrophages and giant cells. Phagocytosis of disrupted elastic lamina was not seen although fragments of the latter appear to be the target of giant cells. The vascular lumen is reduced to a narrow cleft by fibroblastic proliferation in the intima, but rarely becomes completely occluded.

The granulomatous inflammatory reaction is preceded by an acute necrotising phase with exudation of fibrin into the vessel wall. In the later stages of the disease the damaged wall of the vessel is repaired by fibrosis and regeneration of muscle cells.

Laboratory diagnosis

Sedimentation rate: in most cases, the erythrocyte sedimentation rate (ESR) is greatly increased, often above 50 mm in the first hour (Westergren). This simple test is particularly valuable in cases presenting with ocular symptoms, but without headache or palpable thickening of the temporal arteries.

Temporal artery biopsy: biopsy from the same side as the involved eye should be taken in all suspected cases and sectioned at several levels as unaffected 'skip' areas may occur. Although the arteries do not appear diseased clinically, this is not a contra-indication since histological evidence of the disease may be found in such tissue. A negative biopsy does not necessarily exclude giant cell arteritis.

Relationship to polymyalgia rheumatica

Giant cell arteritis involving the cranial arteries occurs in a minority of cases of polymyalgia rheumatica. This is typically a disease of elderly women which is characterised by pain and morning stiffness in the muscles of the neck, shoulders and pelvic girdle. There is often malaise, fever, mental depression, anorexia and loss of weight. The ESR is high. Involvement of the ophthalmic artery or its branches occasionally causes blindness.

Immunological aspects

Antinuclear antibody titres are often raised in both giant cell arteritis and polymyalgia rheumatica thus apparently relating them to other connective tissue disorders thought to have an autoimmune basis. Evidence of deposition of immunoglobulin in the arterial wall is inconclusive. The infiltrating lymphocytes have been identified as T-cells which play a central role in granulomatous inflammation.

TOXIC OPTIC NEUROPATHY

Visual failure due to damage to the optic nerve has been reported following numerous agents including metallic salts, organic solvents, alcohols and various drugs such as ethambutol. The mode of action of these agents is generally unknown. In some cases the damage is dose-dependent, in others it is apparently idiosyncratic. A relationship between serum zinc levels and toxic neuropathies has been established, but little is known of the pathogenetic processes involved.

Methyl alcohol poisoning

In acute methyl alcohol poisoning, irreversible visual failure occurs as a result of demyelination of the nerve. The damage in the CNS is caused by incomplete oxidation in the liver of methyl alcohol to formaldehyde.

Tobacco amblyopia

Loss of vision may occur in smokers, especially elderly pipe smokers. The visual defect is most marked with red and green targets. The probable underlying cause of the condition is inability to detoxify cyanide present in tobacco smoke by conjugation with sulphur to form thiocyanate. Recovery follows after giving up smoking or treatment with hydroxocobolamin, a compound present in commercially available vitamin B12 which has an affinity for cyanide. Inorganic sulphate, high protein diet and, in some cases, folic acid and vitamin B6 have also proved effective, presumably by rectifying the deficiency in sulphur-containing amino acids needed for physiological detoxification of cyanide. The mechanism by which the demyeliation in the optic nerve is produced is not known.

Other causes

Visual loss due to damage to the optic nerve is seen in starvation, vitamin B complex deficiencies and pernicious anaemia. The mechanism involved is probably essentially similar to that which occurs in tobacco amblyopia. Indeed, some cases of tobacco amblyopia may well be nutritional deficiency due to self neglect.

DEGENERATIVE DEPOSITS

Drüsen

Drüsen are hyaline masses varying in size from 50–750 μm in diameter found in the pre-laminar part of the optic nerve (Fig. 13.5). They may be single or multiple and are commonly asymptomatic. The highest reported incidence in post-mortem studies is 20.4 per 1000.

Microscopically, drüsen show concentric lamination and stain positively by the PAS method. They always contain calcium and sometimes iron.

The pathogenesis of drüsen is unknown. They may be associated with minor local morphological abnormalities.

Giant drüsen

Giant drüsen are a separate entity and result from the calcification of astrocytic hamartomas of the nerve head which may occur in tuberous sclerosis (Chapter 15).

Corpora amylacea

Corpora amylacea ('brain dust') are rounded bodies usually located close to the pia in grey matter and around blood vessels in white matter. They are stained by iodine, methyl violet, and PAS, and react positively for glycogen with Best's carmine. Electron microscopy shows they are formed in the processes of fibrous astrocytes.

Corpora arenacea

Corpora arenacea (psammoma bodies) are laminated basophilic bodies found in the pia arachnoid. Similar structures are sometimes found in meningiomas. Both types of body increase in number with age and are of no practical importance.

MYOPIC DEFORMATION

In degenerative myopia progressive stretching of the sclera at the posterior pole results in the exit of the nerve through the sclera becoming increasingly oblique. At the same time the retina and its pigmented epithelium and the choroid are retracted from the margin of the nerve head on the temporal side thus exposing a crescent of sclera which appears white ophthalmoscopically. On the nasal side the retina and choroid overlap the margin of the nerve head so that the disc appears blurred ophthalmoscopically (Fig. 13.6).

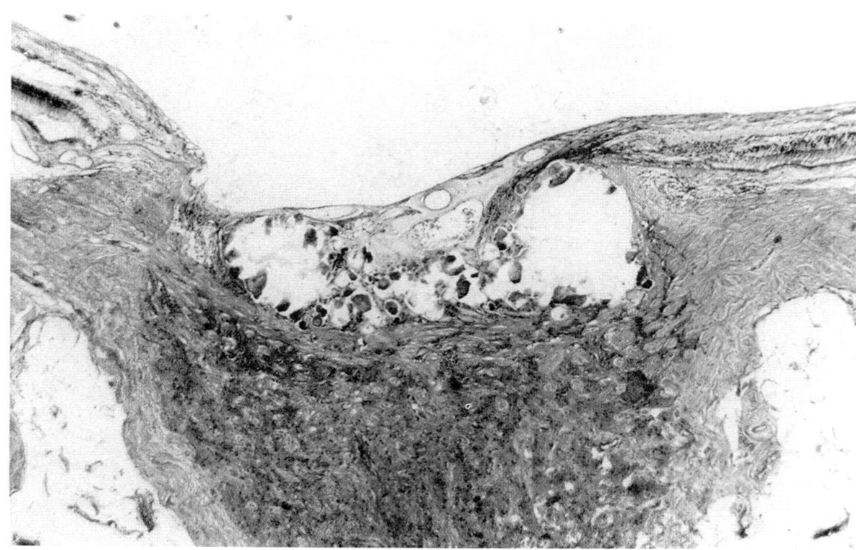

Fig. 13.5 Calcified drüsen of the optic nerve head which have shattered during sectioning.

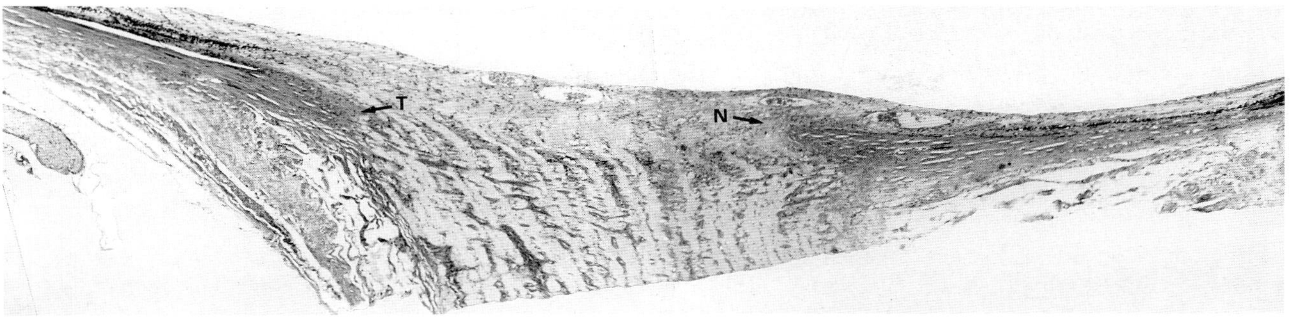

Fig. 13.6 Optic nerve head in myopia. Deformation of nerve and peripapillary atrophy of retina. Arrows indicate scleral margins, N = nasal, T = temporal.

TUMOURS OF THE OPTIC NERVE AND ITS SHEATHS

Meningiomata

Meningiomata arise from arachnoid cells on the deep surface of the dura and from arachnoid prolongations into the dura (arachnoid granulations). It is often difficult to be sure of the exact origin of intraorbital meningiomata and it is always wise to assume that they have an intracranial component.

Age incidence and prognosis

Meningiomata occur more commonly in women than in men and are usually apprehended at about 40 years of age. They grow slowly and are curable by adequate excision, but are not radiosensitive. Even after incomplete removal, recurrent growth is usually slow. Primary intraorbital meningiomata originating from the optic nerve sheath are, however, exceptional in that some of the patients have been under 20 years of age at the time of surgery. The prognosis for these young patients is poor since there is a strong tendency for recurrent growth and intracranial extension.

Types

For convenience they may be grouped as follows:

1 Intracranial meningiomata: the majority of meningiomata encountered in the orbit are secondary invaders which arise intracranially often from the sphenoidal ridge and enter the orbit either through the bone or less commonly along the subarachnoid space surrounding the optic nerve. Meningiomata in the anterior cranial fossa may break into the orbit through its roof.

2 Primary intraorbital meningiomata: a minority of meningiomata originate from the optic nerve sheath from whence they may infiltrate forwards in the subarachnoid space to the back of the globe. They occasionally penetrate the globe to appear in the nerve head or choroid.

3 Intracanalicular meningiomata: these arise within the optic canal, are encapsulated and tend to encircle and adhere to the optic nerve.

4 Meningiomata having no apparent connection with the optic nerve are occasionally found in the orbit and these are thought to arise from ectopic meningeal tissue.

Effects

1 Pressure on the optic nerve causes slow atrophy of the fibres, congestive swelling of the nerve head, vascular stasis in the retina and visual failure. Primary tumours of the nerve sheath eventually break out of the sheath and invade the orbit.

2 Pressure on the cranial nerves, usually the third, less often the fourth and sixth causes paralysis of the extraocular muscles. Disturbed sensation due to pressure on the fifth cranial nerve is less common.

3 Pressure on or infiltration of the extraocular muscles may also cause limitation of ocular movement.

4 Invasion of contiguous bones induces radiologically detectable hyperostoses often of considerable size.

5 Expansion within the orbit either of the meningioma or, more commonly, by hyperostotic growths causes proptosis. Meningiomata occasionally fill the orbit and invade the paranasal sinuses.

Clinical presentation

The mode of presentation can be broadly classified according to the site of origin:

1 Meningiomata on the medial third of the sphenoidal ridge cause visual defects and optic atrophy before exopthalmos.

2 Meningiomata on the middle and lateral thirds of the sphenoidal ridge induce exopthalmos as a result of local hyperostosis first and nerve pressure later.

3 Primary meningiomata of the intraorbital nerve sheath cause visual loss. Proptosis, lid oedema and chemosis

occur later. There is an afferent pupillary defect and papilloedema or atrophy of the nerve head. Shunt vessels are often present in the nerve head.

4 Intracanalicular meningiomata cause early visual failure and proptosis is unusual.

Gross appearance

Meningiomata outside the optic nerve are reddish-grey nodular circumscribed growths while those within its dural sheath form spindle shaped or diffuse thickenings.

Microscopic structure

The diversity of structure exhibited by menigiomata has led to complicated histological classifications. In the orbit, two principal types may be recognised of which the meningotheliomatous is the commoner.

Meningotheliomatous tumours are composed of polygonal cells with poorly defined cytoplasmic boundaries divided into lobules of uneven size by fibrovascular strands. The cells have homogeneous, stringy or granular cytoplasm and large spheroidal nuclei exhibiting a fine chromatin network (Fig. 13.7). Well developed desmosomes are present between contiguous cells and this may help in the differentiation of atypical cases from other fibrocytic tumours.

Psammomatous tumours are characterised by whorls and eddies of elongated cells in the centre of which may be a small vessels or a hyaline or laminated calcified sphere (psammoma body). These spheres result from the degeneration of the central cells in the whorl and are the same as corpora arenacea naturally present in the arachnoid of older persons.

Gliomata

Clinical aspects

Gliomata of the optic nerve may constitute up to 6% of orbital tumours. Few of those which cause ocular symptoms and signs are confined to the intraorbital extent of the optic nerve, so that any consideration of orbital gliomas must necessarily be made in the wider context of optic gliomas involving the visual pathways. They belong to the group of benign astrocytic gliomata which occur most commonly in the cerebellum in children, but differ from other members of the group in that about 25% of cases are associated with neurofibromatosis (Chapter 15). The incidence of optic nerve gliomata in neurofibromatosis has been put at about 5%, although, if clinically silent tumours are taken into consideration, it may be as high as 15%. Those associated with neurofibromatosis tend to arise in childhood and preferentially affect the nerve. The tumours may occasionally be multicentric (Lewis *et al.*, 1984).

Many gliomata of the anterior visual pathways are indolent tumours which tend to enlarge during the patient's early life and then become static. They resemble hamartomata in that they do not seem to have the capacity for unlimited growth. In a recent series, the mean survival time was 17 years for tumours of the optic nerve and 19 years for those of the chiasma (Rush *et al.*, 1982).

Characteristically, the patient is an infant or young child with visual loss or proptosis, but it is important to recognise that some patients with optic gliomata retain good vision indefinitely. When the tumour involves the optic chiasma and adjacent areas of the third ventricle, the clinical picture may be dominated by hypothalamic

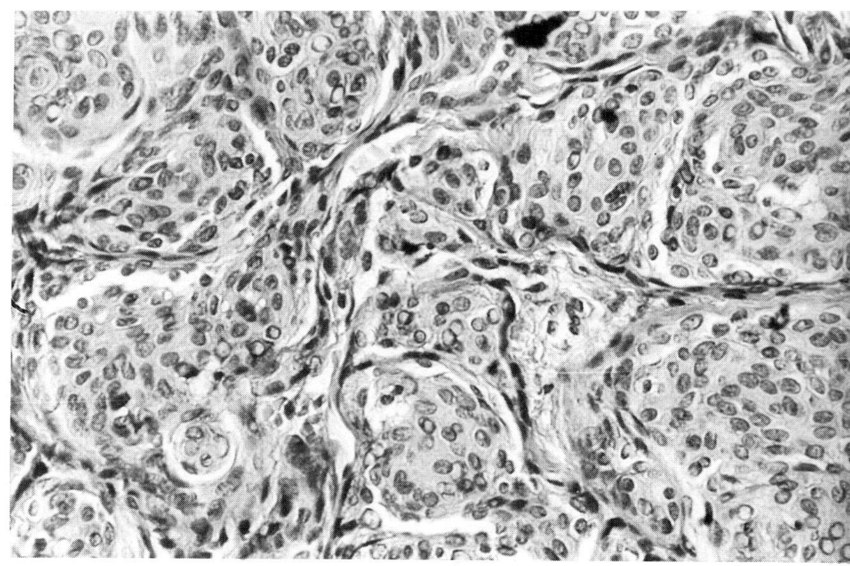

Fig. 13.7 Meningotheliomatous meningioma of optic nerve sheath showing characteristic lobulation.

signs. Not all gliomas of the optic nerve conform to this benign pattern however. Occasionally, and more commonly in adults than in children, anaplastic and invasive astrocytomas are encountered which progress to blindness, intracranial extension and early death.

Pathological aspects

Gliomata in the optic nerve originate from the supportive gial cells. At first there is a diffuse proliferation of glial cells within the existing framework of the nerve, which remains readily recognisable. However, in time the proliferating cells extend through the pial sheath and provoke a hyperplastic response by the arachnoidal cells which form a separate layer. This in turn is invaded until the glioma fills the dural sheath to form a fusiform or rounded elastic growth around the nerve (Fig. 13.8a & b), which usually remains identifiable. The glioma does not transgress the dura, but may infiltrate forwards to the lamina cribrosa and occasionally penetrates into the retina or choroid. More commonly, extension is towards the brain, through the optic foramen, causing radiologically demonstrable erosion of its margin.

Microscopically, the majority of orbital gliomata are composed entirely of stellate and piloid (hair-like) astrocytes (Fig. 13.8c), though some may show an admixture of oligodendrocytes.

Stellate astrocytes have large oval nuclei with punctate chromatin and one or more nucleoli. Their cytoplasm is abundant and extends into spidery processes which join with those of contigous cells to form a meshwork, the spaces of which contain a mucoid substance.

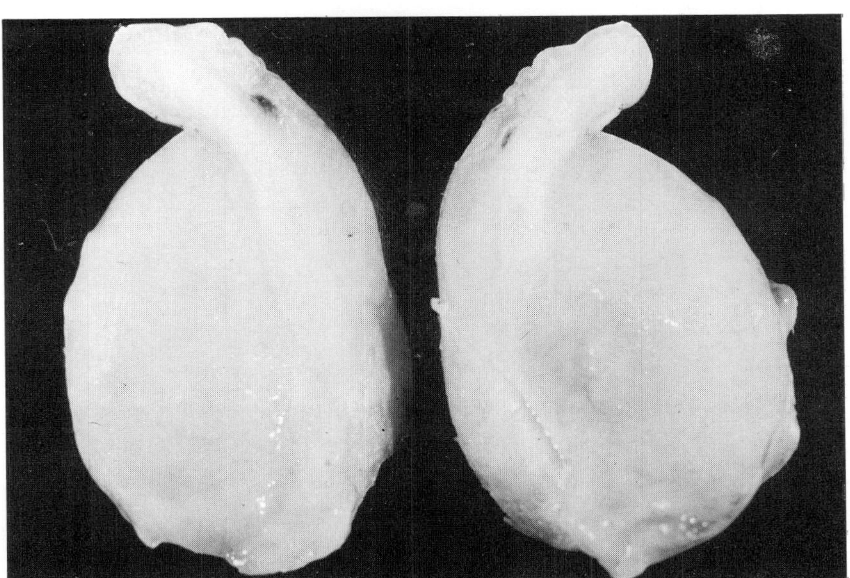

Fig. 13.8 Optic nerve glioma. (a) Macroscopic appearance showing characteristic fusiform tumour confined within the dural sheath. The chiasmal margin is inferior.

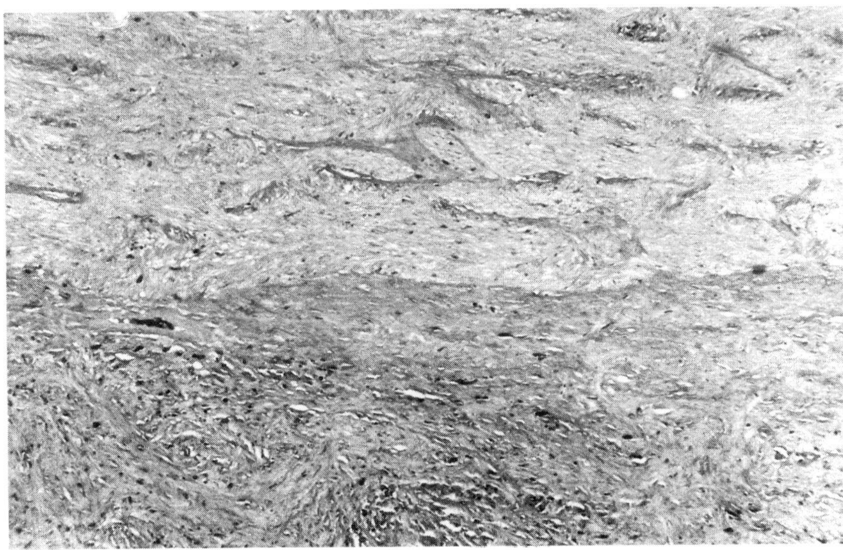

Fig. 13.8 (b) Low power showing boundary between tumour within optic nerve (upper half) and in the arachnoid sheath. Note how the fibrous septa which separated the nerve bundles are preserved in the optic nerve. Masson trichrome (×62).

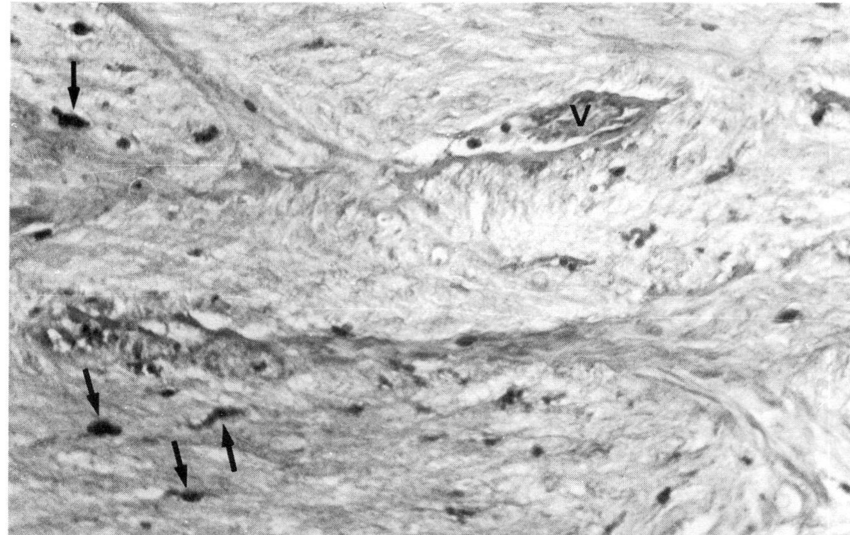

Fig. 13.8 (c) Detail of growth within the nerve showing the orderly arrangement of the astrocytic fibres between the septa. The tendency of the fibres to attach perpendicularly to blood vessels is also evident. V = vessel. Arrows indicate some of the numerous Rosenthal fibres. Masson trichrome (×320).

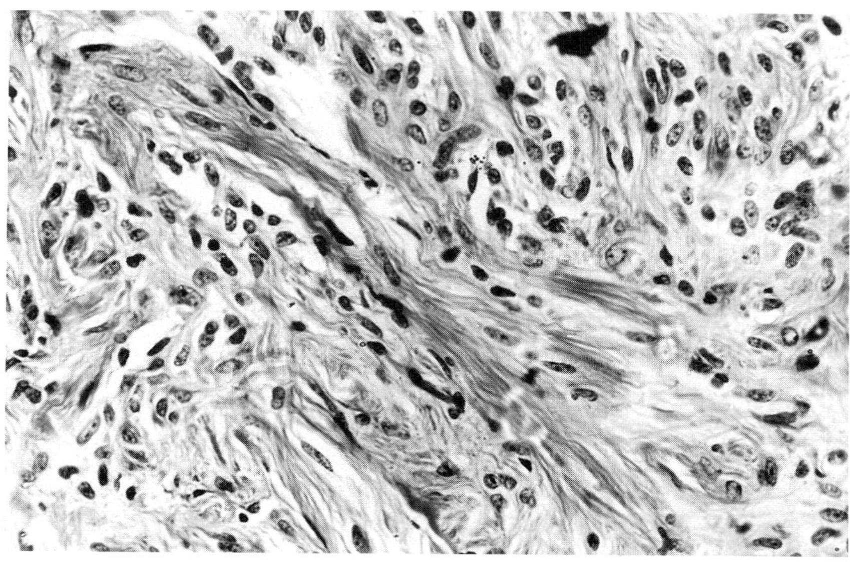

Fig. 13.8 (d) Typical pilocytic structure. The hair-like fibres of the piloid astrocytes are clearly seen.

A characteristic feature, not seen in any adult type astrocytomata, is the presence of numerous Rosenthal fibres. These appear as elongated masses which stain red in Masson's trichrome. By electron microscopy they are seen as dense homogeneous material within the processes of the tumour astrocytes.

The vessels of the tumour are generally of the non-fenestrated type found in the CNS, but fenestraed vessels have also been reported.

Melanocytomata

Lesions composed entirely of large densely pigmented rounded cells occur occasionally in the optic nerve head of eyes with heavily pigmented fundi. They are identical to magnocellular naevi seen in the uveal tract (Chapter 8). They form small jet-black nodules situated centrally in the nerve head. Where they overlap the margin of the nerve head, they exhibit a striated or feathery edge due to infiltration of naevus cells among the nerve fibres. They rarely cause any visual disturbance, but occasionally enlarge slowly, infiltrate the retina and optic nerve and induce optic atrophy.

Secondary tumours

Direct invasion

The optic nerve may be invaded directly by tumours of the eye, orbit or brain. Of these, retinoblastoma is the most important. Invasion of the nerve and extension into the brain is common and fatal when it occurs (Chapter

11). Intraocular malignant melanomata only occasionally invade the nerve (Chapter 8).

Blood-borne metastases

Metastatic deposits from carcinomata usually of breast or lung occur, but are uncommon. Leukaemic infiltration is common and may be asymptomatic.

BIBLIOGRAPHY

General

Blackwood, W. & Corsellis, J. A. N. (1976) *Greenfield's Neuropathology*. Arnold, London.

Structure and function

Awai, T. (1985) Angioarchitecture of intraorbital part of human optic nerve. *Japanese Journal of Ophthalmology* **29**, 79–98.

Lieberman, M. F., Maumenee, A. E. & Green, W. R. (1976) Histologic studies of the vasculature of the anterior optic nerve. *American Journal of Ophthalmology* **82**, 405–423.

Zhao, Y. & Li, F. (1987) Microangioarchitecture of optic papilla. *Japanese Journal of Ophthalmology* **31**, 147–159.

Papilloedema

Hayreh, S. S. (1978) Fluids in the anterior part of the optic nerve in health and disease survey of ophthalmology **23**, 1–25.

Tso, M. O. M. & Fine, B. S. (1976) Electron microscopic study of human papilloedema. *American Journal of Ophthalmology* **82**, 424–438.

Wirtschafter, J. D., Rizzo, F. J. & Smiley, B. C. (1975) Optic nerve axoplasm and papilloedema *Survey of Ophthalmology* **20**, 157–189.

Atrophy, neuritis and neuropathy

Campbell, W. I. (1983) Doyne lecture. The significance of optic neuritis. *Transactions of the Ophthalmological Society of the UK* **103**, 230–246.

Foulds, W. S. (1981) in *The Molecular Basis of Neuropathology*, eds A. N. Davison & R. H. S. Thompson. Arnold, London.

Hughes, B. (1962) Indirect injury of the optic nerves and chiasma. *Bulletin of the Johns Hopkins Hospital,* **111**, 96–125.

Johnston, P. B., Gaster, R. N., Smith, V. C. & Ramesh, C. T. (1979) A clinicopathological study of autosomal dominant optic atrophy. *American Journal of Ophthalmology* **88**, 868–875.

Kwittken, J. & Barest, H. D. (1958) The neuropathology of hereditary optic atrophy (Leber's disease); the first complete anatomic study. *American Journal of Pathology* **34**, 185–207.

Levy, J. & Chatfield, R. K. (1969) Optic atrophy following eyelid injury. *British Journal of Ophthalmology* **53**, 49–52.

Perkin, G. D. & Rose, F. C. (1979) *Optic Neuritis and its Differential Diagnosis*. Oxford University Press, Oxford.

Sullivan, G. (1969) Optic atrophy after seemingly trivial trauma. *Archives of Ophthalmology* **81**, 159–161.

Walsh, F. B. (1966) Pathological–clinical correlations. I. Indirect trauma to the optic nerves and chiasm. II. Certain cerebral involvements associated with defective blood supply. *Investigative Ophthalmology* **5**, 433–449.

Ischaemic optic neuropathy

Hayreh, S. S. (1974) Anterior ischaemic neuropathy. I. Terminology and pathogenesis. *British Journal of Ophthalmology* **58**, 955–963.

Henkind, P., Charles, N. C. & Pearson, J. (1970) Histopathology of ischaemic optic neuropathy. *American Journal of Ophthalmology* **69**, 78–90.

Cranial arteritis

Albert, D. M., Ruchman, M. C. & Keltner, J. L. (1976) Skip areas in temporal arteritis. *Archives of Ophthalmology* **94**, 2072–2077.

Albert, D. M., Searl, S. S. & Craft, J. L. (1982) Histological and ultrastructural characteristics of temporal arteritis. The value of the temporal artery biopsy. *Ophthalmology* **89**, 1111–1126.

Chess, J., Albert, D. M., Bhan, A. K., Paluck, E. I., Robinson, N., Collins, B. & Kaynor, B. (1983) Serologic and immunopathologic findings in temporal arteritis. *American Journal of Ophthalmology* **96**, 283–289.

Cohen, D. N. & Smith, T. R. (1974) Skip areas in temporal arteritis: myth versus fact. *Transactions of the American Academy of Ophthalmology and Otolaryngology* **78**, OP 772–783.

Cullen, J. F. & Coleiro, J. A. (1976) Ophthalmic complications of giant cell arteritis. *Survey of Ophthalmology* **20**, 247–260.

Hinzpeter, E. N. & Naumann, G. (1976) Ischaemic papilloedema in giant-cell arteritis. Mucopolysaccharide deposition with normal intraocular pressure. *Archives of Ophthalmology* **94**, 624–628.

Reinecke, R. D. & Kuwabara, T. (1969) Temporal arteritis. I. Smooth muscle involvement. *Archives of Ophthalmology* **82**, 446–453.

Degenerative deposits

Friedman, A. H., Gartner, S. & Modi, S. S. (1975) Drüsen of the optic disc. A retrospective study in cadaver eyes. *British Journal of Ophthalmology* **59**, 413–421.

Friedman, A. H., Beckerman, B., Gold, D. H., Walsh, J. B. & Gartner, S. (1977) Drüsen of the optic disc. *Survey of Ophthalmology* **21**, 375–390.

Mullie, M. A. & Sanders, M. D. (1985) Scleral canal size and optic nerve head drüsen. *American Journal of Ophthalmology* **99**, 356–359.

Sacks, J. G., O'Grady, R. B., Choromokos, E. & Leestma, J. (1977) The pathogenesis of optic nerve drüsen. A hypothesis. *Archives of Ophthalmology* **95**, 425–428.

Tumours

Davis, F. A. (1940) Primary tumours of the optic nerve (a phenomenon of von Recklinghausen's disease). *Archives of Ophthalmology* **23**, 735–821 and 957–1022.

Hoyt, W.P. & Baghdassarian, S. A. (1969) Optic gliomata of childhood. *British Journal of Ophthalmology* **53**, 793–798.

Karp, L. A., Zimmerman, L. E., Borit, A. & Spencer, W. (1974) Primary intraorbital meningiomas. *Archives of Ophthalmology* **91**, 24–28.

Lewis, R. A., Gerson, L. P., Axelson, K. A., Riccardi, V. M. & Whitford, R. P. (1984) Von Recklinghausen neurofibromatosis. II. Incidence of optic gliomata. *Ophthalmology* **91**, 929–935.

Miki, H. & Hirano, A. (1975) Optic nerve glioma in an 18-month child. *American Journal of Ophthalmology* **79**, 589–595.

Rush, J. A., Younge, B. R., Campbell, R. J. & MacCarty, C. S. (1982) Optic glioma. Long-term follow-up of 85 histopathologically verified cases. *Ophthalmology* **89**, 1213–1219.

Wright, J. E. (1977) Clinical presentation and management of primary optic meningiomas. *Transactions of the American Academy of Ophthalmology and Otolaryngology* **83**, 617–625.

Zimmerman, L. E. & Garron, L. K. (1962) Melanocytoma of the optic disc. *International Ophthalmology Clinics* **2**, 431–440.

Chapter 14 Tumours of the orbit

INTRODUCTION

Because the orbit has a rigid bony wall, expanding lesions within it usually result in proptosis of the globe. Such lesions are both diverse and uncommon. It has been estimated that only four to five patients per million of the population per annum require orbital surgery (Wright, 1979). Secondary orbital changes related to dysthyroid disease are the commonest cause of proptosis. Such proptosis is usually bilateral, but even unilateral proptosis is more often attributable to thyroid dysfunction than to any other cause.

Orbital tumours and other expanding lesions are conveniently listed under the following sub-headings:

1 Inflammatory lesions such as 'pseudotumours' and mucocoeles.
2 Lymphoid hyperplasias and lymphomata (Chapter 16).
3 Vascular tumours and abnormalities.
4 Cysts.
5 Teratoma and choristoma.
6 Embryonal and mesenchymal tumours.
7 Fibrous and osseous lesions.
8 Secondary tumours.
9 Lesions of the lacrimal gland.
10 Tumours of optic nerve, brain and dural sheaths (Chapter 13).
11 Tumours and tumour-like lesions of peripheral nerve sheaths (Chapter 15).

The relative frequency of expanding lesions of the orbit varies somewhat in different published series due to such factors as the type of clinic, diagnostic methods used, etc. However, it is clear that those most commonly encountered fall into the the first four categories.

Though modern non-invasive clinical procedures have greatly improved diagnostic precision in the orbit, biopsy is still essential in many cases and it is important that an adequate specimen is obtained. Crushing between forceps blades must be avoided and the specimen fixed properly for both light and electron microscopy.

INFLAMMATORY DISEASES

Inflammatory pseudotumour is the name in common use for expanding lesions in the orbit which simulate neoplasms in their mode of presentation but are in fact inflammatory lesions. Although among the commoner causes of exophthalmos, they are for the most part of unknown aetiology and obscure pathogenesis. Except in the case of specific granulomata and mucocoeles, the pathologist can often do no more than exclude the presence of a true neoplasm. Interpreting inflammation in rather a broad sense, the following entities can be recognised:

1 Sclerosing inflammatory lesions.
2 Lipogranulomata.
3 Wegener's granulomatosis.
4 Specific granulomata.
5 Chronic myositis.
6 Graves' ophthalmopathy.
7 Mucocoeles.

Sclerosing inflammatory lesions

Pseudotumours consisting chiefly of fibrous tissue are not uncommonly encountered. They are hard and dense and presumably represent the end result of a chronic inflammatory process. A sparse patchy infiltrate of plasma cells is present together with scattered aggregates of lymphocytes often with germinal centres. Eosinophils are often seen in the infiltrate. Evidence of vasculitis is not uncommon and occasional giant cells may be present. Various features are illustrated in Fig. 14.1. The cause of the inflammation usually remains undiscovered.

Lipogranulomata

Fat necrosis due to trauma or bacterial infection may result in lipogranuloma formation. The fat cells are ruptured and the fat runs into globules which provoke a macrophagic and giant cell reaction. The macrophages become foamy due to ingested lipid and the local capillaries show obliterative endothelial proliferation. In time the granulomatous cellular infiltration is replaced by lymphocytes and plasma cells and progressive dense fibrosis occurs. The appearance is then indistinguishable from the sclerosing type. Indeed, it is not uncommon to see evidence of fat necrosis in sclerosing inflammatory lesions in the absence of any history of trauma or infection.

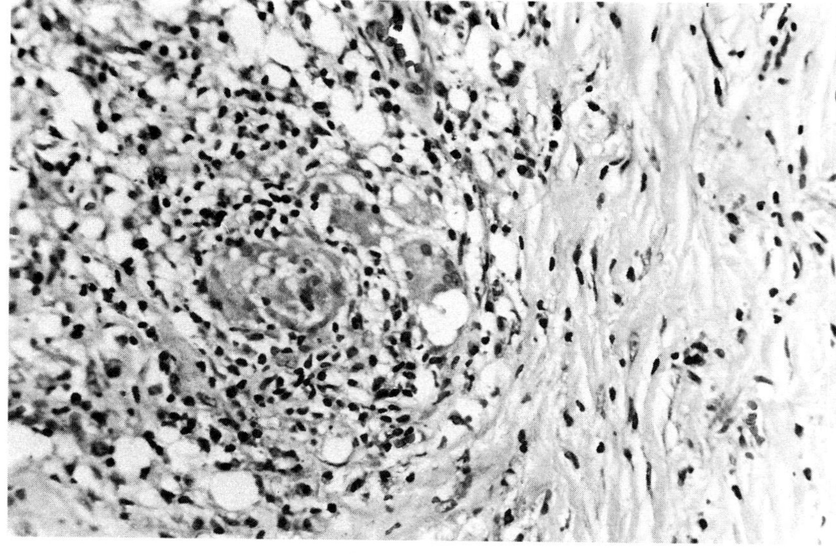

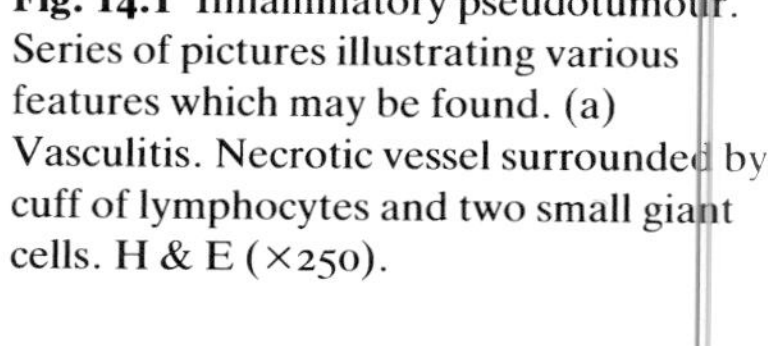

Fig. 14.1 Inflammatory pseudotumour. Series of pictures illustrating various features which may be found. (a) Vasculitis. Necrotic vessel surrounded by cuff of lymphocytes and two small giant cells. H & E (×250).

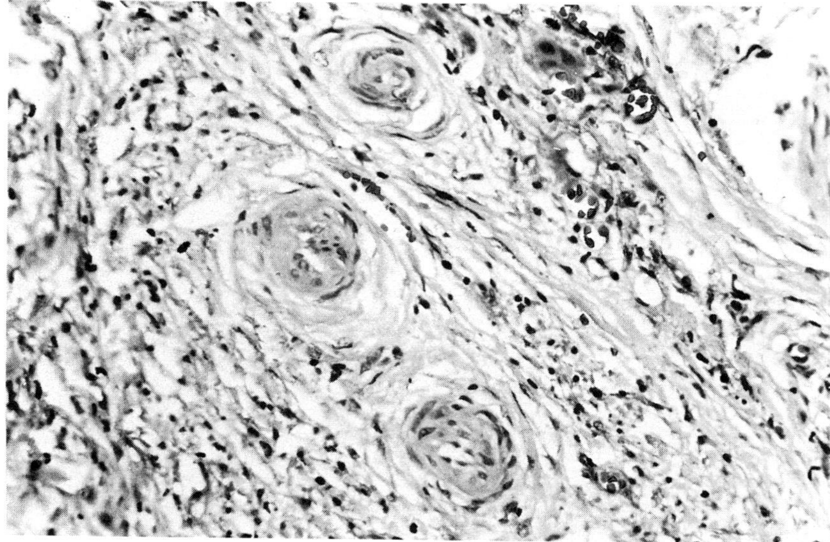

Fig. 14.1 (b) Sclerosed vessels in fibrous stroma lightly infiltrated with lymphocytes and plasma cells. H & E (×250).

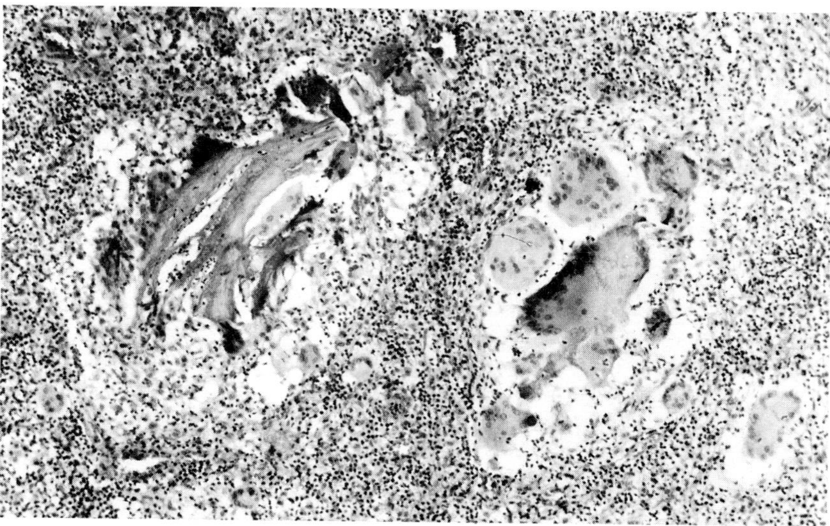

Fig. 14.1 (c) Inflammatory granulomatous reaction to unidentified matter. Large multinucleate cells can be seen. H & E (×160).

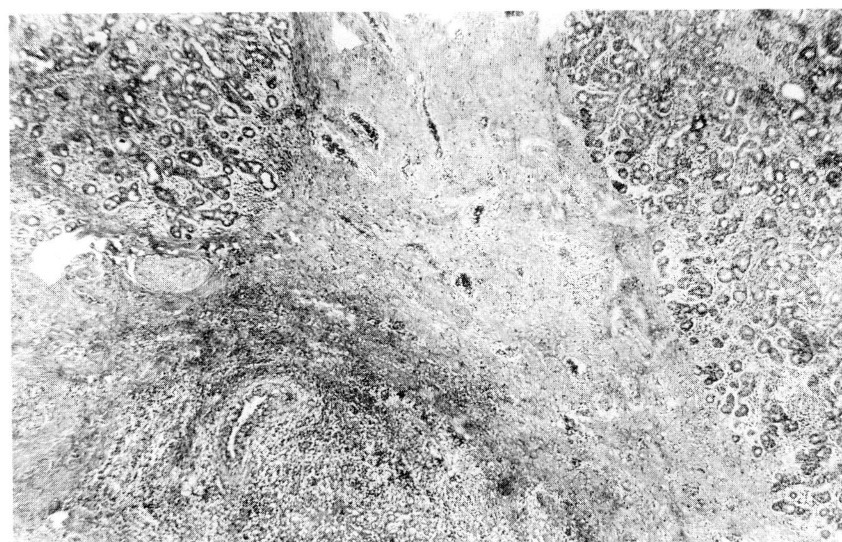

Fig. 14.1 (d) Fibrosis and chronic inflammatory infiltration disrupting the lacrimal lobules. H & E (×38).

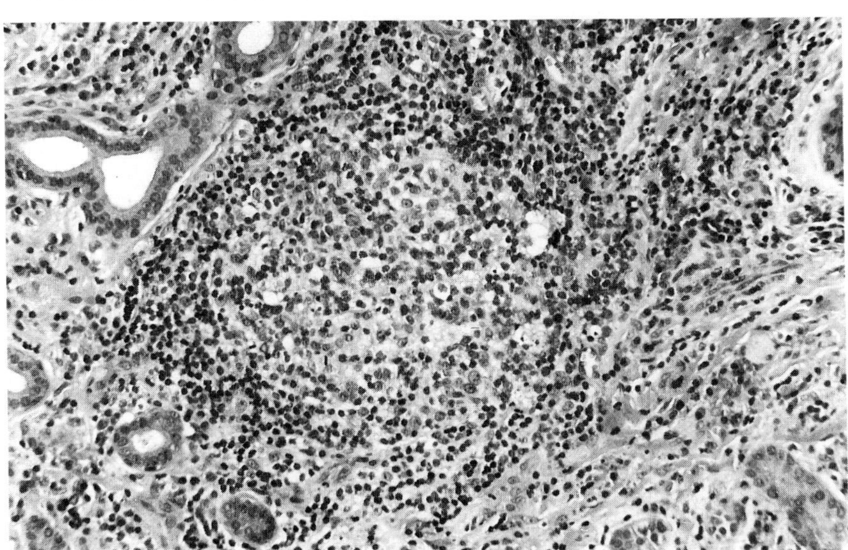

Fig. 14.1 (e) Lymphoid germinal centre in pseudotumour involving lacrimal gland. H & E (×160).

Wegener's granulomatosis

Wegener's granulomatosis is a disease of obscure aetiology characterised by the development of necrotising giant cell granulomata at first in some part of the upper respiratory tract and later in the lungs. This is accompanied by polyarteritis affecting the pulmonary systemic vasculature. Death is usually the result of renal failure due to renal arteritis and necrotising glomerulitis. Although the presenting granuloma is most often in in the nose or sinuses, it may occasionally be in the ear or orbit, and orbital signs may precede systemic manifestations. Microscopically the granulomata exhibit tissue necrosis, necrotising vasculitis and a variable infiltration by plasma cells, eosinophils, histiocytes and multinucleate giant cells. Sometimes the disease may be limited to bilateral infiltration of the orbit without involvement of the upper respiratory tract. Marginal ulceration of the cornea and necrogranulomatous scleritis are other ocular manifestations of Wegener's granulomatosis (Chapter 5).

Specific granulomata

These are the inflammatory response to tubercular and syphilitic infections, fungi and parasites such as microfilaria or nematode larvae. Sarcoid granuloma should be considered as well as reaction to haemorrhage or the contents of a ruptured dermoid cyst. Sarcoidosis is rare except in the lacrimal gland and, when it occurs, tends to affect an older than normal age group. It is among this group of conditions that biopsy of the orbital tissues is most likely to yield a definite diagnosis (Fig. 14.2).

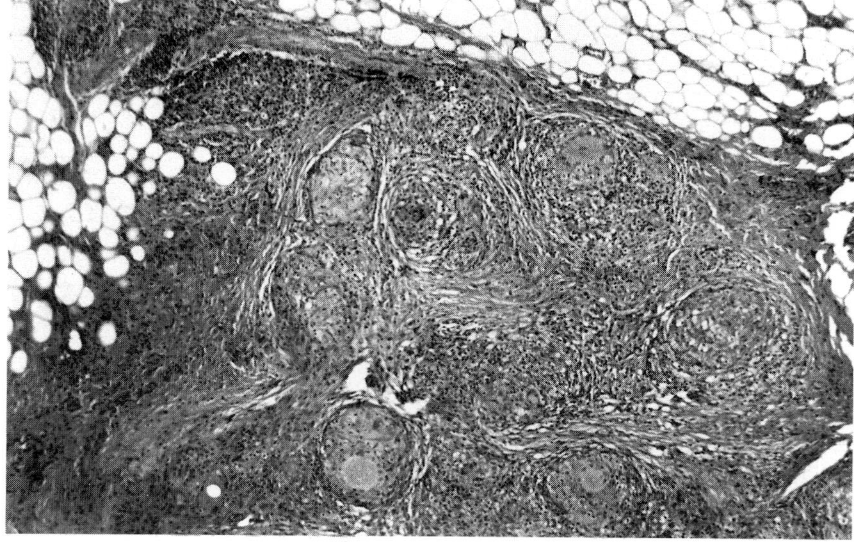

Fig. 14.2 Sarcoidosis. (a) Low power showing follicular infiltrate in orbital fat. H & E (×62).

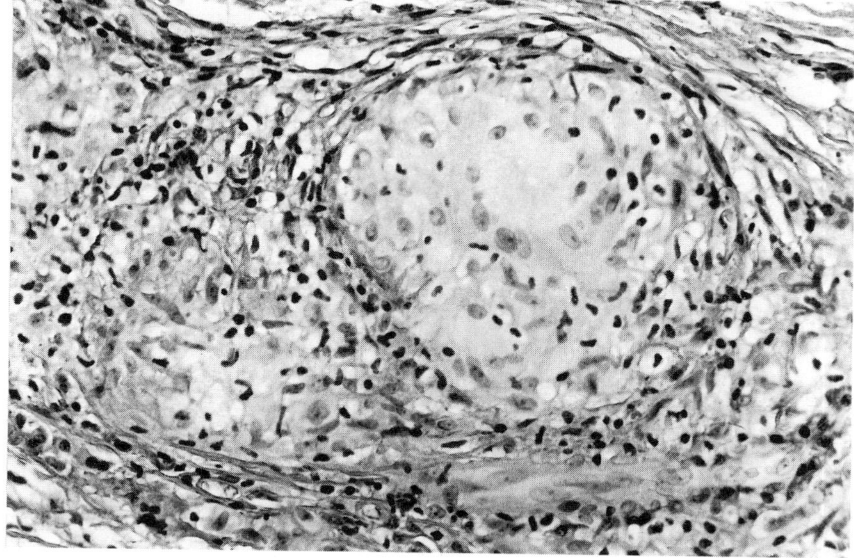

Fig. 14.2 (b) High power to show typical follicle of giant and epithelioid cells. H & E (×260).

Chronic myositis

Painless oedema of the lids, exophthalmos and diplopia are the common symptoms and the extraocular muscles are pale, enlarged and firm. Oedema, lymphocytic infiltration and even follicle formation are seen in one or more of the extraocular muscles with a variable inflammatory involvement of the surrounding connective tissues. Destruction of the muscle cells is followed by fibrosis.

Graves' ophthalmopathy

In this disease there is a marked and sometimes rapid increase in the volume of the orbital tissues due to an accumulation of glycosaminoglycan, the hygroscopic properties of which result in water retention in the orbital fat and connective tissue of the extraocular muscles. The muscles become grossly swollen by interstitial oedema and lymphocytic infiltration (Fig. 14.3). In time this leads to degeneration of the muscle cells, fibrosis and contracture. An increase in the number of tissue mast cells has also been noted. The appearances thus closely resemble chronic myositis and distinction may only be made on the basis of clinical examination and laboratory investigation.

The pathogenesis of Graves' ophthalmopathy is obscure. Long-acting thyroid stimulator (LATS) was at

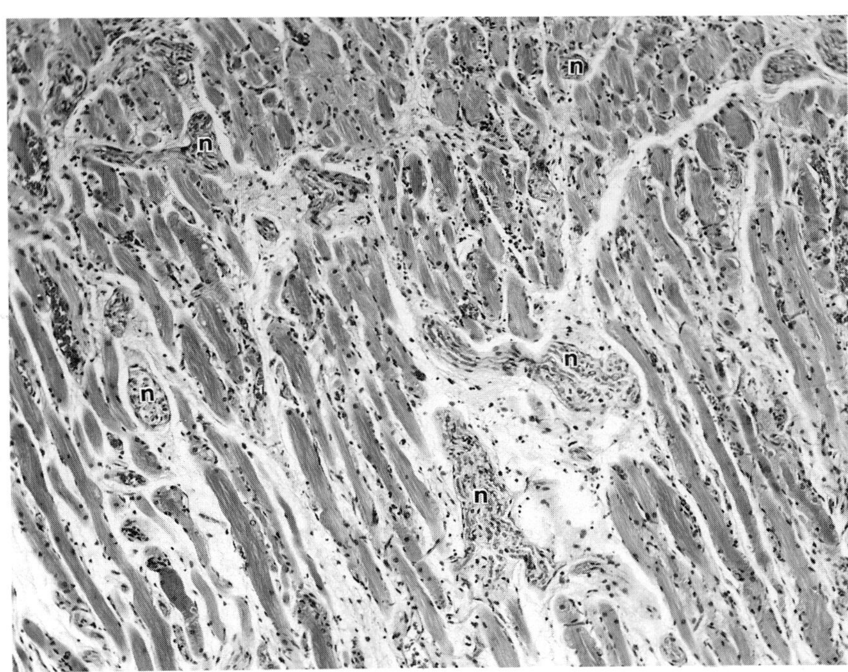

Fig. 14.3 Ophthalmopathy in Graves' disease. (a) Diffuse interstitial mononuclear infiltrate in patient with Graves' disease. Numerous nerve fibres (n) characteristic of extraocular muscles. H & E (×95). (Reproduced with permission from Campbell, 1984.)

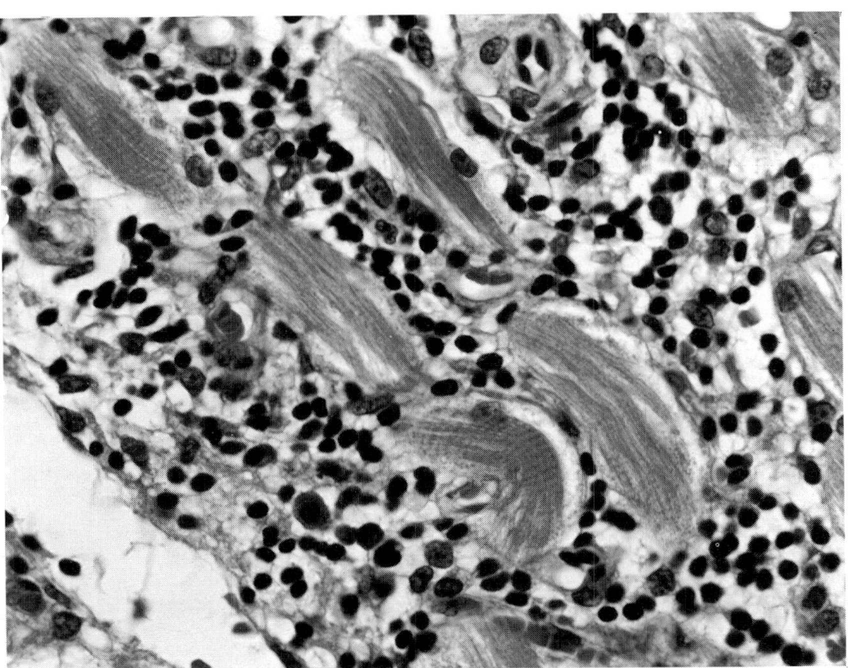

Fig. 14.3 (b) Mononuclear cells (lymphocytes and plasma cells) in close association with striated extraocular muscle. H & E (×610). (Reproduced with permission from Campbell, 1984.)

one time thought to be the humoral factor responsible, but is present in only 50–60% of patients and titres do not correlate with either the ophthalmopathy or the thyrotoxicosis. Thyroid stimulating immunoglobulins (TSI) have been found in the sera of over 90% of cases of Graves' disease, but TSI levels show no relationship with the ophthalmopathy.

Mucocoeles

Though mucocoeles occur in infancy, especially with cystic fibrosis, they are commonest in middle age. Most arise from the frontal or ethmoidal sinuses. They are lined by pseudostratified columnar epithelium in which goblet cells are present.

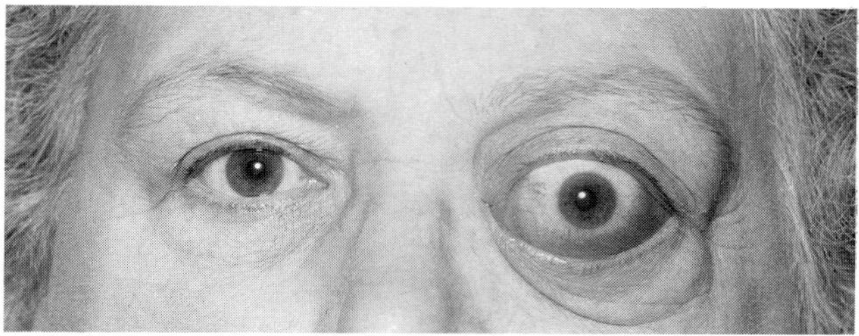

Fig. 14.4 Cavernous haemangioma of orbit. (a) Clinical photograph of patient prior to removal of tumour. (Picture by courtesy of Mr R. Dalgleish.)

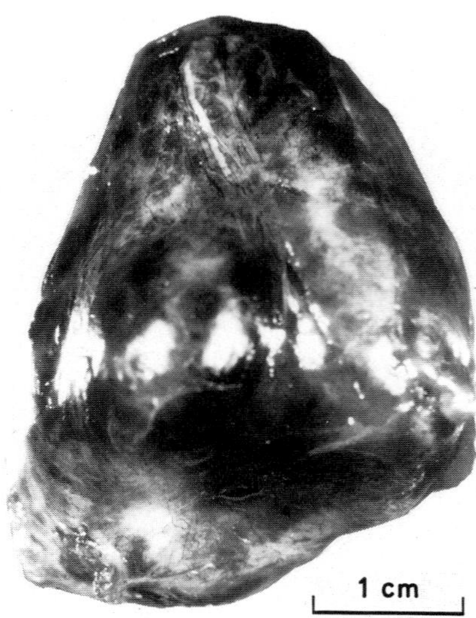

Fig. 14.4 (b) Macroscopic picture of tumour removed from the patient. The lower part of the tumour was in contact with the globe.

VASCULAR TUMOURS AND ABNORMALITIES

Haemangiomata

Haemangiomata are amongst the commonest orbital tumours. Although they are often not manifest clinically until adult life, the majority result from developmental errors of vaso-formative tissue and are thus tumour-like malformations (hamartomata). These, unlike true neoplasms, lack the power of unlimited, disproportionate growth, but become stationary after reaching their maximum size, often at a time when bodily growth stops. Malignant vascular noplasms of the orbit are exceedingly rare.

Cavernous haemangiomata

The majority of orbital haemangiomata are of cavernous type and typically present in adults of middle age (Fig. 14.4). They frequently lie within the muscle cone forming encapsulated, lobulated and often pulsatile tumours which induce a painless reducible proptosis. Thrombosis of the sluggish blood, haemorrhage or infection may cause a sudden increase in size. Calcification of the thrombus may lead to the formation of phleboliths.

Histologically, cavernous haemangiomata show wide, endothelial-lined channels separated by fibrous septa of varying thickness in which aggregations of haemosiderin granules and macrophages are seen. Frequently some capillary formation is also evident. Lymphocytes and sometimes lymphoid follicles are often present in the stroma.

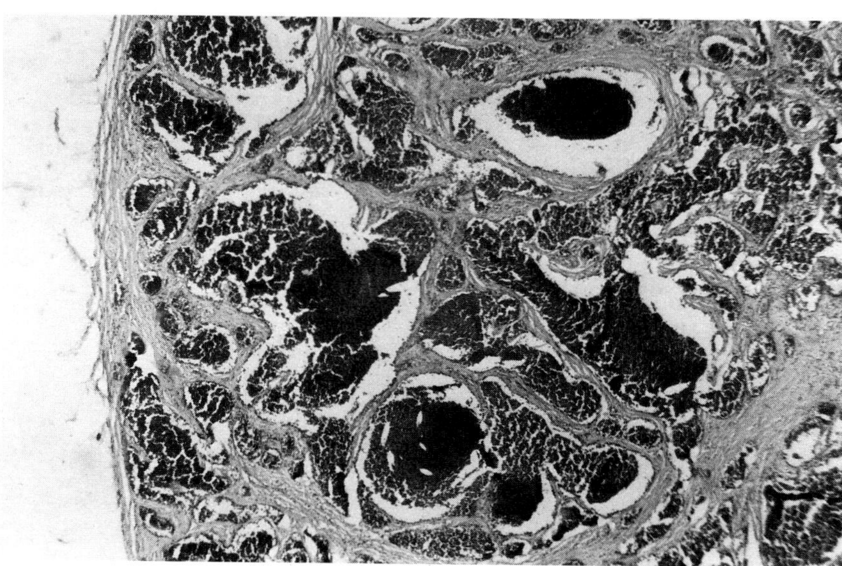

Fig. 14.4 (c) Photomicrograph showing the large vascular spaces with intervening fibrous septa. Masson trichrome (×38).

Benign haemangioendotheliomata

These are less common than the cavernous type and more often involve the anterior part of the orbit. They are not infrequently associated with similar malformations on the face or lid. They grow more rapidly and extensively and are poorly circumscribed. For these reasons, patients often present for treatment in infancy or childhood.

Histologically, benign haemangioendotheliomata are composed of closely packed masses of primitive endothelial cells with little evidence of capillary formation in haematoxylin and eosin preparations. Silver impregnation, however, shows the reticulin framework of numerous small vessels in the solid areas. Rapid increase in size, diffuseness and lack of encapsulation, undifferentiated cytology and a tendency to local recurrence after incomplete removal may suggest angiosarcoma, but this diagnosis is rarely justified in children. They do not metastasise and frequently regress spontaneously by sclerosis over a period of years. This sclerotic process, to which all haemangiomas are prone, is a progressive stromal fibrosis possibly in response to repeated small haemorrhages. Haemosiderin granules, foreign body giant cells and foam cells are frequently found in the stroma and ossification may occur. The ripening fibrous tissue gradually obliterates the vessels and the angiomatous nature of the tumour may be so obscured that it is mistaken for a xanthoma or a granuloma.

Capillary haemangiomas, which also occur in children, differ from haemangioendotheliomata in that the organization of the vasoformative tissue has progressed to the development of capillaries which dominate the histological picture. Capillary haemangiomata also tend to undergo spontaneous regession in time.

Haemangiopericytomata

Haemangiopericytomata are uncommon tumours of pericytes which occur in adults. The pericytes which proliferate between normal endothelial cells, are individually invested by argyrophilic reticulin fibres, but, in contradistinction to benign haemangioendotheliomata, no framework of small vessels is formed. Metastasis is uncommon, but local recurrence is a troublesome complication.

Racemose or plexiform haemangiomata

Racemose and plexiform haemangiomata are rare and usually occur in adults. They are composed of large tortuous arteries and veins. They often extend forwards so that the plexiform tangle of vessels is visible through the bulbar conjunctiva. Such haemangiomata may pulsate in time with the heart beat and tend to enlarge progressively causing pressure atrophy of surrounding structures including orbital bones.

Arteriovenous fistulas

Although the majority of arteriovenous fistulas are acquired vascular deformations due to trauma, they are included here because they may present clinically in a similar manner to orbital haemangiomata, especially those of the racemose variety. Carotid-cavernous fistulas are the commonest type encountered and the majority of these result from fracture through the base of the skull. Blood under arterial pressure is directed into the ophthalmic veins dilating them into tortuous trunks and causing a variable degree of papilloedema, orbital congestion and chemosis, and in a minority of cases, pulsating exophthalmos. The most constant feature of this condition is a bruit.

Carotid-cavernous fistulas may also develop spontaneously especially in women of middle age and over, when they are attributed to the bursting of a saccular carotid aneurysm into the cavernous sinus. This portion of the artery seems particularly liable to aneurysmal dilatations which presumably occur at points of developmental weakness in the arterial wall.

Lymphangiomata

Lymphangiomata are uncommon, benign, slowly progressive tumours of the lymph vascular system. They may affect the superficial adnexal structures alone, but lesions extending from the adnexa into the orbit or affecting the orbit alone are commoner. They are usually present at birth and progress slowly until early adulthood when growth usually ceases. The superficial lesions are of cosmetic significance alone. Haemorrhage into the deeper lesions may cause acute proptosis and compression of the optic nerve.

Histologically, lymphangiomata typically show thin-walled vascular channels containing serous fluid in a diaphanous fibrous stroma. The fluid contains lymphocytes and often a variable number of erythrocytes. Some of the vascular channels may show pericytes and smooth muscle fibres in their walls and smooth muscle fibres may be scattered through the stroma. Secondary changes from repeated excision or haemorrhage may dominate the picture.

CHAPTER 14

CYSTS

Dermoid and epidermoid cysts

Dermoid cysts

Dermoid cysts result from the continued growth of ectoderm buried beneath the surface along lines of ectodermal closure (sequestration dermoids). In the orbit these run between the inner and outer angles along the lower rim. The majority of dermoid cysts occur at the upper and outer or upper and inner angles. Very occasionally deeply placed dermoid cysts behind the globe are encountered.

Dermoid cysts form smooth tense ovoid swellings not fixed to the skin but often attached to underlying bone which may be excavated or even absent so that the cyst adheres to the dura. Some cysts are dumb-bell in shape with intra- and extraorbital portions connected through a bony hole.

Histologically, dermoid cysts are lined by epidermis surrounded by dermal connective tissue in which are pilosebaceous follicles and sometimes sweat glands. Sebum, keratin and hairs make up the pultaceous contents. Escape of the contents into the tissue excites an intense granulomatous reaction dominated by foreign body giant cells and foam cells. In sections, foreign body giant cells and macrophages sometimes partially replace the lining epidermis. If incompletely removed, dermoid cysts will recur.

Dermoid cysts of the type just described are unrelated to the benign cystic teratomata commonly found in the gonads, mediastinum, retroperitoneum and presacral region which are also sometimes known as 'dermoid cysts'.

Epidermoid cysts (cholesteatoma, pearly tumour)

Though also resulting from embryonic ectodermal sequestration, these cysts differ from dermoid cysts in having a simple epidermal lining without hair follicles or supportive dermal tissue. They contain mainly laminated keratin and cholesterol, but no hairs. Epidermoid cysts are rather common in the cranial cavity, but rare in the orbit where they are found in the roof beneath the periorbita.

Cephalocoeles

A cephalocoele is a herniation of brain into the orbit through a congenital defect in the orbital wall. The wall of the hernial sac may consist of meninges alone (meningocoele) or may include brain (meningoencephalocoele).

Cysts associated with microphthalmos

Microphthalmic eyes may be associated with cysts formed by the protrusion of retinal tissue through a defect in the foetal fissure of the globe (Chapter 17).

ECTOPIC BRAIN

Isolated ectopic brain usually consisting mainly of glia, but containing occasional neurones and sometimes peripheral nerves has occasionally been reported as a cause of proptosis. The lesions are choristomata unassociated with cephalocoeles and cause only local problems (see Newman *et al.*, 1986).

TERATOMATA

Teratomata are tumours containing tissue derived from all three germ layers. They are rare, but often rapidly growing congenital orbital tumours. Most are composed predominantly of epithelium, skin and appendages, and connective tissue, muscle, cartilage or bone. Such tumours in the orbit should perhaps be regarded as choristomata rather than true teratomata (Jensen, 1969). Malignancy is extremely rare.

EMBRYONAL AND MESENCHYMAL TUMOURS OF MUSCLE

Rhabdomyosarcomata

Rhabdomyosarcomata are thought to originate in embryonic mesenchyme which is either prospective muscle or capable of differentiating into muscle. They occur most commonly in the urogenital tract (sarcoma botryoides) and in the head and neck where the site of predilection is the orbit. Rhabdomyosarcoma is the commonest primary malignant tumour of the orbit in children, but is very rare in adults. The average age of onset of is 7 to 8 years.

In most cases, rapidly progressive exophthalmos is the presenting sign, but the neoplasm may first form a mass in the eyelid or beneath the conjunctiva. At first surgery, orbital rhabdomyosarcomas may appear deceptively discrete and seem to 'shell out' cleanly.

Routine radiological and laboratory investigations are usually negative. As far as possible, other rapidly growing orbital tumours of childhood must be excluded. These include benign infantile haemangioendotheliomata, leukaemic infiltrates and secondary neuroblastomata. Haemangioendotheliomata have a florid phase of growth simulating malignancy, but this commonly occurs maximally in the first 6 months of life when rhabdomyosarcomata are rare. Blood and bone marrow examinations will help to exclude leukaemia, while secondary neuroblastomatous deposits often occur first in orbital bones with consequent radiological evidence of bone destruction. A biopsy of the tumour should be examined as soon as possible.

Microscopic appearances

The constituent cells range from primitive mesenchymal cells to myoblasts in varying stages of differentiation. The latter may be round, stellate, spindle shaped or strap-like and sometimes form bizarre giant cells. Nuclei are hyperchromatic and sometimes located at one end of the cell to give a tadpole-like appearance. Cytoplasm is eosinophilic and often abundant. The cells may be sparsely distributed in an oedematous stroma or lie in compact clusters; they may form a syncytium or be arranged in bands. Sometimes an alveolar pattern is simulated. The degree of differentiation may vary in different parts of the tumour, but they can broadly be classified as embryonal (undifferentiated) or differentiated.

The cytoplasm of the strap-like cells in the differentiated tumours is stained brick-red with Masson's trichrome stain (myoglobin) and contains diastase-sensitive, PAS-positive material (glycogen). It may appear stringy due to longitudinal fibrils or it may be banded by cross-striations which are rendered more obvious by staining with phosphotungstic acid haematoxylin (Fig. 14.5a). Careful search of multiple sections may be necessary to reveal cross-striations because cells showing them are seldom numerous. They can be found in approximately 50% of cases, but their demonstration is not essential for diagnosis. By electron microscopy, parallel arrays of myofibrils are found in many cells (Fig. 14.5b), though formation of Z bands is less easy to demonstrate. Positive immunohistochemical reactions to the muscle type intermediate filament proteins myoglobin, myosin, desmin and vimentin can be demonstrated (Hirashima *et al.*, 1986).

Prognosis

Surgical treatment gives a 3 year survival rate of about 25%, though most fatal cases die within a year as a result of local spread to the brain and metastatic spread mainly to lungs and bones. Combined treatment with radiotherapy and chemotherapy appears more promising.

Smooth muscle tumours

Both leiomyomata and their malignant counterpart, leiomyosarcomata, are rare in the orbit.

Granular cell myoblastomata

Granular cell myoblastomata are rare, usually benign, tumours of uncertain histogenesis which have been reported in the orbit (Morgan, 1976). They are composed of clusters and ribbons of rounded or polygonal cells with small central nuclei and cytoplasm crammed with coarse eosinophilic granules. Although benign, they are not encapsulated and tend to infiltrate adjacent structures like a naevus.

ALVEOLAR SOFT PART SARCOMATA

Alveolar soft part sarcomata are rare tumours of soft tissues of uncertain histogenesis which occasionally occur

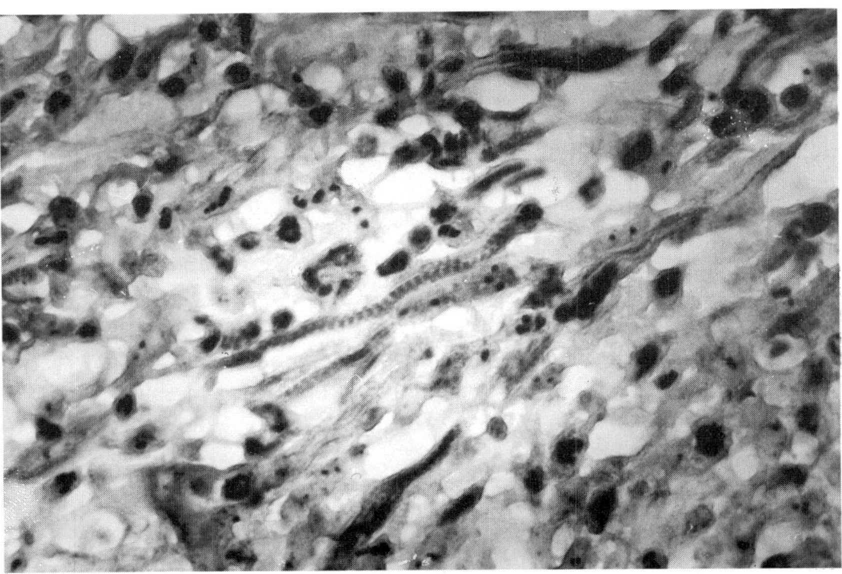

Fig. 14.5 Rhabdomyosarcoma. (a) High power light photomicrograph of elongated rhabdomyoblasts showing cross striation.

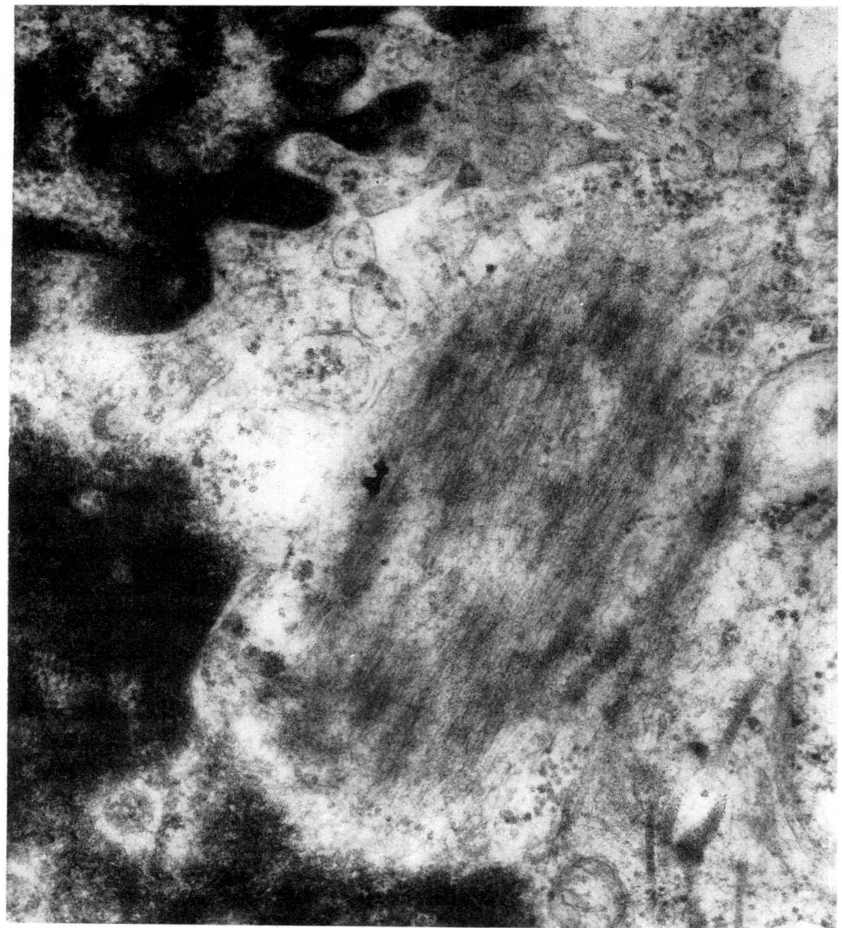

Fig. 14.5 (b) Electron micrograph showing clump of myofibrils within a cell. (×19750).

in the orbit. In a recent series of 17 cases (Font *et al.*, 1982), most patients were under 40 years of age.

The tumours are well circumscribed macroscopically. Microscopically they are composed of clusters of rounded or polygonal cells arranged in a pseudoalveolar pattern (Fig. 14.6). In many cases, the cells contain PAS-positive, diastase resistant crystalline structures which by electron microscopy have a periodicity of 9–10 nm which are pathognomonic.

In the series cited, eight patients were alive and well for follow-up periods of 4 to 16 years. Two died of metastatic disease 14 and 21 years after surgery. A further case had metastases at the time of death from intercurrent disease.

FIBROUS, HISTIOCYTIC AND OSSEOUS LESIONS

Ossifying fibromata (Margo *et al.*, 1985), fibrous dysplasia (Moore *et al.*, 1985) and fibrosarcomata (Weiner *et al.*, 1983) may rarely affect the orbit and aneurysmal bone cysts and chondrosarcomata have occasionally been observed. Several lesions that deserve brief description under this heading are post-irradiational sarcomata, histiocytomata and the histiocytosis-X group.

Post-irradiational sarcomata

A considerable number of cases of sarcoma of the orbit have now been reported following radiotherapy for retinoblastoma. The most common type of tumour is an osteogenic sarcoma, although some fibrosarcomata and other mesenchymal tumours and and occasional carcinoma have also occurred. The latent period between radiotherapy and the appearance of the second tumour is usually between 5 and 25 years. The prognosis is poor.

Fibrous histiocytomata

Fibrous histiocytomata of the orbit have generally been regarded as rare, but Font and Hidayat (1982), have collected 150 cases. The tumours are composed of tangled masses of spindle cells (Fig. 14.7) in which cartwheel (storiform) patterns are commonly seen. Some-

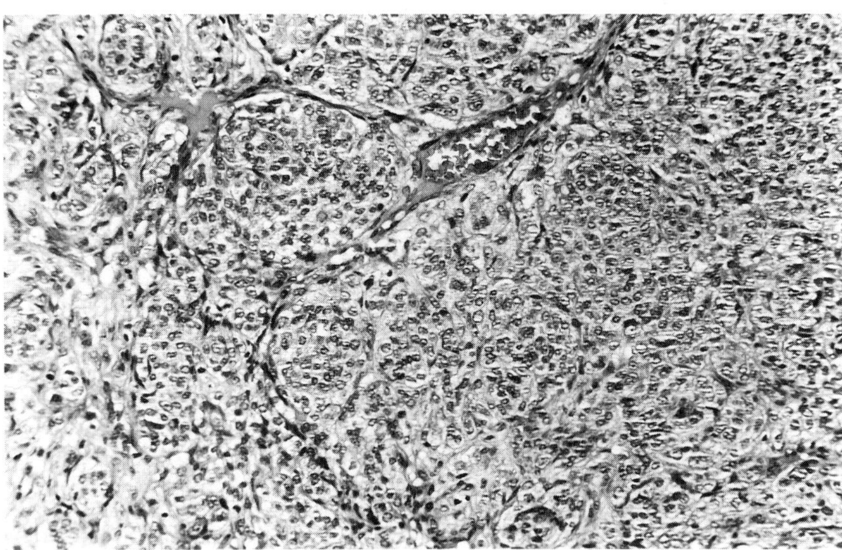

Fig. 14.6 Alveolar soft part sarcoma. Area showing typical arrangement of the cells into compact lobules. H & E (×210).

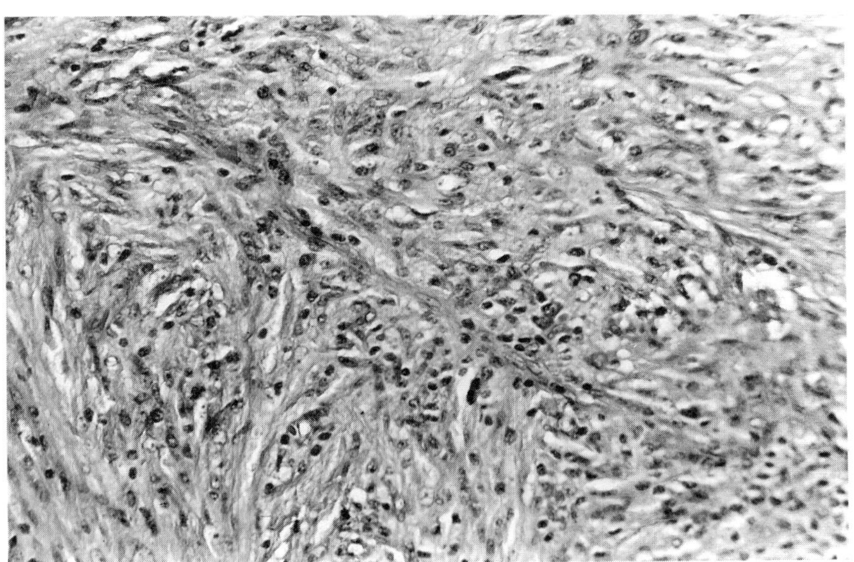

Fig. 14.7 Fibrous histiocytoma. Typical tangled mass of interweaving spindle cells. H & E (×250).

times there is an admixture of lipid-laden histiocytes. There may be pleomorphism and mitotic activity and the tumours can cause serious local problems, but rarely become malignant and metastasise. Most patients have been in middle age.

Histiocytosis-X

Histiocytosis-X comprises a group of three conditions:

1 Letterer–Siwe disease.
2 The Hand–Schuller–Christian syndrome.
3 Eosinophilic granuloma of bone.

In these conditions, apparently benign histiocytes progressively infiltrate soft tissues and bone. The histiocytes contain characteristic Birkbeck granules which appear as rod-shaped organelles by electron microscopy and are derived from Langerhans cells. This distinguishes the group from juvenile xanthogranuloma. In eosinophilic granuloma there is an admixture of eosinophils with the histiocytes. Involvement of the orbit may be the presenting feature in Letterer–Siwe disease and eosinophilic granuloma. In the latter, the disease may be localised to the orbit. The conditions exhibit a wide range of behaviour from the diffuse rapidly fatal condition in infants (Letterer–Siwe disease) to benign solitary lesions in adolescents or young adults.

SECONDARY ORBITAL TUMOURS

Secondary tumours occur in the orbit as a result either of direct invasion from locally situated primary tumours or indirect spread through the bloodstream from more remotely situated primaries. Diffuse malignant diseases such as myelomatosis and leukaemia may also involve the orbit.

Direct invasion

Nasal and nasopharyngeal carcinomata

Carcinomata of the nose and paranasal sinuses account for nearly one third of all secondary orbital tumours. They are commonly of the squamous cell type although transitional cell, anaplastic carcinomata and adenocarcinomata also occur. Most nasopharyngeal carcinomata, on the other hand, are anaplastic and frequently exhibit an intimate mixture of epithelial and lymphoid cells (lymphoepithelial carcinomata). These neoplasms often occur in relatively young patients, often under 30 years of age, and are particularly common in the Mongolian races. They are characterised by early metastases to regional lymph nodes, often from a small symptomless primary growth, and high radiosensitivity.

Malignant nasopharyngeal tumours infiltrate and destroy adjacent structures thereby inducing diverse symptoms and signs:

1 Nasal symptoms: obstruction, discharge and recurrent epistaxes.

2 Oral symptoms due to occlusion of the Eustachian tube: clicking, tinnitus, deafness and pain in the ear.

3 Neuro-ophthalmic symptoms can be the first symptoms of the disease as the neoplasm may enter the middle cranial fossa via the foramen lacerum to press upon and infiltrate cranial nerves III to VI. If the tumour grows upwards and forwards it damages the optic nerve and may enter the orbit through the superior orbital fissure. The results of such infiltration are weakness and paralysis of extraocular muscles, visual impairment, papilloedema or optic atrophy, exophthalmos and trigeminal neuralgia.

Basal and squamous cell carcinomata

Neglected basal and squamous cell carcinomata of the eyelid will eventually invade the orbit.

Malignant melanomata

Choroidal melanomata reach the orbit via the scleral emissary canals or occasionally via the arachnoidal sheath of the optic nerve. Extrascleral extension at enucleation is unusual unless the eye was blind, especially from an old injury which may mask local symptoms. Primary orbital melanomata occur, but are very rare and usually arise as a complication of blue naevi or oculodermal melanocytosis (see Dutton *et al.*, 1984).

Retinoblastomata

Retinoblastomata may reach the orbit via the optic nerve or scleral emissary canals. Such extension greatly worsens the prognosis.

Blood-borne secondaries

Secondary carcinomata

Approximately 10% of all secondary orbital tumours are metastatic carcinomata, of which the majority originate from breast or lung. Metastasis to the orbit occurs considerably less frequently than metastasis to the uveal tract.

Secondary neuroblastomata

Metastatic neuroblastomata are rare tumours found in young children and derived from primary growths in the adrenal medulla or sympathetic ganglia. Metastatic deposits occur in the orbital bones or the orbital soft tissues or both. Radiological evidence of destructive and reactive lesions in the bones of the orbit or skull is present in the majority of cases. Extension of the tumours into the orbital tissues results in exophthalmos, oedema of and haemorrhage into the conjunctiva and lids, and paresis of extraocular muscles. Calcification may be detectable in the orbital mass and there may be increased urinary excretion of vanillyl mandelic acid, a metabolite of adrenalin. Sections show diffuse neoplastic infiltration of the orbital tissue by primitive round or oval neural cells resembling lymphoblasts. Occasionally these cells form small rosettes enclosing a tangle of delicate neurofibrils (Homer Wright rosettes) or exhibit maturation to ganglion cells (ganglioneuroblastoma).

Myeloid leukaemias

The orbit is a site of predilection for myeloid leukaemic infiltrations. When such infiltration of the orbital bones and soft tissues occurs it usually does so late in the disease. Occasionally, however, and particularly in children, an orbital tumour is the first manifestation of acute myeloid leukaemia, occurring at a time when the child is still clinically well. Biopsies from such tumours show a dense infiltration by mononuclear cells which are difficult to categorise. Presumptive evidence that they belong to the granulocyte series may be obtained by noting the presence of eosinophilic myelocytes which are easily recognised in sections. Confirmation of their identity may be obtained by special staining and electron microscopy (Fig. 14.8).

Fig. 14.8 Granulocytic leukaemia presenting as orbital mass. (a) Light microscopic appearance of the tumour showing large cells with indented nuclei containing a large nucleolus. H & E (×620).

Fig. 14.8 (b) (*Below*) Electron micrograph showing typical myeloid character of the cells. (×15 900). Before electron microscopy was carried out the case was thought to be an immunoblastic lymphoma. The bone marrow showed leukaemic transformation 6 months after presentation.

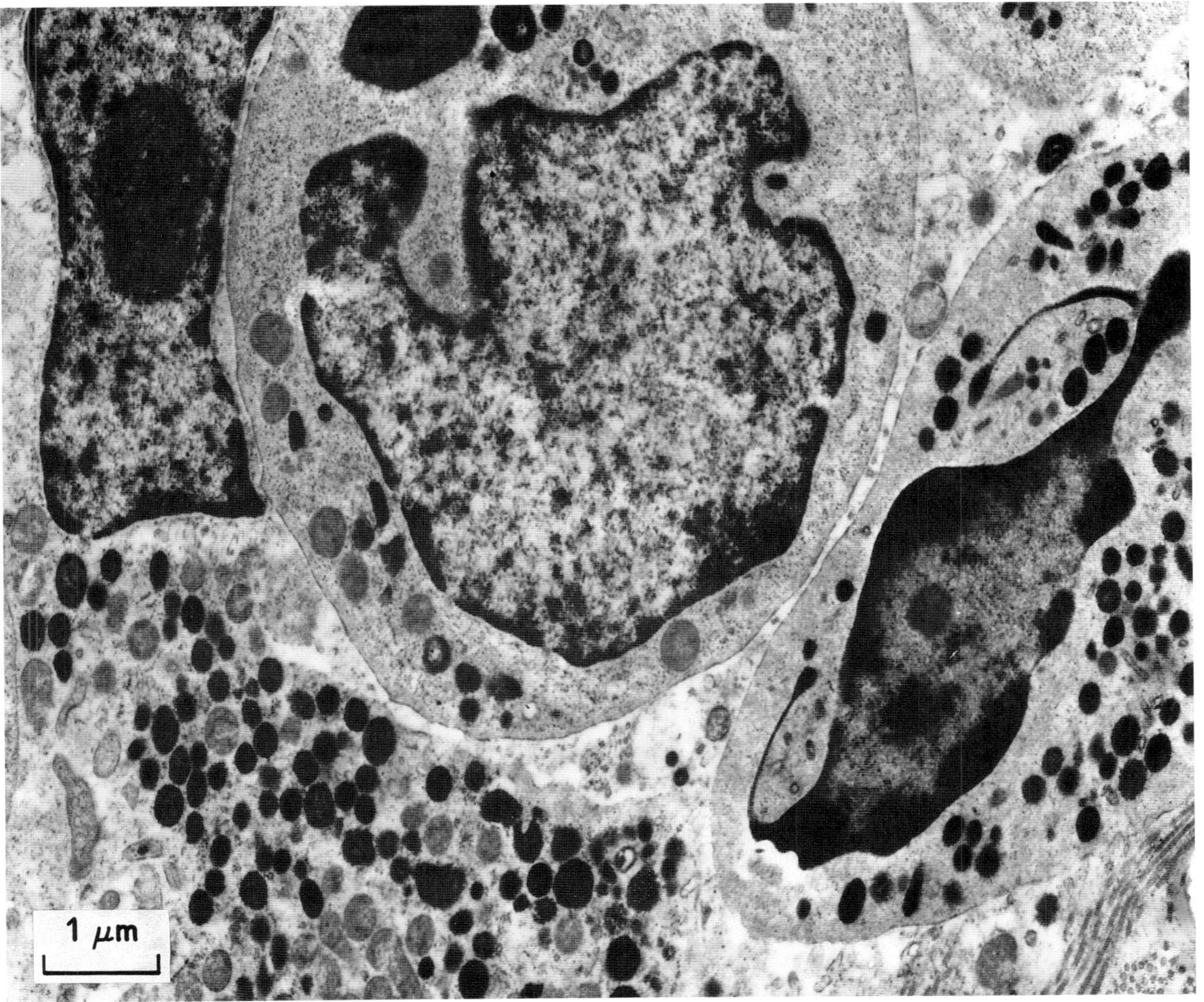

Myelomatosis

Orbital involvement in myelomatosis is uncommon, but proptosis, diplopia and visual impairment can be an initial manifestation of the disease.

Amyloid may be deposited in the orbital bones in myelomatosis. Local deposits of amyloid of sufficient size to cause proptosis also occur in the absence of myelomatosis or any other form of systemic amyloidosis. The nature of these is uncertain, but they usually contain plasma cells and possibly represent 'burnt out' local plasmacytomata (see Lucas *et al.*, 1981).

LACRIMAL APPARATUS

Lacrimal gland tumours

Only 50% of expanding lesions arising in the lacrimal gland or immediately adjacent tissues are neoplasms derived from lacrimal epithelium. Of the remaining 50%, the great majority are non-neoplastic conditions such as reactive lymphoid hyperplasias or lymphomata (Chapter 16) or inflammatory lesions involving the lacrimal gland.

Primary epithelial neoplasm of the lacrimal gland are almost unknown in childhood and rarely, if ever, bilateral at any age. The presence of an expanding lesion in the lacrimal area in a child should suggest the possibility of a dermoid cyst, eosinophilic granuloma or fibrous dysplasia (juvenile ossifying fibroma).

Biopsy is usually necessary to establish a diagnosis. Unfortunately, this makes the recurrence of a benign mixed tumour much more likely and may well worsen the already poor prognosis for malignant tumours.

Slightly more than 50% of all epithelial tumours of the lacrimal gland are pleomorphic adenomata, while a further 25–30% are adenoid cystic carcinomata. Mucoepidermoid tumours, so called because they contain both mucussecreting cells and squamous cells, may infiltrate locally and occasionally metastasise. Although common in the parotid they are very rare in the lacrimal gland.

Pleomorphic adenomata (benign mixed tumours)

Benign mixed tumours of the lacrimal gland occur most commonly in men in the fourth decade of life. They form solitary growths with a greyish white, moist or slimy, lobulated cut surface and a pressure pseudocapsule which may be incomplete or microscopically penetrated by the tumour. Prognosis is good if the whole lacrimal gland is removed without capsular rupture. Recurrences may sometimes occur many years after initial surgery. Histological structure is very varied and both epithelial and stromal components are involved (Fig. 14.9).

Epithelial component: the epithelial component is derived from both the epithelial and myoepithelial cells of the lacrimal ducts. They are characteristically cuboidal with prominent oval nuclei and form poorly defined islands with irregular outlines, slender branching strands, cysts, ducts and acini. Mitotic figures are not seen. From the margins of such formations the neoplastic cells sprout and spray out into the stroma and in the process become elongated or stellate and are detached from their source. The tumour cells may develop into both basal and squamous cells; they may also form small epidermoid knots and epidermal cysts packed with laminated keratin.

Stromal component: the peculiar and usually abundant stroma in which the epithelial formations are embedded varies in appearance. In some areas it is blue and mucoid, in others chondroid, while elsewhere it is fibrous or hyalinised. There is evidence that the chondroid type of stroma originates from neoplastic myoepithelial cells. In addition, true cartilage and even bone may develop in the stroma; this is brought about by metaplasia of connective tissue cells.

Carcinomata in pleomorphic adenoma (malignant mixed tumours)

These tumours results from carcinomatous change in a pleomorphic adenoma. Microscopically, areas characteristic of pleomorphic adenoma are associated with a carcinomatous component which may constitute most of the neoplasm or form only a small part of it. The malignant component may have features of any of the types of carcinoma which occur in the lacrimal gland. Multiple sections from different parts of the growth are essential to make sure that malignant areas are not missed.

Adenoid cystic carcinomata

Clinical features: adenoid cystic carcinomata occur most frequently in adults of either sex in the fourth decade of life. Prognosis is poor. Five year survival is of the order of 20–30%. The tumour is responsive to radiotherapy, but not radio-curable. The slow but remorseless natural evolution of these carcinomata is characterised by:

1 Infiltration into contiguous bones which induces radiologically detectable hyperostosis.

2 Spread along perineural and intraneural lymphatic channels which often causes pain. These spaces provide a ready passage into adjacent soft tissues and bone.

3 Invasion anteriorly and subconjunctivally into the lid and posteriorly into the orbital tissues and eventually into the base of the brain.

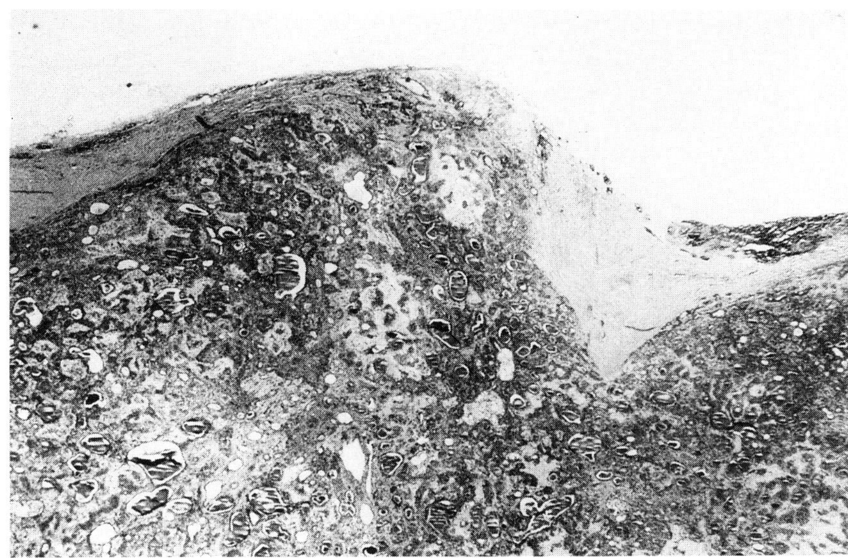

Fig. 14.9 Benign mixed tumour of lacrimal gland. (a) Low power showing thick fibrous capsule through which the tumour has, however, ruptured.

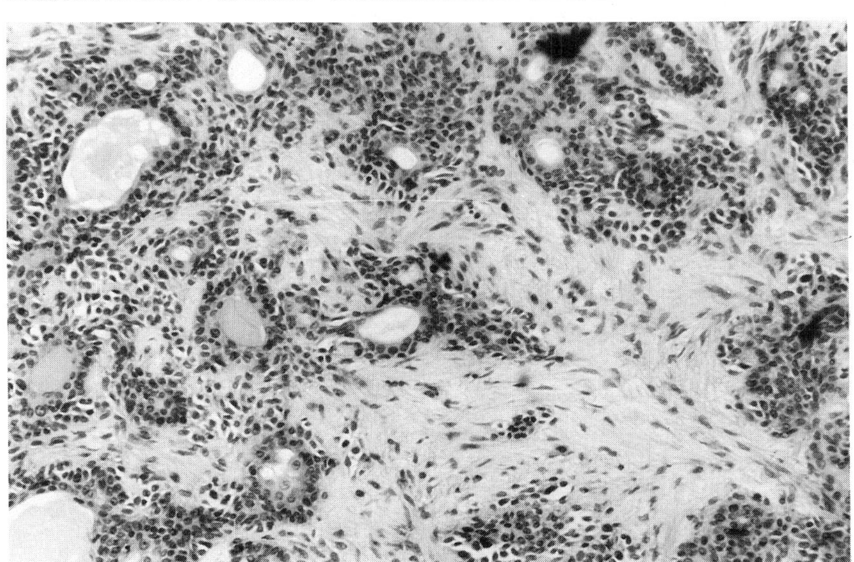

Fig. 14.9 (b) Higher power showing typical acini with two tiers of cells.

4 Metastasis to pre-auricular and cervical lymph nodes.
5 Blood-borne metastasis to lung, bone and skin may occur as a late complication.

Microscopic features: adenoid cystic carcinomata consist of a mosaic of lobules and anastomosing cords of myoepithelial cells with hyperchromatic nuclei and scanty cytoplasm. Cells in mitosis are often numerous. Within the lobules mucoid material collects in sharply defined round spaces producing a cribriform appearance ('Swiss cheese pattern') which is typical. In some tumours the lobules are more solidly cellular while in others duct-like structures lined by cuboidal cells and containing PAS-positive secretion are an additional and prominent feature. There is a close resemblance to adenoid cystic basal cell carcinomata and confusion in diagnosis is possible in a specimen in which anatomical relationships have been lost (Fig. 14.10).

Tumours with a predominantly cribriform pattern appear to be associated with longer survival (Lee *et al.*, 1985).

Other carcinomata

Under this heading are included relatively rare forms of carcinoma including adenocarcinomata, squamous cell and mucoepidermoid carcinomata as well as undifferentiated carcinomata in which the character and arrangement of the cells do not permit classification.

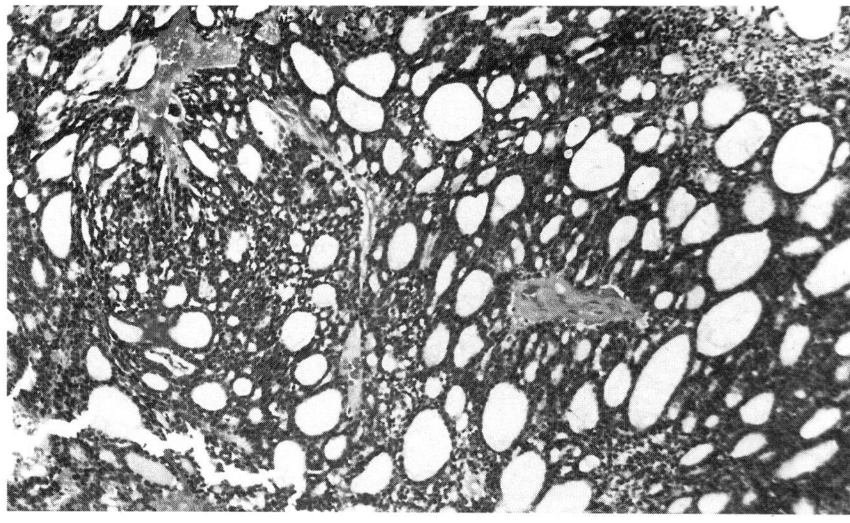

Fig. 14.10 Adenoid cystic carcinoma of lacrimal gland. (a) Cribriform ('Swiss cheese') pattern. H & E (×95).

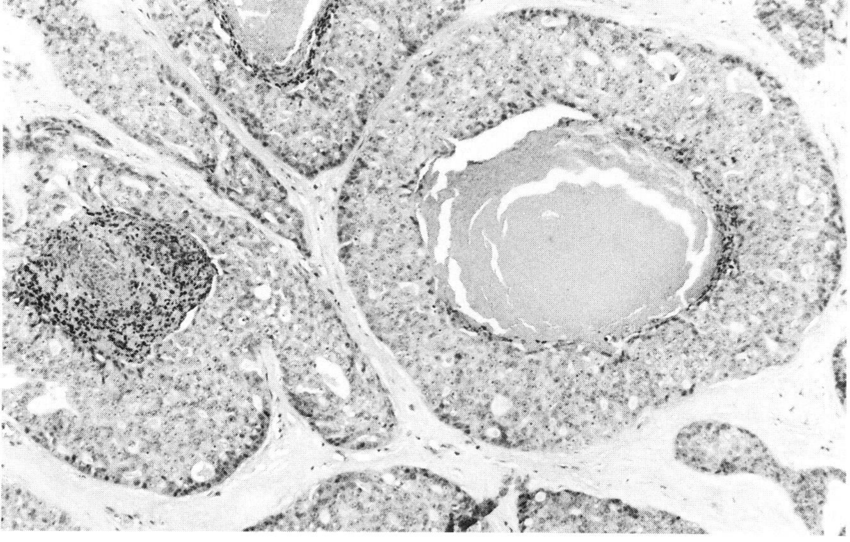

Fig. 14.10 (b) More solid lobules of cells with necrotic centres. H & E (×95).

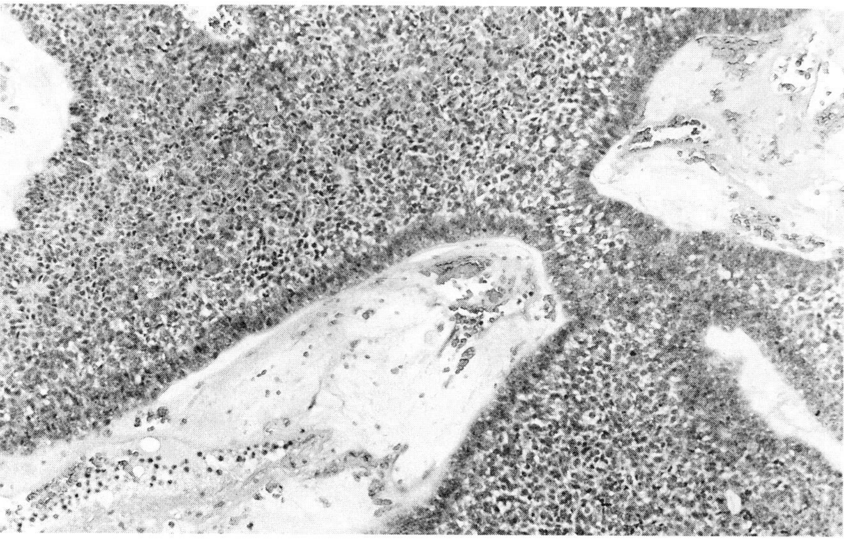

Fig. 14.10 (c) Area showing 'basaloid' appearance. H & E (×95).

Tumours of the lacrimal drainage system

Neoplasms of any kind are rare in the lacrimal drainage system. The majority are papillomata or carcinomata which resemble those arising from the comparable pseudostratified columnar epithelium of the nose and paranasal sinuses.

Papillomata

Papillomata are typically exophytic growths projecting into the lumen of the sac, but some exhibit infolding of the epithelium into the underlying stroma-inverted papillomata. The epithelium is usually transitional in type and consists of elongated columnar and fusiform cells among which are mucus-secreting goblet cells. Squamous metaplasia occurs and some papillomas may be entirely squamous cell. Such papillomata are benign, but may recur if not completely removed. Epithelial dysplasia, carcinoma *in situ* and actual malignant transformation may, however, occur.

Carcinomata

Carcinomata of the sac may be undifferentiated, transitional, squamous cell or occasionally adenoid in type. They commonly show a papillary structure.

Chronic dacryocystitis

Chronic dacryoadenitis comprises a range of conditions from dacryops due to ductal obstruction in which inflammatory changes are minimal, to sclerosing pseudotumour with well-marked inflammatory changes.

Chronic dacryocystitis

As a result of repeated inflammatory episodes presumably related to obstruction of the duct, the wall of the sac becomes thickened and fibrotic and is diffusely infiltrated with a mixture of inflammatory cells. Formation of lymphoid follicles with germinal centres is often conspicuous and goblet cells are usually numerous in the lining epithelium. The lumen contains mucopurulent material.

The lacrimal gland in Sjögren's syndrome

In most cases of Sjögren's syndrome the lacrimal and salivary glands are not enlarged. They show lymphocytic infiltration, progressive fibrosis and atrophy. Occasionally, however, infiltration by lymphocytes and plasma cells may be so massive that enlargement occurs. Mention must also be made of a particular form of lymphoid hyperplasia called the benign lymphoepithelial lesion of Godwin which sometimes occurs in the lacrimal and salivary glands. It may be a manifestation of rheumatoid disease and shows an inconstant association with Sjögren's syndrome. Microscopically the glands exhibit intense lymphocytic infiltration which almost entirely replaces the secreting acini. The epithelial and myoepithelial cells of the intralobular ducts proliferate to form cellular islands in a sea of lymphocytes. Progressive hyalinisation of the islands occurs due to deposition of basement membrane material around and between the component cells. These changes have long been recognised as Miculiczs' syndrome. Unfortunately, the eponym has also been applied to cases of simultaneous enlargement of lacrimal and salivary glands from any cause and now has no specific pathological connotation.

Sarcoidosis of the lacrimal gland

Sarcoidosis is the most common specific granuloma to involve the lacrimal gland where it causes painless enlargement which may be unilateral or bilateral. The enlargement may be asymptomatic or there may be decreased tearing. Simultaneous involvement of the salivary glands may thus produce a picture resembling Sjögren's or Miculiczs' syndromes. If there is an associated uveitis, the combination is known as Heerfordt's syndrome.

Biopsy sections should be examined carefully to exclude the presence of acid-fast bacilli and a histological diagnosis of sarcoidosis not accepted until supported by other clinical, radiological and laboratory evidence.

BIBLIOGRAPHY

General

Blodi, F. C. (1975) Unusual orbital tumours and their treatment. *Modern Problems in Ophthalmology* **14**, 565–588.

Boniuk, M., ed. (1964) In *Ocular and Adnexal Tumours*, Section IV. C. V. Mosby Co., St Louis.

Jakobiec, F. A., ed. (1978) In *Ocular and Adnexal Tumours*, Section V. Aesculapius Publishing Co., Birmingham, Ala.

Jakobiec, F. A. & Tannenbaum, M. (1975) Classification of orbital tumours based on electron microscopy. *Modern Problems in Ophthalmology* **14**, 330–343.

Jones, I. S. & Jakobiek, F. A., eds (1979) *Diseases of the Orbit*. Harper & Row, Hagerstown.

Porterfield, J. F. (1962) Orbital tumours in children: a report on 214 cases. *International Ophthalmology Clinics* **2(2)**, 319–335.

Reese, A. B. (1971) Expanding lesions of the orbit. *Transactions of the Opthalmological Society of the UK* **91**, 85–104.

Reese, A. B., ed. (1976) In *Tumours of the Eye*, 3rd edn., pp 303–466. Harper & Row, Hagerstown.

Rootman, J., Quenville, N. & Owen, D. (1984) Recent advances in pathology as applied to orbital biopsy. *Ophthalmology* **91**, 708–718.

Wright, J. E. (1979) Introduction to symposium on orbital tumours. *Transactions of the Ophthalmological Society of the UK* **99**, 216–219.

Zimmerman, L. E. (1973) Orbital tumours in children. *Medical Problems in Ophthalmology* **14**, 305.

Inflammatory diseases

Chavis, R. M., Garner, A. & Wright, J. E. (1978) Inflammatory orbital pseudotumour. A clinicopathologic study. *Archives of Ophthalmology* **96**, 1817–1822.

Garner, A. (1973) Pathology of pseudotumours of the orbit. *Journal of Clinical Pathology* **26**, 639–648.

Spalton, D. J., Graham, E. M., Page, N. G. R. & Sanders, M. D. (1981) Ocular changes in limited forms of Wegener's granulomatosis. *British Journal of Ophthalmology* **65**, 553–563.

Sarcoidosis

Benedict, W. L. (1949) Sarcoidosis involving the orbit. Report of two cases. *Archives of Ophthalmology* **42**, 546–550.

Collinson, J. M. T., Miller, N. R. & Green, W. R. (1986) Involvement of orbital tissues by sarcoid. *American Journal of Ophthalmology* **102**, 302–307.

Leino, M., Tuovinen, E. & Romppanen, T. (1982) Orbital sarcoidosis. A case report. *Acta Ophthalmologica* **60**, 809–814.

Graves' ophthalmopathy

Campbell, R. J. (1984) Pathology of Graves' ophthalmology. In *The Eye and Orbit in Thyroid Disease*, pp 25–32. Raven Press, New York.

Gorman, C. A., Waller, R. R. Waller & J. A. DyerGorman, C. A., Waller, R. R. & Dyer, J. A., eds (1984) *The Eye and Orbit in Thyroid Disease*, Raven Press, New York, 1984.

Sergott, R. C. & Glaser, J. S. (1981) Graves' ophthalmopathy. A clinical and immunological review. *Survey of Opthalmology* **26**, 1–21.

Vascular tumours and abnormalities

Iliff, W. J. & Green, W. R. (1979) Orbital lymphangiomas. *Ophthalmology* **86**, 914–929.

Jones, I. S. (1959) Lymphangiomas of the ocular adnexa: an analysis of 62 cases. *Transactions of the American Opthalmological Society* **57**, 602–665.

Rootman, J., Hay, E., Graeb, D. & Miller, R. (1986) Orbital-adnexal lymphangiomas. A spectrum of haemodynamically isolated vascular hamartomas. *Ophthalmology* **93**, 1558–1570.

Searl, S. S. & Ni, C. (1982) Haemangiopericytoma. *International Ophthalmology Clinics* **22(1)**, 141–162.

Ectopic brain

Newman, N. J., Miller, N. R. & Green, W. R. (1986) Ectopic brain in the orbit. *Ophthalmology* **93**, 268–272.

Teratomata

Garden, J. W. & McManis, J. C. (1986) Congenital orbital-intracranial teratoma with subsequent malignancy: case report. *British Journal of Ophthalmology* **70**, 111–113.

Jensen, O. A. (1969) Teratoma of the orbit. *Acta Ophthalmologica* **47**, 317–327.

Levin, M. L., Leone, C.R. & Kincaid, M. C. (1986) Congenital orbital teratomas. *American Journal of Ophthalmology* **102**, 476–481.

Primary tumours

Ashton, N. & Morgan, G. (1965) Embryonal sarcoma and embryonal rhabdomyosarcoma of the orbit. *Journal of Clinical Pathology* **18**, 619–714.

Dutton, J. J., Anderson, R. L., Schelper, R. L., Purcell, J. J. & Tse, D T. (1984) Orbital malignant melanoma and oculodermal melanocytosis: report of two cases and review of the literature. *Ophthalmology* **91**, 497–507.

Font, R. L., Jurco III, S. & Zimmerman, L. E. (1982) Alveolar soft-part sarcoma of the orbit: a clinicopathologic analysis of seventeen cases and a review of the literature. *Human Pathology* **13**, 569–579.

Forrest, A. W. (1962) Tumours following radiation about the eye. *International Ophthalmology Clinics* **2(2)**, 543–553.

Grant, G. D., Shields, J. A., Flanagah, J. C. & Horowitz, P. (1979) The ultrasonographic and radiological features of a histologically proven case of alveolar soft part sarcoma of the orbit. *American Journal of Ophthalmology* **87**, 773–777.

Harry, J. (1975) Pathology of rhabdomyosarcoma. *Modern Problems in Ophthalmology* **14** 325–329.

Hirashima, S., Matsushita, Y. & Sameshima, M. (1986) Orbital rhabdomyosarcoma: case report with immunohistochemical detection of muscle cell type intermediate type filament proteins. *Japanese Journal of Ophthalmology* **30**, 461–471.

Knowles II, D. M., Jakobiec, F. A., Potter, G. D. & Jones, I.S. (1976) Ophthalmic striated muscle neoplasms. *Survey of Ophthalmology* **21**, 219–261.

Morgan, G. (1976) Granular cell myoblastoma of the orbit. *Archives of Ophthalmology* **94**, 2135–2142.

Nuutinen, J., Karja, J. & Sainio, P. (1982) Epithelial second malignant tumours in retinoblastoma survivors. A review and report of a case. *Acta Ophthalmologica* **60** 133–140.

Porterfield, J. T. & Zimmerman, L. E. (1962) Rhabdomyosarcoma of the orbit: a clinicopathologic study of 55 cases. *Virchows Archives of Pathological Anatomy* **335**, 329–344.

Sauborn, G. E., Valenzuela, R. E. & Green, W. R. (1979) *American Journal of Ophthalmology* **87**, 371–375.

Soloway, H. (1966) Radiation-induced neoplasms following curative therapy for retinoblastoma. *Cancer* **19**, 1984–1988.

Vigstrup, J. & Glenthøj, A. (1982) Leiomyoma of the irbit. *Acta Opthalmologica* **60**, 992–997.

Weiner, J. M. & Hidayat, A. A. (1983) Juvenile fibrosarcoma of the orbit and eyelid. A study of five cases. *Archives of Ophthalmology* **101**, 253–259.

Wharam, M., Beltangady, M., Hays, D., Weyn, R. I., Ragab, A., Soule, E. I., Teft, M. & Maurer, H. (1987) Localised orbital rhabdomyosarcoma. An interim report of the Intergroup Rhabdomyosarcoma Study Committee. *Ophthalmology* **94**, 251–254.

Fibrous, histiocytic and osseous lesions

Baghdassarian, S. A. & Shammas, H. F. (1977) Eosinophilic granuloma of orbit. *Annals of Ophthalmology* **9**, 1247–1257.

Donoso, L. A., Magargal, L. E. & Eiferman, R. A. (1982) Fibrous dysplasia of the orbit with optic nerve decompression. *Annals of Ophthalmology* **14**, 80–83.

Font, R. L. & Hidayat, A. A. (1982) Fibrous histiocytoma in the orbit: a clinico-pathologic study of 150 cases. *Human Pathology* **13**, 199–209.

Krishnan, M. M., Kawatra, V. K., Ratnaker, C., Rao, V. A. & Vehath, A. J. (1987) Ocular malignant fibrous histiocytoma: clinical and histopathological characteristics. *British Journal of Ophthalmology* **71**, 864–866.

Margo, C. E., Ragsdale, B. D., Perman, K. I., Zimmerman, L. E. & Sweet, D. E. (1985) Psammomatoid (juvenile) ossifying fibroma of the orbit. *Ophthalmology* **92**, 150–159.

Momoeda, S. & Ishikawa, Y. (1976) Eosinophilic granuloma of the orbit: report of a case and some ultrastructural findings of histiocytes in the lesion. *Japanese Journal of Ophthalmology* **20**, 119–124.

Moore, A. T., Buncic, J. R. & Munro, I. R. (1985) Fibrous dysplasia of the orbit in childhood. Clinical features and management. *Ophthalmology* **92**, 12–20.

Rodgrigues, M., Furgiuele, F. P. & Weinreb, S. (1977) Malignant fibrous histiocytoma of the orbit. *Archives of Ophthalmology* **95**, 2025–2028.

Secondary tumours

Davis, J. L., Parke II, D. W. & Font, R. L. (1985) Granulocytic sarcoma of the orbit. *Ophthalmology* **92**, 1758–1762.

Ferry, A. P. & Font, R. L. (1975) Carcinoma metastatic to the orbit. *Modern Problems in Ophthalmology* **14**, 377–381.

Fratkin, J. D., Shammas, H. F. & Miller, S. D. (1978) Disseminated Hodgkin's disease with bilateral orbital involvement. *Archives of Ophthalmology* **96**, 102–104.

Amyloid deposits

Knowles II, D. M., Jakobiec, F. A., Rosen, M. & Howard, D. (1979) Amyloidosis of the orbit and adnexae. *Survey of Ophthalmology* **19**, 367–383.

Lucas, D. R., Knox, F. & Davies, S. (1981) Apparent monoclonal origin of lymphocytes and plasma cells infiltrating ocular adnexal amyloid deposits: report of 2 cases. *British Journal of Ophthalmology* **66**, 600–606.

Nehen, J. K. (1979) Primary localized amyloidosis. *Acta Ophthalmologica* **57**, 287–295.

Tumours of lacrimal apparatus

Ashton, N. (1973) Epithelial tumours of the lacrimal gland. *Modern Problems in Ophthalmology* **14**, 306–323.

Font, R. L. & Gamel, J. W. (1980) Adenoid cystic carcinoma of the lacrimal gland. A clinicopathologic study of 79 cases. In *Ocular Pathology Update*, ed. D. H. Nicholson, pp 227–283. Masson, New York.

Harry, J. & Ashton, N. (1968) The pathology of tumours of the lacrimal sac. *Transactions of the Ophthalmological Society of the UK* **88**, 19–35.

Lee, D. A., Campbell, R. J., Waller, R. R. & Ilstrup, D. M. (1985) A clinicopathologic study of primary adenoid cystic carcinoma of the lacrimal gland. *Ophthalmology* **92**, 128–134.

Ni, C., D'Amico, D. J., Fan, C. Q. & Kuo, P. K. (1981) Tumours of the lacrimal sac: a clinicopathologic analysis of 82 cases. *International Ophthalmology Clinics* **22(1)**, 121–140.

Nicholson, D. H., ed. (1980) Tumours of the lacrimal gland. In *Ocular Pathology Update*, pp 271–275. Masson, New York.

Ryan, S. J. & Font, R. L. (1973) Primary epithelial neoplasms of the lacrimal sac. *American Journal of Ophthalmology* **76**, 73–88.

Wright, J. E. (1982) Factors affecting the survival of patients with lacrimal gland tumours. *Canadian Journal of Ophthalmology* **17**, 3–9.

Witschel, H. & Zimmerman, L. E. (1981) Malignant mixed tumour of the lacrimal gland. A clinicopathologic report of two unusual cases. *Albrecht von Graefes Archiv für Klinische Ophthalmologie* **216**, 327–337.

Sjögren's syndrome

Font, R. L., Yanoff, M. & Zimmerman, L. E. (1967) Benign lymphoepithelial lesion of the lacrimal gland and its relationship to Sjögren's syndrome. *American Journal of Clinical Pathology* **48**, 365–376.

Ryan, S. J. & Font, R. L. (1973) Primary epithelial neoplasms of the lacrimal sac. *American Journal of Ophthalmology* **76**, 73–88.

Williamson, J., Gibson, A. A. M., Wilson, T., Forrester, J. V., Whaley, K. & Dick, W. C. (1973) Histology of the lacrimal gland in keratoconjunctivitis sicca. *British Journal of Ophthalmology* **57**, 852–858.

Chapter 15 Neural tumours and phacomatoses

PHACOMATOSES

The phacomatoses comprise a number of syndromes in which various organ systems, particularly the eye, central nervous system and skin, are affected by tissue malformations (hamartia) or hamartomata. The term phacoma was devised to indicate a mother spot or birthmark (see Font & Ferry, 1972). Since neurofibromatosis is the commonest and most important disease in this group it is convenient to include in this chapter a note on the structure of peripheral nerves and a description of neurilemmomata.

STRUCTURE OF PERIPHERAL NERVES

A knowledge of the structure of peripheral nerves is helpful in understanding the derivation of some of the lesions described in this chapter.

A large peripheral nerve consists of several separate fascicles bound in a layer of loose connective tissue (epineurium). Each fascicle contains numerous nerve fibres enclosed in a thin, tough, lamellated outer fibrous sheath (perineurium) which resists longitudinal stretching. Small nerves, e.g. ciliary nerves, consist of a single fascicle with its perineural sheath. The nerve fibres within a fascicle are embedded in a network of fine fibrils (endoneurium) which condenses to form an endoneural tube around each fibre. Some or all the endoneural fibrocytes may, like Schwann cells, be derived from the neural crest.

There is a plexus of small blood vessels in the perineurium and these acquire a perineural sheath as they enter the endoneurium. A functional blood–nerve barrier comparable to the blood–brain barrier has been demonstrated.

Each myelinated nerve fibre consists of an axon and a myelin sheath provided by Schwann cells. The axon is a prolongation of the cytoplasm of a neurone and contains mitochondria and many fine filaments. The myelin sheath is periodically interrupted along its length by apparent constrictions (nodes of Ranvier) which are boundaries between individual Schwann cells. In the process of myelination, the Schwann cells rotate around the long axis of the axon, wrapping it in successive layers of lipid-rich plasmalemmal membrane. During this process, most of the cytoplasm is squeezed from between the plasmalemmal membranes. The myelin sheath thus consists of a double layer of these membranes and has a spiral form when seen in section under the electron microscope. A small amount of Schwann cell cytoplasm remains in several locations such as around the cell nucleus. Unmyelinated nerve fibres, which have only a trace of covering myelin, are in general smaller and up to 12 or more may be enclosed in the cytoplasm of a single Schwann cell.

NEURILEMMOMATA (SCHWANNOMATA)

Neurilemmomata are benign tumours which originate from the neuroectodermal Schwann cells of peripheral nerves. Neurilemmomata commonly arise centrally in the spinal and cranial nerve roots, e.g. acoustic neuroma, whereas neurofibromata are most frequently of cutaneous distribution,. Though not common in the ocular field, they occur in the lids, conjunctiva and orbit. In the orbit they may be intraconal or extraconal.

Neurilemmomata are usually solitary, but about 20% occur in association with neurofibromatosis when they are often multiple. They grow slowly and expansively from within the perineurium to form rubbery circumscribed, encapsulated, spherical or fusiform tumours eccentric to their nerve of origin, the fibres of which are spread out over the surface. The centre of the tumour is often cystic. Neurilemmomata exhibit two main and contrasting cellular patterns both of which are usually present in the same tumour (Fig. 15.1):

1 *Antoni A:* elongated cells lie side by side in rows or palisades or form interlacing bundles and whorls. Abundant reticulin fibres pass between the cells to form zones free of nuclei between the palisades. Cross-sections of the cells show each to be surrounded by a delicate collagenous membrane reinforced by fine reticulin fibrils. The cells and fibres may be arranged in nodules (Verocay bodies) which have been likened to enlarged Wagner–Meissner tactile corpuscles.

2 *Antoni B:* cells of various sizes form a loose meshwork often with abundant intercellular spaces containing watery or bluish mucoid fluid. Cyst formation occurs and fatty change results in the appearance of aggregates of foam cells.

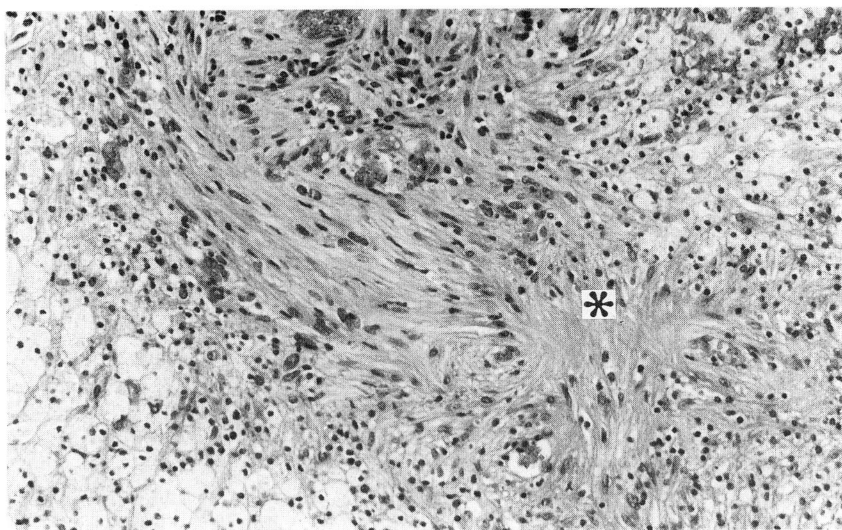

Fig. 15.1 Neurilemmoma. Note the foam cells which which are particularly conspicuous in an Antoni Type B area in the bottom left. Regimentation of the Antoni type A fibres is evident in the centre of the picture with the formation of a Verocay body (asterisk). H & E (×160).

Hyalinised small arteries with argyrophilic fibres in their walls are often seen in neurilemmomata.

NEUROFIBROMATOSIS

Solitary neurofibromata sometimes occur in the orbit and lids without other evidence of disease, but many of the neurofibromata encountered in ophthalmic practice are part of generalised neurofibromatosis.

Neurofibromatosis is an hereditary disease characterised by widespread hyperplasia and neoplasia of the supportive tissue of the whole nervous system both central and peripheral including the autonomic system. The disease is transmitted by an autosomal dominant gene with a high mutation rate. Penetrance is also high, but expression is very variable so that abortive and incomplete forms of the disease are common. The influence of the gene falls mainly on the sheath tissues of the peripheral nerves, to a lesser extent on the supportive glia of the central nervous system and least often on the leptomeninges. When peripheral lesions are numerous and gross, few lesions are found in the central nervous system and the converse is also true. In general terms, therefore, neurofibromatosis manifests itself either in a peripheral form or in a central form and the two tend to be mutually exclusive. For descriptive purposes, the protean expressions of the disease fall conveniently into three categories:

1 Peripheral manifestations.
2 Central manifestations.
3 Ocular manifestations.

Peripheral manifestations

Peripheral neurofibromata are the commonest manifestation of the disease and occur anywhere along the course of the peripheral and autonomic nerves from their roots to their terminals in the skin or viscera. They do not apparently occur on purely motor nerves (P. O. Yates, personal communication.) These tumours may be divided into several descriptive categories which are all manifestations of the same process of nerve sheath proliferation.

Cutaneous neurofibromata

Cutaneous neurofibromata commonly appear as multiple small soft nodules which are frequently associated with *café au lait* spots in the overlying epidermis. Mollusca fibrosa are usually larger and present as soft, projecting, sometimes pedunculated growths in the skin.

Plexiform neurofibromata

Plexiform neurofibromata are formed as a result of a nerve and its branches undergoing diffuse thickening and sometimes becoming beaded. The tortuous tangled fibres can be felt under the skin.

Elephantiasis neuromatosa

Elephantiasis neuromatosa results from a diffuse proliferation of sheath tissue throughout long segments of nerves in their course from the spine to their terminals. Such proliferation is often gross in degree and, being associated with thickened, redundant, hairy and pigmented skin, results in most unsightly deformations sometimes of whole limbs or large segments of the body surface.

Osseous lesions

Osseous lesions occur when intra-osseous nerves are affected by the neurofibromatous process. They may result in destruction or hypertrophy of bone.

Microscopic structure

Neurofibromata are composed of thin elongated cells with comma-shaped nuclei arranged in interlacing cords, whorls and eddies or just haphazardly. Collagen fibres are abundant and characteristically wavy. The growth is pierced by nerve fibres either singly or in fasicles (Fig. 15.2). Oedema is common, inducing a reticular pattern. Mast cells are present scattered through the stroma.

The tumours are characteristically diffuse and unencapsulated and the nerve fascicles, whether seen in transverse or longitudinal section, appear to have undergone expansion and thickening by a diffuse proliferation of all their sheath tissues including both Schwann cells and the fibrocytes of the endoneurium and perineurium. This proliferation may be confined within the perineural sheath or extend beyond it into the adjacent tissues.

Central manifestations

Most of the central manifestations of neurofibromatosis are beyond the scope of this book; however, include:

1 Neurilemmomata of the cranial and spinal nerve roots.
2 Tumours of the brain, cord and meninges:
  (i) Meningiomata, often multiple.
  (ii) Ependymomata, especially in the central canal of the spinal cord.

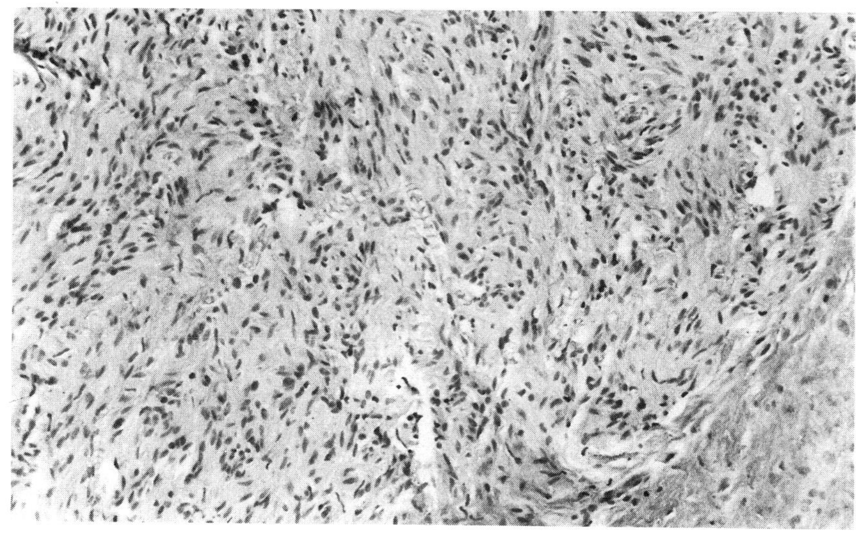

Fig. 15.2 Neurofibroma. (a) Low power showing rather ill-defined arrangment into bundles. H & E (×160).

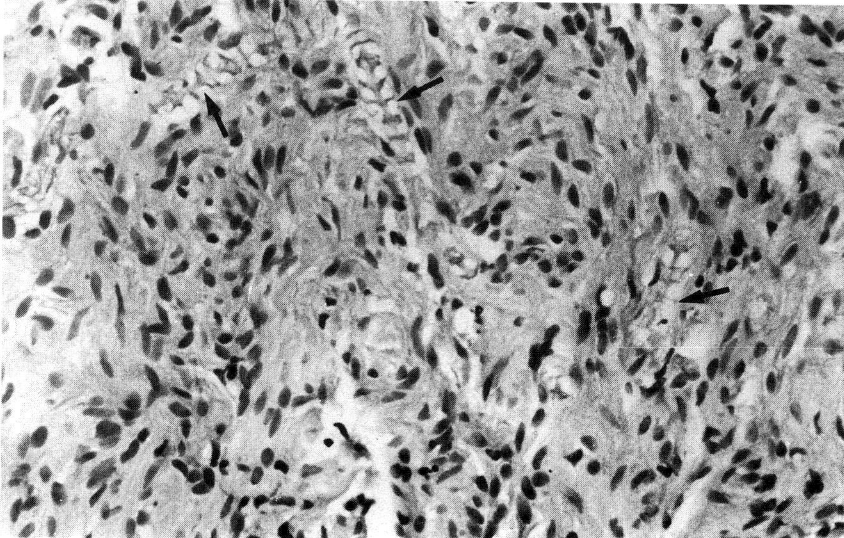

Fig. 15.2 (b) Higher power. The comma-shape of many of the nuclei and the presence of myelinated nerve twigs (arrows) is better appreciated. H & E (×300).

(iii) Astrocytomata of the third ventricle, cerebrum, cerebellum, brain stem and spinal cord.
(iv) Astrocytomata of the optic nerve and retina.

Ocular manifestations

Eyelids

1 *Plexiform neurofibromata:* this is the most characteristic lesion which also occurs as a solitary tumour unassociated with generalised neurofibromatosis. The growth may be present at birth and sometimes extends into the orbit or over the fronto-temporal area of the face. The overlying skin may be thick, coarse and redundant. Microscopically the thickened nerve fasicles appear to be expanded from within by proliferation of endoneurium and Schwann cells and circumscribed without by thickened perineurium which merges into surrounding connective tissue (Fig. 15.3).
2 *Mollusca fibrosa:* these are commonly multiple and may grow into the lid margin causing trichiasis. They are soft, lobulated and often pedunculated. Microscopically, nerve fibres may be difficult to find and the whole tumour consists of fibrocytes and interlacing collagen fibres so that distinction from a simple fibroma may be impossible.

Orbit

1 *Osseous lesions:* destruction of orbital bones is a frequent ocular manifestation. Bony hypertrophy, more particularly of the superior orbital magin, is less common. Defects in the orbital roof may allow transmission of arterial pulsations while herniation of brain substance into the orbit may lead to exophthalmos.
2 *Orbital plexiform neuromata:* may also cause exophthalmos, but is less common. As already noted, the growth may be congenital and part of an extensive malformation involving the nerves of the lids and adjacent area of the face.

Optic nerve

Infants and children with gliomata of the anterior visual pathways (Chapter 13) should be suspected of harbouring the abnormal gene which makes its possessor subject to neurofibromatosis in later childhood or adolescence. In early childhood, the only evidence of this propensity may be *café au lait* spots on the skin and a significant family history.

Uveal tract

In recent studies (Lewis & Riccardi, 1981; Huson *et al.*, 1987), Lisch nodules on the iris have been observed clinically in over 90% of cases and naevus-like lesions in the choroid in 30–50% of cases. Lisch nodules are raised and transparent and microscopically are seen to be composed of melanocytes.

The uveal tract is sometimes involved in a neurofibromatous thickening of the ciliary nerves. The whole tract is closely packed by small elongated and sometimes pigmented cells arranged in lamellae lying parallel to Bruch's membrane. Groups of neurones (ganglion cells) (Fig. 15.4) and small ovoid lamellated fibrous bodies like tactile corpuscles are often visible while melanocytic naevi may be present in the iris and choroid. The ovoid bodies are not really sensory nerve endings, but peripheral nerves expanded by Schwann cell hyperplasia (Kurosawa & Kurosawa, 1982).

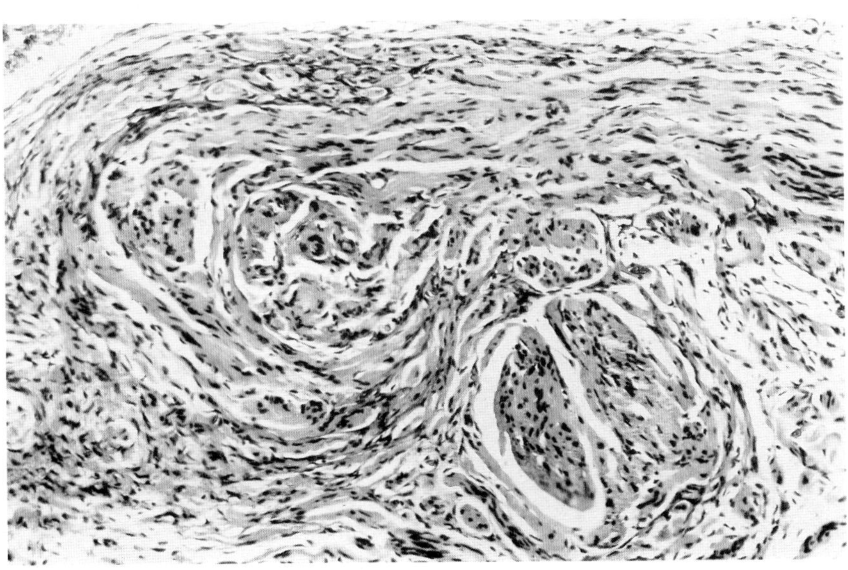

Fig. 15.3 Plexiform neurofibroma. Bundles of nerve fibres are surrounded by proliferated nerve sheath. H & E (×160).

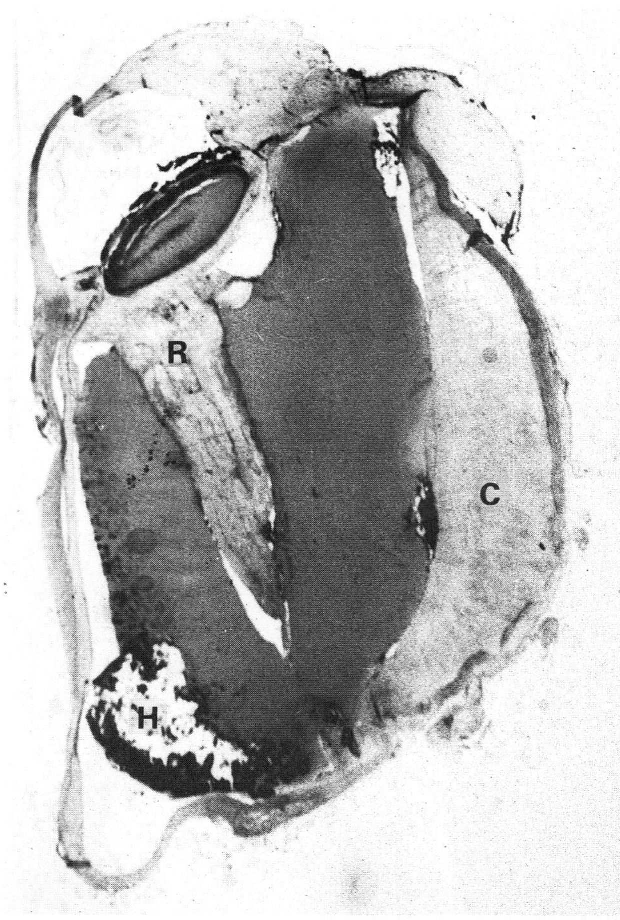

Fig. 15.4 Gross involvement of eye in 'neuromatosa' type of case. (a) Low power. There is gross thickening of the conjunctiva and choroid (C). The retina (R) is detached and there is a subretinal haemorrhage (H).

Glaucoma resulting in buphthalmos is a common complication. The cause is often obscure although malformation or deformation of the angle is evident in some cases.

Malignant neurilemmomata (Schwannomata)

Malignant neurilemmomata in the orbit, conjunctiva and lids are rare. Some examples have occurred in young children and have been regarded as manifestations of neurofibromatosis. It has been stated that malignancy supervenes in 10–15% of cases of neurofibromatosis and, although this figure is probably high, the possibility remains a definite risk for a patient on reaching adult life. Malignant change is indicated clinically by:

1 Accelerated growth in a previously quiescent tumour.
2 Multiple recurrences after excision.
3 The appearance of distant metastases in the lungs and other viscera and very occasionally in the regional lymph nodes.

Microscopically, malignancy is indicated by:

1 Increasing cellular anaplasia and pleomorphism with the appearance of polyhedral epithelioid cells and giant cells.
2 Enhanced mitotic activity.
3 Infiltration into adjacent tissue.

Progressive loss of those distinctive features of cell form and arrangement which indicate a neural origin means that malignant nerve sheath tumours often come to resemble other fibrosarcomata in their histological detail.

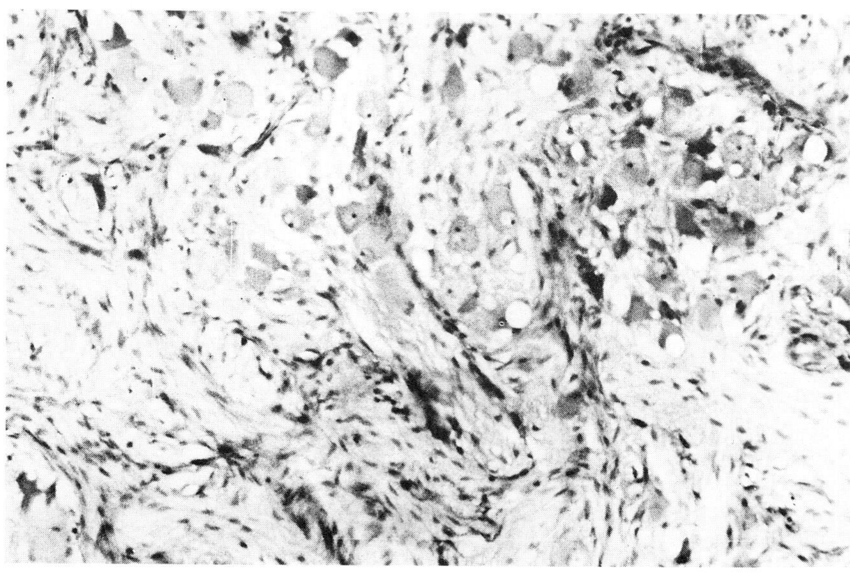

Fig. 15.4 (b) High power of choroidal lesion. Note presence of neurones resembling those found in sympathetic ganglia.

TUBEROSE SCLEROSIS

Retina

Retinal tumours are occasionally encountered as a manifestation of Bourneville's tuberose sclerosis (4% of cases). They are often multiple and appear as yellowish-white or grey tumours which may be large and protuberant or, more commonly, small, flat and disseminated. The question as to whether they are tumour-like glial malformations (hamartomata) or benign astrocytomata of fibrillary or giant-celled type remains unsettled. Tuberose sclerosis is a dysgenetic syndrome which is transmitted as an irregular dominant by an abnormal gene with a high degree of penetrance, but variable power of expression so that incomplete forms of the syndrome are not uncommon. This is important in diagnosis because, in the absence of the classical triad of angiofibroma on the face, epilepsy and mental deficiency further evidence of the disease may be found as described below.

Central nervous system

The multiple widespread glial tubers which are a major manifestation of this disease may be demonstrated by biopsy. They are tumour-like glial malformations (hamartomata) composed mainly of pleomorphic asrocytes including giant forms. Calcification in the tubers leads to nodular cerebral calcification developing during childhood usually in the region of the basal ganglia and round the third and lateral ventricles.

Skin

There may be plaques of thickened nodular skin usually located in the lumbar region and described as resembling goose-flesh, morocco leather or shagreen. Leucoderma and alopecia of the scalp occur and multiple subungual fibromata may be a prominent feature.

Viscera

1 Yellowish-white or reddish angiomyolipomatous masses in the renal cortex causing haematuria or a palpable mass may be found, usually in young adults. These are frequently multiple and bilateral and occur in 75% of all cases of tuberose sclerosis. Whether they are true tumours or tumour-like malformations is uncertain. Sarcomatous change with metastases occasionally develops.
2 Malformations of the myocardium with prominent accumulation of gycogen-like substance in the muscle fibres (so-called rhabdomyomata). Fifty per cent of patients with this manifestation die in the first year of life and 85% before puberty.
3 Nodular cystic foci of connective tissue, smooth muscle and blood vessel overgrowth in the lungs causing dyspnoea.

ANGIOMATOSIS RETINAE

Angiomatosis retinae is a rare hereditary disease most commonly manifesting itself in males in the second and third decades of life by the development of retinal haemangiomata in one or both eyes. Transmission is by a dominant gene, but penetrance may be incomplete and the power of expression is often variable. A familial tendency is evident in 20% of cases. In approximately 25% of cases, angiomatosis retinae is part of a wider defect involving the brain and sometimes also the viscera (von Hippel–Lindau disease). In the brain there are subtentorial cystic haemangiomata, most commonly in the cerebellum and less frequently in the medulla and spinal cord. The pancreas, suprarenals and kidneys may contain congenital cysts. In the kidney there may also be single or multiple hypernephroma-like growths and phaeochromocytomata may occur in the adrenal medulla and sympathetic chain.

There is disagreement as to whether the angiomata should be regarded as tumour-like malformations (hamartomata) or true tumours (haemangioblastomata). They do not metastasise, but the retinal angiomata may very occasionally be sufficiently aggressive to invade the choroid and sclera and perforate the globe.

The retinal haemangiomata which may be single or multiple, are often at the periphery, but may occur at the posterior pole and involve the optic nerve. They form yellowish-red, rounded tumours supplied by large tortuous vessels from the optic nerve head. Haemorrhage from the lesions is variable in amount, but retinal exudates are a constant feature of the disease and form circinate figures, a macular star or woolly masses in the fundus. In time, glial proliferation may overwhelm the angiomatous elements. Eventually, retinal detachment, secondary glaucoma, cataract and phthisis bulbi supervene. If the eye is retained for many years, bone may ultimately form as it often does in long retained, unabsorbed haemorrhages in the subretinal space. The ophthalmoscopic appearances may closely simulate those of Coats' disease, but the latter has no hereditary or familial tendency, is almost always unilateral and is a purely ocular disease without CNS or other associations.

Microscopically the tumours show some areas in which there is a fine meshwork of capillary vessels lined by plump endothelial cells with nests of foamy stromal cells between the capillaries while other areas consist of poorly canalised masses of endothelial cells and pericytes with admixed stromal cells (Fig. 15.5). Fibrous astrocytes are also numerous and electron microscopy has

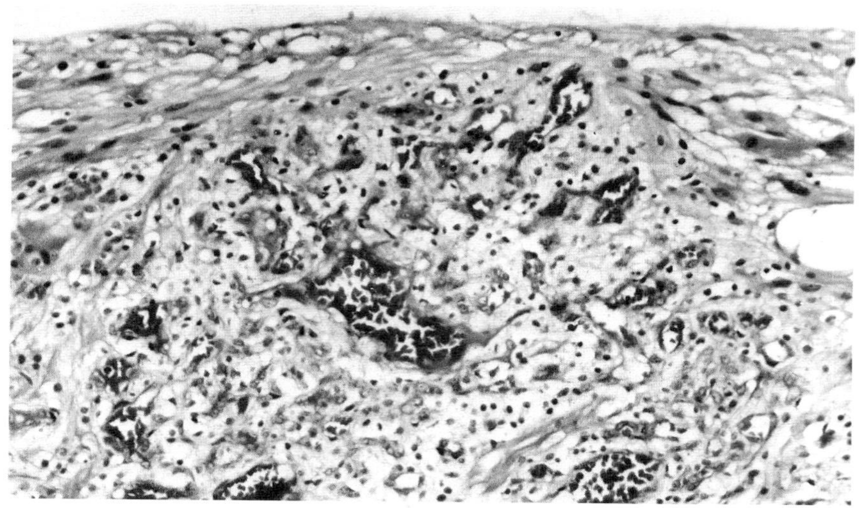

Fig. 15.5 Angiomatosis retinae. Clusters of proliferated capillaries with intervening foam cells (lipidised glial cells). Masson trichrome (×160).

shown that the stromal cells are lipidised fibrous astrocytes (Jakobiec *et al.*, 1976).

In the neighbouring retina there are thin-walled vascular spaces and abnormally large feeder vessels often with relatively thick muscular walls.

Numerous pools of serum, old and recent haemorrhages and cholesterol crystal profiles surrounded by foreign body giant cells are invariably present because of the leaky nature of the angiomatous capillaries.

STURGE–WEBER SYNDROME

The Sturge–Weber syndrome classically consists of the triad of naevus flammaeus, leptomenigeal haemangioma and homolateral glaucoma, but in contrast to the other phacomatoses, there is no clearcut herditary pattern.

Naevus flammaeus

This 'port-wine' stain is present at birth and usually involves the facial area supplied by the first and second divisons of the trigeminal nerve. The area supplied by the third division is affected less often. Histologically the lesion is characterised by large dilated capillaries in the dermis which should not be confused with capillary haemagiomata.

Central nervous system involvement

The intracranial haemangiomata are of racemose type and most commonly located in the meninges overlying the occipital lobe. The underlying cerebral cortex may be poorly developed. Varying degrees of mental deficiency are common.

It is noteworthy that involvement of the central nervous system occurs only if the territory of the first division of the trigeminal nerve is affected (Yates, 1987).

Ocular involvement

Glaucoma: occurs in the eye on the affected side. In about 60% of cases the onset is early enough to result in buphthalmos. In some cases, the glaucoma is due to hypoplasia of the angle similar to that occurring in other types of congenital glaucoma or to anterior peripheral synechiae. However, sometimes no anatomical cause is demonstrable, but recent work has suggested that there may be premature ageing of the trabecular meshwork/Schlemm's canal complex in the late onset cases (Cibis *et al.*, 1984).

Choroidal haemangioma: about 40% of cases have a solitary choroidal haemangioma of the cavernous type. Indeed, 50% of reported case of choroidal haemangioma have been in cases of Sturge–Weber syndrome.

Heterochromia of the iris: the iris may be more deeply pigmented on the side of the facial lesion.

ARTERIO-VENOUS MALFORMATIONS IN THE RETINA

(Arterio-venous aneurysm; racemose haemangioma; Wyburn–Mason syndrome)

Developmental angiomatous malformations consisting of enlarged tortuous arteries and veins may occur in one part of the retina or involve almost its whole extent. Usually an arterio-venous connection is detectable; either an artery and vein join at the end of their course without an intervening capillary bed or they communicate via an anomalous vessel. In many cases there is a similar malformation of the ipsilateral midbrain vessels in the distribution of the middle cerebral arte.y. In such cases the tangle of vessels usually extends in a continuous skein via the optic nerve, chiasma and optic tract to the dorsum of the midbrain. The optic foramen may in consequence be considerably enlarged. Part of the vascular malformation may be in the orbit with resulting proptosis and pulsation of the globe. There is sometimes an associated facial haemangioma.

The majority of patients are children or young adults, most of whom have diminished visual acuity. Homonymous hemianopia, oculomotor paralysis, hydrocephalus and hemiplegia are attributable to the intracranial part of the malformation.

Microscopically, many of the aberrant retinal vessels have an arterial structure and some show aneurysms. Veins with thickened collagenous walls are also recognisable. The retina may be almost wholely replaced by vessels, or show only a few tortuous vessels and slight cystic degeration and gliosis. In the optic nerve and brain, arteries predominate and these often show structural abnormalities particularly of their muscle coats which may be thinned to allow aneurysmal dilatation or thickened into nodules. In the optic nerve and tract the nerve fibres may suffer ischaemic death leaving only glia.

ATAXIA TELANGIECTASIA
(Louis–Barr syndrome)

In this rare condition, which usually becomes manifest in early childhood, the most consistent ocular finding is telangiectasia of the bulbar conjunctiva, but impairment of eye movements is common. The telangiectasia subsequently involves the skin of the face, ears and extensor surfaces of the extremities.

Mental retardation is common. In cases coming to autopsy, the cerebellum showed atrophy, loss of Purkinje cells and gliosis. There was softening and gliosis of the cerebrum and and demyelination of the white matter.

There is lymphoid hypoplasia with impaired immune responses and cases are particularly susceptible to respiratory infections, leukaemia and malignant lymphoma (see Harley *et al.*, 1967).

BIBLIOGRAPHY

General

Font, R. L. & Ferry, A. P. (1972) The phakomatoses. *International Ophthalmology Clinics* **12**, 1–50.

Neurilemmoma

Rootman, J., Goldberg, C. & Robertson, W. (1982) Primary orbital schwannomas. *British Journal of Ophthalmology* **66**, 194–204.

Neurofibromatosis

Bolthauser, E., Fueler, U. & Kilchofer, A. (1985) Iris hamartomas as diagnostic criterion in neurofibromatosis. *Annals of Neurology* **18**, 415–416.

Huson, S. (1987) The different forms of neurofibromatosis. *British Medical Journal* **294**, 1113–1114.

Huson, S., Jones, D. & Beck, L. (1987) Ophthalmic manifestations of neurofibromatosis. *British Journal of Ophthalmology* **71**, 235–238.

Klein, R. M. & Glassman, L. (1985) Neurofibromatosis of the choroid. American Journal of Ophthalmology **99**, 367–368.

Kurosawa, A. & Kurosawa, H. (1982) Ovoid bodies in choroidal neurofibromatosis. *Archives of Ophthalmology* **100**, 1939–1941.

Lewis, R. A. & Riccardi, V. M. (1981) von Recklinghausen neurofibromatosis. Incidence of iris hamartomata. *Ophthalmology* **88**, 348–354.

Perry, H. D. & Font, R. L. (1982) Iris nodules in von Recklinghausen's neurofibromatosis. *Archives of Ophthalmology* **100**, 1635–1640.

Rubenstein, A. A., Bunge, R. P. & Housman, D. E., eds (1986), Neurofibromatosis. *Annals of New York Academy of Sciences* **145**.

Tuberose sclerosis

Ramsay, R. C., Kinyoun, J. L., Hill, C. W., Aturaliya, U. P. & Knobloch, W. H. (1979) Retinal astrocytoma. *American Journal of Ophthalmology* **88**, 32–36.

Angiomatosis retinae

Hardwig, P. & Robertson, D. M. (1984) Von Hippel–Lindau disease: a familial, often lethal, multi-system phakomatosis. *Ophthalmology* **91**, 263–270.

Jakobiec, F.A., Font, R. L. & Johnson, F. B. (1976) Angiomatosis retinae. An ultrastructural study and lipid analysis. *Cancer* **38**, 2042–2056.

Sturge–Weber syndrome

Cibis, G. W., Tripathi, R. C. & Tripathi, B. J. (1984) Glaucoma in Sturge–Weber syndrome. *Ophthalmology* **91**, 1061–1071.

Jakobiec, F. A., Font, R. L. & Johnson, F. B. (1976) Angiomatosis retinae. An ultrastructural study and lipid analysis. *Cancer* **38**, 2042–2056.

Morgan, G. (1963) Pathology of the Sturge–Weber syndrome. *Proceedings of the Royal Society of Medicine* **56**, 14–15.

Arteriovenous malformations

Davis, W. S. & Thumin, M. (1956) Cavernous haemangioma of the optic disc and retina. *Transactions of the American Academy of Ophthalmology and Otolaryngology* **60**, 217–218.

Ataxia telangiectasia (Louis–Barr syndrome)

Harley, R. D., Baird, H. W. & Craven, E. M. (1967) Ataxia telangiectasia. Report of seven cases. *Archives of Ophthalmology* **77**, 582–592.

Chapter 16 Lymphoid hyperplasias and lymphomata

INTRODUCTION

The lymphoid aggregations which occur in the orbit and conjunctiva present practical and theoretical difficulties. The occurrence of such lesions in the conjunctiva is not surprising since there is an indigenous population of lymphoid cells, but it is less easy to understand why they should occur in the orbit which has no such indigenous population, except in the lacrimal gland. There may, however, be a special B-cell subset which homes preferentially to the orbit (Lazzarino *et al.*, 1985). The appearance and general behaviour of conjunctival and orbital lesions is essentially similar. The borderline between true tumours in which the ocular adnexal lesion is the first manifestation of a systemic process and so-called reactive lymphoid 'pseudotumours' which remain localised is blurred and a distinction cannot always be made, especially by routine histological methods. However, the wider use of thin sectioning, electron microscopy, immunological and other methods of identifying cells more precisely allows hope that this situation is changing. Thus, T-lymphocytes can be identified by, for example, cytochemically demonstrable acid α-naphthyl acetate esterase activity and B-lymphocytes can be categorised on the basis of heavy and light chain immunoglobulin determinates. This enables the cell population to be defined in terms of proportion of T- and B-cells. The range and reliabilty of monoclonal antibodies which enable much more detailed categorisation of both T- and B-lymphocytes into different sub-groups is continuously being extended. Unfortunately, in some cases, especially large cell lymphomata, surface markers may be lacking. Monoclonality of the B-lymphocyte population can be inferred if there is gross distortion in the ratio of $\kappa:\lambda$ labelled cells from the normal 65:35. The identification of small clones amounting to as few as 2–5% of cells in an infiltrate is now possible by the use of genetic probes which detect the rearrangemnt of DNA sequences (Jakobiec *et al.*, 1987)

Notwithstanding these technical advances, it is still necessary to discuss lymphoid lesions in the three categories:

1 Reactive hyperplasias (pseudotumours).
2 Indeterminate lesions.
3 Malignant lymphomata.

Within the last few years the use of special techniques such as those referred to earlier has led to a complete revision of the classification of malignant lymphomata. This is because some cells originally thought on morphological grounds to be non-lymphoid are, in fact, lymphocytic in origin.

Older classifications were thus inaccurate and have have been replaced by a confusing variety of immunologically based classifications, none of which is entirely satisfactory. There is, indeed, considerable difficulty in achieving consistency in diagnosis. It must, moreover, be remembered that the classifications were developed for nodal lymphomata, although the principles appear to be applicable to extranodal lymphoma.

It is beyond the scope of this book to discuss the merits of the various classifications, but all agree on certain basic principles. Malignant lymphomata may be divided into the two main groups:

1 Non-Hodgkin's lymphoma.
2 Hodgkin's lymphoma.

The vast majority of ocular adnexal lymphomata are of the non-Hodgkin type.

REACTIVE HYPERPLASIAS (PSEUDOLYMPHOMATA)

Reactive lesions consist predominantly of small lymphocytes, but there is a variable admixture of plasma cells, histiocytes, macrophages and sometimes eosinophils. The presence of normal germinal centres is an indication that the lesion is likely to remain localised. Proliferating capillaries with thick endothelial lining are common, but also occur in lymphomata.

Reactive epibulbar lymphoid hyperplasia may occasionally be associated with massive lymphoid infiltration of the uvea.

Local recurrence after treatment may occur and Jakobiec *et al.* (1979) found that nearly 20% of lesions in this category had spread beyond the orbit within 5 years.

INDETERMINATE LYMPHOID LESIONS

These lesions usually consist almost entirely of mature lymphocytes, but may show worrying cytologic characteristics such as the presence of immature cells. Germinal centres, if present, tend to be poorly preserved (Fig. 16.1). It is virtually impossible by histological examination of a biopsy to determine whether the hyperplasia is a benign local condition or is the initial manifestation of lymphoma or even lymphatic leukaemia. In about 25–40% of cases prolonged follow-up will finally witness the emergence of unequivocal malignant lymphoma months or even years later (Morgan & Harry, 1978; Jakobiec *et al.*, 1979).

Eosinophilic PAS-positive glycoprotein inclusions (Dutcher bodies) in the nuclei of the infiltrating cells were noted by Morgan (1975) and Morgan and Harry (1978) only in tumours which did not disseminate, but, as such bodies are also seen in multiple myeloma as well as Waldenstrom's macroglobulinaemia, cases in which they occur should have quantitative serum electrophoresis (Jakobiec *et al.*, 1979).

NON-HODGKIN'S LYMPHOMATA

Classification

Non-Hodgkin's lymphomata may be sub-divided initially according to their cell of origin:

1 T-lymphocytic.
2 B-lymphocytic.
3 Histiocytic.

Recent classifications of non-Hodgkin's lymphomata have further sub-divided them according to growth pattern and the stage of maturation of the predominant cell. During normal maturation in lymph nodes, both T- and B-lymphocytes undergo morphological changes, especially to the nucleus. The small dense nucleus associated with the circulating lymphocyte enlarges. The chromatin becomes peripherally distributed and the nucleus

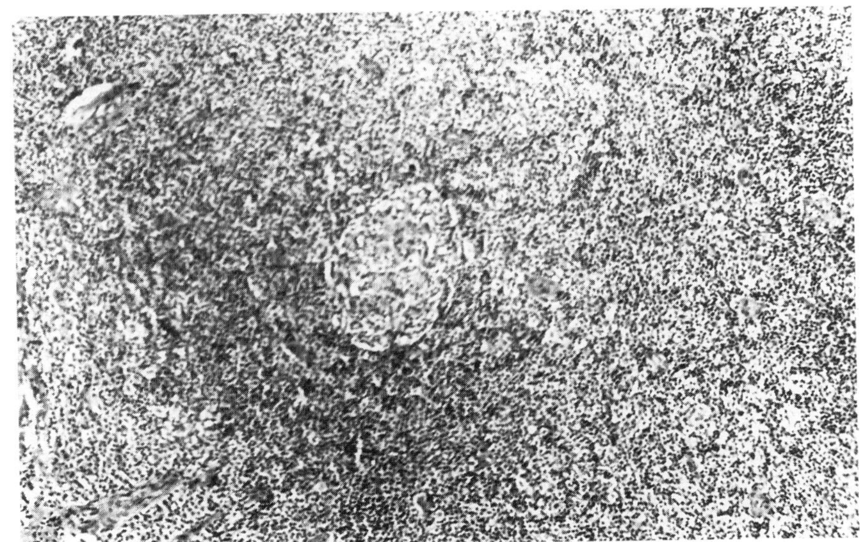

Fig. 16.1 Borderline lymphoid hyperplasia. (a) Low power showing germinal centre surrounded by small lymphocytes. H & E (×98).

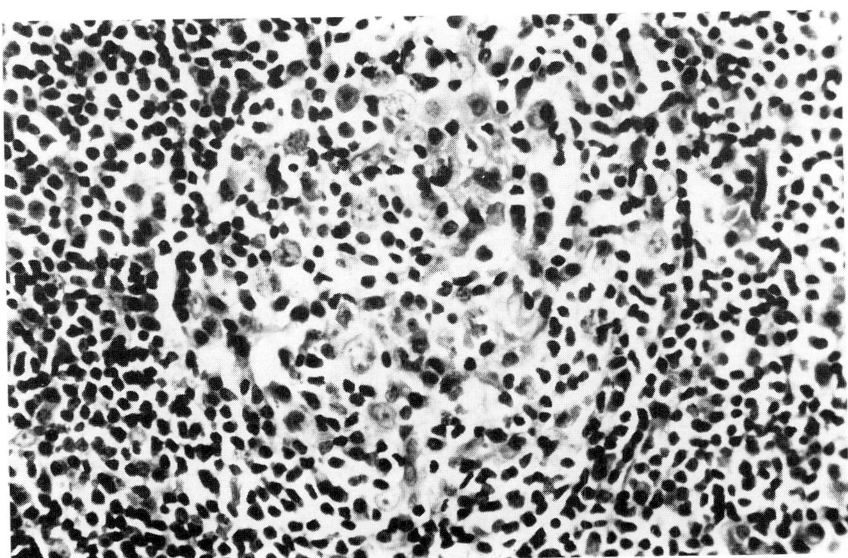

Fig. 16.1 (b) High power of germinal centre. H & E (×400). This lesion recurred locally.

appears pale. Nucleoli develop and infolding of the nuclear membrane occurs so that the nucleus may appear rounded, cleaved or convoluted. Distinct stages can be recognized in this process and have been given descriptive names, e.g. large or small, cleaved or non-cleaved or names which imply origin and maturity, e.g. centroblastic or centrocytic. Classification on the basis of cell maturity is somewhat comparable to that of leukemias.

In general, the larger the nucleus of the predominant tumour cell and the further its morphology deviates from that of the small lymphocyte the more malignant the tumour.

Follicular lymphomata

Maturation of B-lymphocytes usually occurs in germinal centres of lymph nodes and some B-cell lymphomata retain a nodular pattern of growth (Fig. 16.2). Care must be taken not to confuse the follicular differentiation with the formation of true germinal centres which, as already noted, occurs in benign hyperplasias.

Diffuse lymphomata

Diffuse lymphomas show no nodular pattern and have a significantly worse prognosis than follicular lymphomas of comparable cell type. They may be B- or T-cell in origin.

Large cell lymphomata ('reticulosarcomata')

It is probable that most of the tumours which were formerly classified as 'reticulosarcoma' or 'histiocytic lymphoma' are in fact lymphomata of B-cell origin,

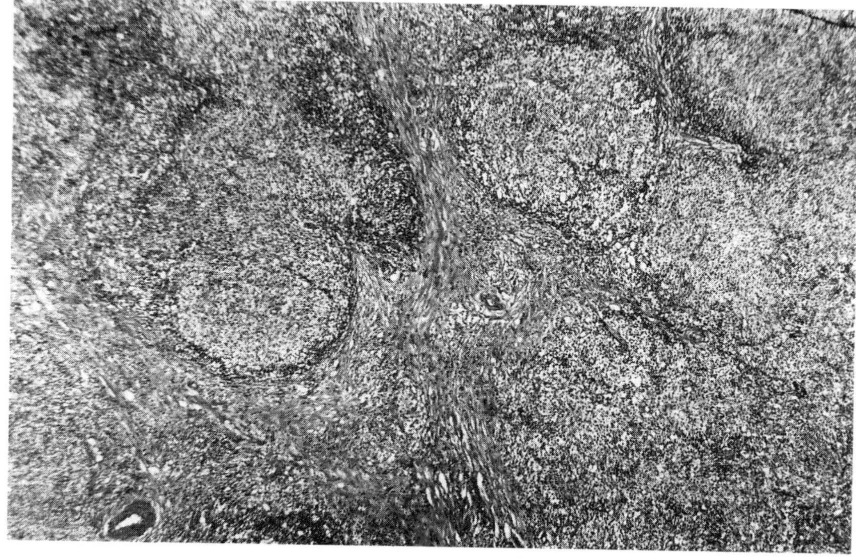

Fig. 16.2 Follicular lymphoma. (a) Low power showing follicular arrangement. H & E (×41).

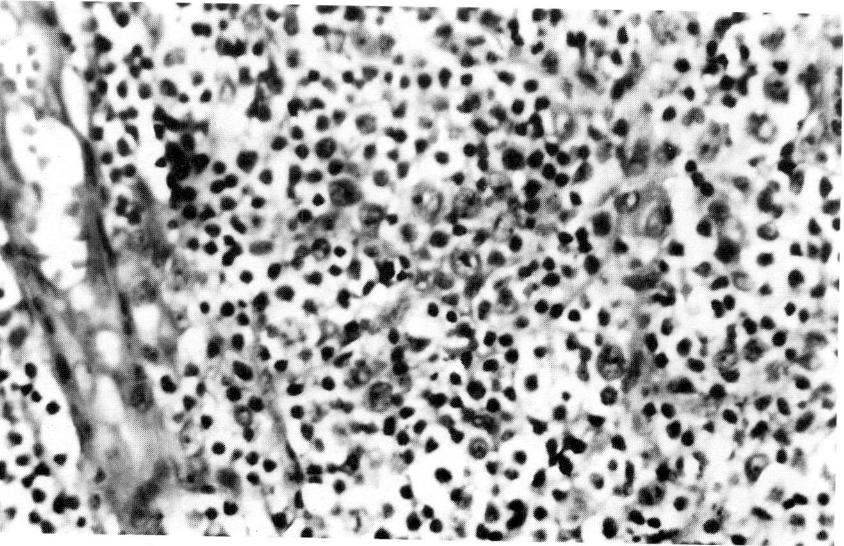

Fig. 16.2 (b) High power to show presence of large cells with conspicuous nucleoli amongst the small lymphocytes. A capillary with high endothelium is present on the left hand side of the picture. H & E (×400).

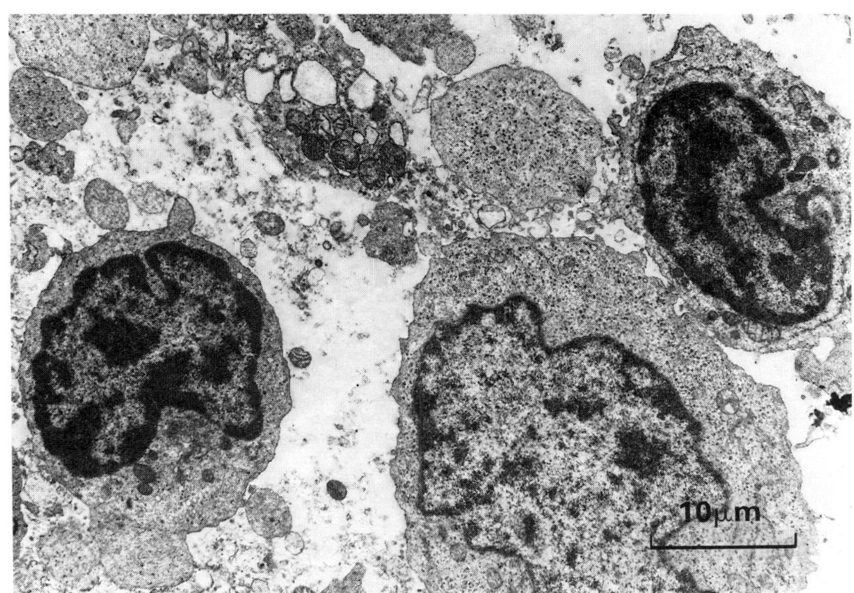

Fig. 16.2 (c) Electron micrograph showing two small lymphocytes with well marked nuclear indentation and a larger immature cell with folds in nuclear nuclear membrane and conspicuous lack of cytoplasmic organelles. This case recurred locally and subsequently spread to pre-auricular lymph nodes.

although the cells do not always carry surface markers. The tumour is composed of large cells with abundant pale cytoplasm, distinct cell borders and oval or indented nuclei with peripherally situated nuclear chromatin and conspicuous nucleoli as described above (Fig. 16.3). Less than 1% of these tumours are now thought to be true histiocytic lymphomata.

The uveal tract may occasionally be infiltrated by lymphomata and it is usually this type of lymphoma which is responsible. Clinical presentation may be as uveitis (masquerade syndrome).

Plasmacytomata

Some 'large cell' B-lymphomata show plasmacytoid differentiation to a degree which justifies the category of extra-medullary plasmacytoma. They are commoner in extranodal sites than in lymphomata arising in lymph nodes.

Burkitt's lymphomata

This is a lethal form of B-cell lymphoma which has a high incidence among native children in certain parts of Africa and New Guinea. In Africa most cases occur in a broad zone across the middle of the continent but within this zone the tumour does not occur in very dry areas nor at elevations above 1640 m where the minimum temperature falls below 15.6°C. The same strict relationship to altitude and temperature has not been observed in New Guinea. A small number of cases have been recorded in Europe and America.

The geographical distribution of the disease has suggested that it is caused by an insect-borne virus. Cell lines cultured from Burkitt's lymphoma carry herpes-like virus (Epstein–Barr, EB, virus) which is also closely associated with infectious mononucleosis, but there is as yet no proof that this or any other virus is the cause of Burkitt's lymphoma. The concentration of cases in areas where malaria is hyperendemic suggests a link between lymphomata, EB virus and malaria. The nature of this inter-reaction is unknown, but it has been postulated that continuous stimulation and stress exerted by malarial parasites on the lymphoid tissues might render them susceptible to neoplastic transformation in the presence of EB virus.

Lymphatic leukaemia

Overspill of tumour cells into the blood sometimes occurs, especially in small cell lymphomata. Confusion can thus occur between lymphomata and chronic lymphatic leukaemia, especially if the leukaemic cells invade lymph nodes. The distinction is, in effect, artificial and prognosis is not affected.

Clinical manifestations

Malignant lymphomata may occur at any age, but are predominantly a disease of middle and advanced life and males are affected twice as often as females. They usually arise multifocally in lymph nodes and extranodal lymphoid tissue and metastasize via lymphatic and blood channels to all parts of the body. Occasionally, however,

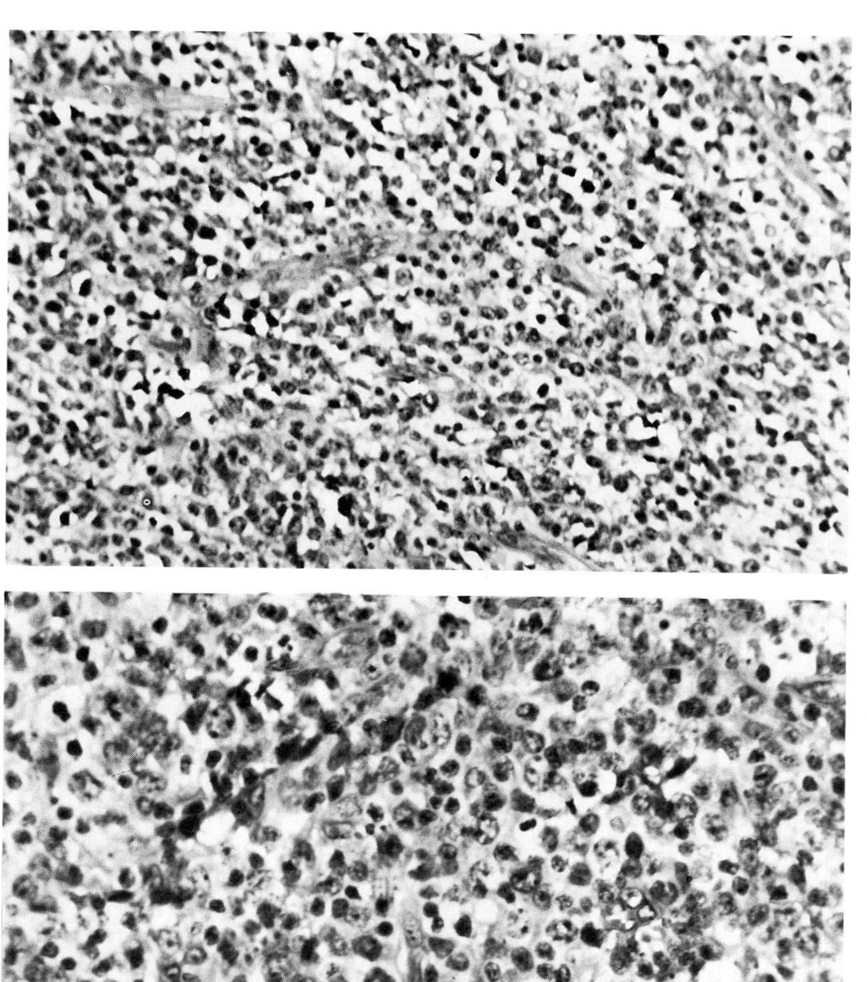

Fig. 16.3 Large cell lymphoma. (a) Low power showing unorganised cells passing through which can be seen capillaries with high endothelium. H & E (×150).

Fig. 16.3 (b) High power to show pleomorphic nature of tumour with numerous large cells. H & E (×390). This case responded to radiotherapy, but developed a carcinoma of breast 4 years after presentation.

they appear first in sites where they attract early attention, e.g. orbit, lacrimal gland, lacrimal sac, conjunctiva, lids, tonsils and cervical glands.

The presenting symptoms of orbital lymphomata are exophthalmos or an orbital mass. Lymphomata presenting in the fornices are firm, smooth, long and sausage-shaped, while those arising in the lacrimal gland tend to present subconjunctivally in constrast to lacrimal epithelial tumours which present under the skin of the lid. A rather distinctive clinical picture results from simultaneous bilateral lymphomatous infiltration of the lids, conjunctivae and orbits.

From the foregoing, it is clear that any case which presents clinically as a potential ocular adnexal lymphoma should be investigated for evidence of possible manifestations of the lesion elsewhere. Such manifestations may indeed be more accessible for biopsy than an orbital deposit.

IMMUNOLOGICAL CONSIDERATIONS

The extensive studies by Jakobiec and his colleagues (see Jakobiec *et al.*, 1987), have done much to improve our understanding of the relationship between 'reactive lymphoid hyperplasia' and 'non-Hodgkin's lymphoma'. These have shown that, in the former, T-cells predominate (50–70%) and that the B–cell population is polyclonal. There is often an excess of T-helper over T-suppressor cells and this may promote clonal expansions of B-cells which usually, however, remain localised to the orbit. Reactive lymphoid hyperplasia thus appears to be a benign, but unstable, lesion. The indeterminate lesions may possibly be compared to carcinoma *in situ* or pre-invasive melanocytic lesions.

MORTALITY

Five year mortality rates of 6%, 19% and 58% respectively were found by Jakobiec *et al.* (1979) classified as 'reactive' , 'atypical' and 'malignant' in their series of 66 cases of orbital lymphoid hyperplasia. Of 98 cases of indeterminate lymphocytic orbital and conjunctival tumours followed up by Morgan and Harry (1978), 24 were dead within 7 years, though not all of generalised malignant lymphoma. While these figures indicate the potentially serious nature even of borderline lesions, most are amenable to treatment by surgery, chemo- and radiotherapy or a combination of such methods and there have been advances in their management in the last decade.

HODGKIN'S LYMPHOMATA

Although they are the commonest primary tumours of lymphoid tissue, Hodgkin's lymphomata only rarely involve ocular adnexae. Tumours in the orbit, lids and lacrimal gland are the more usual manifestations, but these are rarely, if ever, the first evidence of the disease in the body. Corneal infiltrations, keratitis, episcleritis and uveitis have also been recorded. In the early stages of its evolution, the neoplastic tissue in the orbit may be mistaken both clinically and histologically for a chronic inflammatory reaction and the likeness to an inflammatory condition may be heightened by the simultaneous neoplastic involvement of the nasal sinuses.

Hodgkin's lymphoma is notable for its many histological variants. The essential neoplastic elements are multinucleate Sternberg–Reed cells and mononuclear cells with similar nuclear features. Intimately associated with these and in quite variable proportions are lymphocytes, neutrophils, eosinophils and histiocytes which often form the bulk of the tumour.

BIBLIOGRAPHY

Classification of lymphomata

Henry, K., Bennett, M. H. & Farrer-Brown, G. (1978) Classification of the non-Hodgkin's lymphomas. In *Recent Advances in Pathology*, eds P. P. Anthony & N. Woolf, pp 275–302. Churchill Livingstone, Edinburgh.

Nathanwi, B. N. (1979) A critical analysis of the classifications of non-Hodgkin's lymphomas. Cancer **44**, 347–384.

NCI Non-Hodgkin's Lymphoma Classification Project Working Committee (1985) Classification of non-hodgkin's lymphoma. Reproducibility of major classification systems. *Cancer* **53**, 91–95.

Ocular lymphomata

Corriveau, C., Easterbrook, M. & Payne, D. (1986) Lymphoma simulating uveitis (masquerade syndrome). *Canadian Journal of Ophthalmology* **21**, 144–149.

Garner, A. & Chavis, R. M. (1979) Lymphoid pseudotumour of the orbit. *Transactions of the Ophthalmological Society of the UK* **99**, 231–233.

Jakobiec, F. A., Iwamoto, T. & Knowles II, D. M. (1982) Ocular adnexal tumours, correlative ultrastructural and immunologic marker studies. *Archives of Ophthalmology* **100**, 84–98.

Jakobiec, F. A., Iwamoto, T., Patell, M. & Knowles II, D. M. (1986) Ocular adnexal monoclonal lymphoid tumours with a favourable prognosis. *Ophthalmology* **93**, 1547–1557.

Jakobiec, F. A., McLean, I. & Font, R. L. (1979) Clinicopathologic characteristics of orbital lymphoid hyperplasia. *Ophthalmology* **86**, 948–966.

Jakobiec, F. A., Neri, A. & Knowles II, D. M. (1987) Genotypic monoclonality in immunophenotypically polyclonal orbital lymphoid tumours. A model of tumour progression in the lymphoid system. *Ophthalmology* **94**, 980–994.

Kleener, J. (1977) Lymphoma and other lymphoid lesions of the orbit (II). *Acta Ophthalmologica* **55**, 549–560.

Knowles II, D. M., Jakobiec, F. A. & Halper, J. P. (1979) Immunological characterization of ocular adnexal lymphoid neoplasms. *American Journal of Ophthalmology* **87**, 603–619.

Lazzarino, M., Morra, E., Rosso, R., Brusamolino, E., Pagnucco, G., Castello, A., Ghisolfi, A., Tafi, A., Zennaro, G. & Bernasconi, C. (1985) Clinicopathologic and immunologic characteristics of non-Hodgkin's lymphomas presenting in the orbit. A report of eight cases. *Cancer* **55**, 1907–1912.

Levy, R., Warnke, R., Dorfman, R. F. & Haimovich, J. (1977) The monoclonality of human B-cell lymphomas. *Journal of Experimental Medicine* **145**, 1014–1028.

Morgan, G. (1971) Lymphocytic tumours of the conjunctiva. *Journal of Clinical Pathology* **24**, 585–595.

Morgan, G. (1975) Lymphocytic tumours of the orbit. *Modern Problems in Ophthalmology* **14**, 355–360.

Morgan, G. & Harry, J. (1978) Lymphocytic tumours of indeterminate nature: A 5-year follow-up of 98 conjunctival and orbital lesions. *British Journal of Ophthalmology* **63**, 381–383.

Ryan, S. J., Zimmerman, L. E. & King, F. M. (1972) Reactive lymphoid hyperplasia. An unusual form of intraocular pseudotumour. *Transactions of the American Academy of Ophthalmology and Otolaryngology* **76**, 652–670.

van der Gaag, R., Koornneef, L., van Heerde, P., Vroom, Th. M., Pegels, J. H., Feltkamp, C. A., Peeters, H. J. F., Gillissen, J. P. A., Bleeker, G. M. & Feltkamp, T. E. W. (1984) Lymphoid proliferations in the orbit: malignant or benign? *British Journal of Ophthalmology* **68**, 892–900.

Chapter 17 Congenital anomalies

INTRODUCTION

Malformations which affect the eye either alone or as part of a syndrome are extremely numerous. Some of those which affect predominantly one component tissue of the eye have already been mentioned in the appropriate chapter. The present chapter catalogues a number of more complex abnormalities. The eye(s) alone may be affected or the ocular abnormalities may form part of a generalised syndrome.

There may be a recognised pattern of inheritance or an association with chromosomal abnormalities. Some are presumably due to interference with develoment by an unknown agent or virus. In general, most abnormalities, whatever their cause result from an interplay in varying proportions of three pathogenetic processes:

1 Simple retardation or suppression of growth and/or differentiation.
2 Aberrant growth and development.
3 Failure of fusion of the foetal cleft.

An account of the normal development of the human eye is beyond the scope of this book and reference should be made to larger works or original papers (e.g. O'Rahilly, 1975). The consideration of a particular abnormality in the context of normal develoment may give an indication as to which stage in development genetic or other factors began to operate.

It should also be noted that remnants of the vascular pupillary membrane attached to the collarette are commonly present in newborn infants.

Post-mortem changes which may cause confusion are swelling of the cornea, indentation of the posterior surface of the lens and folding of the central retina.

ANOPHTHALMOS, MICROPHTHALMOS AND COLOBOMATA

Anophthalmos

True anophthalmos in which the primary optic vesicle either fails to develop or undergoes complete regression is extremely rare and usually bilateral.

Microphthalmos

True microphthalmos (nanophthalmos) must be distinguished from shrinkage of a once normal eye as a result of disease or injury (phthisis bulbi). Cases in which the eye is small, but apparently normal, are rare and usually unilateral. Such eyes are commonly hypermetropic and

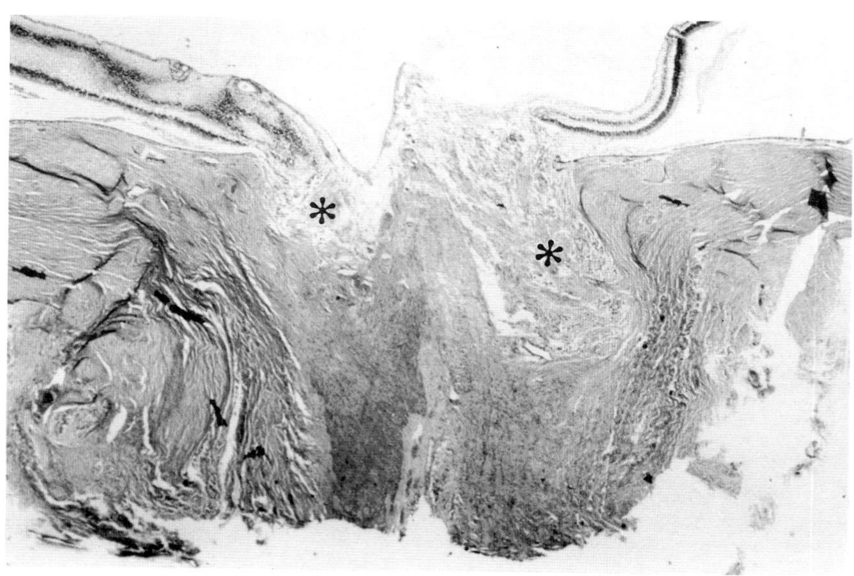

Fig. 17.1 Coloboma of optic nerve (from case of CHARGE syndrome). The entrance to the coloboma is indicated by asterisks. Because, in this case, there was a persistent hyaloid artery the out-pouching appears to have two pockets at this level. Retina can be seen in the superficial part of the ectasia on the left. The remaining space contains mainly glia. H & E (×20). (Specimen by courtesy of Miss J. Duvall.)

susceptible to angle closure glaucoma. More often there are other abnormalities, especially colobomata. Inheritance may be autosomal recessive or dominant.

Colobomata

Colobomata may show an irregular dominant pattern of inheritance and are frequently bilateral. A typical coloboma results from a failure of the foetal cleft to close completely during development and is thus located infero-nasally. There is a defect in the retina and choroid which may be localised or, in complete colobomata, extend from the optic nerve forwards as a triangular or oval area to involve the ciliary body and iris. This appears ophthalmoscopically as a white area often with pigmented edges. The sclera is usually ectatic in the affected area and is covered by an often rather tenuous layer of nondescript cells derived from retina and choroid.

Coloboma of the ciliary body is usually part of a more generalised coloboma. There is a defect in the ciliary processes and ciliary muscle. On either side of the defect, the ciliary processes are, however, hyperplastic.

Typical coloboma of the iris may, as already noted, form part of a larger defect. It may also, however, occur in atypical positions and can vary from a small notch in the pupillary border to a substantial gap involving the sphincter pupillae and sometimes a corresponding defect in the zonule and notch in the lens.

Coloboma of the optic nerve head (Fig. 17.1) is usually part of a wider coloboma, but occasionally occurs in the absence of a wider defect. In a typical case, the inferior part of the nerve head is affected. The cribiform plate is displaced upwards and posteriorly and a pouch of ectatic dural sheath and sclera lined by retinal and neural remnants or glia is formed inferiorly.

Heterotopic tissues such as smooth muscle , adipose tissue, lacrimal tissue, bone and cartilage are sometimes seen in association with colobomata. Atypical colobomata of sclera and iris may also occur in association with corneal choristomata (Fig. 17.2a–c).

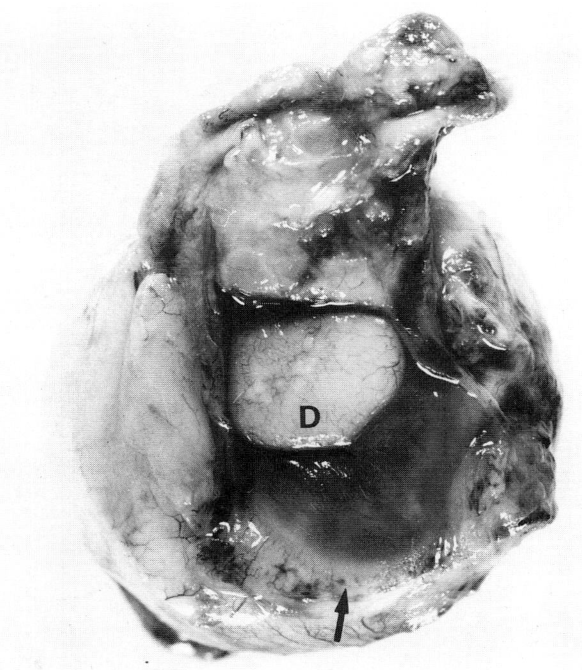

(a)

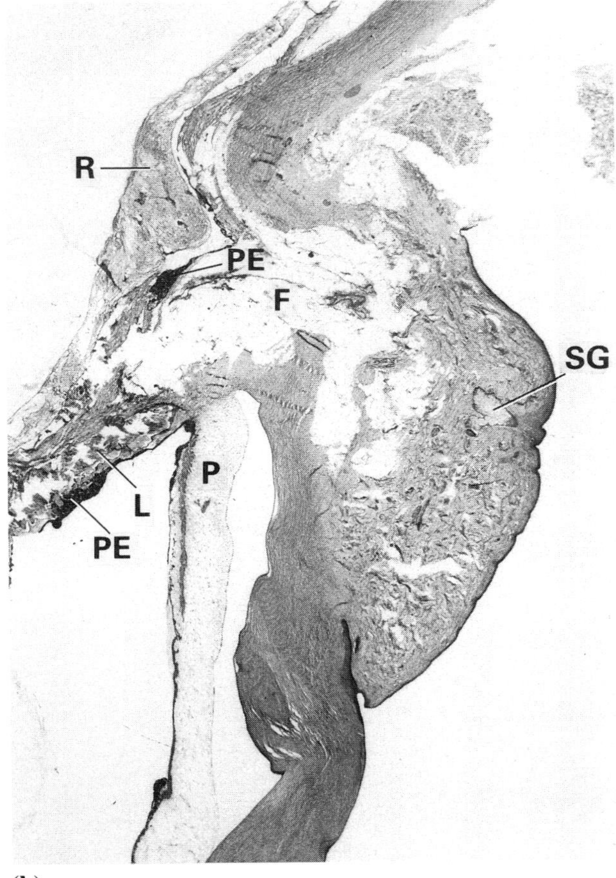

(b)

Fig. 17.2 Corneal dermoid with underlying atypical coloboma of sclera, iris and ciliary body. (a) Macroscopic picture of eye. D = dermoid. Limbus inferiorly indicated by arrow. (b) Section through dermoid showing underlying limbal scleral defect occupied by adipose tissue (F) which is adherent to retina (R), the inferior pupillary border of the iris inferiorly (P) and a calcified lens rudiment posteriorly (L). No ciliary processes could be identified at this level and there is irregular proliferation of pigmented epithelium (PE) around the lens rudiment. A sebaceous gland (SG) can just be made out in the dermoid.

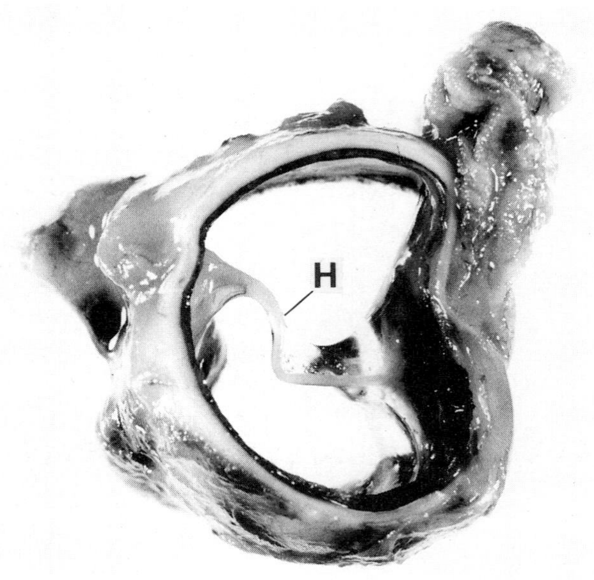

Fig. 17.2 (c) Lateral view showing thick fibrous cord (H) derived from a persistent hyaloid artery terminating anteriorly on a cap of fibrous tissue on the posterior surface of the lens rudiment.

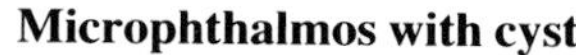

Microphthalmos with cyst

Sometimes a cyst arises at the margin of a colobomatous defect posteriorly. Such a cyst may undergo progressive enlargement and the relative size of cyst and eye varies greatly. The eye itself may show other gross abnormalities or may be relatively normal. Since the cyst is initially an expansion of the primary optic vesicle it is lined by retinal rudiments and communicates with the subretinal space. Secondary communication with the vitreous space is, however, common. The sclera usually extends around the cyst and the choroid may partially line the scleral sac. However, the scleral envelope may become tenuous and glial hyperplasia is a common feature as in the example illustrated (Fig. 17.3). The hyperplastic glia may contain neuroepithelial rosettes (Fig. 17.3c).

Occasional cysts arise in a position remote from the foetal fissure, presumably due to extrusion of a knuckle of retina from the optic vesicle.

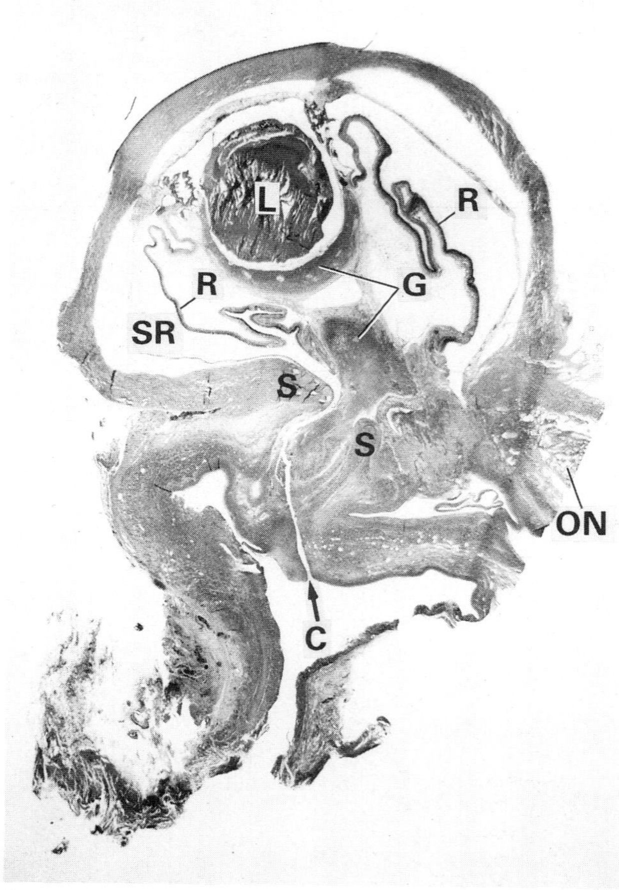

(a)

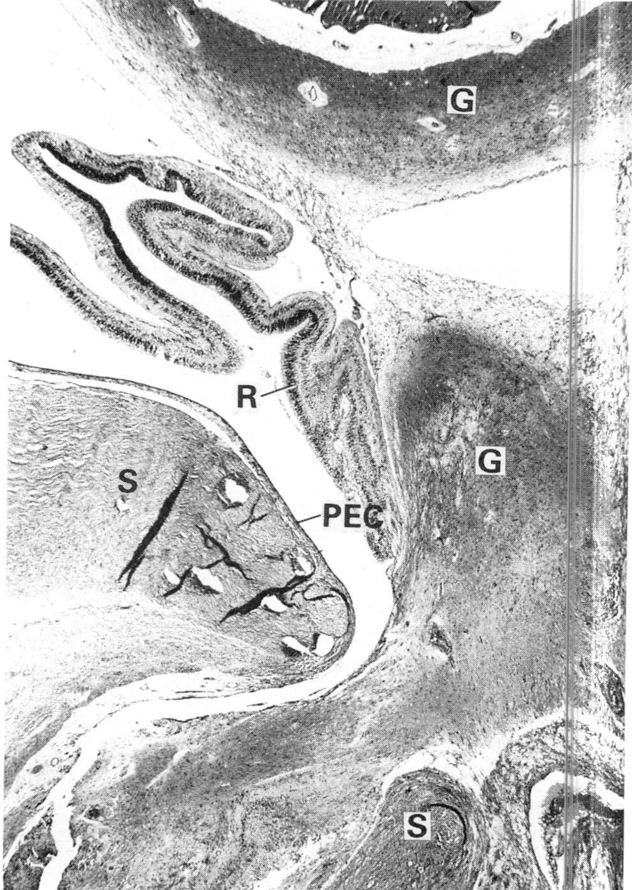

(b)

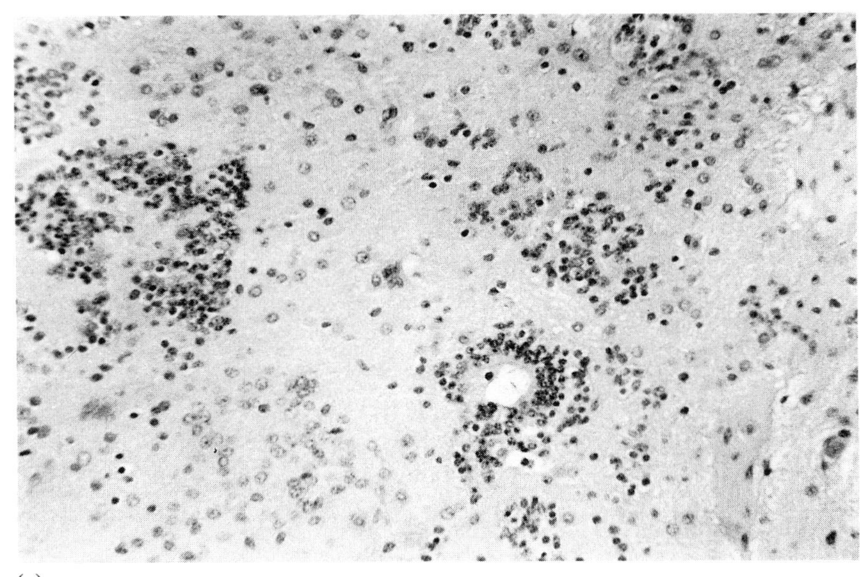

(c)

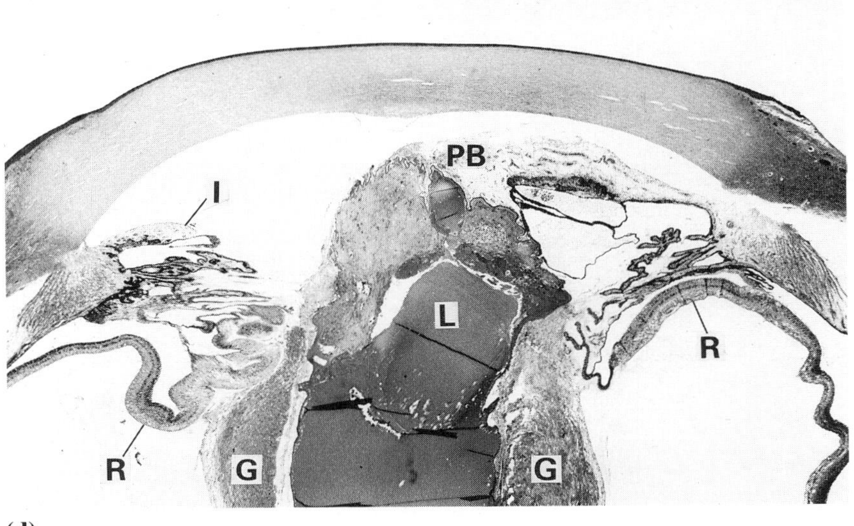

(d)

Fig. 17.3 Microphthalmos with cyst. The specimen was removed from a healthy female child of 4 months with increasing proptosis. The other eye was normal. (a) (*Opposite*) Low power showing masses of hyperplastic glia (G) forming a crescent around the misshapen, cataractous and partially calcified lens (L) and related to the optic nerve head (ON = optic nerve). The latter glial mass protrudes through a gap in the sclera together with folds of retina (R). The cyst was ruptured during removal and an artifical channel (arrow) can be seen entering the channel connecting cyst (C) with subretinal space (SR). The wall of the cyst is composed of hyperplastic glia. The sclera extends to enclose the cyst, but tapers off to become unidentifiable. H & E. (b) (*Opposite*) Scleral gap (S = sclera) in more detail. Pigmented epithelium and choroid (PEC) can be seen extending over the lip of the scleral gap. H & E. (c) Detail of the cyst wall showing its glial nature. A neuroepithelial rosette is present. H & E (×160). (d) Anterior part of globe. Section through deeper level showing partial coloboma of iris (I). The pupillary border (PB) on the other side is adherent to the misshapen cataractous lens (L). The ciliary processes are hyperplastic, particularly on the side of the coloboma and indrawn together with peripheral retina (R) to become attached to the glia (G) partially enveloping the lens.

SYNDROMES ASSOCIATED WITH MICROPHTHALMOS AND COLOBOMATA

Many syndromes have been recorded in which microphthalmos and colobomata occur. These include:

1 Oligophrenia with microphthalmos.
2 Microphthalmos with polydactyly.
3 Microphthalmos with hare lip and cleft palate.
4 Various facial dystrophies including:
  (i) Mandibulofacial dysostosis.
  (ii) Oculo-auricular dysplasia (Goldehaar's syndrome).
  (iii) Mandibulo-oculo-facial dyscephaly (bird-face).
5 Trisomy 13–15 (Patau's syndrome).
6 Trisomy 18 (Edwards' syndrome).
7 CHARGE association (see below).
8 Triploidy.
9 Partial 18 monosomy.

Trisomy 13–15 (Patau's syndrome)

Ocular defects ranging from congenital cataract to anopthalmia are a feature of 13–15 trisomy (see Apple *et al.*, 1970). In a minority of cases, gross ocular derangement is associated with multiple malformations in other organs including cerebral dysgenesis, arrhinecephaly, septal heart defects, cleft lip and palate, hydronephrosis and polydactyly. The condition is rare, sometimes familial and has a high mortality. Both eyes

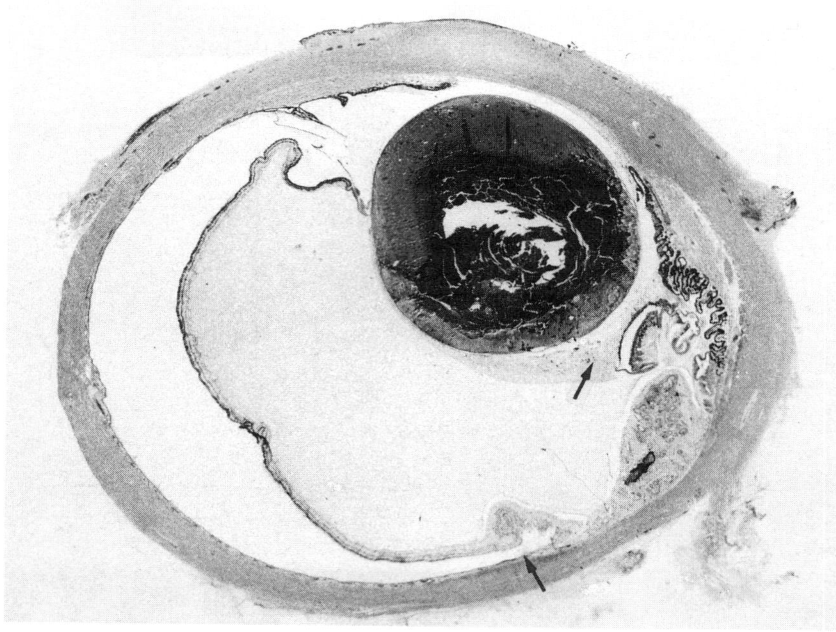

Fig. 17.4 Microphthalmic eye from a case of 47XY−13 Trisomy which was born after 36 weeks gestation and lived 1.5 hours. (a) Low power of globe. The anterior chamber has hardly formed and there is a coloboma inferiorly affecting iris and choroid. The lens is rounded and cataractous and there is a retrolenticular mass of cellular fibrous tissue. The areas shown in more detail are indicated by arrows. Masson trichrome.

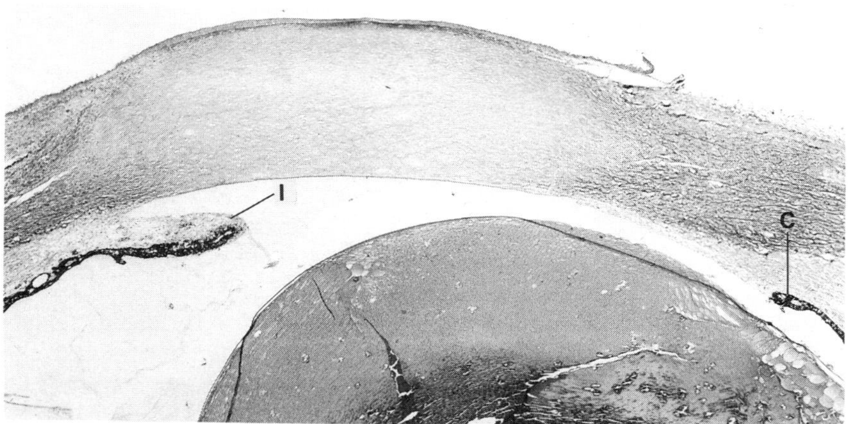

Fig. 17.4 (b) Anterior part of globe (slightly deeper level). The iris (I) is incompletely cleaved and there is a coloboma of the iris inferiorly (C). H & E.

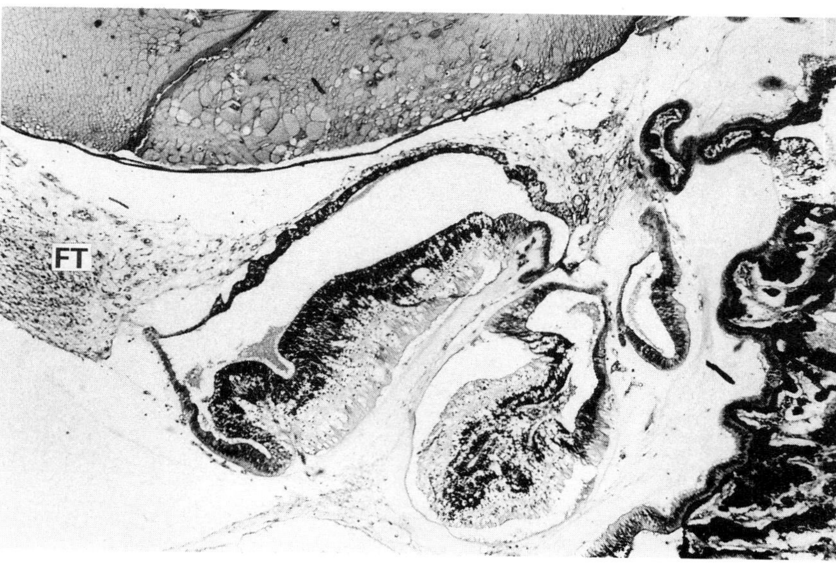

Fig. 17.4 (c) Detail of ciliary region showing erratic proliferation and attachment to the retrolenticular fibrous tissue (FT). The equatorial lens fibres are swollen. H & E (×38).

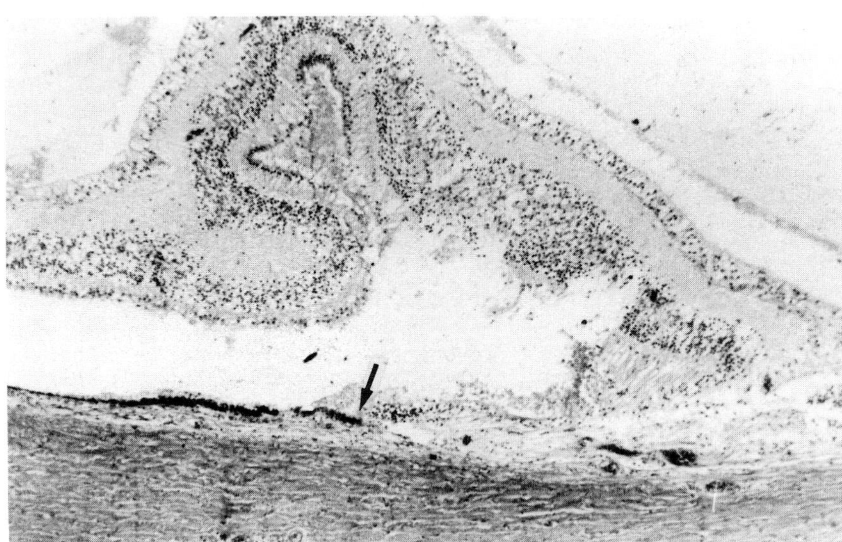

Fig. 17.4 (d) Anterior margin of choroidal coloboma. Note swelling of pigmented epithelium at margin (arrow). Masson trichrome (×64).

show some or all of the following features (Fig. 17.4):

1 A retrolental mass of vascularised connective tissue which sometimes contains a nodule of cartilage. This connective tissue passes laterally through a coloboma of the ciliary body and merges with the sclera. There may be an associated coloboma of the iris. The uveal defects may be missed unless serial sections are taken. The retrolental connective tissue occasionally contains dendritic melanocytes.

2 Dysplasia of the retina, which is folded to form branching tubules that are composed of elements of the outer retinal layers and open into the subretinal space. This malformation probably results from the aimless growth of developing sensory retina which occurs when it becomes separated from the retinal pigmented epithelium. The latter may be absent in the vicinity of a coloboma.

3 Retarded develoment of the anterior segment resulting in hypoplasia of the iris and malformed filtration angles which may result in glaucoma.

4 Congenital cataract.

CHARGE association

CHARGE is an acronym for *C*oloboma, *H*eart disease, *A*tresia choanae, *R*etarded development, *G*enital hypoplasia and *E*ar malformations. Four of these features need to be present to justify the diagnosis (see Duvall *et al.*, 1987).

OCULORENAL SYNDROMES

A number of well-established syndromes relate the eye to the kidney. These include:

1 Lowe's syndrome (oculocerebrorenal syndrome).

2 Aniridia with Wilms' tumour.

3 Alport's syndrome (see Chapter 9).

4 Various tapetoretinal degenerations associated with cystic kidneys.

PERSISTENT HYPERPLASTIC PRIMARY VITREOUS

While a retrolental mass of cellular fibrous tissue occurs in eyes with other defects as noted above, it is also not uncommonly seen as a sole unilateral abnormality usually in a slightly small eye. Both sexes are equally affected and there is no clear mode of inheritance. Although the basic defect is present at birth, leucoria may not be observed for some months.

The pathological manifestations (Fig. 17.5) are a cellular fibrous mass on the posterior aspect of the lens into which the hyaloid artery arborises. In individual sections, only small lengths of the hyaloid artery may be evident. The posterior lens fibres show cataractous changes and the posterior capsule of the lens may be ruptured. The ciliary processes are drawn inward and often attached to the retrolental mass. The *pars plana ciliaris* is narrowed and may sometimes be absent so that the peripheral retina is inserted directly into the ciliary processes or occasionally to the margin of the retrolental mass.

The anterior chamber may be shallow and the chamber angle immature. Raised intraocular pressure complicates some cases, but immaturity of the angle is not often associated with glaucoma.

The retina becomes detached in a proportion of cases by retinal traction either from preretinal glial strands or attachment of the peripheral retina to the retrolental mass and organisation of recurrent vitreous haemorrhages from ruptured hyaloid vessels.

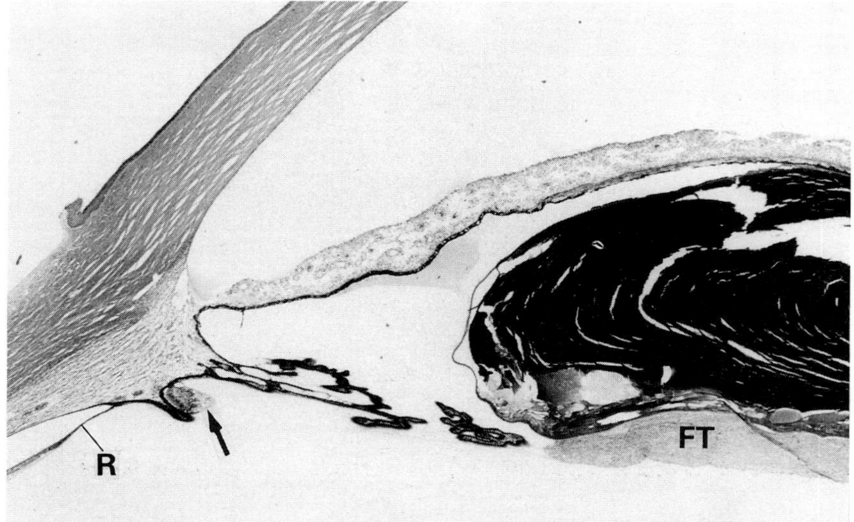

Fig. 17.5 Persistent hyperplastic primary vitreous. Child aged 6 months in whom a white reflex had been noticed since 4 weeks after birth. (a) Anterior segment. Note forward position of retina (R) due to shortening of the pars ciliaris and indrawing of ciliary processes to the retrolental fibrous tissue (FT). A small focus of aberrant retinal differentiation is seen on a ciliary process (arrow). Masson trichrome.

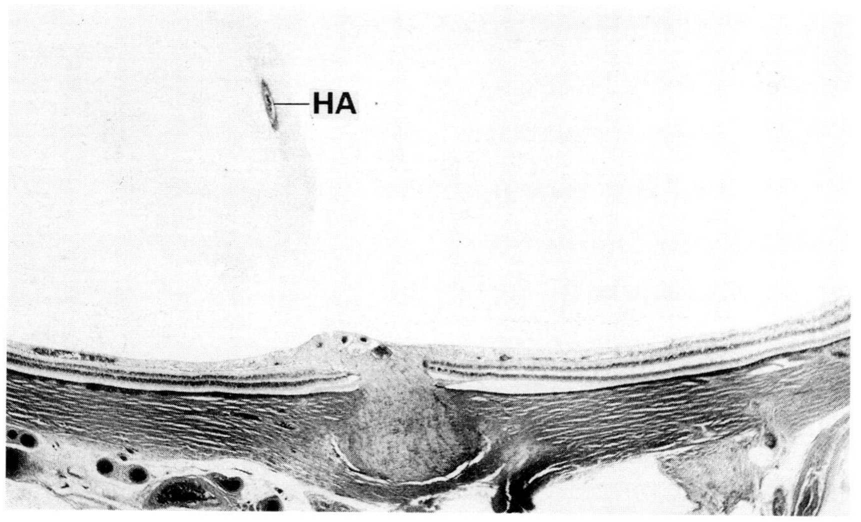

Fig. 17.5 (b) Posterior part of globe. A short length of hyaloid artery (HA) can be seen traversing the vitreous space at this level. Masson trichrome.

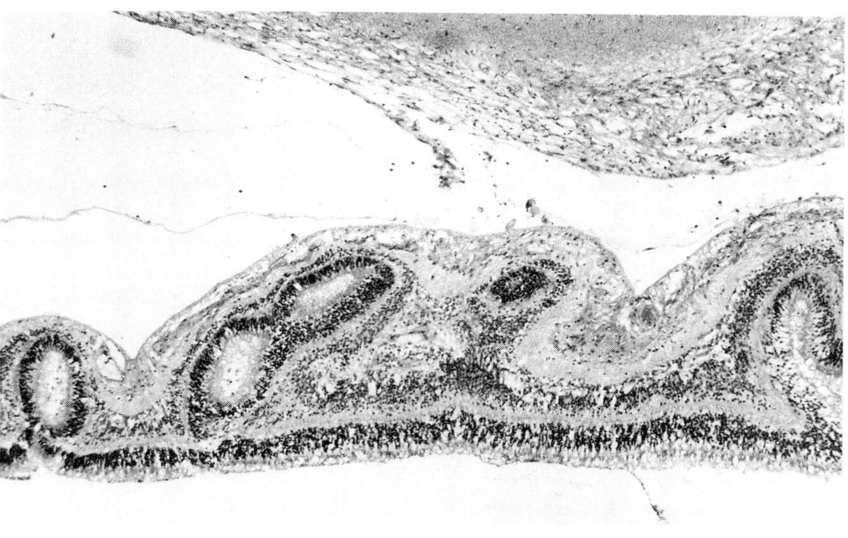

Fig. 17.6 Retinal dysplasia. Retina showing dysplastic folds comprising all layers (same case as Fig. 17.3). H & E (×41).

The condition was considered to represent persistence of the posterior part of the vascular tunica of the lens and the hyaloid system with hyperplasia of mesodermal elements of the primary vitreous, but it is clear that this is an oversimplification which overlooks the participation of retinal glia in the pathogenesis (Blodi, 1972; Manschot, 1958).

ANOMALIES OF THE RETINA

Retinal dysplasia

Retinal dysplasia is characterised by the formation of abnormal structures known as retinal rosettes (Fig. 17.6). They are commonly seen in association with other intraocular abnormalities and occasionally as an isolated feature in otherwise normal eyes. The rosette is the appearance in cross section of a tunnel or tube of retina. Such dysplastic rosettes should not be confused with the rosettes seen in retinoblastomas. A dysplastic rosette comprises one or more layers of cells linked by terminal bars which form a membrane resembling the external limiting membrane of the retina and continuity can be traced between this membrane and the external limiting membrane of the retina so that there is communication between the lumen of the rosette and the subretinal space. When the rosette is composed of a single layer of cells, the constituent cells are derived from the outer nuclear layer. Rosettes containing several layers of cells may include cells of the inner nuclear layer. Rosettes seen in retinoblastomata are, by contrast with dysplastic rosettes, sections of spherules of cells and continuity between the lumen of the rosette and the subretinal space is never demonstrable.

The lethal autosomal recessive Walker–Warburg (HARD ± E) syndrome associates retinal dysplasia with disordered brain development (*H*ydrocephalus, *A*gyria, *R*etinal *D*ysplasia with or without an *E*ncephalocoele) (see Donnai & Farndon, 1986). However, similar brain defects have been reported with anterior chamber defects and hypoplasia of the optic nerve without retinal dysplasia (Attia *et al.*, 1986)

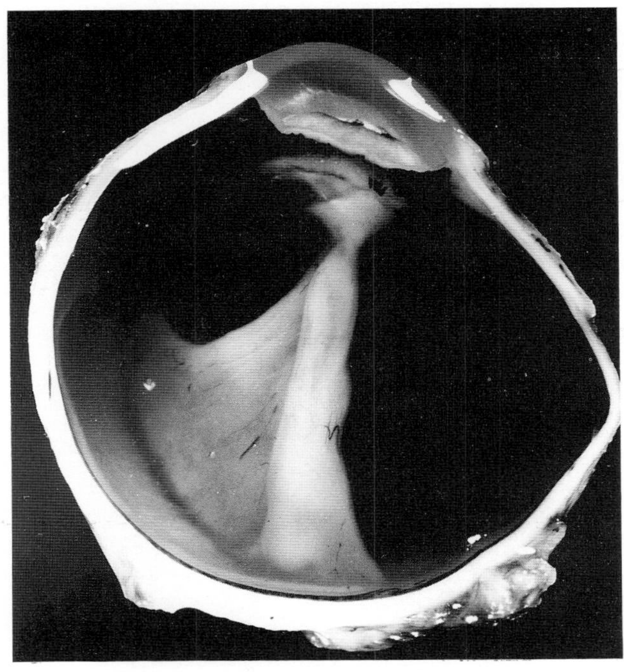

Fig. 17.7 Retinal fold. Irritable blind eye since birth which was enucleated at age 3.5 years. (a) Macroscopic picture showing thick central column of retina extending to posterior aspect of a malformed lens with crescentic fold of retina extending to the equator of the globe.

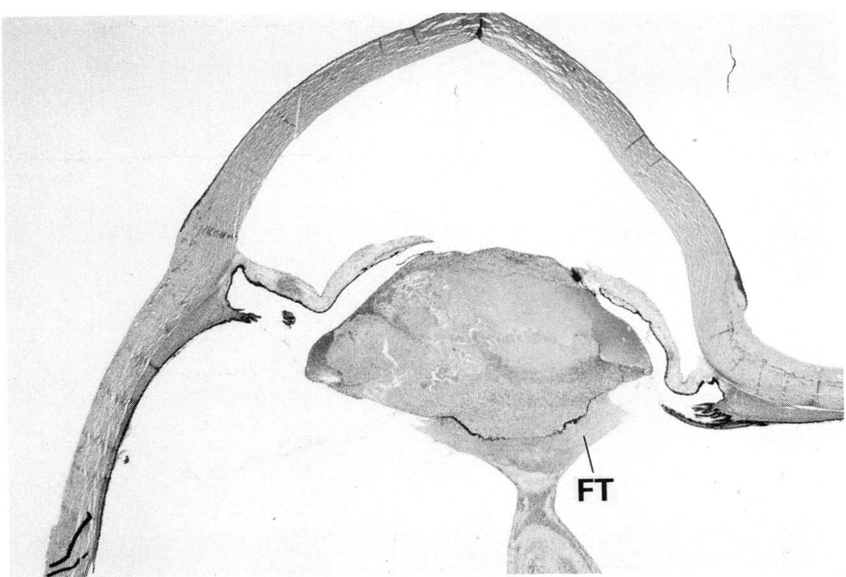

Fig. 17.7 (b) Anterior part of globe showing anterior part of globe. The fold is attached to a mass of retrolenticular fibrous tissue (FT). Indrawing of ciliary processes is evident on one side. PAS/tartrazine.

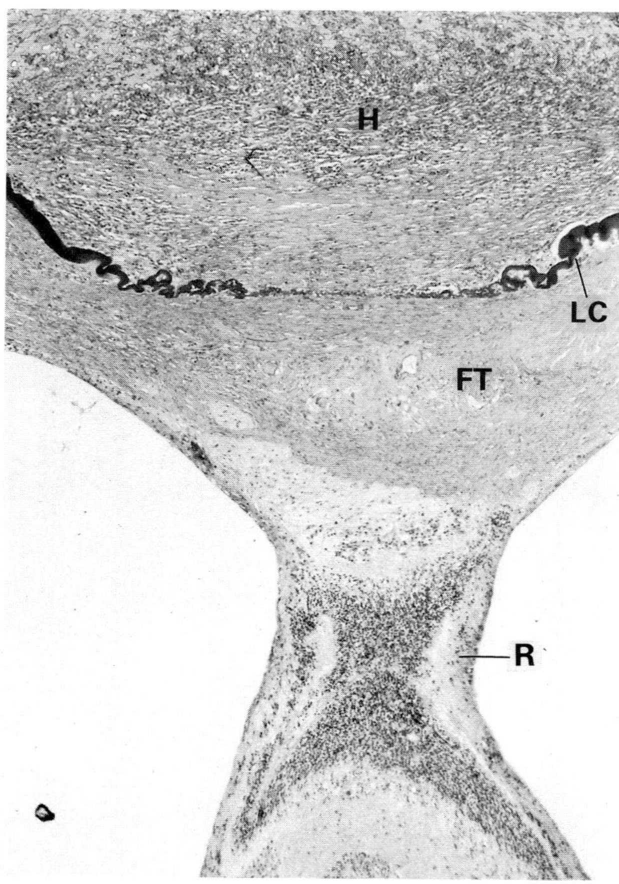

Fig. 17.7 (c) Detail of attachment of retinal fold (R) to retrolenticular fibrous tissue (FT). The lens capsule (LC) is thickened, but defective posteriorly and haemorrhage has occurred into the lens. The haemorrhage (H) is in process of organisation. PAS/tartrazine (×41).

Congenital (falciform) retinal fold

A congenital retinal fold occurs most commonly in one or both eyes of full-term male infants and may be inherited as a recessive character. A crescentic fold of retina extends from the optic nerve head to the equator of the lens where there may be a local opacity. Remnants of hyaloid vessels are found in the fold and features associated with persistent hyperplastic primary vitreous sometimes present in the anterior segment.

A variant of the typical condition is illustrated in Fig. 17.7. In this, the retinal fold is actually attached to persistent hyperplastic primary vitreous at the posterior pole.

ANTERIOR CHAMBER CLEAVAGE SYNDROME

This is a convenient term for a group of rare abnormalities of the cornea, iris and lens which have overlapping features that enable them to be arranged in a logical stepwise sequence of increasing complexity according to which combination of such features is manifest (Fig. 17.8). This aids understanding and avoids the use of too many cumbersome or eponymous names for minor variants. The features fall into two groups:

1 Peripheral.

(i) Prominent Schwalbe's ring (posterior embryotoxon).

(ii) Strands of iris to Schwalbe's ring.

(iii) Hypoplasia of the iris stroma.

2 Central.

(i) Defect in Desçemet's membrane and the corneal endothelium with overlying corneal opacity.

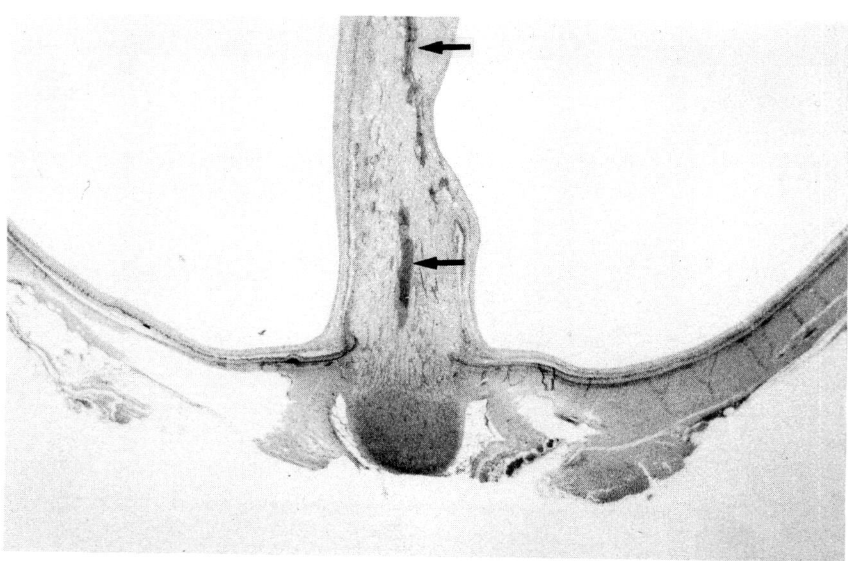

Fig. 17.7 (d) Posterior part of globe showing how the central column comprises grossly elongated optic nerve head within the retinal fold. Large central vessels (arrows) are present in the optic nerve. PAS/tartrazine.

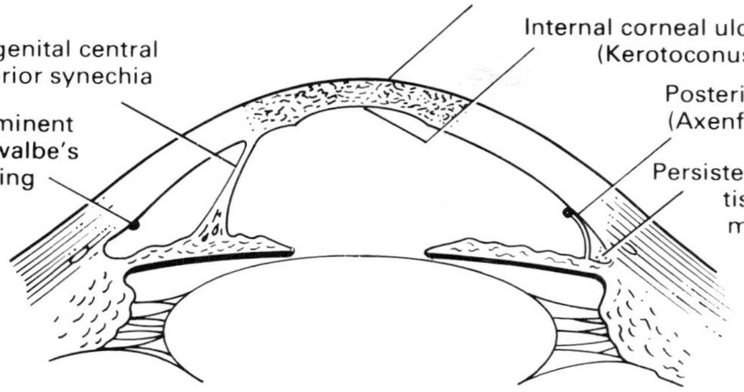

Fig. 17.8 Anterior cleavage syndrome. Diagram illustrating step-ladder classification proposed by Reese and Ellsworth (*Archives of Opthalmology* **75**, 307–318. Copyright 1966, American Medical Association).

Table 17.1 Anomalies included in the anterior cleavage syndrome. Reproduced with permission from Mullaney, 1984.

Posterior embryotoxon	Prominent Schwalbe's line
Axenfeld's anomaly	Prominent Schwalbe's ring with iris strands to ring
Rieger's anomaly	Prominent Schwalbe's ring with iris strands to ring
Iridogoniodysgenesis	Prominent Schwalbe's ring with iris strands to ring Hypoplasia of anterior iris stroma
Posterior keratoconus	Posterior corneal depression
Peter's anomaly (3 groups)	1 Posterior corneal defect and leucoma 2 With iris adhesions to leucoma margin 3 With apposition of lens to leucoma

(ii) Inconstant components such as central irido-corneal adhesions, apposition of lens with cornea and scleralisation of the cornea (Fig. 17.9).

Cases may present with peripheral or central anomalies alone or combinations of both. Developmental glaucoma commonly affects cases of all groups. Different combinations may be seen in the two eyes of one individual or in different members of the same family and systemic abnormalities may be present. The combinations seen in the well-known eponymous conditions which may be placed in this category are given in Table 17.1.

Four hypotheses have been advances to account for the central abnormalities seen in Peters' anomaly (see Waring *et al.*, 1975; Mullaney, 1984).

1 Failure of the mesodermal cells forming the cornea to migrate centrally thus leaving a posterior central corneal defect.

2 Failure of the lens vesicle to separate from the surface ectoderm so that a keratolenticular adhesion persists.

3 Secondary anterior displacement of the lens–iris diaphragm by a retro-lenticular mass such as persistent hyperplastic primary vitreous.

4 Multiple origin: either the second or third mechanism may operate. There are accordingly two types of case — primary or secondary.

RARE SYNDROMES WHICH MAY PRESENT WITH A RETROLENTAL MASS

Norrie's disease

This rare recessive X-linked hyaloideoretinal dysplasia results in congenital blindness in both eyes. The eyes are often of normal size but may be smaller or larger than normal. The anterior chamber is usually shallow and the iris often atrophic. Posterior adhesions may be present at birth or develop during the early months of life together with anterior adhesions and ectropion of the iris pigment epithelium. The lens is clear at first and behind it is a mass of vascular connective tissue. The retina, which is often totally detached, exhibits marked disorganisation, loss of neural cells and glial proliferation. Encysted haemorrhages are sometimes present in its inner layers and there may be marked overgrowth of the retinal pigmented epithelium. The optic nerve is atrophic.

In the course of time, corneal opacities develop, the retina is reduced to glial scar tissue, bone forms in the choroid and subretinal space and the eyes shrink so that the histological picture becomes indistinguishable from that following severe endophthalmitis. Some patients are mentally retarded while others become deaf later in life.

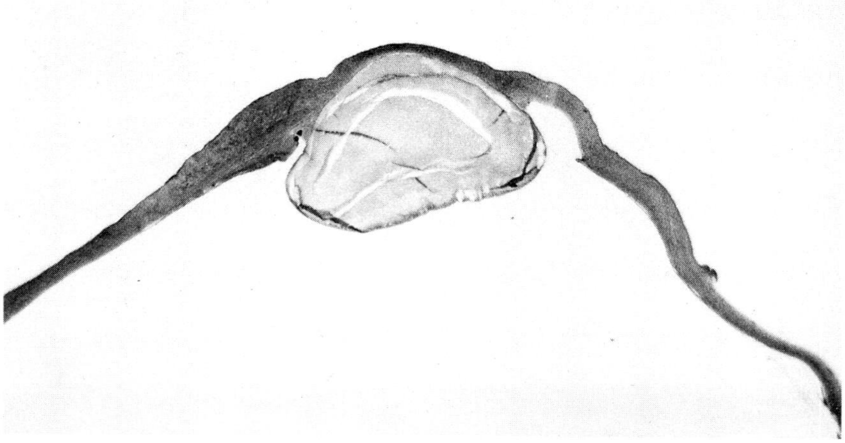

Fig. 17.9 Anterior cleavage syndrome. Complete failure of development of anterior chamber. (a) Showing lens in apposition to small cornea. PAS/tartrazine.

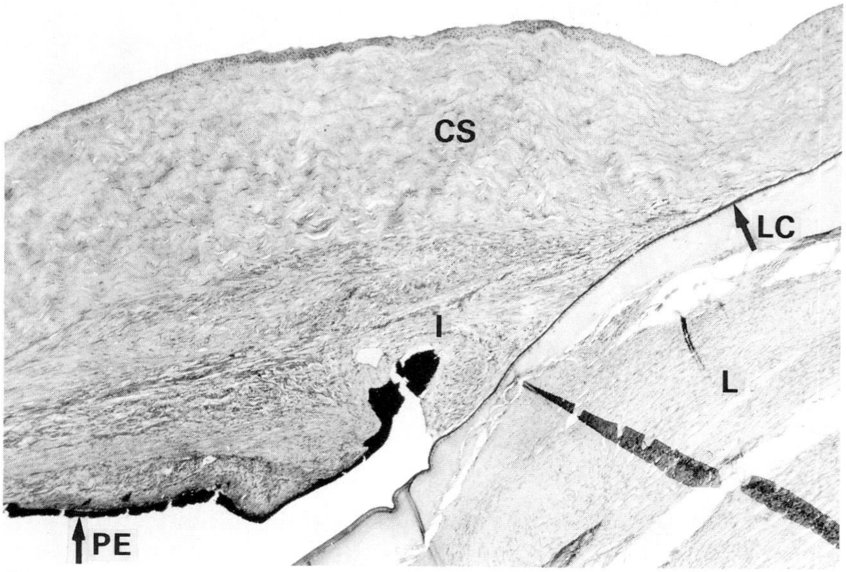

Fig. 17.9 (b) & (c) Detail of corneal periphery. The iris stroma merges with the posterior corneoscleral stroma (CS) and the pupillary border (I) is also adherent to lens (L). The pigmented epithelium of the iris (PE) is attenuated. The peripheral cornea is imperfectly differentiated from the sclera. No endothelium or Desçemet's membrane could be demonstrated and the lens capsule (LC) is in apposition with the posterior corneal stroma. PAS/tartrazine.

(b)

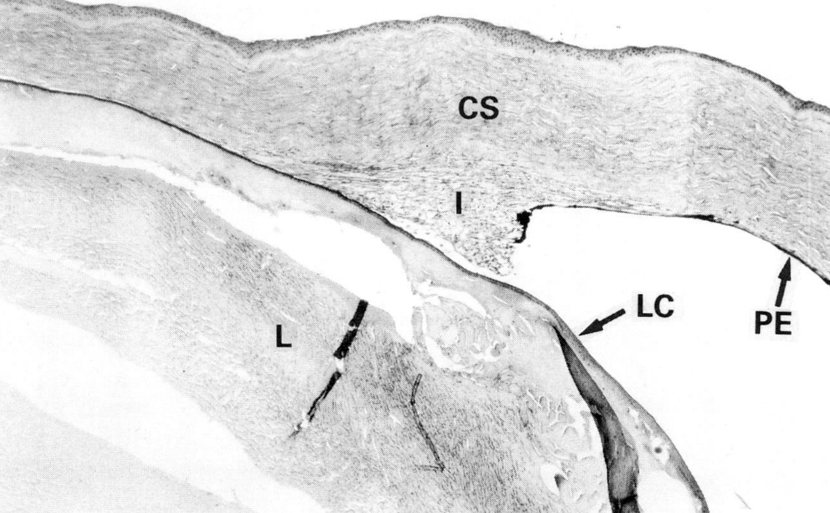

(c)

Incontinentia pigmenti

Incontinentia pigmenti (Bloch–Sulzberger syndrome) is a rare disease of female infants thought to be an X-linked dominant which is characterised by recurrent vesicular and bullous skin eruptions. On healing, these leave pigmented lines and blotches on the trunk and limbs. In 25% of cases there are associated ocular lesions including retinal detachment and intraocular haemorrhage which may result in an organised retrolental fibroglial mass. Cataract and corneal opacities may also be present.

SPHEROPHAKIA AND DISLOCATION OF THE LENS

Marfan's syndrome

Marfan's syndrome (dystrophia mesodermalis congenita hypoplastica) is generally inherited as an autosomal dominant with rather variable penentrance. Although the manifestations may be extremely diverse they commonly comprise ocular, skeletal and cardiovascular abnormalities.

Ocular abnormalities

Dislocation of the lens is an essential feature. It is usually bilateral, upwards and outwards in direction and incomplete (Plate 5). The lens itself is usually small and globular (spherophakia). The chamber angle may show persistance of mesodermal tissue and dense pectinate remnants are common. The iris stroma is hypoplastic and the dilator pupillae sometimes deficient (Fig. 17.10a & b). Pigmentation of the posterior layer of the pigmented epithelium may be segmentally reduced. Numerous more severe ocular defects have also been reported in occasional cases.

Skeletal abnormalities

The bones of the limbs are long and thin and fingers and toes show the characterisic arachnodactyly. Dolichocephaly usually results in the face being long and thin. Kyphoscoliosis affects over half the cases.

Cardiovascular abnormalities

These include persistent foramen ovale, transposition of the great vessels, aneurysms and coarctation or hyplasia of the aorta. Rupture of a dissecting aneurysm is a common cause of death.

Weill–Marchesani's syndrome

This syndrome (sometimes known as dystrophia mesodermalis congenita hypertrophica) is much rarer than Marfan's and a consistent mode of inheritance is not fully

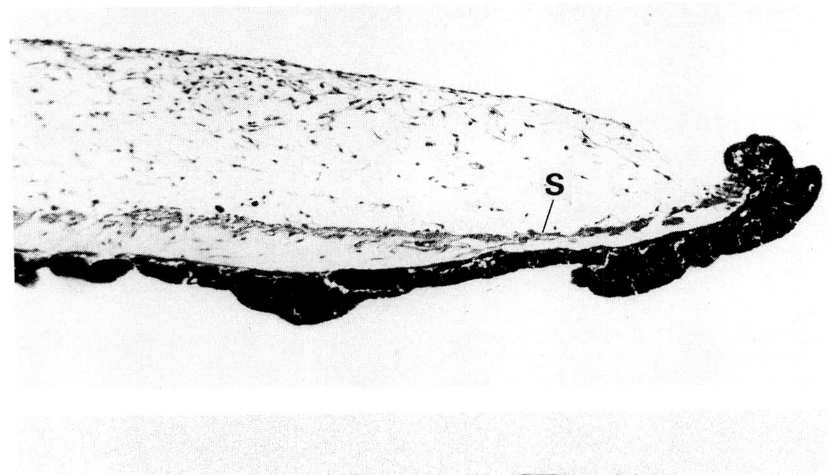

Fig. 17.10 Marfan's syndrome. (a) Pupillary border of iris showing atrophic stroma and poorly developed sphincter pupillae (S). PAS/tartrazine (×93).

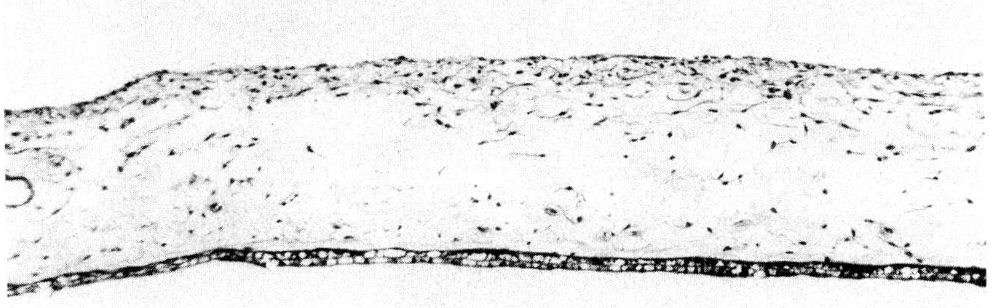

Fig. 17.10 (b) Peripheral iris showing double layer of pigmented epithelium and no evidence of a dilator pupillae. PAS/tartrazine (×93).

established. By contrast with Marfan's, affected persons are short and stumpy with spade-like hands.

Ocular abnormalities

High myopia is common because of the spherophakic lens. Dislocation of the lens is common and usually downwards and inwards. Degenerative changes in the suspensory ligament produce a thick PAS-positive coating on the ciliary processes resembling that seen in homocystinuria. Secondary glaucoma is common.

Homocystinuria

Homocystinuria is due a deficiency of cystathione synthetase so that there is an inability to convert homocysteine to cystathione. A build-up of homocystine results. Inheritance is thought to be by an autosomal recessive gene. Patients are usually fair and may be mentally retarded and have skeletal abnormalities. Reduced platelet survival time results in arterial thrombosis and other thromboembolic problems.

Ocular abormalities

The lens becomes dislocated infero-nasally or into the anterior chamber. Histologically a thick PAS-positive coating of filamentous material is seen on the ciliary processes. The coating consists of zonular remants composed mainly of short filaments in total disarray.

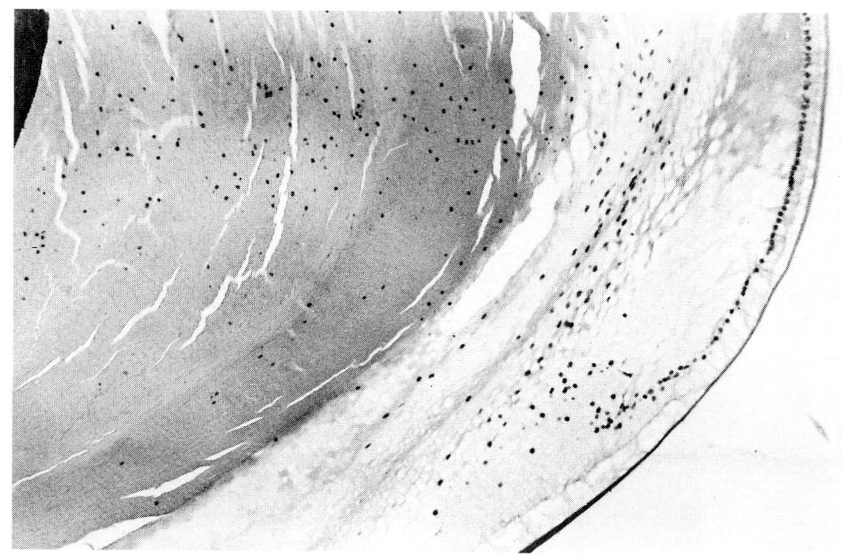

Fig. 17.11 Rubella syndrome. (a) Lens. Equator showing lens bow with nuclei extending into nucleus. PAS/tartrazine (×94). (Specimen by courtesy of Dr J. L. S. Smith.)

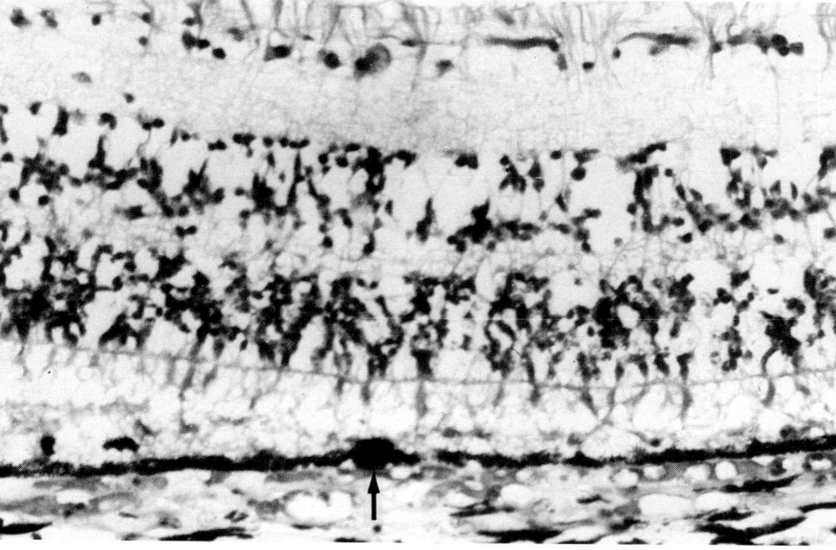

Fig. 17.11 (b) Retina showing swollen pigmented epithelial cell adjacent to an area of atrophy (arrow). Masson trichrome (×260).

RUBELLA SYNDROME

The commonest, but by no means the only congenital lesions attributable to intrauterine infection by the rubella virus are cardiac malformations, ocular defects, mental retardation and deafness. Maternal infection in the first trimester of pregnancy results in virus localisation in embryonic cells causing death of cells and disturbances of normal tissue development. The ocular component of the rubella syndrome comprises cataract, glaucoma, iris defects and pigmentary retinopathy. The globe is somewhat smaller than normal, but is not severely microphthalmic.

1 Congenital cataracts are present in one or both eyes. The lens is rounded and its sclerosed nucleus contains nucleated fibres. A variable degree of cortical necrosis is evident, but the lens capsule and subcapsular epithelium are more or less normal and there is no migration of the lens epithelium over the posterior surface of the lens such as commonly occurs in other congenital cataracts (Fig. 17.11a). Virus can persist in the lens for at least 3 years after birth. Cataract surgery during this time may be complicated by a viral endopthalmitis.

2 Glaucoma is presumed to be the result of maldevelopment of the filtration angle in which the iris root does not separate from the meshwork, while the angle recess and ciliary processes are displaced anteriorly. Ciliary muscle may be found inserted into the trabeculae of the meshwork instead of onto the sceral spur.

3 The iris shows hypoplasia of the dilator muscle and sometimes of the sphincter as well. There may be a nongranulomatous iridocyclitis and focal necrosis of the pigmented epithelium of the iris and ciliary body accompanied by phagocytosis of the dispersed melanin granules. Pigmentary retinopathy is manifest by alternating areas of atrophy and hypertrophy (Fig. 17.11b) of the pigmented epithelium which produce the so-called pepper and salt fundus seen clinically.

BIBLIOGRAPHY

General

Duke-Elder, S. (1964) Congenital deformities, normal and abnormal development. In *System of Ophthalmology*, vol. III, Parts 1 & 2. Henry Kimpton, London.

Mann, I. (1973) *Developmental Abnromalities of the Eye*. Cambridge University Press, Cambridge.

Mullaney, J. (1984) Normal development and developmental anormalies of the eye. In *Pathobiology of the Eye*, eds A. Garner & G. Klintworth, pp 443–552. Dekker, New York.

O'Rahilly, R. (1975) The prenatal development of the human eye. *Experimental Eye Research* **21**, 93–112.

Anophthalmos, microphthalmos and coloboma

Cogan, D. G. (1978) Coloboma of the optic nerve with overlay of peripapillary retina. *British Journal of Ophthalmology* **62**, 347–350.

Font, R. L. & Zimmerman, L. E. (1971) Intrascleral smooth muscle in coloboma of the optic nerve disc. *American Journal of Ophthalmology* **72**, 452–458.

Mullaney, J. (1978) Complex sporadic coloboma. *British Journal of Ophthalmology* **62**, 384–385.

Waring III, G. O., Roth, A. M. & Rodrigues, M. M. (1976) Clinicopathologic correlation of microphthalmos with cyst. *American Journal of Ophthalmology* **82**, 714–721.

Syndromes associated with microphthalmos and coloboma

Apple, D. J., Holden, J. D. & Stallworth, B. (1970) Ocular pathology of Patau's syndrome with an unbalanced D/D translocation. *American Journal of Ophthalmology* **70**, 383–390.

Attia, M. F. D., Burn, J., McCarthy, J. H., Purohit, D. P. & Milligan D. W. A. (1986) Warburg (HARD ± E) Syndrome without retinal dysplasia: case report and review. *British Journal of Ophthalmology* **70**, 742–747.

Cogan, D. G. & Kuwabara, T. (1964) Ocular pathology of the 13–15 Trisomy syndrome. *Archives of Ophthalmology* **72**, 246–253.

Donnai, D. & Farndon, P. A. (1986) Walker–Warburg syndrome (Warburg syndrome, HARD ± E syndrome). *Journal of Medical Genetics* **23**, 200–203.

Duvall, J., Miller, S. L., Cheatle, E. & Tso, M. O. M. (1987) Ocular changes in a syndrome of multiple congenital anomalies. A histopathological study. *American Journal of Ophthalmology* **103**, 701–705.

James, P., Karseras, A. G. & Wybar, K. C. (1974) Systemic associations of uveal coloboma. *British Journal of Ophthalmology* **58**, 917–921.

Maskett, S., Galioto, F. M. & Best, M. (1970) Anophthalmia, multiple abnormalities, and unusual karyotype. *American Journal of Ophthalmology* **70**, 381–383.

Warburg, M & Mikkelsen, M. (1963) A case of Bartholin–Patau's syndrome. With a review of the ophthalmic literature. *Acta Ophthalmologica* **41**, 321–334.

Yanoff, M., Rorke, L. B. & Niederer, B. S. (1970) Ocular and cerebral abnormalities in chromosome 18 deletion defect. *American Journal of Ophthalmology* **70**, 391–402.

Oculorenal syndromes

Brownstein, S., Kirkham, T. H. & Kalousek, D. (1976) Bilateral renal agenesis with multiple congenital anomalies. *American Journal of Ophthalmology* **82**, 770–774.

Garner, A., Fielder, A. R. & Stevens, A. (1982) Tapetoretinal degeneration in the cerebro-hepato-renal (Zellweger's) syndrome. *British Journal of Ophthalmology* **66**, 422–431.

Ginsberg, J., Buchino, J. J., Menefee, M., Ballard, E. & Husain, I. (1979) Multiple congenital ocular abnormalities with agenesis of the urinary tract. *Annals of Ophthalmology* **11**, 1021–1079.

Haddard, R., Font, R. L. & Friendly, D. S. (1976) Cerebrohepatorenal syndrome of Zellweger. *Archives of Ophthalmology* **94**, 1927–1930.

Peterson, W. S. & Albert, D. M. (1974) Fundus changes in hereditary nephropathies. *Transactions of the American Academy of Ophthalmology and Otolaryngology* **78**, 762–271.

Persistent hyperplastic primary vitreous

Blodi, F. C. (1972) Preretinal glial nodules in persistence and hyperplasia of primary vitreous. *Archives of Ophthalmology* **87**, 531–534.

Font, R. L., Yanoff, M. and Zimmerman, L. E. (1969) Intraocular adipose tissue and persistent hyperplastic primary vitreous. *Archives of Ophthalmology* **82**, 43–50.

Haddad, R., Font, R. L. & Reeser, F. (1978) Persistent hyperplastic primary vitreous. A clinicopathologic study of 62 cases and review of the literature. *Survey of Ophthalmology* **23**, 123–134.

Jensen, O. A. (1968) Persistent hyperplastic primary vitreous. *Acta Ophthalmologica* **46**, 418–429.

Manschot, W. A. (1958) Persistent hyperplastic primary vitreous. special reference to preretinal glial tissue as a pathological characteristic and to the development of the primary vitreous. *Archives of Ophthalmology* **59**, 188–203.

Pruett, R. C. (1975) The pleomorphism and complications of persistent hyperplastic primary vitreous. *American Journal of Ophthalmology* **80**, 625–629.

Reese, A. B. (1955) Persistent hyperplastic primary vitreous. Jackson Memorial Lecture. *Transactions of the American Academy of Ophthalmology and Otolaryngology* **59**, 271–286.

Wegener, J. K. & Sogarrd, H. (1968) Persistent hyperplastic primary vitreous with resorption of the lens. *Acta Ophthalmologica* **46**, 171–175.

Wolter, J. R. & Flaherty, N. W. (1959) Persistent hyperplastic vitreous. *American Journal of Ophthalmology* **47**, 491–503.

Anomalies of retina

Boniuk, M. & Hittner, H. (1975) Congenital retinal disinsertion syndrome. *Transactions of the American Academy of Ophthalmology and Otolaryngology* **79**, 827–834.

Lahav, M., Albert, D. M. & Wyand, S. (1973) Clinical and histopathologic classification of retinal dysplasia. *American Journal of Ophthalmology* **75**, 648–667.

Anterior cleavage syndrome

Kivlin, J. D., Fineman, R. N., Crandall, A. S. & Olson, R. J. (1986) Peters' anomaly as a consequence of genetic and nongenetic syndromes. *Archives of Ophthalmology* **104**, 61–64.

Reese, A. B. & Ellsworth, R. M. (1966) The anterior cleavage syndrome. *Archives of Ophthalmology* **75**, 307–318.

Townsend, W. M., Font, R. L. & Zimmerman, L. E. (1974) Congenital corneal leucoma. 3. Histopathologic findings in 13 eyes with noncentral defects in Desçemet's membrane. *American Journal of Ophthalmology* **77**, 400–412.

Waring, G. O. III, Roth, A. M. & Rodrigues, M. M. (1975) Anterior cleavage syndrome. A stepladder classification. *Survey of Ophthalmology* **20**, 3–27.

Norrie's disease

Warburg, M. (1966) *Norrie's Disease. A Congenital Progressive Oculo-Acoustico-Cerebral Degeneration.* Translated from the Danish by A. Rousing. G. Asboe-Hansen, Copenhagen.

Spherophakia and dislocation of the lens

Henkind, P. & Ashton, N. (1965) Ocular pathology in homocystinuria. *Transactions of the Ophthalmological Society of the UK* **85**, 21–37.

Jensen, A. D., Cross, H. E. & Paton, D. (1974) Ocular complications in the Weill–Marchesani Syndrome. *American Journal of Ophthalmology* **77**, 261–269.

McGavic, J. S. (1966) Weill–Marchesani syndrome — brachymorphism and ectopia lentis *et pupillae*. *American Journal of Ophthalmology* **62**, 820–823.

Ramsey, M. S., Daitz, L. D. & Beaton, J. W. (1975) Lens fringe in homocystinuria. *Archives of Ophthalmology* **93**, p. 318.

Ramsey, M. S. & Dickson, D. H. (1975) Lens fringe in homocystinuria. *British Journal of Ophthalmology* **59**, 338–342.

Ramsey, M. S., Fine, B. S., Shields, J. A. & Yanoff, M. (1973) The Marfan syndrome. A histopathologic study of ocular findings. *American Journal of Ophthalmology* **76**, 102–116.

Ramsey, M. S., Fine, B. S. & Yanoff, M. (1972) The ocular histopathology of homocystinuria. A light and electron microscopic study. *American Journal of Ophthalmology* **74**, 377–385.

Rubella syndrome

Boniuk, M. & Zimmerman, L. E. (1967) Ocular pathology in the rubella syndrome. *Archives of Ophthalmology* **77**, 455–473.

Gregg, N. M. (1941) Congenital cataract following German measles in the mother. *Transactions of the Ophthalmological Society of Australia* **3**, 342–345.

Gregg, N. M. (1944) Further observations on congenital defects in infants following maternal rubella. *Transactions of the Ophthalmological Society of Australia* **4**, 119–131.

Roy, F. H., Hiatt, R. L., Korones, S. B. & Roane, J. (1966) Ocular manifestations of the congenital rubella syndrome. Recovery of virus from affected infants. *Archives of Ophthalmology* **75**, 601–607.

Chapter 18 Accidental and surgical trauma

The effects of injuries to the eye are conveniently considered under three headings.

1 *Contusion*. This may result either from direct force applied to the globe or from indirect force as in head injuries, explosions, etc.

2 *Perforation of the corneoscleral envelope*.

3 *Intraocular foreign bodies*. These may be inert substances, irritant metal or organised materials.

Obviously, in many cases all three effects will be involved. Only a limited account of this very extensive subject can be given here and reference should be made to larger works.

EFFECTS OF CONTUSION

Hyphaema

Hyphaema is one of the most important results of contusion, though it does, of course, also occur in perforating injuries or simply from the rupture of new vessels on the anterior surface of the iris.

The eye has a considerable capacity for clearing blood from the anterior chamber via the outflow pathway, but, when the haemorrhage is large or recurrent, the blood may clot in the anterior chamber. Organisation of this clot by granulation tissue leads to the formation of adhesions between the iris, cornea and lens. These may result in secondary angle closure and occlusion and/or seclusion of the pupil.

After large haemorrhages into the anterior chamber, cholesterol may crystallise from the plasma and become the focus of a foreign body giant cell reaction. Eventually, the whole anterior chamber may be filled with scar tissue.

Hyphaema in the presence of raised intraocular pressure and damage to the cornea leads to blood staining of the cornea. This apparently occurs through local defects in Desçemet's membrane and focal damage to the endothelium. Microscopically, there are no red cells in the cornea but the lamellae and interlamellar spaces are packed with innumerable ovoid and spherical eosinophilic refractile granules containing haemoglobin. These slowly disintegrate. The breakdown products and released haemosiderin are taken up by keratocytes. The latter show extensive degenerative changes. Removal of the breakdown products of haemoglobin is believed to be by diffusion and occurs very slowly.

On the cornea

Post-traumatic corneal rings (traumatic annular keratopathy) seen after the cornea is struck by small projectiles are the result of local endothelial damage (see Stulting *et al.*, 1986).

On the iris

Direct or indirect contusion of the eye may cause a radial split through the pupillary border of the iris or detachment of the iris root from the ciliary body (iridodialysis) following which the ciliary processes may adhere to the corneoscleral trabecular meshwork.

If the haemorrhage is small, the blood is washed away in the aqueous stream and the iris tear remains unhealed. Larger haemorrhages, however, usually clot and organise so that the iris defect is bridged by scar tissue. At the same time, adhesions may develop between the iris, lens and cornea and a capillary vascular membrane may form on the anterior surface of the iris. Bleeding from the delicate new vessels leads to recurrent hyphaema and the iris stroma may become stained yellowish-brown with haemosiderin. A wedge of iris may be forced back into the circumlental space (recession of the iris) while, if the zonular fibres are ruptured, the iris may be retroverted against the ciliary body (inversion of the iris).

On the ciliary body

Contusions of the globe cause tears in the ciliary stroma and muscle, and rupture of the ciliary processes. These are frequently followed by severe haemorrhage which spreads into the vitreous and posterior and anterior chambers. The ciliary muscle may be completely torn away from the scleral spur (cyclodialysis) with rupture of the anterior ciliary vessels in the suprachoroidal space. Tears through the anterior aspect of the ciliary body often rupture branches of the major circle of the iris and thus result in massive hyphaema. Tears through the anterior part of the ciliary muscle may also result in angle recession. Subtle secondary changes in the recessed angle sometimes lead insidiously to the development of 'post-contusion angle deformity glaucoma' (Chapter 12). Contused limbal lacerations are frequently complicated by a 'contre-coup' tear in the angle on the opposite side of the globe (Fig. 18.1).

Damage to the ciliary muscle or its nerve supply may result in cycloplegia. Although secondary glaucoma is the common outcome of ciliary body injuries, the opposite state of hypotony occasionally develops when contusion results in such extensive haemorrhage into and disruption of the ciliary body that aqueous secretion is severely diminished.

On the lens

Dislocation

Contusion of the lens may rupture the zonular fibres and dislocate the lens either into the anterior chamber or into the vitreous.

A lens dislocated anteriorly may be arrested in and block the pupil or become completely displaced into the anterior chamber. In either case it obstructs aqueous outflow and results in a rapid rise in intraocular pressure. Glaucoma also follows posterior dislocation of the lens, but its onset may be delayed for years. In many instances, the cause of the glaucoma is not the dislocated lens itself, but the traumatic recession of the anterior chamber angle already described.

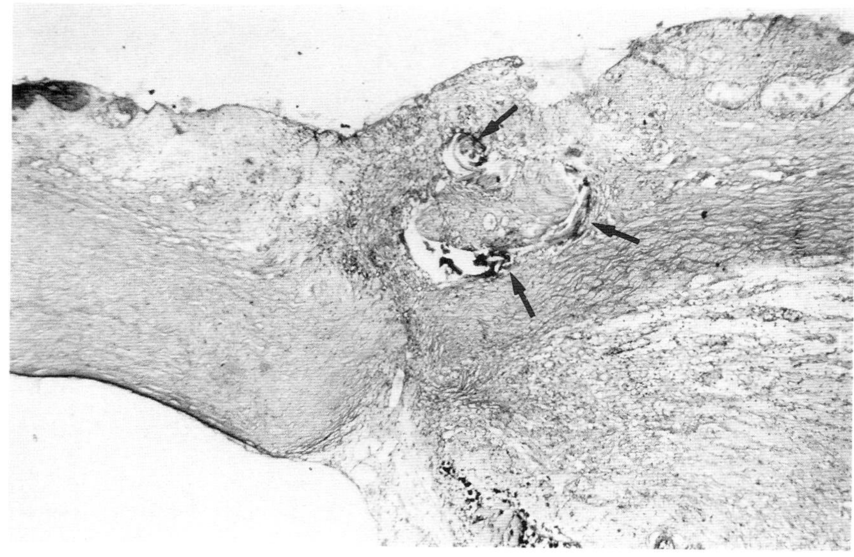

Fig. 18.1 'Contre-coup' injury to angle. (a) Contused limbal laceration. Suture profiles (arrows) are visible. PAS/tartrazine (×41).

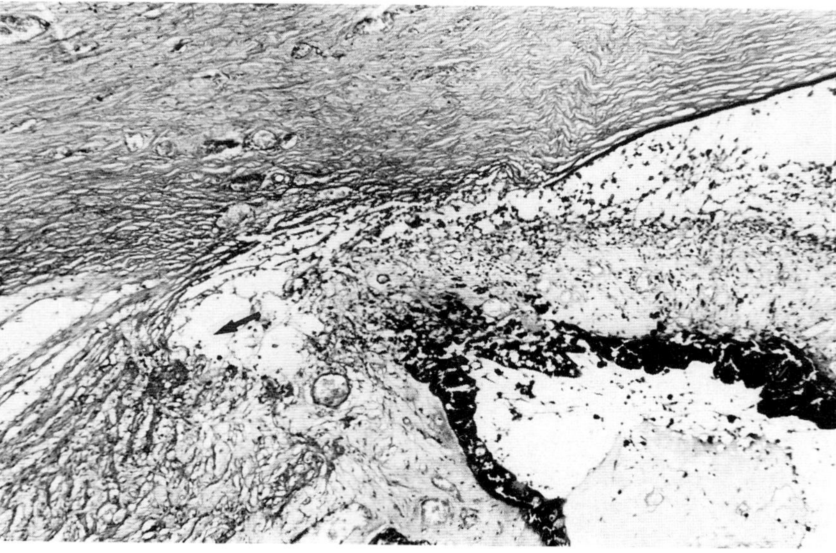

Fig. 18.1 (b) Chamber angle on opposite side of globe showing tear through root of iris into anterior part of ciliary muscle (arrow). PAS/tartrazine (×64).

Contusional cataract

Cataract may develop in either dislocated or undislocated lenses following contusion, usually without rupture of the capsule. The lens opacity commonly develops at the posterior pole and takes the form of a rosette due to the forcible separation of the suture lines between the lens fibres.

On the vitreous

Haemorrhage may occur into the vitreous or between the posterior face of the vitreous and the internal limiting membrane of the retina. Blood within the vitreous may take months to clear and organisation accompanied by the formation of epiretinal fibroglial membranes results in traction detachment of the retina.

On the retina

Commotio retinae

Contusion of the eye sometimes results in commotio retinae, a condition characterised by widespread oedema of the retina with scattered haemorrhages which usually resolves without permanent damage. The pathogenesis of commotio retinae is not fully understood, but its immediate cause appears to be vasoparalysis of the small retinal vessels which slows blood flow and allows the escape of plasma into the retinal tissues. The oedema gradually subsides, but loss of neuronal elements and photoreceptors and pigment proliferation may give an end picture resembling retinitis pigmentosa (Chapter 10).

Apart from direct trauma, retinal haemorrhages may also result from severe indirect trauma such as violent shaking (Fig. 18.2).

The effects of retinal haemorrhages vary considerably according to their size and location. Small retinal haemorrhages absorb completely or leave only a few haemosiderin-laden macrophages around the local vessels. Superficial haemorrhages may rupture into the vitreous and provoke local new vessel formation. Haemorrhages from the peripheral retina sometimes seep forwards into the anterior vitreous face and become organised to form a cyclitic membrane which will subsequently result in a traction detachment of the retina.

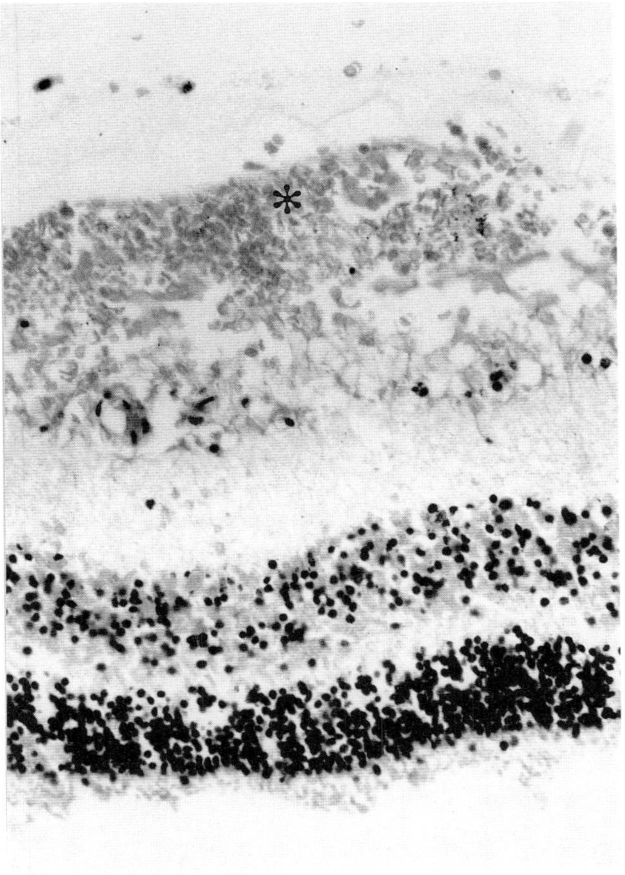

Fig. 18.2 Retinal haemorrhages due to indirect trauma. Male child aged 3 months was shaken violently and died with subdural and subarachnoid haemorrhages. The intra-retinal haemorrhage affects all layers, but is particularly marked deep to the internal limiting membrane (asterisk). Rupture into the vitreous was seen in places. H & E (×280). (Specimen by courtesy of Dr E. Tapp.)

Macular hole

Following contusion, retinal oedema restricted to the macular area sometimes develops. The fluid collects mainly in the outer plexiform layer, but also in the outer nuclear layer and subretinal space. Although the oedema subsides in 3 to 4 weeks, there is often residual damage and some loss of central vision. There is local degeneration of the photoreceptors and some pigmented epithelial cells die while others proliferate. Empty spaces which probably contained watery fluid may be seen in the outer plexiform layer in the macular area. These may coalesce to form a relatively large cyst. If the thin inner wall of such a cyst ruptures, a macular hole is formed, the margins of which are sometimes bound down to a fibrous scar containing proliferated pigment (Fig. 18.3).

Peripheral breaks

Contusion may also result in retinal tears or disinsertion of the retina at the ora serrata allowing fluid from the vitreous to accumulate behind the retina and detach it (Fig. 18.4).

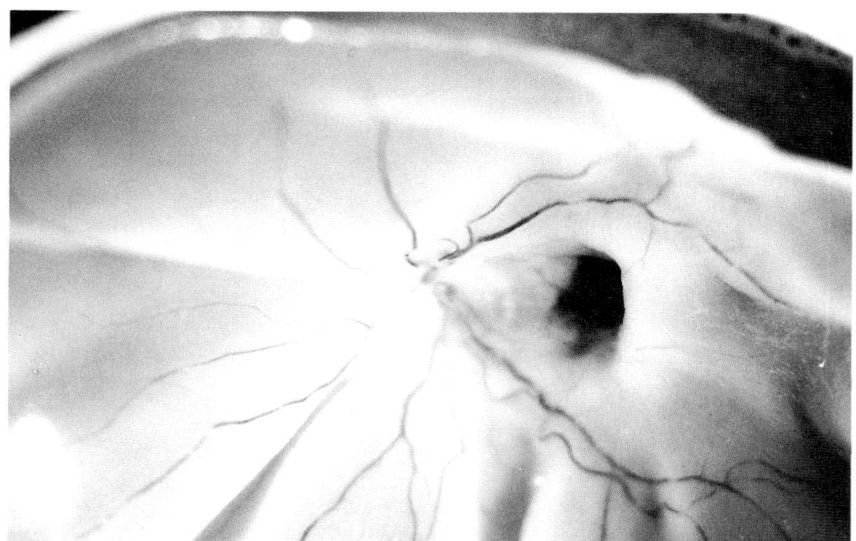

Fig. 18.3 Macular hole following trauma. The patient was punched in the eye and sustained a hyphaema and dislocation of lens. Removal of the lens was followed by a vitreous hamorrhage. When this cleared, a large inferior detachment and macular pigmentation were observed. The angle was deeply recessed. The eye became glaucomatous and was removed 9 months after injury. (a) Macrocopic picture showing macular hole with retina billowing around it.

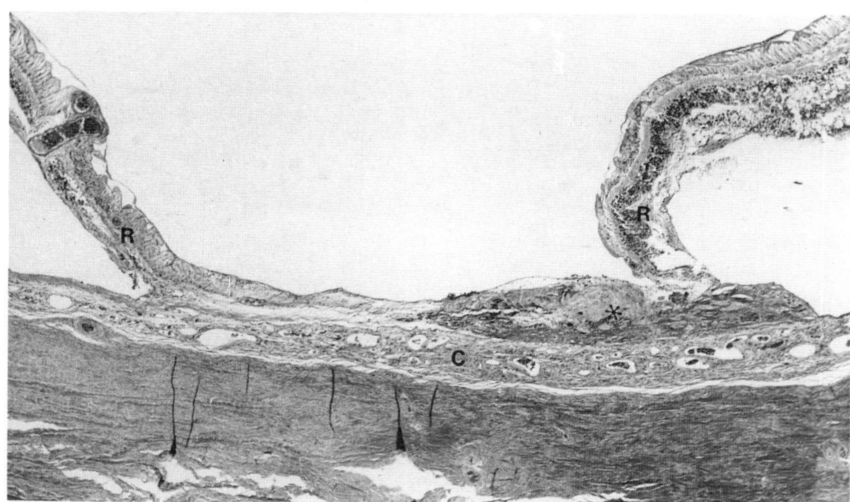

Fig. 18.3 (b) Low power microscopy of section through hole. The margins of the hole in the retina (R) are bound down to a fibrous scar (asterisk) on Bruch's membrane in which there is some pigment proliferation. C = choroid. Masson trichrome.

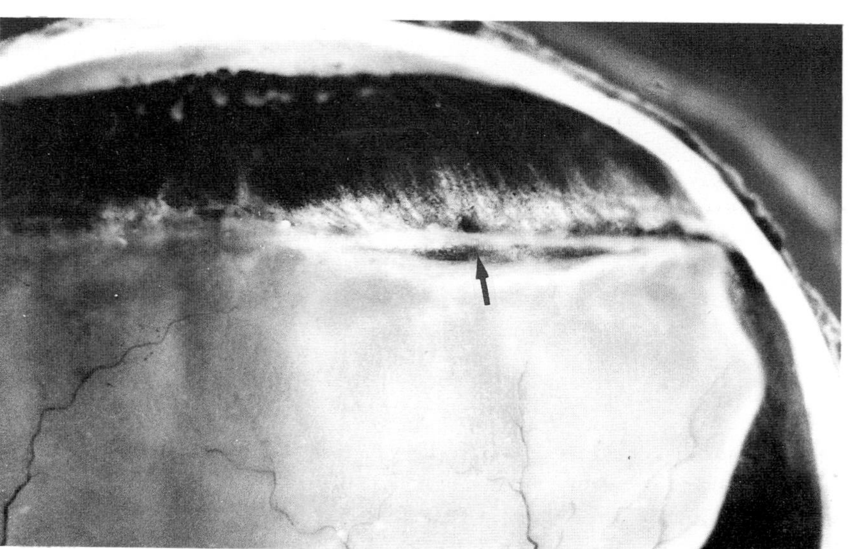

Fig. 18.4 Peripheral traumatic retinal break. The patient was kicked in the eye at football and, despite subsequent loss of vision, did not seek advice for nearly 6 months. The eye was enucleated 2 years later when blind and painful. This appeared to be due to raised intraocular tension resulting from contusional recession of the drainage angle. (a) Macroscopic picture of break (arrow) in nasal calotte.

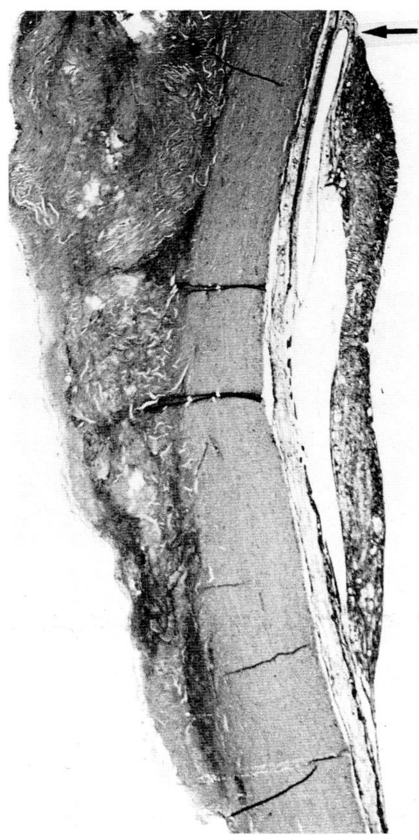

Fig. 18.4 (b) Section of calotte showing that the anterior margin of the break, which was several millimetres posterior to the ora, has become reflected forwards and sealed to the pars plana (arrow). H & E.

On the choroid

Haemorrhages following contusion of the choroid may spread into the suprachoroidal space and detach the choroid from the sclera or break through a rupture in Bruch's membrane into the subretinal space. Microscopically, such areas of choroidal injury and haemorrhage are seen later as localised plaques of scar tissue in the choroid or suprachoidal space or on the inner surface of Bruch's membrane beneath a span of atrophic retina. Some proliferation of the pigmented epithelium occurs and pigmented cells are incorporated into the scar. The end result may thus resemble a disciform scar (Chapter 10).

Rupture of the globe

The contusional force may be sufficent to rupture the corneoscleral envelope. This occurs at the point of impact or on the opposite side of the globe or at a site of weakness elsewhere such as the equatorial or limbal sclera. Staphylomatous areas or old scars are particularly liable to rupture as a result of a blunt injury. Extensive loss of intraocular contents, gross haemorrhage and eventual phthisis bulbi are the rule in such cases.

PERFORATING INJURIES

Wounds which perforate the corneoscleral envelope are for obvious reasons more commonly anterior than posterior.

Simple anterior wounds

Small punctures or lacerations through the cornea, which are uncomplicated by infection, significant loss of tissue or damage to intraocular structures, unite by first intention as do surgical wounds and the margins of corneal grafts. The following is the sequence of events after uncomplicated corneal wounding:

1st day: the edges of the wound swell with oedema and are soon sealed together by fibrin clot. Within 1–3 hours an epithelial migration or slide from the edges of the wound begins. The nuclei of the basal cells in the vicinity of the wound become arranged with their long axes radial to the wound. These cells flatten out as they slide over to cover the defect with a thin layer on which full thickness epithelium is built up later. The fact that only cells in the vicinity of the wound participate in this migration suggests a chemotactic stimulus from injured cells. After a refractory period of several hours, the initial cellular migration is reinforced by a wave of mitotic activity in the adjacent corneal epithelium. The epithelium at first plugs the anterior part of the wound, but is later displaced to the surface as fibroblasts close the underlying gap. Keratocytes within 300 μm of the wound degenerate, creating an acellular zone around the wound. Polymorphs appear in the wound area attracted from the limbal vessels by chemotactic factors released by damaged tissue (Chapter 1).

If the wound is close to the limbus, the defect may initially be partly covered by conjunctival epithelium complete with goblet cells. This is later replaced by normal corneal epithelium unless the superficial layers of the cornea become vascularised in which case it may persist for many months.

2nd–6th day: undamaged keratocytes in the vicinity of the wound multiply and migrate into the acellular zone where they are transformed into fibroblasts. Other fibroblasts are derived from macrophages which migrate into the wound area from the limbal vessels. By the sixth day the anterior half of the wound is sealed by fibroblasts.

9th–14th day: tropocollagen fibres appear among the

fibroblasts sealing the wound. It seems that important stimuli to connective tissue formation emanate from regenerating epithelial cells on the surface of the wound.

The corneal endothelial cells now form a complete cover over the posterior aspect of the wound. This is accomplished mainly by migration from beyond the margins of the wound since human corneal endothelial cells have little proliferative capacity.

Normal stromal ground substance contains an abundance of keratan sulphate, but this largely disappears from the wound area and is replaced by freshly synthesised chondroitin sulphate.

Thereafter the fibroblasts mature into fibrocytes which align themselves into laminae while the endothelial cells form a new span of Desçemet's membrane. Bowman's membrane never regenerates and its blunt, severed margins may be identified microscopically years after injury. Regeneration of the severed corneal nerves occurs from their proximal ends between the 3rd and the 30th day. The severed distal ends rapidly degenerate and disappear.

Complicated anterior wounds

The healing process just described is modified when the wound is ragged and there are complications such as substantial loss of tissue, infection, retained foreign matter or prolapse of uveal tissue, lens matter or vitreous.

In such cases, wound healing is dominated by inflammatory cell infiltration, vascular ingrowth from the limbus, granulation tissue formation and serious corneal scarring. Adhesions form between the wound and the iris, lens and vitreous. In addition, any concurrent damage to intraocular structures and haemorrhage within the globe will, even in the absence of infection, result in intraocular scarring. Eventually, cataract, retinal detachment and secondary glaucoma ensue and the globe shrinks.

Suprachoroidal haemorrhage sometimes follows perforating injuries or surgical wounds and may be massive enough to detach the whole choroid and balloon it forwards to force the retina, vitreous and lens through the wound (expulsive haemorrhage).

Injured eyes are subject to chronic persistent or episodic endophthalmitis due in some instances to recurrent haemorrhages from intraocular granulation tissue. Complicating intraocular suppuration, sympathetic ophthalmitis and lens-induced endophthalmitis have already been discussed (Chapters 2 and 4).

Post-operative or post-traumatic intraocular suppuration may be due to exogenous fungal infection introduced at the time of injury or operation. Typically there is a latent period after the injury varying from several days to several months before the onset of iridocyclitis followed by the formation of a pupillary membrane and localised abscesses in the anterior vitreous or on the surface of the inferior ciliary processes. *Candida*, *Aspergillus* and *Cephalosporium* are among the many fungi identified.

On the institution of antibiotic and steroid therapy, there is a characteristic rapid initial improvement followed after 2–3 weeks by progressive uncontrolled endophthalmitis necessitating enucleation. In many cases, an aetiological diagnosis cannot be made until the fungus is found in sections or cultures from the enucleated eye.

Epithelial ingrowths, implantations and cysts

Epithelial ingrowths: faulty apposition of wound edges or delayed healing after surgical or accidental injuries allows corneal or limbal epithelium to grow through the wound into the anterior chamber. This complication was commoner after cataract extraction than following accidental wounds of the cornea, but is now rarely seen.

The epithelium forms a stratified layer of variable thickness along the posterior surface of the cornea, over the filtration angle and along the anterior surface of iris (Fig. 18.5a). Sometimes the epithelium spans the anterior chamber on existing fibrous adhesions to form a cyst containing watery fluid. Occasionally, the epithelium grows round the pupillary border of the iris onto its posterior surface and spreads over the equator of the lens and zonular fibres.

Microscopically, prickle cells and, occasionally, goblet cells may be identified in the ingrown epithelium.

Epithelial implants: accidental and operative perforations of the globe or foreign bodies sometimes carry minute fragments of corneal or limbal epithelium or lid epidermis or cilia with attached epidermal cells into the eye. This may result after some weeks, months or even years in the formation of epithelial implantation cysts (Fig. 18.5b). These cysts, which are usually on the iris, tend to increase gradually in size and may eventually cause glaucoma.

Many such cysts have thin transparent walls of stratified squamous epithelium and contain watery fluid. Occasionally, there is a deposit of desquamated squamous cells which moves with movements of the head. Less often the implant develops into a solid cellular mass, the centre of which undergoes necrosis with the release of fat and cholesterol and the formation of a central cavity.

Posterior wounds

Perforating wounds through the posterior sclera are less common than wounds of the anterior segment and

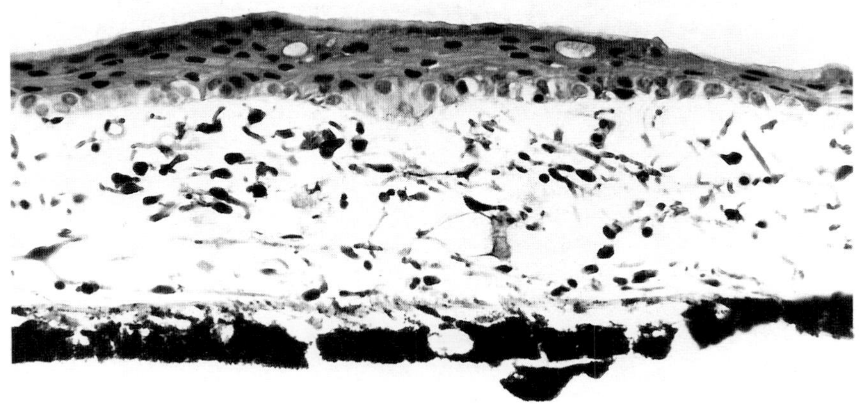

Fig. 18.5 Epithelium in anterior chamber. (a) Epithelial ingrowth. Layer of stratified squamous epithelium containing goblet cells on anterior surface of iris. Extensive spread of epithelium had occurred in the anterior part of the globe which was enucleated 12 years after injury. Details of the injury are not recorded. H & E (×320).

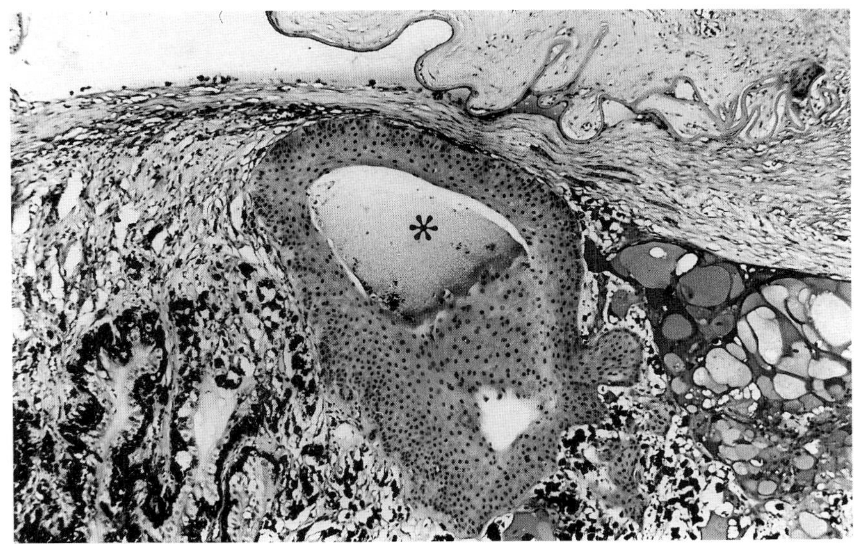

Fig. 18.5 (b) Epithelial implantation cyst (asterisk) in disorganised anterior segment. Note convoluted Desçemet's membrane and fibrous layer covering the implant and a lens remnant. Globe enucleated 4.5 months after the patient fell onto a metal tube causing an annular laceration involving lids and extending across the central cornea.

most commonly occur on the temporal side. Small puncture wounds, even when they enter the vitreous may result in no more than minor local scarring. Large wounds complicated by loss of vitreous and haemorrhage lead to extensive scar formation, retinal detachment as a result of vitreous organisation and eventual shrinkage of the globe.

INTRAOCULAR FOREIGN BODIES

The effects of foreign bodies retained in the eye depend on the following factors:

1 Entry site and position in eye.
2 Size and number.
3 Type (composition).
4 Amount of tissue destruction and haemorrhage.
5 Introduction of infective agents.
6 Time for which they are retained.

Entry site and position in eye

Most foreign bodies enter the eye through the cornea, limbus or anterior sclera. In general terms, foreign bodies in the anterior segment excite less reaction than those in the posterior while those in the lens excite least reaction at all.

Foreign bodies in the anterior segment: in the anterior segment, the foreign matter may lodge inferiorly as a result of gravity and initiate an iridocyclitis of variable severity and eventually become encapsulated. Foreign bodies which enter the iris or ciliary body cause haemorrhage and inflammation which, even in the absence of infection, may eventually lead to atrophy of the globe.

Foreign bodies in the lens: diffuse opacification of the lens quickly follows the impaction of a foreign body in it (traumatic cataract). Occasionally, if the capsular wound is small and can be sealed by fibrin or adherent iris, the subcapsular epithelium covers the defect and only a local lens opacity results. Once sealed within the lens, even noxious materials such as copper or iron exert little deleterious effect on the rest of the eye.

Foreign bodies in the posterior segment: foreign bodies entering the posterior segment are usually metallic splinters travelling at high speed. Most commonly they enter through the cornea, iris and lens or directly through the sclera. A particle may be arrested in the vitreous before falling to the bottom of the globe or ricochet off the retina before coming to rest. Sometimes it passes completely through the globe into orbit.

In its passage, the fragment may cut a permanent hole in the iris, slice the lens in two and damage the retina and choroid so that extensive haemorrhage results. The point of impact in the retina and choroid often becomes a focus of scarring when fibrous bands radiate along the track of the missile and out into the vitreous.

Types of foreign body

For descriptive purposes, intraocular foreign bodies may be divided into three types:

1 Inert substances.
2 Irritant metals.
3 Organised materials.

Inert substances

Inert substances such as gold, silver, stone, clay, coal, glass, rubber and many plastics cause no specific reaction in the eye attributable to their composition. In the anterior chamber, they may lie quietly for an indefinite time, becoming encapsulated by a process of slow fibrosis which may also lead to the formation of adhesions between the iris, cornea and lens. Sometimes their presence is signalled by a limited area of persistent corneal oedema corresponding to an area of endothelium damaged by the foreign body. In the posterior segment, inert substances slowly induce opacification and liquefaction of the vitreous, localised retinal atrophy with secondary gliosis and fibroglial proliferation. Traumatic haemorrhage and infection apart, such substances cause mechanical irritation of variable degree depending largely on their size and location.

Liquid golf ball cores

Cutting up golf balls is a well recognised hazard usually to children because the core of many contains a slurry under high pressure which spurts out with considerable force. The principal constituent of the slurry is barytes with a variable amount of muscovite or hydromuscovite which may impart a dark colour. The crystals penetrate the bulbar conjunctiva to form a pool in the substantia propria (see Chapter 5).

Irritant metals

Among the irritant metals, iron and copper produce the most serious effects in the eye. Lead is better tolerated, but this is of little comfort to a patient whose eye has been irrevocably damaged by an airgun pellet.

Iron foreign bodies

Tool fragments composed of iron and steel are among the commonest intraocular foreign bodies and, in most cases, they have sufficient velocity to reach the posterior segment of the eye. They are often sterilised by frictional heat so that complicating infection is rare.

Retained iron, especially soft iron, gradually disintegrates and very small particles have been known to disppear completely in the course of a few years.

If the fragment is rapidly encapsulated in organising blood clot or lies within the lens or cornea, the products of decomposition tend to be deposited mainly in its immediate vicinity (direct siderosis). If, however, it remains unclothed or lies free, as, for example, on the surface of the retina, general dissemination of iron occurs throughout the eye. Such generalised siderosis, which imparts a rusty appearance to the ocular tissues, is most commonly the result of an iron fragment in the posterior segment.

The chemistry of siderosis is not fully understood, but it is probable that the constant current which passes postero-anteriorly through the globe leads to an electrolytic dissociation of the metal and its dissemination in ionic form. The ions enter the tissue cells and combine with protein to form insoluble complexes which interfere with cell metabolism. Simple diffusion of soluble iron products, e.g. iron oxide, most probably occurs as an additional process.

Microscopically, the distribution of iron is very variable according to the composition, size and location of the foreign body, its degree of encapsulation and the time for which it has been retained. Iron deposits are found preferentially in the retina, the ciliary and lens epithelia and the iris stroma, but almost every ocular tissue may become impregnated with resultant heterochromia, cataract, atrophy and depigmentation of the ciliary epithelium and secondary glaucoma. The cause of this glaucoma is not always obvious since the angle may remain open, but deposition of iron salts in the meshwork probably leads to degeneration and sclerosis. In the lens the deposits are seen as 'rust spots' deep to the anterior capsule (Fig. 18.6a).

In H & E preparations, iron is seen in three principal forms:

1 The foreign body itself is black or dark grey and often has a yellow crust. Nearby, for example in the surrounding scar tissue or retina, black or yellow fragments which have broken away from the main mass are seen.

2 Small intracellular golden-brown granules are found both in the vicinity of the foreign body and widely disseminated in the retina, iris, trabecular meshwork and sometimes in the corneal substantia. These granules may be found in macrophages as well as in tissue cells.

3 Extremely fine brown granular iron is seen at high magnification in the cytoplasm of tissue cells, particularly those of the ciliary and lens epithelia and retina, which is likely to be gliosed. There is often also a diffuse light-brown staining which cannot be resolved into granules.

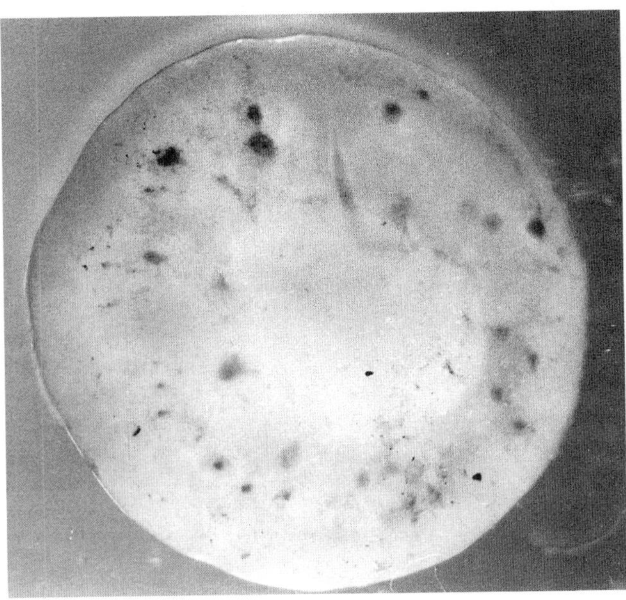

Fig. 18.6 Siderosis of lens. (a) Macroscopic appearance of siderotic deposits.

All these forms of iron are well demonstrated in formalin-fixed siderotic eyes by Perls' stain (Fig. 18.6b and Appendix IV). Haemosiderin (hydrated ferrous oxide combined with protein) also gives Perls' reaction, but melanin, of course, does not. Eyes impregnated with haemosiderin after prolonged retention of large amounts of blood present a histological picture similar to that resulting from a retained foreign body except, of course, that there is no foreign body and the iron staining is accompanied by blood clot and often cholesterol crystals.

Copper foreign bodies

The introduction of relatively pure copper into the eye is immediately followed by profuse suppuration. This dramatic reaction is due to chemical irritation since it can be induced experimentally by introducing copper aseptically into either the anterior or posterior segment. Alloys containing less than 85% copper cause a less severe chronic non-granulomatous inflammatory reaction.

The foreign body may disintegrate, but usually becomes encapsulated in fibrous tissue, which probably reduces the dissemination of copper in the globe. A greenish-blue peripheral ring develops in and about Desçemet's membrane. On focal illumination of the lens, a brilliantly coloured green or red iridescent sunflower cataract is seen on and beneath the anterior capsule while brightly refringent particles are are found on the zonular fibres, in the aqueous and vitreous and on the surface of the retina.

Copper can be demonstrated in tissues by spectrophotometry and by staining with rhodamine or rubeanic acid. Such studies have demonstrated the metal mainly in the fibrous capsule and in macrophages around the

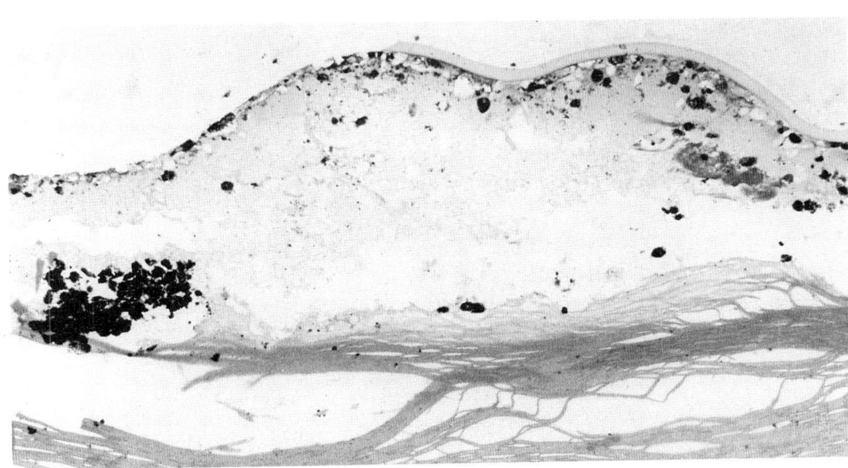

Fig. 18.6 (b) Section showing the deposits lying deep to the lens capsule. Perls' stain (×100).

foreign body. It may also be found in Desçemet's membrane, in the vitreous and in the internal limiting membrane of the retina and in reactive retinal glia in the vicinity of a foreign body.

Organised materials

The most important foreign bodies in this category are wood and cilia, but caterpillar setae also deserve mention.

Wood

Flying splinters of chopped wood or thorns from bushes or trees brushing across the face do not, as a rule, have sufficient velocity to penetrate far into the eye and are, therefore, most commonly found either in the cornea or in the anterior chamber.

Such bodies may carry pyogenic organisms into the eye and thus result in panophthalmitis or a more limited suppuration either in the anterior segment or vitreous. Less often, saprophytic fungi or yeasts are carried into the eye where they propagate slowly in a torpid vitreous abscess.

In the absence of infection, the fragment may become the centre of a granulomatous reaction dominated by epithelioid macrophages and numerous foreign body giant cells. Sometimes there is a virtual absence of reaction for several weeks or even months or years, but in all such cases a delayed inflammatory rection is to be anticipated.

Cilia

An eyelash is occasionally driven into the anterior segment and less often into the posterior segment at the time of surgical or accidental perforation of the globe or may be carried in by a foreign body. Frequently the cilium excites little or no reaction (Fig. 18.7) and may remain indefinitely floating free in the anterior chamber or becoming adherent to the iris. Alternatively, it may excite a foreign body giant cell reaction. Oddly enough, suppuration following the entry of an eyelash is uncommon.

Caterpillar setae

Certain widely distributed species of hairy caterpillars possess fine setae which are both poisonous and covered in spiny barbs. Apart from the possibility of introducing microbial infection, they are capable of causing severe irritation. The effect of the spiny barbs is that the setae are propelled through the ocular integumenta by flexional movements during versions. The setae may also migrate within the globe and result in endophthalmitis (ophthalmia nodosa). Movement ceases within the globe when the setae have become coated in exudate or the spines blunted by enzymatic degradation (see Steele *et al.*, 1984).

COMPLICATIONS OF CATARACT SURGERY

Removal of the lens causes profound changes in the hydrodynamics of the eye. The lens and zonule act as a barrier between anterior and posterior segments and when it is removed saccadic eye movements can set up turbulences in the aqueous and pools of liquefied vitreous. The destabilising effect of intracapsular cataract extraction is greater than that of extracapsular and has a higher incidence of complications such as corneal decompensation, cystoid macular oedema and retinal detachment which have been related to disturbances in internal hydrodynamics. Other complications, which are directly attributable to misadventures occurring at operation, must first be considered. Whilst from a surgical point of view such complications are commonly considered according to the time at which they arise, the pathological consequences may not be seen for months or years. They may indeed be difficult to recognise in a painful blind eye removed long after surgery.

Operative complications

A sound cataract scar which has healed with good apposition of the wound edges may be quite inconspicuous (Fig. 18.8). The external aspect is often marked by slight in-dipping of the limbal conjunctival epithelium. The stromal extent usually shows a few capillaries cut in cross-section. The gap in Desçemet's membrane is small and may be sealed by a new thin layer of membrane.

Faulty wound closure

Faulty apposition results in failure of reformation of the anterior chamber after operation and hypotony. If it is not rectified, healing by second intention occurs and a weak scar results which may stretch (Fig. 18.9) or even rupture.

Remnants of lens capsule, globules of vitreous or part of the iris may all become incarcerated in the wound.

Epithelial ingrowth may occur (q.v.) Microbial infection is an increased risk.

Haemorrhage

Minor bleeding may occur into the anterior chamber,

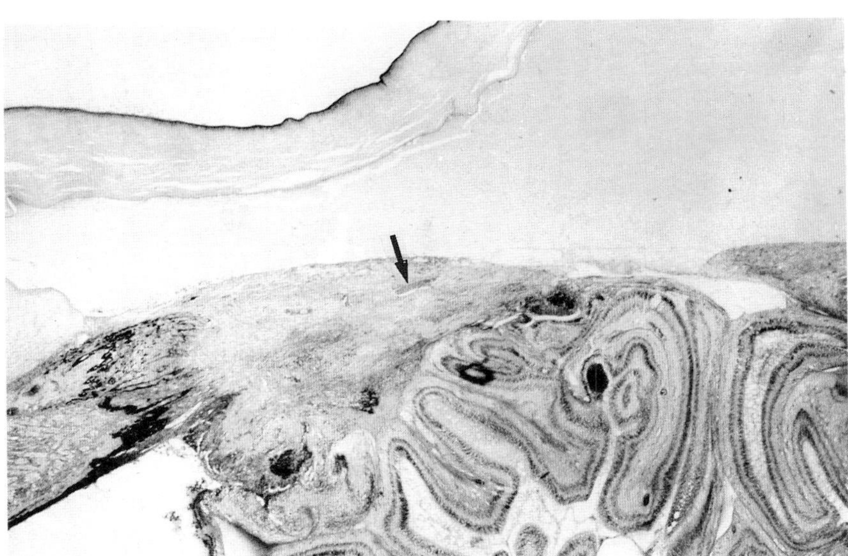

Fig. 18.7 Fragment of in-driven cilium. (a) Low power showing position of fragment (arrow) in fibrous tissue attaching bunched up, detached retina to ciliary processes. H & E (×20).

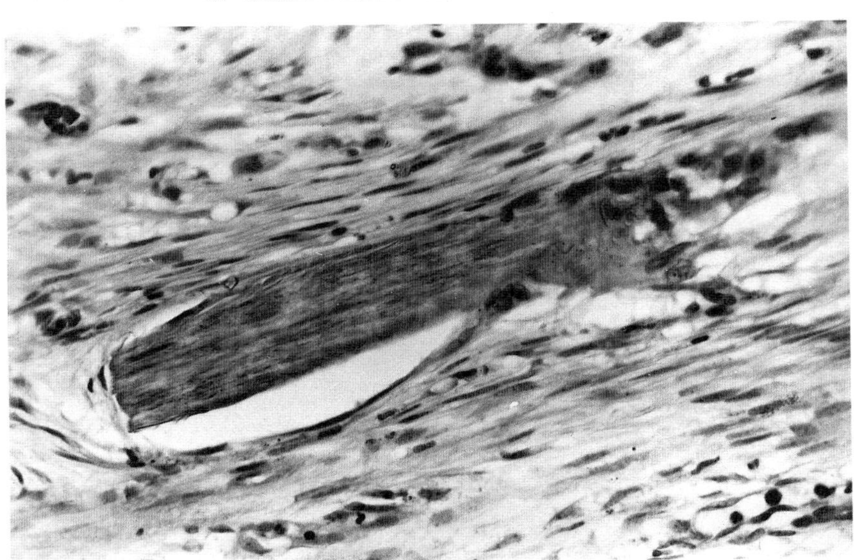

Fig. 18.7 (b) Higher power showing fragment embedded in fibrous tissue with minimal cellular reaction. H & E (×160).

usually from the iridectomy site. This is not usually a serious problem. Blood remaining in the anterior chamber is organised and eventually forms a layer of hyaline fibrous tissue.

Massive bleeding occasionally occurs into the potential suprachoroidal space which is suddenly expanded with the result that the choroid pushes forwards expelling the intraocular contents through the wound. Such expulsive haemorrhages result in loss of the eye. The source of the bleeding can rarely be identified in the resulting pathological specimen. Expulsive haemorrhage is more likely to occur in the presence of faulty wound closure.

Unplanned rupture of lens

Unplanned rupture of the lens capsule may, as already mentioned, result in capsular remnants becoming incarcerated in the wound (Fig. 18.10). The contents may set up an inflammatory reaction in the eye.

Vitreous loss

Rupture of the anterior face of the vitreous with entry of vitreous into the anterior chamber may damage the endothelium and eventually result in corneal oedema. Entrapping of strands of vitreous in the wound which subsequently become organised leads to traction on the retina.

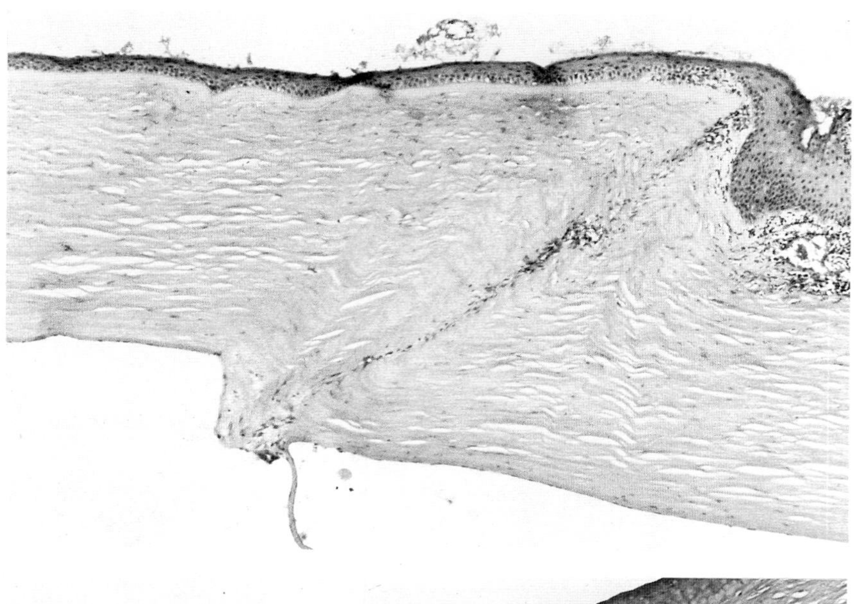

Fig. 18.8 Cataract section scars. (a) A recent scar. The globe was enucleated a month after cataract extraction because of a melanoma. The scar is sound, but there is a small flap of Desçemet's membrane. H & E (×64).

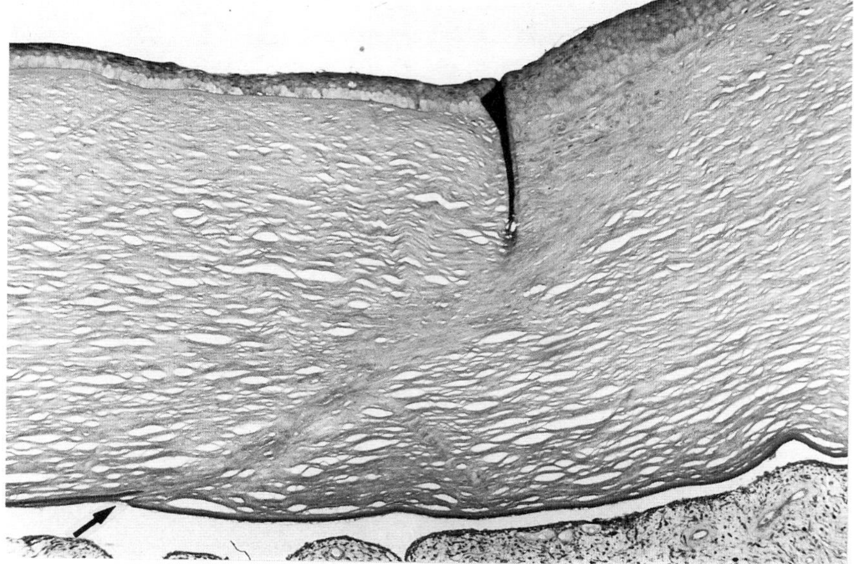

Fig. 18.8 (b) An old scar. The globe was enucleated because of a traumatic limbal rupture which did not involve the cataract scar from an operation 8 years previously. Note small gap in Desçemet's membrane (arrow). The anterior chamber is flat and there is a factitious crease in the section. PAS/tartrazine (×90).

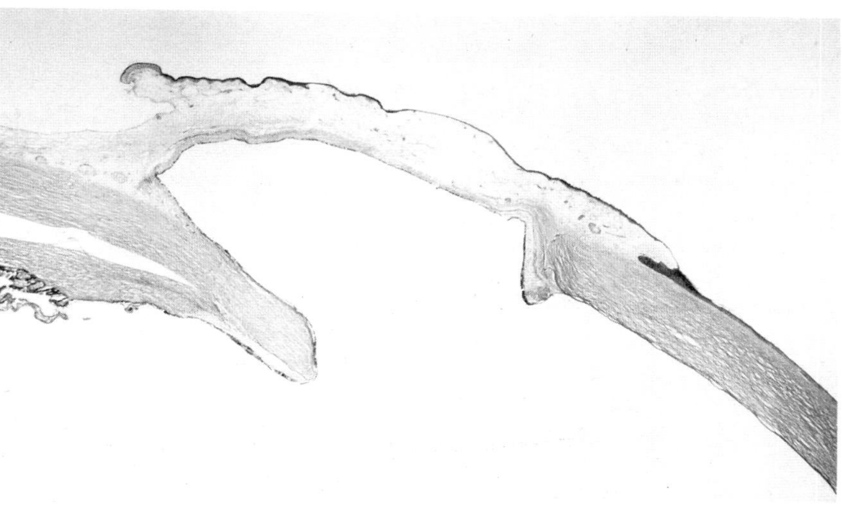

Fig. 18.9 A cataract section which has given way to form a cystoid scar lined by remnants of iris. An operation 11 years previously was complicated by prolapse of ciliary body. There was a coloboma of choroid and iris. PAS/tartrazine (×20).

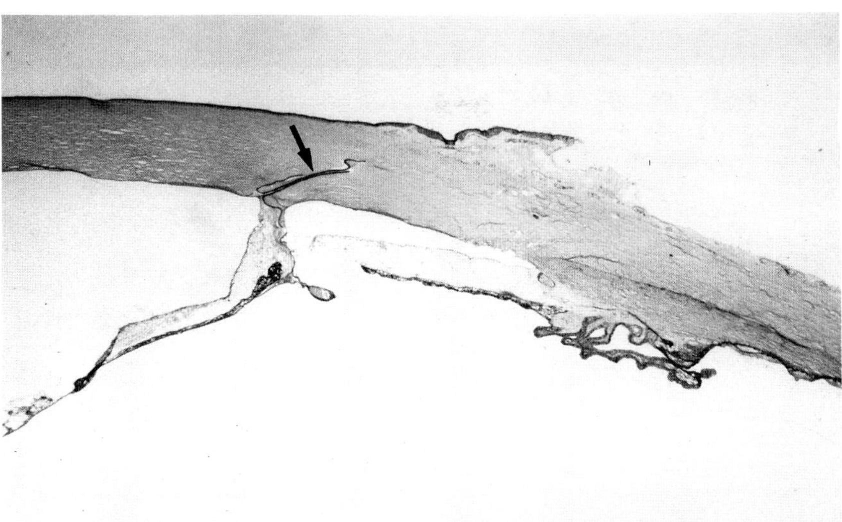

Fig. 18.10 Incarceration of lens capsule (arrow) in a scar from cataract section. The capsule ruptured during delivery of the lens 13 years previously. PAS/tartrazine (×20).

Detachment of Desçemet's membrane

Minor separations of Desçemet's membrane are not uncommon. Occasionally a substantial area may become detached and may, indeed, remain unnoticed (Fig. 18.11).

General complications

Under this heading are considered various complications many of which have already been mentioned in passing because they are directly related to the operative complications already discussed.

'After cataracts'

Lens epithelium retained in the eye following extracapsular surgery is capable of proliferation, especially in young people. Large globular cells are formed which stain homogeneously with eosin and Congo red and are sometimes nucleated. These are referred to as Elschnig's pearls. They are thought to represent attempted regeneration of lens fibres.

Sometimes the anterior and posterior parts of the lens capsule become apposed centrally while at the periphery residual cortex and proliferated epithelial cells persist so that a doughnut-shaped structure known as Soemmering's ring is formed (Fig. 18.12).

Infection

Suppurative or fungal endopthalmitis is a rare complication to which reference has already been made as it is more likely to occur in the presence of faulty wound closure, especially if there is also iris prolapse.

Inflammation

Sympathetic ophthalmitis is a rare complication of cataract surgery (see Chapter 4), particularly if iris prolapse is present. Lens-induced endophthalmitis may occur with extracapsular extraction, planned or unplanned.

Bullous keratopathy

Persistent corneal oedema may result from:
1 Endothelial trauma during surgery from instruments, chemical agents or foreign matter.
2 Exacerbation of pre-existing corneal disease, particularly Fuchs' dystrophy.
3 Aphakic glaucoma (see below).
4 Vitreous adhesions.
5 Detachment of Desçemet's membrane.
6 Uveitis.

Cystoid macular oedema

Cystoid macular oedema is due to a breakdown in the blood–retina barrier (Chapter 10). Nearly 50% of eyes subjected to cataract surgery may be clinically affected. Experimentally, it has been shown that breakdown of the blood–brain barrier at the level of the retinal pigmented epithelium is a regular consequence of cataract surgery (Tso & Shih, 1977).

The use of high intensity instruments at operation has also been called into question (see Chapter 10). Other probable local contributory factors are:
1 Disturbances in intraocular hydrodynamics to which reference has already been made. Vitreous loss increases the incidence of cystoid macular oedema.
2 Retinal phlebitis which has been shown by histological

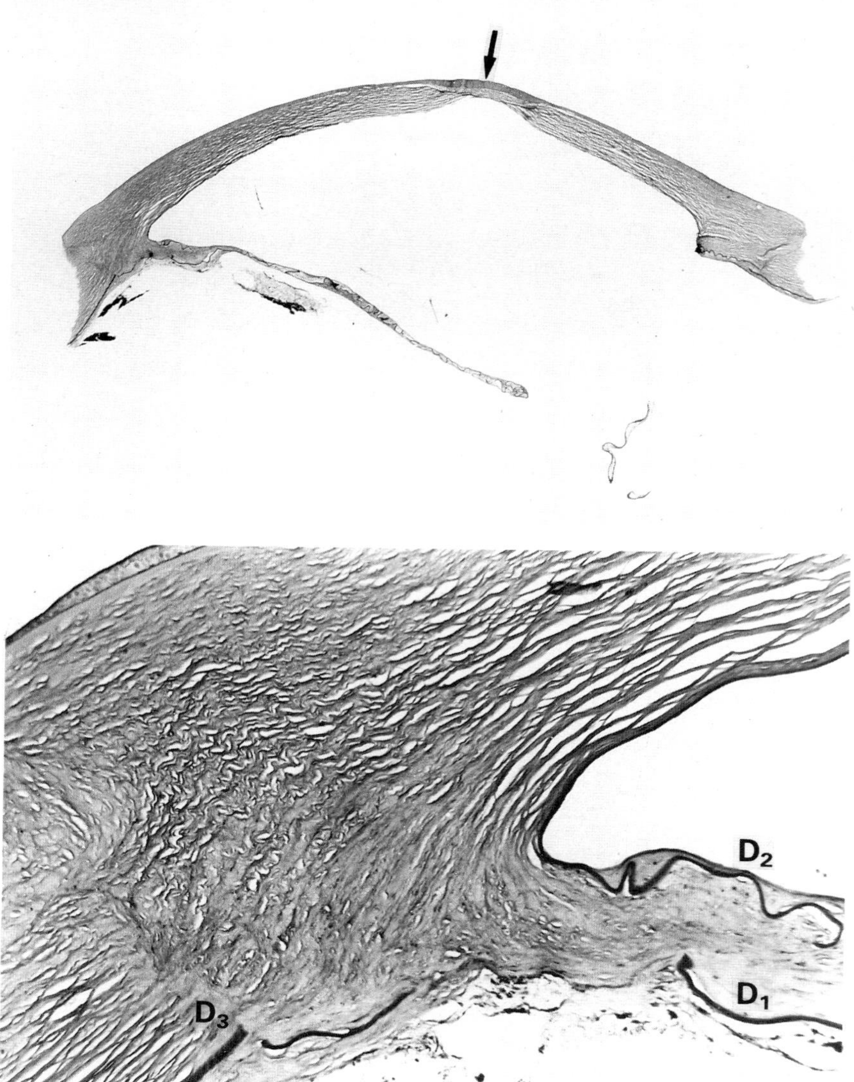

Fig. 18.11 Detachment of Desçemet's membrane. Intracapsular cataract extraction and implantation of a Binkhorst lens was followed by decompensation for which a perforating keratoplasty was performed. The graft eventually ulcerated and a further keratoplasty with removal of lens implant was carried out. (a) Low power showing profile of membrane formed of Desçemet's membrane and a thin layer of associated fibrous tissue. This is attached to scar resulting from an earlier keratoplasty at which it presumably became detached. The scar from the ulcer is seen in the axial part of the cornea (arrow) and there are small fragments of iris and ciliary processes near the site of attachment. PAS/tartrazine.

Fig. 18.11 (b) Detail of site of attachment. D1 = Desçemet's membrane presumed to have been left behind from the original keratoplasty. D2 = Desçemet's membrane of the second graft. D3 = host Desçemet's membrane. PAS/tartrazine (×95).

examination to have a significant incidence in enucleated aphakic eyes in which cystoid macular oedema is present (Martin *et al.*, 1977).

3 Systemic diseases such as diabetes mellitus and hypertension also increase the incidence of cystoid macular oedema.

Aphakic detachment

Most detachments occur within 6 months of cataract surgery and, in the great majority, a retinal break is found (Fig. 18.13). Such breaks tend to be more peripheral than those found in phakic eyes.

Vitreous loss at operation increases the probability of retinal detachment occurring, presumably because of increased traction at the vitreous base.

Vitreo-retinal traction

If vitreous remains attached to the wound or incarcerated in it, bridging of the gap in Desçemet's membrane is inhibited and the endothelium tends to spread over the vitreous and lay down baement membrane material on it. At the same time the vitreous becomes organised. There are usually associated adhesions to the iris. Subsequent vitreo-retinal traction results in detachment of the retina. Such a mechanism can often be recognised in painful blind enucleated aphakic eyes.

Aphakic glaucoma

Pupillary block is liable to occur if a leaky wound allows the anterior face of the vitreous to become adherent to

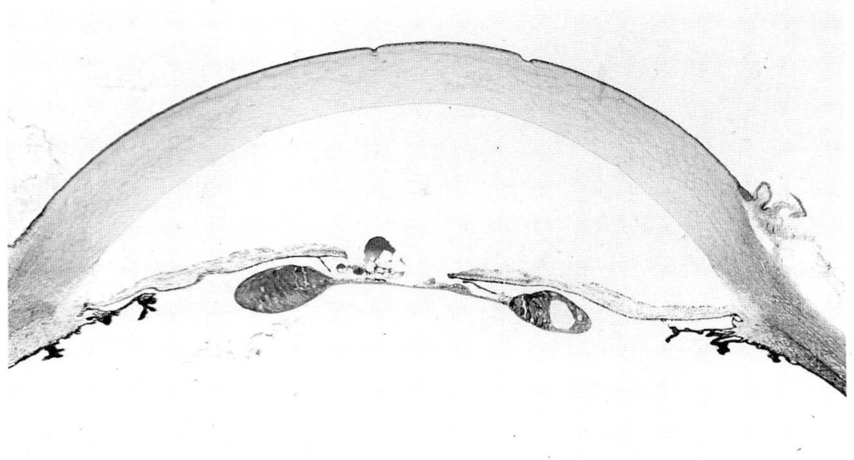

Fig. 18.12 Soemmering's ring following needling for a congenital cataract (case obtained post-mortem). (a) Low power showing profile of annular lens remnant. H & E.

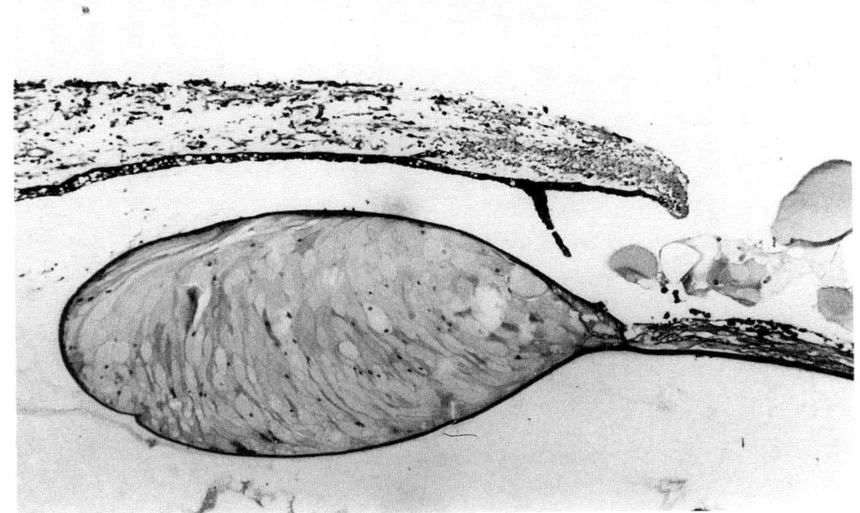

Fig. 18.12 (b) Higher power to show swollen lens fibres enclosed in capsule. PAS/tartrazine (×63).

the iris and any surgical apertures in it.

Secondary angle closure due to the formation of anterior peripheral synechiae as a result of a persistent flat anterior chamber post-operatively is probably the most important cause of aphakic glaucoma.

Excessive fibrosis in the anterior chamber may occur around poorly closed wounds in which iris or lens capsule etc. has become incarcerated, especially if hyphaema also occurs. This results in the formation of extensive anterior synechiae and sometimes a fibrous membrane covering the iris and extending across the pupil (Fig. 18.14).

Epithelialisation of the anterior chamber is uncommon (q.v.). Glaucoma from gradual covering of the drainage angle by a layer of epithelium and occurs late. Sometimes the epithelial layer is seen covering the false angle in aphakic glaucoma with secondary angle closure.

Epithelial implantation at the time of surgery may result in the formation of cysts on the anterior surface of the iris usually associated with anterior synechia formation which, if extensive, may result in secondary glaucoma.

LENS IMPLANTATION

The number of intraocular lenses implanted is continuing to rise steeply and their widespread use has inevitably opened up a new field of ocular pathology. A bewildering and steadily increasing variety of lenses is in use. The historical evolution of the types in current use is summarised in Table 18.1.

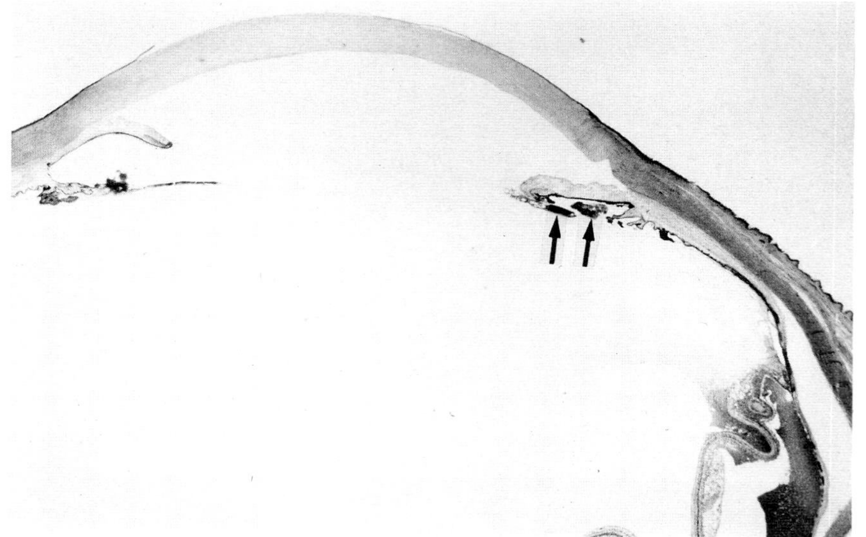

Fig. 18.13 Aphakic detachment with peripheral retinal break. Eye obtained post-mortem. Capsulotomy was followed by removal of lens nucleus 10 months before death. Vitreous prolapse occurred during the latter procedure. (a) Low power showing angle closure with lens remnants (arrows) adherent to posterior surface of iris. Retroflexion of the iris on the side of the break is indicative of vitreous traction. Masson trichrome.

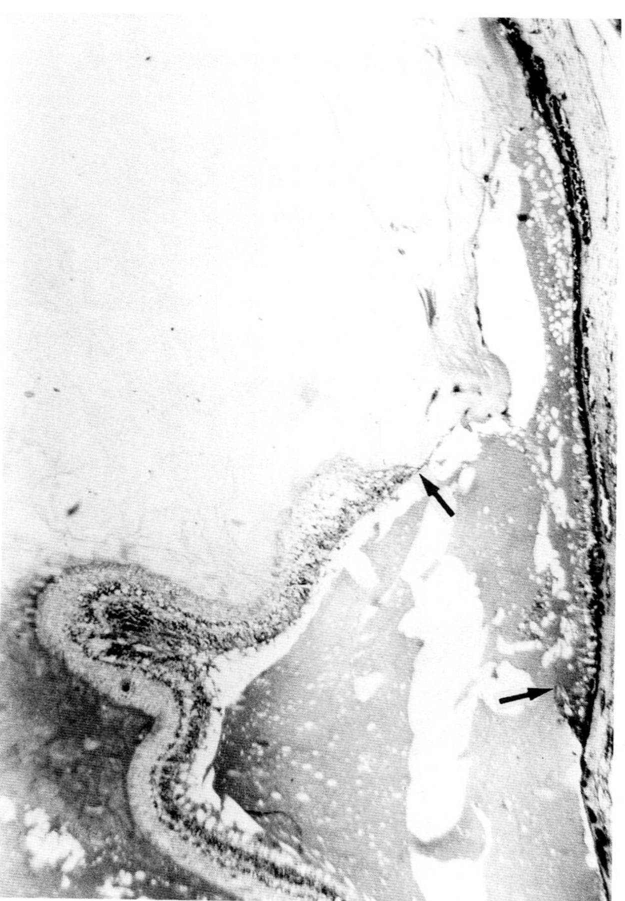

Fig. 18.13 (b) Detail of retinal break (arrows). A vitreous remnant is attached to the retinal margin and proteinaceous fluid is present on both retinal surfaces. Masson trichrome (×44).

Materials used in construction

Optic: in the vast majority of lenses the optic has been polymethyl methacrylate (PMMA) which is biologically inert and has never been proved to undergo degradation in the eye. Glass has occasionally been used (Lynell).

Haptics: many of the earlier designs, including the popular Binkhorst types had nylon haptics. Alarming pictures of surface cracking and flaking soon began to appear (Fig. 18.15). The changes are believed to be due to enzymatic hydrolysis of the amide linkages in the nylon polymer. Serious clinical consequences have rarely been shown to result from these changes, but obviously erosion of surfaces with which they are in contact is likely to be increased.

Nylon was superseded by polypropylene which was believed to be non-biodegradable. However, surface changes have been reported in polypropylene sutures, especially if they are placed in actively metabolising tissue. Degradation from ultra-violet light is also possible, but there is no evidence that this occurs at physiological levels of exposure.

Sterilisation

PMMA cannot be autoclaved so that the most widely used method of sterilisation for surgery is ruled out. Earlier lenses were sterilised by storage in caustic soda which was neutralised by bicarbonate prior to use. However, outbreaks of fungal and bacterial endophthalmitis due to contamination of the neutralising solution led to the introduction of ethylene oxide. Some lenses sterilised in this way resulted in a sterile hypopyon which was originally thought to be due to residual ethylene

Fig. 18.14 Excessive fibrosis of anterior chamber following cataract extraction 7 years previously. The operation was followed by persistent glaucoma and epithelialisation of the anterior chamber was suspected. (a) Low power showing fibrous band extending across anterior surface of iris. Lens remnants are attached to the pupillary border and detached retina is attached to organised vitreous more posteriorly. H & E.

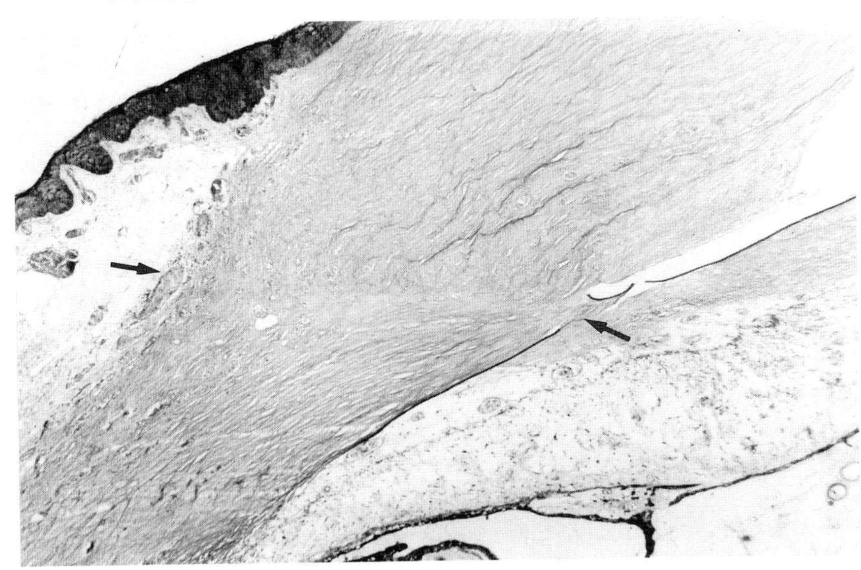

Fig. 18.14 (b) Detail of scar (arrows) which appears sound at this level (a second factitious break is present in Desçemet's membrane anterior to the scar). PAS/tartrazine (×40).

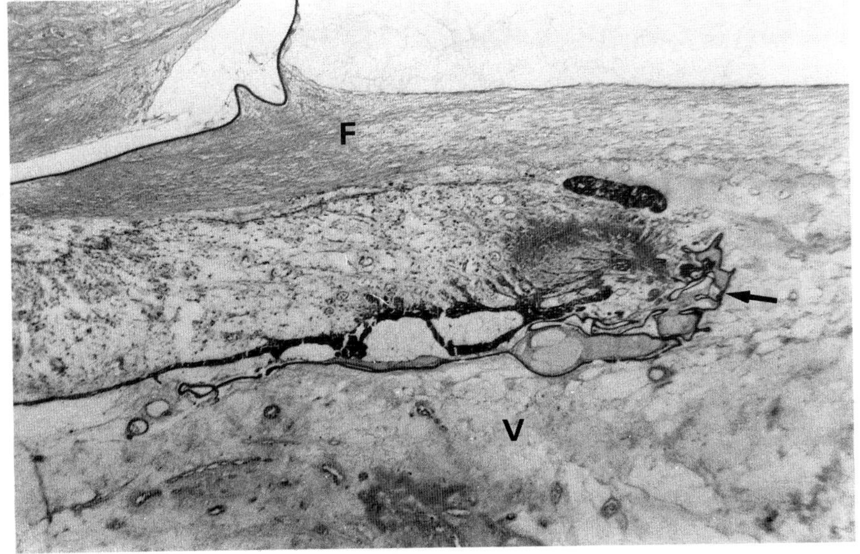

Fig. 18.14 (c) Detail of pupillary border showing iris sandwiched between a thick fibrous layer (F) anteriorly and organised vitreous posteriorly (V). A capsular remnant is adherent to the pupillary border (arrow). PAS/tartrazine (×41).

Table 18.1 Historical evolution of the lens implant (from Apple *et al.*, 1984)

Generation I (1949–54)
Original Ridley posterior chamber lens and early modifications

Generation II (1952–62)
Development of anterior chamber lenses
1 Rigid or semi-rigid
2 Flexible or semi-flexible loops
Closed loops
Open loops

Generation III (1953–70)
Continued development of anterior chamber lenses and introduction of iris-supported lenses

Anterior chamber
1 Rigid or semi-rigid
2 Flexible

Iris-supported
Includes Binkhorst and Fyodorov types

Generation IV (1975 onwards)
Major improvements in microsurgical technique and lens design lens design and re-introduction of posterior lenses

Anterior chamber
1 Rigid or semi-rigid
2 Flexible or semi-flexible loops or footplates
Closed loops
Open loops or footplates
Radial loops

Posterior chamber
1 Rigid (Pearce tripod)
2 Various J- and C-loop patterns

'Universal'
Designed to be placed in anterior or posterior chamber

The numerous eponymous types have been omitted from this classification as these and their relative advantages are discussed in clinical texts.

oxide, but eventually shown to be caused by grinding debris. Presumably, soaking in caustic soda had removed this.

Complications

The complications already noted to occur in cataract surgery also occur in implant surgery and there are additional complications directly related to the presence of the implant.

Dislocation

Dislocation of unsutured lenses due to atonicity of the sphincter pupillae may occur into the anterior chamber or vitreous before adhesions have formed, but excessive fibrosis may occur around a dislocated lens (Fig. 18.16).

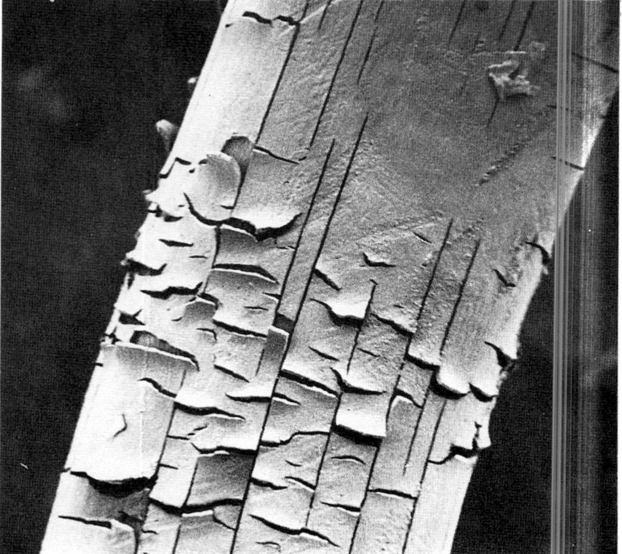

Fig. 18.15 Biodegradation of nylon loop. Cracking and flaking of surface of loop as seen by scanning electron microscopy (×400). Keratoplasty and removal of lens implant were carried out for corneal decompensation. The time for which the lens had been *in situ* is not recorded.

Other complications present as a great variety of clinical syndromes, but the pathological changes can conveniently be considered under the headings of erosion, atrophy, proliferation and inflammation from various causes (Champion *et al.*, 1985).

Erosion

Some erosion where the implant is in contact with ocular tissue is inevitable. Both iris and ciliary epithelium may be affected and there may be pigment dispersion (Fig. 18.17). Deeper erosion into the ciliary body, although giving good anchorage, may result in haemorrhage if the lens has to be removed.

Placing the posterior loops in the capsular bag appears to reduce erosion of the ciliary body and iris (Fig. 18.18). Anterior chamber lenses commonly erode the chamber angle which may become endothelialised.

Atrophy

Corneal endothelium: accelerated endothelial cell loss, which may be due to contact with a loop, is the commonest cause of visual failure after implant surgery, especially with anterior chamber implants. The functional reserve of the corneal endothelium is remarkable and a substantial loss of cells can occur without decompensation resulting (Fig. 18.19). It may be noted that the loss of endothelium is not uniform, being greatest in the

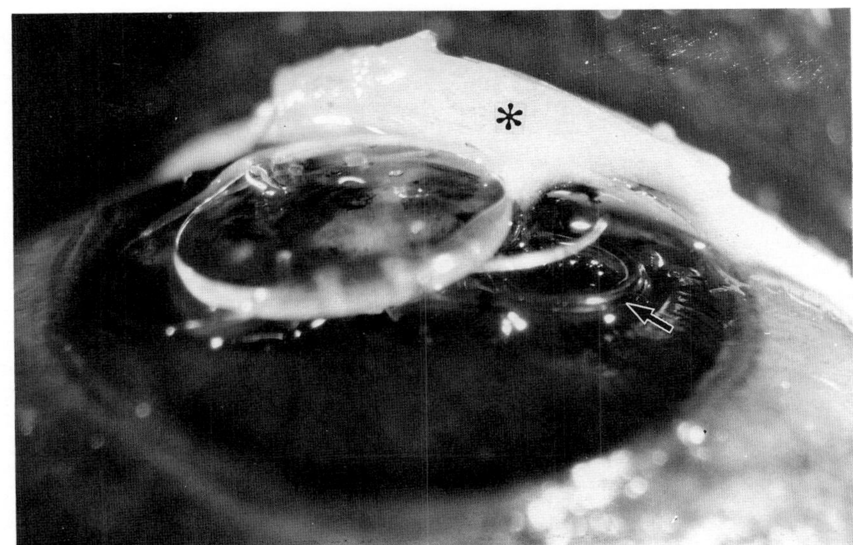

Fig. 18.16 Dislocation of a Binkhorst lens. Insertion of the lens 7 years previously when the patient was 7 years old was complicated by prolapse of vitreous into anterior chamber. (a) Macroscopic view after cutting away cornea. Note massive fibrosis (asterisk) and posterior loop (arrow) anterior to iris.

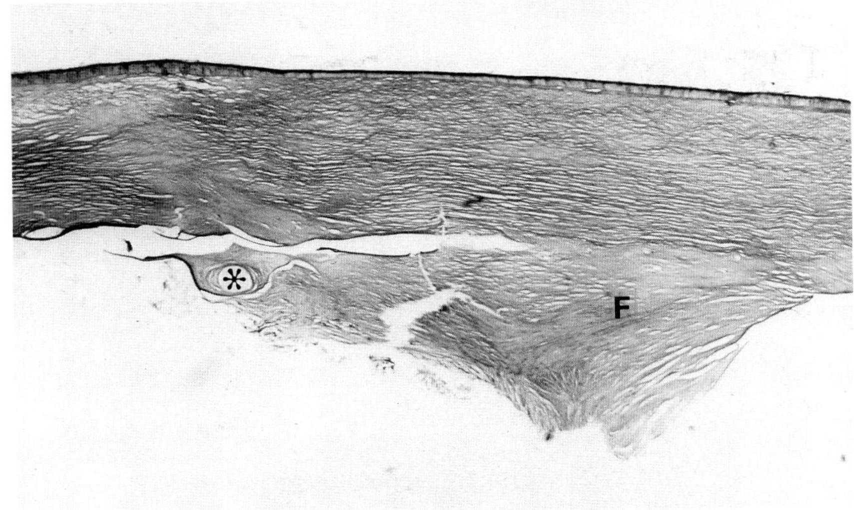

Fig. 18.16 (b) Section showing the massive fibrosis (F) and site where anterior loop was adherent to corneal scar. Loop profile indicated by asterisk. PAS/tartrazine (×40).

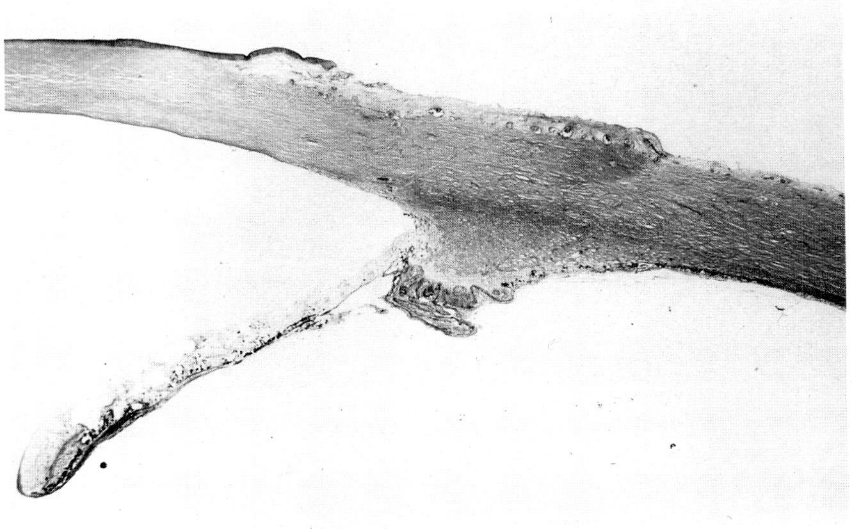

Fig. 18.17 Erosion and atrophy from a Severin lens which had been removed within a year of insertion because of recurrrent attacks of uveitis and glaucoma. The globe eventually became blind and painful and had to be enucleated. The iris is atrophied and there is disruption of pigment epithelium on its posterior surface of iris and on the anterior part of pars plana presumably due to contact with the implant.

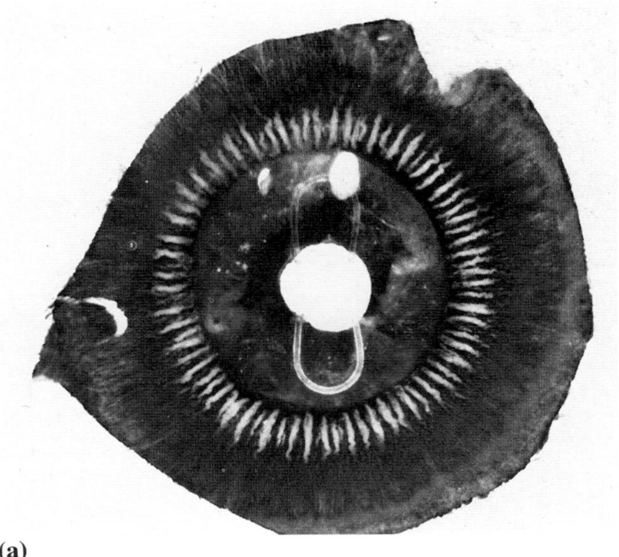

(a)

Fig. 18.18 Binkhorst iridocapsular lens inserted after extracapsular extraction. There were no complications and the eye was obtained post-mortem 2.5 years after surgery. (a) Macroscopic view. Large and small peripheral iridectomies, and upper loop appears to be buried within lens tissue overlying the larger iridectomy. The lower loop appears to lie on lens tissue. (b) Vertical section through through iris, ciliary body and lens remnant. The site where the loop was thought to be located is indicated by an arrowhead. The section passes through the larger peripheral iridectomy (asterisk). (Reproduced with permission from Mullaney, Lucas & Condon, 1985.)

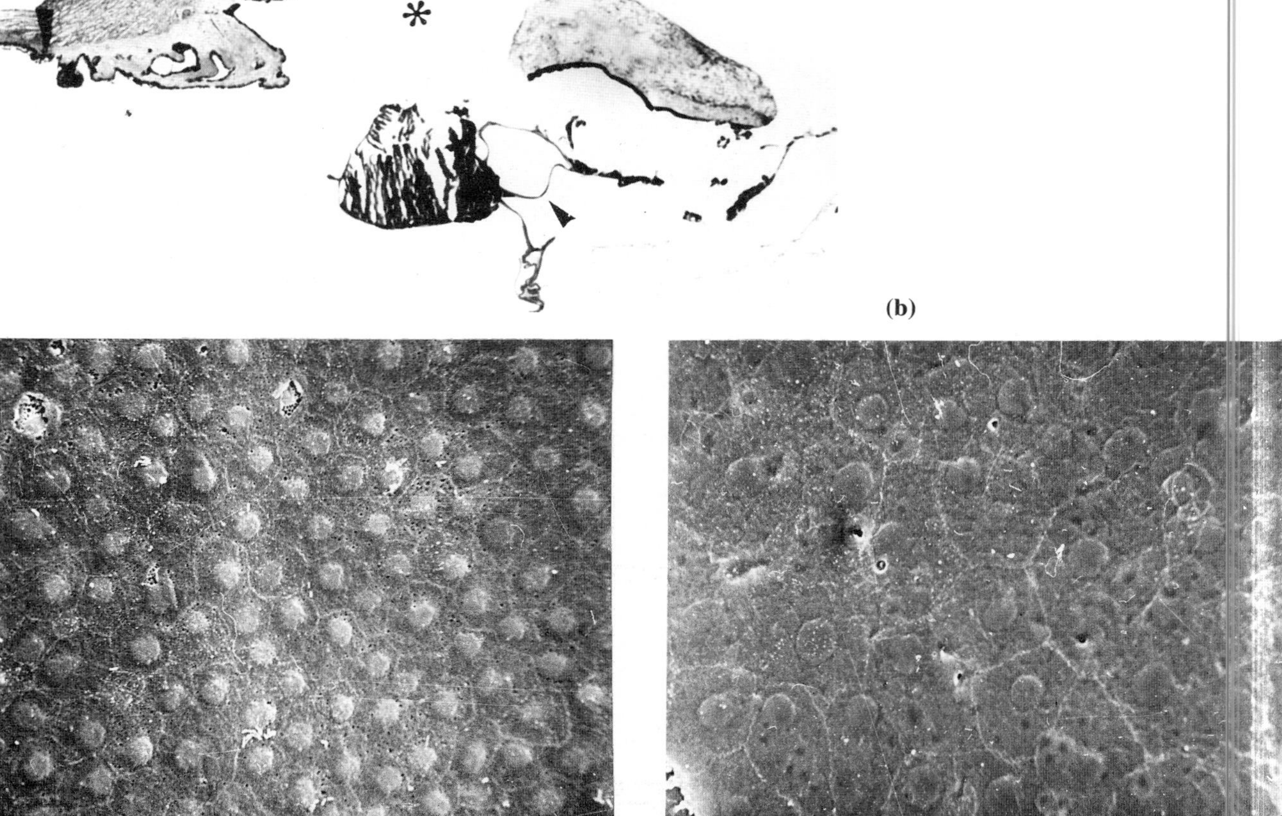

(b)

Fig. 18.19 Depletion of corneal endothelium following lens implantation. Eyes obtained post-mortem from a case in which Binkhorst lens had been *in situ* for 4 years without adverse effects. (a) Unoperated eye showing normal endothelial cell density. Scanning electron micrograph (×530).

Fig. 18.19 (b) Operated eye, upper part of cornea showing marked reduction in endothelial cell density compensated for by enlargement of cells. Scanning electron micrograph (×530).

upper part of the cornea near the surgical incision and grading off towards the lower margin.

Iris: some atrophy of the iris is usual and of little consequence. However, there may also be displacement and compression of the radial iris vessels. New vessels, which are liable to bleed, are then formed.

Proliferative reactions

The commonest type of proliferative reaction is by the lens epithelium when an extracapsular extraction has been carried out. Indeed the formation of 'pseudoconnective tissue' by metaplastic lens capsule is thought to be important in anchoring iridocapsular lenses. Proliferating lens epithelium may grow onto the posterior capsule and cause wrinkling through myoblastic differentiation and contraction. Besides lens epithelium, pigmented cells and connective tissue elements may participate. In the presence of inflammation or haemorrhage, a substantial fibroblastic reaction occurs and the haptics may become bound to the iris (Fig. 18.20).

Inflammatory reactions to the implant

The materials of which the lens is composed are generally thought to be inert, and inflammatory reactions to contaminants on the lens have already been discussed. However, both nylon and polypropylene loops may be capable of activating the C5 fraction of complement *in vitro* and thus generate a chemoctactic factor for polymorphs.

A macrophage-based reaction occurs even to inert foreign matter and a lens implant is no exception. Lenses examined after implantation show macrophages and giant cells on the surface of both loops and optic (Fig. 18.21). These often contain substantial amounts of phagocytosed pigment. The number of these cells appears to reduce with time. It has been suggested that these cells are present in a thin proteinaceous film and tend to facilitate toleration of the lens (see Wolter, 1985). Apparent examples of an immune response to the pseudophakos have only occasionally been reported (Wolter, 1983; Mullaney & Condon, 1985).

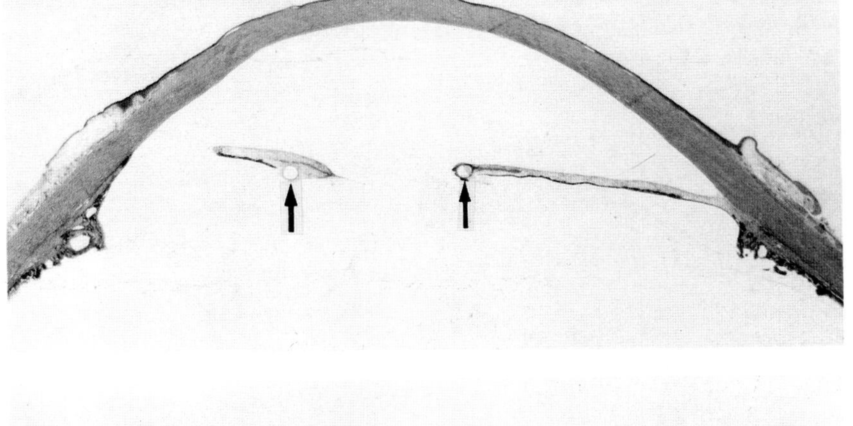

Fig. 18.20 Adhesion of haptics to pupil in a case complicated by vitreous haemorrhage. An intracapsular cataract extraction with insertion of a Binkhorst 4-loop iris-supported lens 10 years previously had been followed by a perfect surgical result, but after 5 years vision began to deteriorate and ultrasonography showed a vitreous haemorrhage. The eye eventually became blind and painful as a result of secondary glaucoma. (a) Low power at level of iridectomy showing profiles of posterior loops (arrows). PAS/tartrazine.

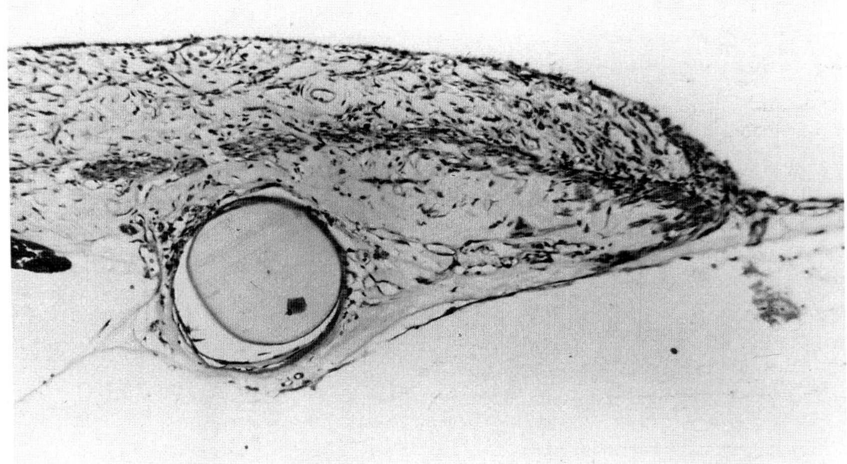

Fig. 18.20 (b) Higher power showing erosion of pigmented epithelium of iris and replacement by vascular connective tissue enveloping loop. After the long interval, it is difficult to identify the cause of the vitreous haemorrhage for certain.

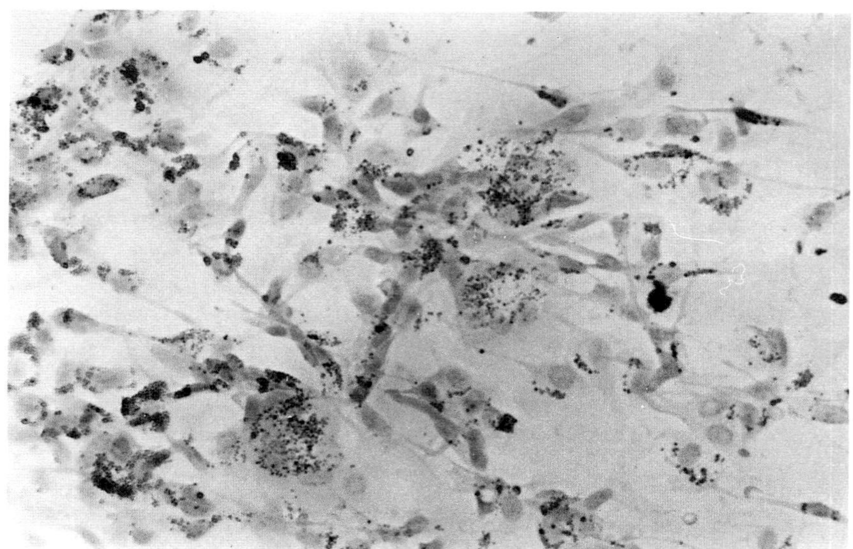

Fig. 18.21 Cells on the optic of a Novaflex lens. Spindly forms and giant cells containing pigment can be recognised, though the optical arrangement does not permit very sharp pictures to be obtained. H & E (×320).

Inflammation caused by mechanical irritation

Surgical manipulation and subsequent chafing of intraocular tissues by the implant probably leads to the release of prostaglandins and other chemical mediators of inflammation such as bradykinins and leukotrienes. Such factors were of more importance in the early days when lenses were larger and less well finished.

Inflammation caused by autoimmune reaction to retained lens matter

With extracapsular surgery, there is a risk of lens-induced endopthalmitis (Chapter 4), but this complication is unusual.

Inflammation caused by infection

Reference has already been made to contamination of neutralising solutions. When such mishaps are excluded, the incidence of infection is no higher with implant surgery.

COMPLICATIONS OF RETINAL DETACHMENT SURGERY

A comprehensive review of the complications of retinal detachment surgery is beyond the scope of this book, but the following may be mentioned:

Infection

1 *Intraocular:* the interior of the globe is fortunately rarely infected by micro-organisms following detachment surgery.

2 *External:* infection of the plombe is, by contrast, common. Microscopically, there is infiltration of the meshwork of the silicone sponge by inflammatory cells of all types and colonies of micro-organisms may also sometimes be seen.

Causes of failure of post-operative retinal function

1 Failure to reposition the retina because:
 (i) The retinal break is not closed.
 (ii) Vitreous traction bands formed, for example, when a detachment follows cataract surgery complicated by prolapse of vitreous into the anterior chamber and incarceration in the wound.
2 Retinal atrophy.
3 Persistent cystoid macular oedema.
4 Preretinal membranes are not uncommon following detachment surgery and cause macular pucker. These membranes may also progress to massive preretinal fibrosis (Chapter 10).
5 Ciliochoroidal effusion.

Intrusion of an encircling band or suture through the sclera

Although the Arruga string has been abandoned in favour of silicone rubber bands, the occasional eye in which a detachment has been treated with such a string still arrives in the laboratory. Such an eye may show erosion of the string through the full thickness of the sclera.

Ischaemia of the anterior segment

Overtightening of the band may cause closure of the

drainage angles and secondary glaucoma or severe ischaemic necrosis of the iris and ciliary body (Fig. 18.22).

Effects of silicone oil

The treatment of complicated detachments by intravitreal silicone oil may result in various late complications of which cataract, glaucoma and retinal changes are the commonest. One case of sympathetic ophthalmitis has been reported (Laroche *et al.*, 1983). Glaucoma is the commonest reason for enucleation.

The oil is inevitably lost during histological processing, but the empty profiles of spaces presumably occupied by oil droplets can be recognised. The oil does not appear to excite an inflammatory reaction, but may induce a fibrocytic reaction.

Cataracts are probably not a direct result of the treatment and are variable in type, though fibrous metaplasia of the lens epithelium is usual. Glaucoma is thought to be due to blockage of the trabecular meshwork by silicone emulsion, though macrophages and pigment deposition are contributory.

Droplet profiles are seen in the retina and in preretinal (Fig. 20.23) and subretinal membranes, sometimes in massive amounts (see Ni *et al.*, 1983). Electron microscopy has shown the oil droplets in preretinal membranes to be in intracytoplasmic membrane-bound vacuoles in cells of glial and pigmented epithelial origin (Bornfeld *et al.*, 1987). Since droplet profiles were not observed when the retina remained attached, it is probable that the oil enters the retina from the subretinal space (Kirchhof *et al.*, 1986). Apart from retina, droplet profiles are also sometimes seen in the iris, ciliary body and optic nerve head.

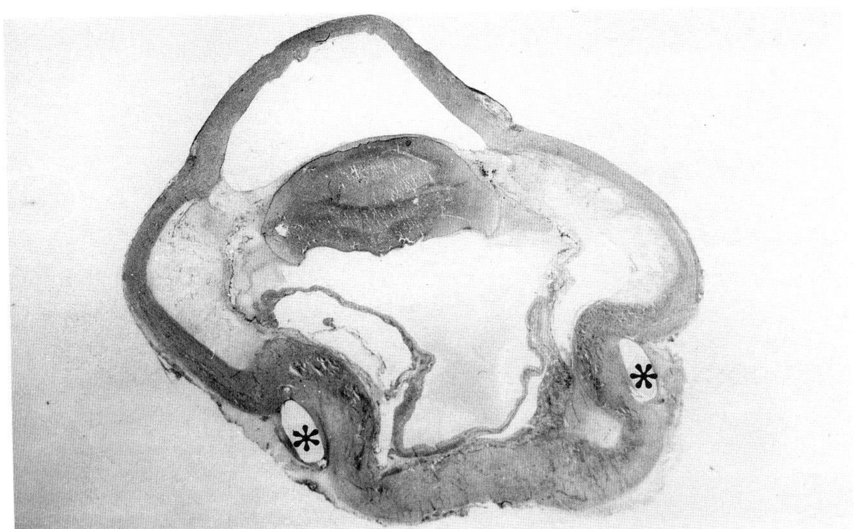

Fig. 18.22 Ischaemia of anterior segment due to overtight encircling bands. (a) The band appears to have caused complete necrosis of anterior segment and slipped posteriorly. PAS/tartrazine.

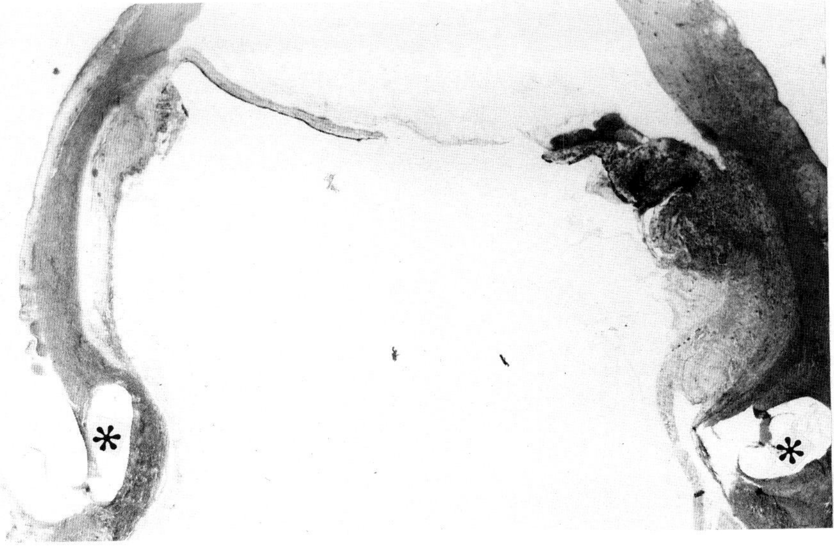

Fig. 18.22 (b) The band appears to have become rotated and intruded somewhat into the sclera (which has torn during sectioning) and caused marked congestion and haemorrhage into the iris and ciliary body superiorly (right hand side). There is a cilichoroidal effusion inferiorly where there is a double band profile, presumably near the buckle. Band profiles indicated by asterisks. H & E.

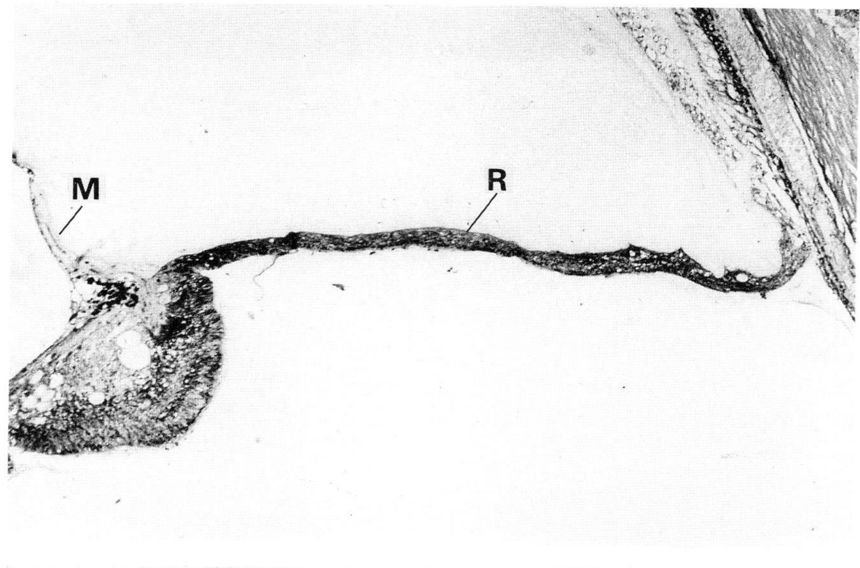

Fig. 18.23 Aphakic detachment unsuccessfully treated with silicone oil injection. (a) Low power showing attenuated peripheral retina (R) and preretinal membrane (M).

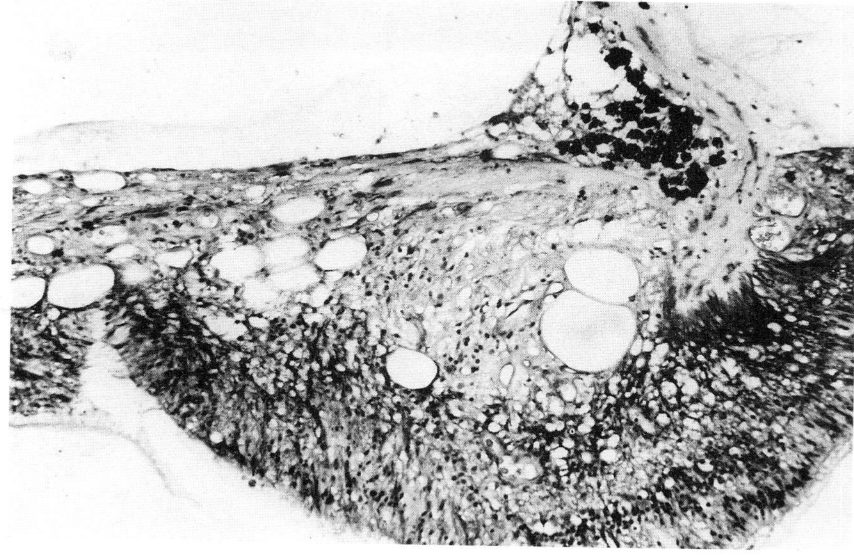

Fig. 18.23 (b) Higher power showing profiles of round, apparently empty. spaces presumed to have contained oil droplets. PAS/tartrazine (×94).

KERATOPLASTY

Keratoplasty may be lamellar or perforating. Lamellar keratoplasty is suitable for diseases or injuries confined to the superficial stroma while penetrating keratoplasty is essential when the deep stroma is affected or when the endothelium is compromised.

A fundamental difference between the two procedures is that the viability of the donor cornea is unimportant in lamellar keratoplasty, but, for a penetrating keratoplasty to succeed, the endothelium must be viable.

The other factors governing success are the quality of the surgery, successful control of infection and post-operative management of the host-versus-graft reaction.

Viability of donor tissue

The first essential is to obtain the donor tissue as soon after death as possible. Since the endothelial cell population declines during life, donors aged under 50 have been advocated, but the evidence is controversial. It may, however, be preferable for the donor to be no older than the recipient.

The medical history of the donor must be considered and freedom from possibly transmissible virus disease such as hepatitis B, AIDS and Jacob–Kreuzfeldt disease established as far as possible. Having obtained the material, it may be stored for a limited period:

1 In a moist chamber at 4°C for several hours. The principal advantage of this method is simplicity.

2 In culture medium, of which the McCarey–Kaufman

formulation is the most popular. The cornea is removed with a rim of sclera. This method is relatively simple and believed to give a marginally longer storage period than the moist chamber. A disadvantage is that the medium can be contaminated without overt signs and reliance must be made on microbial cultures set up at time of placing the material in the medium.

3 In culture medium at 37°C. Again the cornea is removed with a rim of sclera. This method is considerably more complex, but has several advantages:

(i) Microbial contamination is obvious because the medium is maintained in an incubator.

(ii) The endothelium remains in good condition for 2–3 weeks, though it is preferable to use it as soon as possible.

(iii) Time is gained to carry out tests on donor serum to exclude hepatitis and AIDS.

(iv) Time is also gained to undertake tissue matching when this is indicated.

4 Frozen-dried for an indefinite period. The parameters governing successful freeze-drying of cornea have not yet been fully worked out.

Assessment of endothelial viability

1 *Specular microscopy:* it is possible to examine the endothelium directly with a specular microscope either before removal from the donor eye or in certain types of culture chamber.

2 *Dye exclusion:* intact endothelial cells do not permit the entry of dyes such as trypan blue and nitro blue tetrazolium (NBT). Corneas may be used for grafting after exposure to these dyes, but, obviously, this increases the time for which they are stored before use and the amount of handling.

It may be noted in passing that NBT is useful in experimental work, because, if the endothelium is frozen, all the cells that were viable before freezing stain, whereas those which were not viable do not stain.

Survival of donor tissues

Evidence from animal experiments indicates that donor endothelial cells and keratocytes survive for long periods in clear grafts, but there may be gradual replacement of the keratocytes by host cells.

Immunological aspects

A classical host-versus-graft reaction such as occurs with allografts of skin and other organs is seldom seen with corneal allografts. This reaction depends mainly on the sensitisation of the host T-lymphocytes to unshared Type 1 histocompatibilty antigens, which are expressed in all nucleated cells. The Type 2 histocompatibilty antigens, which are expressed in immunocompetent cells are probably required to trigger the reaction. In the eye, the following factors modify the reaction:

1 *Paucity of lymphatic drainage:* unless the host cornea is vascularised, lymphatic drainage from the limbus is minimal. The donor antigens do not, therefore, have ready access to regional lymph nodes.

2 *Variable expression of antigens:* although Type 1 antigens are expressed by all the major cellular components of the cornea, the degree of expression appears to vary considerably, thus it is strongest in the epithelium and weakest in the endothelium and stronger at the periphery than the centre. Hence stripping of the epithelium has been advocated in order to reduce the antigenic burden.

Type 2 antigens are present in the Langerhans cells in the cornea. These are specialised dendritic cells which reside in the epithelium of the cornea and conjunctiva. They are more numerous in the peripheral than in the central cornea.

3 *Drainage via the aqueous pathway:* some donor antigen escapes into the aqueous which passes directly into the bloodstream and thus to the spleen without passing through a lymph node. Such direct entry to the spleen of small quantities of antigen is known to facilitate tolerance.

Notwithstanding these factors, some degree of rejection occurs in at least 10% of corneal grafts and rejection is still the commonest cause of graft failure. Adverse factors which enhance rejection are:

1 Vascularisation of the bed into which the graft is to be placed.

2 Inflammation.

3 Failure of a previous graft for any reason.

In such cases tissue matching is indicated and advances in conservation techniques for the donor tissue now make this feasible.

ABO antigens: the importance of ABO antigens in corneal grafting is controversial.

Humoral factors: when sensitisation of T-lymphocytes is stimulated, there is concomitant triggering of B-lymphocytes to produce antibodies to the Type 1 antigens of the donor tissue. Such antibodies are important in the rejection of transplants of vascularised organs because they attach to vascular endothelium where they activate complement and cause antibody-dependant cell-killing. The role of humoral antibodies in corneal graft rejection is less well established.

Pathological changes in graft rejection

The pathological changes associated with rejection have been worked out in detail on the experimental animal (Polack, 1977).

Vascular ingrowth: blood vessels reach the scar some weeks after operation and there is infiltration of the scar with lymphocytes and plasma cells together with a few polymorphs. A fine network of blood vessels eventually penetrates the graft. The cellular infiltration extends to Descemet's membrane and into the graft stroma.

Epithelium: rejection of the surface epithelium proceeds as an irregular line that can be detected by vital dyes such as methylene blue or Congo red. Scanning electron microscopy shows disruption of the epithelial mosaic and damaged epithelial cells on the graft side of the line and large cells with prominent microvilli on the host side. Possibly the latter are host cells migrating across the graft.

Stroma: keratocytes showed retraction of cell processes and elongation of nuclei and cytoplasm. When in contact with lymphocytes in an area of rejection, they showed more severe cytoplasmic changes including distension of the endoplasmic reticulum, vacuoles, phagocytosed material and dense intracytoplasmic crystalline material. Swelling of the stromal fibres and loss of ground substance was seen in the late stages.

Endothelium: the earliest observed change was destruction of the cells at the periphery of the graft. This was preceded by a line of predominantly lymphocytic infiltration that progressed towards the centre of the graft. Lymphocytes were also observed on the surface of and between endothelial cells. They appeared to have reached the endothelium through the host-graft junction. The endothelial cells were often rounded and, where they were in contact with lymphocytes, showed cytoplasmic densification and loss of cell junctions.

Histopathological aspects of graft failure

For convenience, various histopathological changes have been categorised separately, but they are often seen in combination in failed corneal grafts.

Endothelial deficiency

This is commonly seen and is presumed to be due to poor quality donor material. The endothelium appears greatly attenuated. The lack of cells has to be interpreted with caution as loss by artefact during processing readily occurs. The loss appears much more dramatic if the specimen is examined by scanning electron microscopy. Other changes are secondary. The epithelium is thin and irregular and shows bullous separation from Bowman's membrane. The stroma is oedematous and Desçemet's membrane undulating in profile.

Faulty wound apposition

Poor alignment of the margins of the donor disc with those of the recipient rim may lead to infolding and incarceration of Bowman's layer and Desçemet's membrane. This may result in weak or defective bonding because the host stroma does not unite as readily with these surfaces. A correlation has been established between infolding of Bowman's layer and astigmatism (Fig. 18.24) (Lang *et al.*, 1986). Poor wound apposition has long been thought to be a factor favouring the development rejection.

Vascularisation

Ingrowth of vessels across the scar into the central stroma is a serious risk when the bed is already vascularised and is likely to result in rejection unless the graft is well matched. Other factors known to promote vascularisation are:

1 Persistent oedema.
2 Adherence or incarceration of iris.
3 Silk sutures.

Rejection

Streaming of lymphocytes and plasma cells into the graft along blood vessels may be seen (Fig. 18.25) and histiocytes and giant cells appear in the degenerating graft. However, by the time the specimen becomes available for study, histopathological evidence of rejection may be inconclusive.

Inflammation

Apart from inflammation occurring due to rejection, viral and microbial infections may occur.

1 Herpes simplex. Recurrence in the graft of a herpetic keratitis is a common problem when cases of herpetic keratitis are grafted. It usually starts with deep epithelial ulceration at the host–graft margin and may be associated with rejection. It may indeed often be difficult to differentiate between recurrence and rejection on histopathological grounds. The deep stroma may show a granulomatous reaction to Desçemet's membrane.
2 Infection by bacteria such as *Pseudomonas* and various fungi usually cause ulceration and loss of the graft.

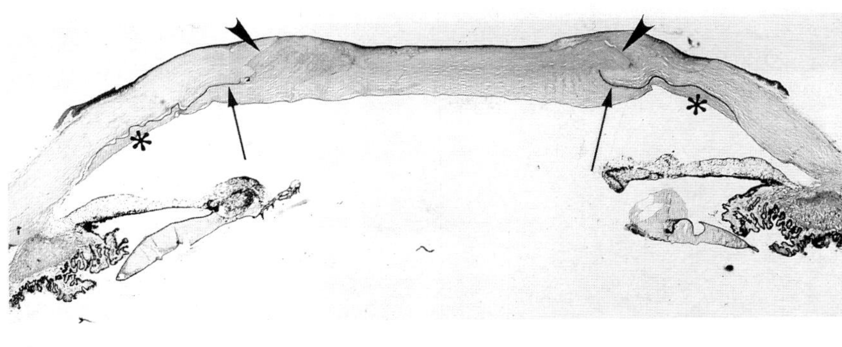

(a)

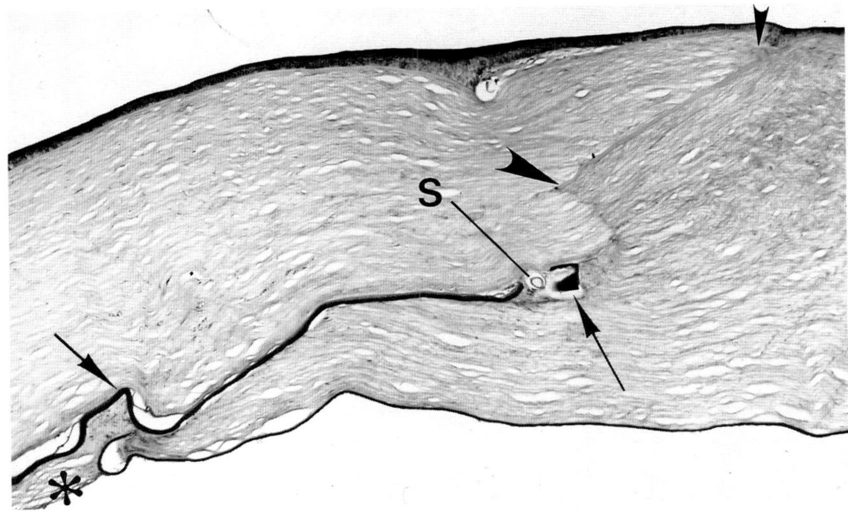

(b)

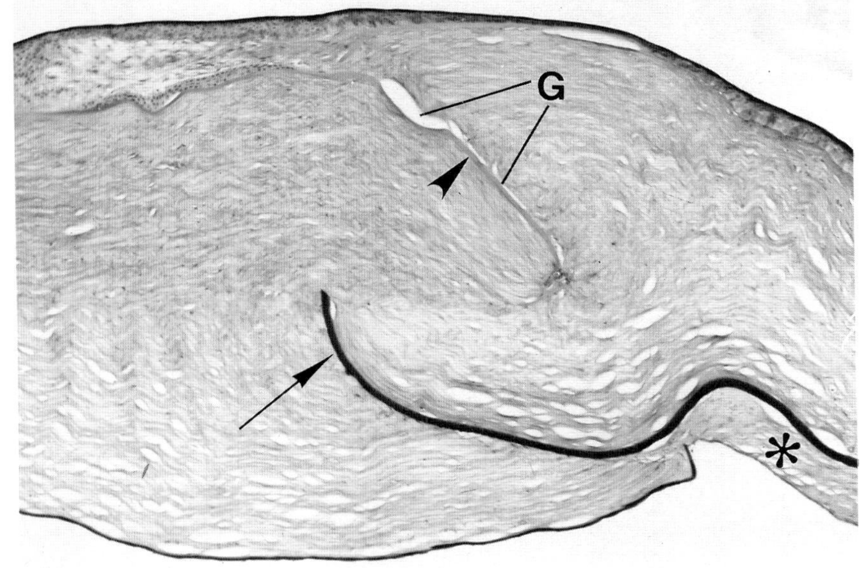

(c)

Fig. 18.24 Mal-apposition of corneal graft. Eye obtained post-mortem from a 70-year old man with congenital syphilis and interstitial keratitis who underwent penetrating keratoplasty, extracapsular cataract extraction and anterior vitrectomy (necessary after a surgical break in the posterior capsule) 8 months before death. (a) Low power view of anterior segment shows keratoplasty scars with overriding of wound edges with Bowman's layer (arrowheads) and incarceration of Desçemet's membrane (arrows). A retrocorneal fibrous tissue layer extends from the wound and covers the remaining recipient cornea (asterisk). Equatorial cataractous lens remnants are present with iridolenticular synechiae superiorly and some exposed lens material inferiorly. PAS (×10). (b) Higher power view of superior keratoplasty wound shows incarcerated Bowman's layer (between arrowheads) and Desçemet's membrane (between arrow). A suture (S) has perforated Desçemet's membrane near trephine margin and a fibrous tissue layer (asterisk) extends from the wound margin onto posterior surface of recipient cornea. Only a small central portion of the wound is void of any incarcerated tissue. PAS (×54). (c) Higher power view of inferior keratoplasty wound shows incarcerated Bowman's layer (arrowhead), Desçemet's membrane (arrow) and retrocorneal fibrous tissue layer (asterisk) on recipient cornea. The wound appears weakened from lack of aherence of donor stroma (to right) to the anterior surface of incarcerated Bowman's layer where there is a gap (G) between the two tissues. PAS (×64). (Published with permission from Lang, C.K., Greene, W.R. & Maumenee, A.E., 1986, *The American Journal of Opthalmology* **101**, 28–40. Copyright by The Opthalmic Publishing Company.)

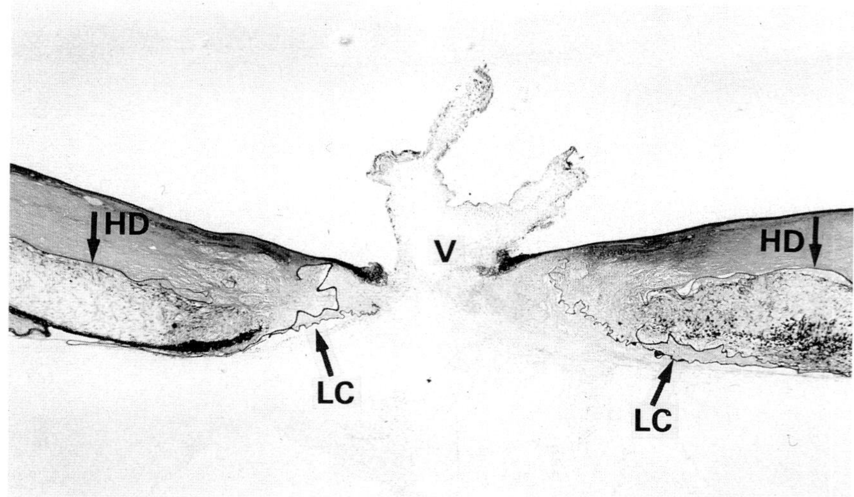

Fig. 18.25 Graft rejection. Case of bilateral keratitis, possibly herpetic. The eye was enucleated 18 months after re-graft for rejection of a previous graft 4.5 years earlier. (a) Low power showing perforation of grafted cornea with prolapse of ruptured lens capsule (LC) and vitreous (V).

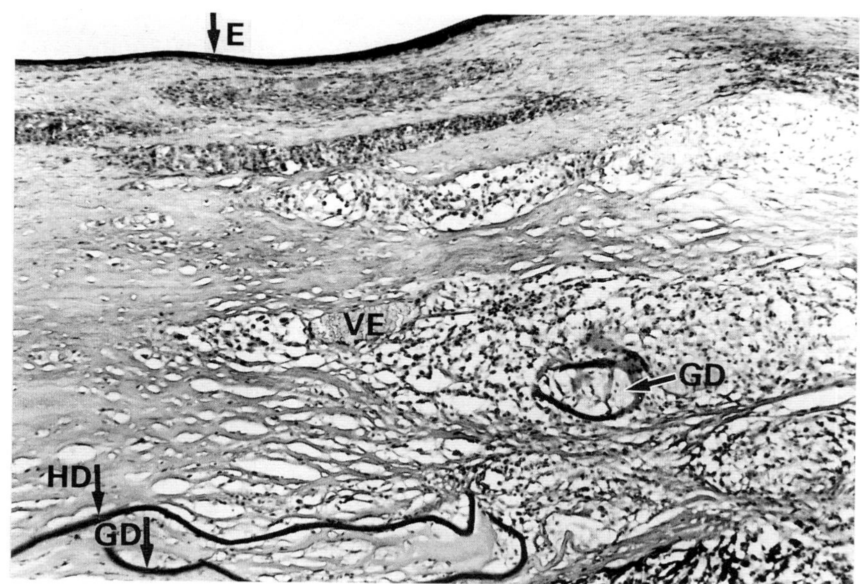

Fig. 18.25 (b) Higher power of graft margin (indicated by bar in (a) showing cells streaming along vessels deep to the host-epithelium (E)). PAS (×95). HD = host Desçemet's membrane; GD = graft Desçemet's membrane; VE = small vessel in deeper stroma.

Infection by low grade pathogens, particularly *Streptococcus viridans*, is less destructive and results in the appearance of branching opacities with a crystalline appearance. The condition has been termed 'infectious crystalline keratopathy', but 'arborescent bacterial keratopathy' is more appropriate (Watson *et al.*, 1988). The organisms probably gain access to the stroma via a suture channel and set up colonies between the superficial stromal lamellae (Fig. 18.26). No cellular reaction to these colonies is seen. The development of the condition appears to be promoted by prolonged application of topical steroids.

Stripping of Desçemet's membrane

Partial stripping of Desçemet's membrane may occur when the buttons are trephined. This is especially likely to occur if scissors are used to complete to incision (Lang *et al.*, 1986). This may result in a broad gap between host and recipient membranes either because of a defect or because the membrane is folded back. Small gaps may be sealed by endothelium and a thin new membrane laid down. Unfortunately, they sometimes become covered by fibroblasts derived from host stroma.

Retrocorneal fibrous membranes

The fibroblastic growth at the host–graft junction may progress centrally and/or peripherally so that a fibrous membrane of variable extent is laid down on the posterior surface of the cornea. Sometimes a thin new endothelial membrane is formed.

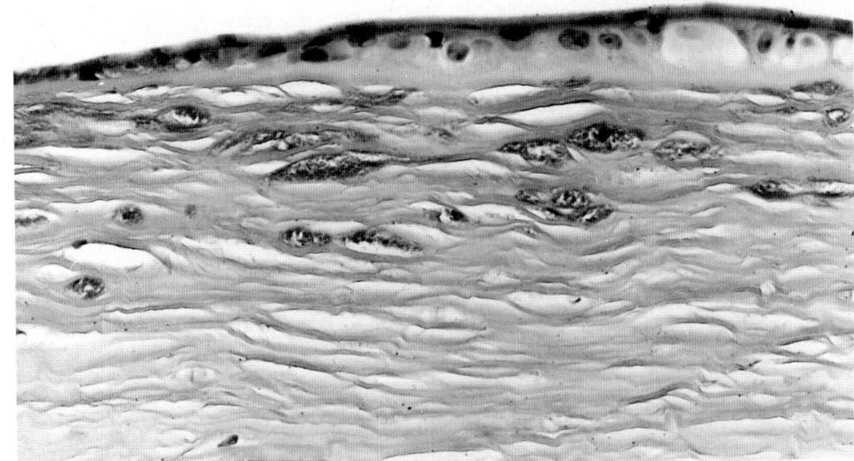

Fig. 18.26 Crystalline keratopathy. Keratoplasty carried out one year previously for aphakic bullous keratopathy. (a) Clumps of bacteria in anterior stroma. Note absence of cellular reaction. The epithelium is flattened and some cells hydropic. H & E (×320).

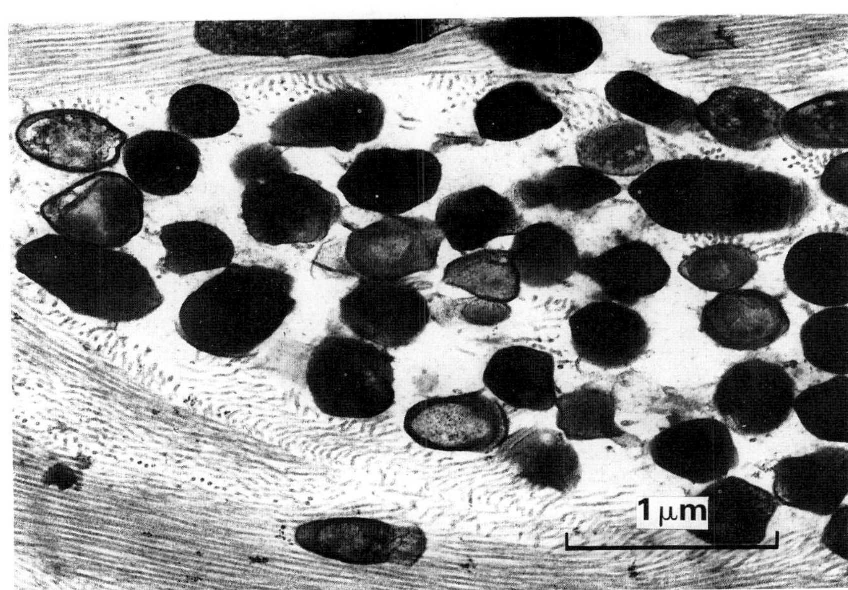

Fig. 18.26 (b) Clumps of bacteria as seen by electron microscopy. The double cell wall can be appreciated in some of the organisms.

Synechiae

Iris or vitreous (in combined procedures) may become adherent to or incarcerated in the wound.

Retrocorneal pigmentation

May be due to proliferation of iris melanocytes or pigmented epithelium or to phagocytosis of pigment by the endothelium.

BIBLIOGRAPHY

Contusion

McDonnell, P. J., Green, W. R., Stevens, R. E., Bargeron, C. B. & Riquelme, J. L. (1985) Blood staining of the cornea. Light microscopical and ultrastructural features. *Ophthalmology* **92**, 1668–1674.

Stulting, R. D., Rodrigues, M. M. & Nay, R. E. (1986) Ultrastructure of traumatic corneal endothelial rings. *American Journal of Ophthalmology* **101**, 156–159.

Intraocular foreign matter

Lucas, D. R., Dunham, A. C., Lee, W. R., Weir, W. & Wilkinson, F. C. F. (1976) Ocular injuries from liquid golf ball cores.

British Journal of Ophthalmology **60**, 740–747.

Rao, N. A., Tso, M. O. & Rosenthal, A. R. (1976) Chalcosis in the human eye. *Archives of Ophthalmology* **94**, 1379–1384.

Steele, C., Lucas, D. R. & Ridgway, A. E. A. (1984) Endophthalmitis due to caterpillar setae: surgical removal and electron microscopic appearances of the setae. *British Journal of Ophthalmology* **68**, 284–288.

Cataract surgery

Binkhorst, C. D. (1980) Corneal and retinal complications after cataract extraction. The mechanical aspect of endophthalmodonesis. *Ophthalmology* **87**, 609–617.

Christensen, L. (1960) Epithelialisation of the anterior chamber. *Transactions of the American Ophthalmological Society* **58**, 284–296.

Henry, M. H., Henry, Louise. M. & Henry, L. M. (1977) A possible cause of chronic cystic maculopathy. *Annals of Ophthalmology* **9**, 455–457.

Jaffé, N. S. (1984) *Cataract Surgery and its Complications*. C. V. Mosby Co. St Louis.

McDonnell, P. J., de la Cruz, Z. C. & Green, W. R. (1986) Vitreous incarceration complicating cataract surgery. A light and electron microscope study. *Ophthalmology* **93**, 247–253.

Martin, N. F., Green, W. R. & Martin, L. F. (1977) Retinal phlebitis in the Irvine–Gass syndrome. *American Journal of Ophthalmology* **83**, 377–386.

Merenmies, L. & Tarkkanen, A. (1977) Causes of enucleation following cataract surgery. *Acta Ophthalmologica* **55**, 347–352.

Smith, J. L. S. (1959) Sequelae of lens extraction. *Transactions of the Ophthalmological Society of the UK* **79**, 677–688.

Tso, M. O. M. & Shih, C-Y. (1977) Experimental macular oedema after lens extraction. *Investigative Ophthalmology and Visual Science* **16**, 381–392.

Lens implantation

Apple, D. J., Mamalis, N., Lotfield, K., Googe, J. M., Novak, L. C., Kavka-van Norman, N., Brady, S. E. & Olson, R. J. (1984) Complications of intraocular lenses. A historical and histopathological review. *Survey of Ophthalmology* **29**, 1–54.

Apple, D. J., Mamalis, N, Steinmetz, L., Loftfield, K., Crandall, A. S. & Olson, R. J. (1984) Phacoanaphylactic endophthalmitis associated with extracapsular cataract extraction and posterior chamber intraocular lens. *Archives of Ophthalmology* **102**, 1528–1532.

Champion, R., McDonnell, P. J. & Green, W. R. (1985) Intraocular lenses. Histopathologic characteristics of a large series of autopsy eyes. *Ophthalmology* **30**, 1–32.

Drews, R. C. (1983) Quality control, and changing indications for lens implantation. *Ophthalmology* **90**, 301–310.

Drews, R. C., Smith, M. E. & Okun, N. (1978) Scanning electron microscopy of intraocular lenses. *Ophthalmology* **85**, 415–424.

Galin, M. A., Turberville, A. W. & Dotson, R. S. (1982) Immunological aspects of intraocular lenses. *International Ophthalmology Clinics* **22**, 227–234.

Irvine, A. R. (1981) Extracapsular cataract extraction and pseudophakos implantation in primates: a clinico-pathologic study. *Ophthalmic Surgery* **12**, 27–38.

Kappelhof, J. P., Vrensen, G. F. J. M., de Jong, P. T. V. M., Pameyer, J. & Willekens, B. (1986) An ultrastructural study of Elschnig's pearls in the pseudophakic eye. *American Journal of Ophthalmology* **101**, 58–69.

Krause, U. & Alanko, H. I. (1986) Dislocated intraocular lens after biodegradation of fixation loops. A case report. *Acta Ophthalmologica* **64**, 338–343.

Krause, U. & Tarkkanen, A. (1980) Histopathology of clinically successful intraocular lens implant. *Acta Ophthalmologica* **58**, 56–62.

McDonnell, P. J., Green, W. R. & Champion, R. (1986) Pathologic changes in pseudophakia. *Seminars in Ophthalmology* **1**, 80–103.

Manschot, W. A. (1974) Histopathology of lenses containing Binkhorst lenses. *American Journal of Opthalmology* **77**, 865–871.

Manschot, W. A. (1978) Mechanism of fixation of two-loop iridocapsular lenses. *American Journal of Ophthalmology* **85**, 465–468.

Mondino, F. J. & Rao, H. (1983) Effect of intraocular lenses on complement levels in human serum. *Acta Ophthalmologica* **61**, 76–84.

Mullaney, J. & Condon, P. I. (1985) Pseudo-phaco anaphylactic endopthalmitis-P.M.M.A. related? *Acta Ophthalmologica* **63**, Suppl. 170, 34–40.

Mullaney, J., Lucas, D. R. & Condon, P. I. (1985) Successful intraocular lens implantation: a histological and scanning electron microscopic study. *Acta Ophthalmologica* **63**, Suppl. 170, 41–49.

Nicholson, D. H. (1982) Occult iris erosion. A treatable cause of recurrent hyphaema in iris-supported intraocular lenses. *Ophthalmology* **89**, 113–120.

Pettit, T. H., Olson, R. J., Foos, R. Y. & Martin, W. J. (1980) Fungal endophthalmitis following intraocular lens implantation. A surgical epidemic. *American Journal of Ophthalmology* **98**, 1025–1039.

Rosen, E. S., Haining, W. M. & Arnott, E. J., eds (1984) *Intraocular Lens Implantation*. C. V. Mosby Co., St Louis.

Turberville, A. W., Galin, M. A., Perez, D. H., Banda, D., Ong, R. & Goldstein, R. M. (1982) Complement activation by nylon- and propylene-looped prosthetic and intraocular lenses. *Investigative Ophthalmology and Visual Science* **22**, 727–733.

Veress, B. & Barkman, Y. (1982) A histomorphological study on the effect of iridocapsular intraocular lens on the iris. *Acta Ophthalmologica* **60**, 821–827.

Wolter, J. R. (1982) Lens implant cytology. *Ophthalmic Surgery* **13**, 939–942.

Wolter, J. R. (1983) Pseudo-anaphylactic endopthalmitis. *Graefe's Archive Ophthalmology* **220**, 160–166.

Wolter, J. R. (1985) Cytopathology of intraocular lens implantation. *Ophthalmology* **92**, 135–142.

Wolter, J. R. (1985) Acellular proteinaceous film on lens implants: a typical reactive situation in complicated cases. *Ophthalmic Surgery* **16**, 242–246.

Detachment surgery

Boniuk, M. & Zimmerman, L. E. (1961) Necrosis of uvea, sclera and retina following operations for retinal detachment. *Archives of Ophthalmology* **66**, 318–326.

Bornfeld, N., El-Hifnawi, El-S. & Laqua, H. (1987) Ultrastructural characteristics of preretinal membranes from human eyes filled with silicone oil. *American Journal of Ophthalmology* **103**, 770–775.

Kirchhof, B., Tavakolian, U., Paulmann, H. & Heimann, K.

(1986) Histopathological findings in eyes after silicone oil injection. *Graefe's Archive for Clinical and Experimental Ophthalmology* **224**, 34–37.

Laroche, L., Pravlakis, C., Saraux, H. & Orcel, L. (1983) Ocular findings following intravitreal silicone injection. *Archives of Ophthalmology* **101**, 1422–1425.

Ni, C., Wang, W-J., Albert, D. M. & Schepens, C. L. (1983) Intravitreous silicone injection. Histopathologic findings in a human eye after 12 years. *Archives of Ophthalmology* **101**, 1399–1401.

Rosengren, B. & Osterlin, S. (1976) Hydrodynamic events in the vitreous space accompanying eye movements. Significance for the pathogenesis of retinal detachment. *Ophthalmologica* **173**, 513–524.

Wilson, D. J. & Green, W. R. (1987) Histopathologic study of the effect of retinal detachment surgery on 49 eyes obtained post mortem. *American Journal of Ophthalmology* **103**, 167–179.

Wilson, W. A. & Irvine, S. R. (1955) Pathologic changes following disruption of the blood supply to iris and ciliary body. *Transactions of the American Academy of Ophthalmology and Otolaryngology* **55**, 501–502.

Keratoplasty

Abbott, R. L. & Forster, R. K. (1979) Determinants of graft clarity. *Archives of Ophthalmology* **97**, 1071–1075.

Batchelor, J. R., Casey, T. A., Gibbs, D. C., LLoyd, D. F., Webb, A., Prasad, S. S. & James, A. (1976) HLA matching and corneal grafting. *Lancet* **i**, 551–562.

Bourne, W. M., Lindstrom, R. L. & Doughman, D. J. (1985) Endothelial cell survival on transplanted human corneas preserved by organ culture with 1.35% chondroitin sulphate. *American Journal of Ophthalmology* **100**, 789–793.

Ehlers, N. & Kissmeyer-Nielsen, F. (1979) Corneal transplantation and HLA compatibility. A preliminary communication. *Acta Ophthalmologica* **57**, 738–741.

Chandler, J. W. (1982) Symposium: pathophysiology of graft failure. Immunology — new approaches. *Cornea* **1**, 281–286.

Foster, C. S. & Allansmith, M. R. (1979) Lack of blood group antigen A on human corneal endothelium. In *Immunopathology and Immunology of the Eye*, eds A. M. Silverstein & M. R. Allansmith, pp 151–156. Masson, New York, 1979.

Fujikawa, L. S., Colvin, R. B., Bhan, A. K., Fuller, T. C. & Foster, C. S. (1982) Expression of HLA-A/B/C and -DR locus antigens on epithelial, stromal, and endothelial cells of the human cornea. *Cornea* **1**, 213–222.

Gorovoy, M. S., Stern, G. A., Hood, C. I. & Allen, C. (1983) Intrastromal noninflammatory bacterial colonisation of a corneal graft. *Archives of Ophthalmology* **101**, 1749–1752.

Hales, R. H. & Spencer, W. H. (1963) Unsuccessful penetrating keratoplasties. *Archives of Ophthalmology* **70**, 805–810.

Harbour, R. C. & Stern, G. A. (1983) Variables in McCarey–Kaufman corneal storage. Their effect on corneal graft success. *Ophthalmology* **90**, 136–142.

Jenkin, M.S., Lempert, S. L. & Brown S. I. (1979) Significance of donor age in penetrating keratoplasty. *Annals of Ophthalmology* **11**, 974–976.

Klareskog, L., Forsum, U., Tjernlund, U. M., Rask, L. & Peterson, P. A. (1979) Expression of Ia antigen-like molecules on cells in the corneal epithelium. *Investigative Ophthalmology and visual science* **18**, 310–313.

Kurz, G. H. & D'Amico, R.A. (1968) Histopathology of corneal graft failures. *American Journal of Ophthalmology* **66**, 184–199.

Lindstrom, R. L., Doughman, D. J., Skelnik, D. L. & Mindrup, E. A. (1986) Minnesota system of corneal preservation. *British Journal of Ophthalmology* **70**, 47–54.

Lang, G. K., Greene, W. R. & Maumenee, A. E. (1986) Clinicopathologic studies of keratoplasty eyes obtained post mortem. *American Journal of Ophthalmology* **101**, 28–40.

Meisler, D. M., Langston, R. H. S., Aaby, A. A., Stern, G. S., Binder, P. S. (1984) Infectious corneal crystalline formation. *Investigative Ophthalmology and Visual Science* **23**, Suppl. 25.

Meisler, D. M., Langston, R. H. S., Naab, T. J., Aaby A. A., McMahon, J. T. & Tubbs, R. R. (1984) Infectious cystalline keratopathy. *American Journal of Ophthalmology* **97**, 337–343.

Morrison, J. C. & Swan, K. C. (1982) Bowman's layer in penetrating keratoplasties of the human eye. *Archives of Ophthalmology* **100**, 1835–1838.

Morrison, J. C. & Swan, K. C. (1983) Desçemet's membrane in penetrating keratoplasties of the human eye. *Archives of Ophthalmology* **101**, 1927–1929.

Ozdemir, O. (1986) A prospective study of histocompatibility testing for keratoplasty in high-risk patients. *British Journal of Ophthalmology* **70**, 183–186.

Polack, F. M. (1977) *Corneal Transplantation*. Grune & Stratton, New York.

Strak, W. J., Taylor, H. R., Bias, W. B. & Maumenee, A. E. (1978) Histocompatibilty (HLA) antigens and keratoplasty. *American Journal of Ophthalmology* **86**, 595–604.

Streilin, J. W. & Kaplan, H. J. (1979) Immunologic privilege in the anterior chamber. In *Immunology and Immunopathology of the Eye*, eds A. M. Silverstein & H. J. Kaplan, pp 174–179. Masson, New York.

Streilin, J. W., Toews, G. B. & Bergstresser, P. R. (1979) Corneal allografts fail to express Ia antigens. *Nature* **282**, 326–327.

Taylor, M. J. & Hunt, C. J. (1985) A new preservation solution for storage of corneas at low temperatures. *Current Eye Research* **4**, 963–973.

Van Horn, D. L. & Schultz, R. O. (1977) Corneal preservation: recent advances. *Survey of Ophthalmology* **21**, 301–312.

Vannas, S. (1975) Histocompatibility in corneal grafting. *Investigative Ophthalmology* **14**, 863–886.

Watson, A. P., Tullo, A. B., Kerr-Muir, M., Ridgway, A. E. A. & Lucas, D. R. (1988) Arborescent bacterial keratopathy (infectious crystalline keratopathy). **Eye** (in press).

Yau, C-W. & Kaufman, H. E. (1986) A medium-term corneal preserving medium (K-Sol). *Archives of Ophthalmology* **104**, 598–601.

Zakov, Z. N., Dohlman, C. H., Perry, H. D. & Albert, D. M. (1978) Corneal donor material selection. *American Journal of Ophthalmology* **86**, 605–610.

Appendix I Examining eye sections

This scheme is based on a handout provided for postgraduate students attending the Manchester FRCS course and is intended to encourage a systematic approach which will ensure that no important pathological changes are overlooked.

Preliminary survey

Establish:

- Size
- Relative proportions of chambers
- Local lesion or diffuse changes

Preliminary categorisation

On the basis of the preliminary survey most eyes can be placed in one of the following categories:

- Tumour present
- End-stage glaucoma
- Old retinal detachment
- Inflammatory condition
- Phthisis bulbi
- Malformation

Tumour present

- Is it primary or secondary?
- Secondary carcinomata occasionally resemble melanomata, but mitotic figures are nearly always more numerous in anaplastic carcinomata than in melanomata. Intracellular pigment should be sought (Masson–Fontana stain)
- Secondary oat-cell carcinoma of lung can simulate retinoblastoma, but is more likely to appear as an examination trap than a diagnostic problem.

Primary tumours

Establish the features listed:

Melanoma

- Size and location
- Predominant cell type
- Mitotic activity
- Degree of pigmentation
- Scleral invasion
- Extrascleral extension
- Presence of necrosis
- Vascular invasion
- Reticulin content (if available)
- Evidence of surgery or other treatment

Retinoblastoma

- Size and location
- Differentiation
- Mitotic activity
- Choroidal invasion
- Invasion of optic nerve
- Vascular staining

Secondary tumours

Carcinoma

- Cell type
- Mitotic activity
- Differentiation, e.g. adenoid, squamous
- Mucus secretion (PAS or mucin stains)
- Think of lung, breast, GI tract and kidney

Others

- All rare, deposits of malignant lymphoma and leukaemic cells occasionally occur

Inflammatory conditions

Establish the following:

- Acute or chronic
- Localisation (anterior, posterior, both, etc.)
- Granulomatous or non-granulomatous or both
- Micro-organisms present (demonstration may require special stains, e.g. Gram, Grocott–Gomori, Ziehl–Neelsen)

Systematic survey

Even if a diagnosis has been made, the eye should be examined systematically looking particularly at the structures listed and for changes which may affect them.

APPENDIX I

Cornea

- Epithelium:

Number of rows of cells, presence of bullae or sub-epithelial pannus (especially at periphery)
- Bowman's membrane:

Evidence of breaks, band keratopathy, etc.
- Stroma:

Thickness (oedema)
Scarring
Vessels
Abnormal deposits (dystrophies)
- Desçemet's membrane (breaks, thickening, excrescences)
- Endothelium (density of cell population, adherent cells, etc.)

Anterior chamber

- Shape and depth
- Adhesions
- Presence of plasmoid aqueous
- Cells, blood, foreign matter

Iris and ciliary body

- Configuration of ciliary muscle (gross refractive errors, congenital glaucoma, post-contusion angle deformity)
- Drainage angle open or closed?
- Meshwork (cells, pigment, etc.)
- Iris (new vessels, atrophy, necrosis, condition of sphincter and dilator muscles)
- Ciliary epithelium (evidence of cryotherapy or diathermy, deposits of pseudoexfoliative debris)

Lens

- Integrity of capsule
- Deposits of pseudoexfoliative debris
- Epithelium intact (presence of subcapsular fibrosis)
- Nuclear bow
- Condition of fibres (evidence of cataract)
- Presence of nuclei along posterior capsule

Retina

- Detachment present, is it genuine or factitious?
- Ganglion cells normal or reduced in number (evidence of glaucoma)
- Visual cells normal or reduced in number
- Condition of retinal vessels (sclerotic changes in post-thrombotic neovascular glaucoma)
- Presence of exudates or haemorrhage
- Pigmented epithelium (proliferative changes, etc.)

Optic nerve

- Cupping
- Atrophy
- Condition of vessels
- Presence of new vessels at margins of nerve head

Choroid

- Bruchs' membrane and choriocapillaris (drüsen, deposits, breaks, etc.)
- Choroidal vessels (atheroma, thrombi)

Appendix II Connective tissue fibres: types of collagen

• A collagen molecule is composed of three polypeptide chains (α-chains) coiled around one another in helical fashion
• Pro-α-chains are polypeptides synthesised within the cell. They have N and C extension peptides which do not assume a helical form
• Pro-collagen is a soluble precursor synthesised within the cell from the pro-α-chains
• Tropocollagen is formed outside the cell by removal of the N and C extension peptidases
• A unit microfibril comprises five collagen molecules staggered with respect to each other by a quarter length. This arrangement gives rise to the regular 64 nm banding of collagen fibres

Table 1 Types of collagen. Reproduced with permission from Catto, 1985.

Type	Molecular form	Tissue
I	Two chains α1 (I)2 One chain α2 (I)	Cornea (dermis, tendon, bone, etc.)
II	Three chains α1 (II)3	Cornea, vitreous, retina (cartilage, intervertebral discs)
III	Three chains α1 (III)3	Cornea, sclera, uvea (blood vessels, lung, liver — takes silver stain as reticulin)
IV	Three chain α1 (IV)3	Basement membranes, not fibrillar, not banded by electron microscopy
V	Two chains α1 (V)2 One chain α1 (V)	Interstitial tissue, basement membranes

• A collagen fibre consists of a variable number of longitudinally arranged microfibrils. The tensile strength depends on co-valent intermolecular cross links
• A number of different, although very similar, α-chains have been identified and there are at least five different types of collagen (Table 1)

Elastic fibres

Elastic fibres are composed of protein and elastin and may be found singly or in sheets, as in arteries. Such sheets have fenestrae and resemble 'expanded metal'. Elastin is amorphous under the electron microscope. It is highly refractile in tissue sctions and may be demonstrated by special stains (Appendix 4). Elastic fibres are normally present in sclera, but not in healthy cornea.

Oxytalan fibres

Oxytalan fibres are filaments 15–20 nm in diameter interspersed with amorphous material. They are digested by elastase only after oxidation.

Bibliography

Bancroft, J. D. & Stevens, A., eds (1982) *Theory and Practice of Histological Techniques*. Churchill Livingstone, New York.

Catto, M. E., (1985) In *Muir's Textbook of Pathology*, 12th Edn, ed. Anderson, J. R., pp 5.1–5.26. Arnold, London.

Lindberg, K. A. & Pinnell, S. R. (1982). In *Pathobiology of Ocular Disease*, vol. 2, ed. Garner, A. & Klintworth, G. K. Dekker, New York.

Appendix III Glycoconjugates

R. W. STODDART

Glycoconjugates are complex molecules in which a sugar is covalently linked to a non-carbohydrate moiety. The two major classes are glycolipids and glycoproteins.

Glycolipids

A class of glycoconjugates in which sugar is linked to lipid. *Glycosphingolipids* form the largest group and, of these, the *glucosphingolipids* are the most common. In glycosphingolipids, galactose or glucose are linked directly to sphingosine or a derivative by a glycosidic bond. The glycosphingolipids are common components of cell surfaces and some intracellular membranes. They are assembled in the Golgi apparatus. The other glycolipids include *glycoglycerolipids* and *glycosylated phosphoinositides*. The latter can anchor heparan sulphate to cell surfaces.

Glycoproteins

A class of glycoconjugate in which carbohydrate is attached to polypeptide by one or more covalent links. Because a simple polypeptide may be linked to several different saccharides, classification is of individual glycopeptides rather than of entire glycoproteins. The *carbohydrate moieties* fall into two general categories:

Oligosaccharides: exhibit non-repeating saccharide sequences of usually fewer than 20 sugar residues. May be branched.

Glycosaminoglycans: exhibit highly repetitive linear saccharide sequences (mucopolysaccharides in old terminology).

The division between glycoprotein oligosaccharides and glycosaminoglycans is not precise. For example, *keratan sulphate* (a repeating polymer of galactose and *N*-acetyl glucosamine) may be regarded as either. Glycoproteins rich in glycosaminoglycans are often referred to as '*proteoglycans*' (not to be confused with 'peptidoglycan' found on bacterial surfaces).

1 *Galactosaminoglycans:* are linear polymers based on a repeating disaccharide sequence which includes *N*-acetyl galactosamine and glucuronic acid (or iduronic acid). They are widely distributed in extracellular matrices and include the chondroitin sulphates and dermatan sulphate.

2 *Glucosaminoglycans:* are linear polymers, but differ from galactosaminoglycans in tending to be more extensively altered after assembly and so come to have non-repetitive disaccharide sequences. The original disaccharide contains *N*-acetyl glucosamine and glucuronic acid. They include heparin and heparan sulphate.

The *glycopeptides* of glycoproteins are classified according to nature of the link between carbohydrate and protein:

(i) *N-linked saccharides:* the sugar is linked via the N atom of the side-arm of asparagine. They occur widely in plants, animals and fungi and share a common core structure. Their synthesis is complicated and begins in the rough endoplasmic reticulum and is continued in the Golgi apparatus. Several types are recognised, among which are:

(a) *High mannose saccharides:* characterised by five to nine α-mannosyl residues at their non-reducing terminals. Phosphorylated forms are common in lysosomal glycoproteins.

(b) *Complex saccharides:* these common forms lack alpha mannosyl terminals and have 'outer chains' attached to the 'core'. There is enormous potential for variation through variation (1) in the number and length of the outer chains, which may be repeating or non-repeating; and (2) in sugar sequences and, hence, in content of helical structure in the outer chains.

(ii) *O-linked saccharides of the mucin type:* are characterised by the presence of a glycoside linkage between α-*N*-acteyl galactosamine and the side chain oxygen atom of serine or threonine. They vary greatly in molecular size and in their content of repeating structures. Some can carry blood group antigens. They are widespread at cell surfaces and in secretory glycoproteins and are synthesised in the Golgi apparatus.

(iii) *O-linked saccharides of the collagen type:* collagen and related glycoproteins such as C1q are characterised by a distinctive type of linkage between galactose and the hydroxyl group of hydroxyproline.

In Type 1 collagen the α1(I) chains have a single disaccharide, while the α2 chains have a monosaccharide and a disaccharide.

(iv) *O-linked saccharides of glycosaminoglycan type:* chondroitin sulphate, dermatan sulphate and heparan sulphate are linked to protein by a distinctive O-linked sequence in which the side chain oxygen atom of serine or threonine is linked to a residue of xylose and thence through two galactosyl residues, to glucuronic acid. It is formed in the Golgi apparatus. Keratan sulphate is not associated with this linkage.

Some saccharides important in the eye

1 Keratan sulphate is a linear polymer based on the re-

peating disaccharide −3 Gal β1, 4 Glc*N*Ac β1-. It differs from most glycosaminoglycans in its linkage sequence and lack of uronic acid and is better regarded as a rather specialised glycoprotein oligosaccharide (q.v.). Each *N*-acetyl glucosamine carries a sulphate ester group attached to the hydroxyl group on C6 'over-sulphated' forms occur in the cornea. Small amounts of other sugars may be present and blood group activity is often expressed.

Cornea contains Type 1 keratan sulphate in which attachment to protein is via an N-linked saccharide. Type 2 keratan sulphate is O-linked via a mucin-type linkage.

2 Chondroitin sulphates: these are a family of galactosaminoglycans in which the disaccharide is modified by sulphation, predominantly of the hydroxyl groups and C4 and C6 of the residues of *N*-acetylgalactosamine. 'Over-sulphated' forms occur. Chondroitin 4-sulphate is the precursor of dermatan sulphate and segments of the polymer chain may be converted to it.

Cornea contains chondroitin sulphate where it probably subserves the same function as keratan sulphate under conditions of oxygen lack (Scott & Haigh, 1988).

3 Dermatan sulphate resembles chondroitin sulphate, but the configuration at C5 of the glucuronosyl residue is reversed after assembly, thus making it an iduronosyl residue.

4 Heparin is a glucosaminoglycan comprising a chain of about 200 repeating disaccharide units. It contains more *N*-sulphate and iduronic acid than in heparan sulphate. It often occurs as the free glucosaminoglycan and is found in connective tissue type mast cells. Some molecules exhibit binding sites for anti-thrombin III and low density lipoprotein.

5 Heparan sulphate is a smaller molecule than heparin (40−80 disaccharide units) and less homogeneous. As a results of modification after polymerisation, its sequences are very variable. It contains less *N*-sulphate and iduronic acid. It is found in extracellular matrices including basement membranes and on the surface of most types of cells. In these locations, it is usually present as proteoglycan rather than free glucosaminoglycan.

6 Hyaluronic acid is a family of montonous linear polymers of disaccharides based on the saccharide −3 *N*-acetyl glucosamine β1, 4 glucuronic acid β1-. The chain length is variable, but normally very long. The molecule has a capacity for self-aggregation which makes accurate determination of the molecular weight difficult. In the vitreous body, the molecules probably contain in excess of 3000 disaccharide units.

Hyaluronic acid is almost entirely extracellular and associated with matrices. There is no evidence of its covalent linkage to protein or lipid. It differs from other mammalian oligo- and polysaccharides in that the molecule grows at the reducing terminal and synthesis is at the cell surface and not in the Golgi apparatus.

Demonstration in tissues

Lectin-binding is now widely used to identify the oligosaccharides of glycoproteins and glycolipids. Lectins are proteins which bind in a chemically specific way to particular oligsaccharides and do so by at least two binding sites. They are of universal occurrence, though most of those used histochemically come from plants. Some lectins bind via terminal sugars and others to internal sugar sequences. They are used in a similar manner to monoclonal antibodies.

Few lectins are known which bind specifically to glycosaminoglycans, but these can be demonstrated in tissues by such methods as the periodic acid−Schiff reaction (Appendix IV).

Bibliography

Horowitz, M. I. & Pigman (1977−78) W. *The Glycoconjugates*, vols 1 & 2. Academic Press, New York.

Lennarz, W. J. (1980) *The Biochemistry of Glycoproteins and Proteoglycans*. Plenum Press, New York.

Scott, J. E. & Haigh, M. (1988) *Journal of Anatomy* **158**, 95−108.

Stoddart, R. W. (1985) *The Biosynthesis of Polysaccharides*. Croom Helm, London.

Appendix IV Common special staining reactions

1 *Periodic acid–Schiff (PAS) reaction:* in this reaction, periodic acid oxidises 1,2 diols to dialdehydes which give a coloured product with an appropriate chromogen such as bleached *p*-rosaniline. Flexible diols, e.g. in sialic acid are attacked first. Many glycolipids and glycoproteins are thus stained, especially those found in mucins and basement membranes. Connective tissue glycosaminoglycans such as chondroitin sulphate, hyaluronic acid and heparan sulphate, which contain uronic acid, react after prolonged oxidation, but keratan sulphate does not. The PAS stain is excellent for microanatomical purposes and was used extensively for illustrating this book. Contrast is improved by the use of tartrazine as a counterstain.

2 *Grocott–Gomori reaction:* chromate oxidises more than 1,2 diols and so will affect 1,3 linked sugars which are unaffected by periodic acid. The reaction product is demonstrated with methenamine silver. The method is mainly useful for demonstrating basement membranes and fungal cell walls which have a high content of carbohydrate, much of it often 1,3 linked.

3 *Basic dyes* such as alcian blue, toluidine blue, safranin and methyl green interact with the acidic groups of saccharides of the glycosaminoglycan group. The pH or salt concentration at which the reaction takes place can be adjusted to differentiate between acidic groups such as carboxyl or sulphate. Metachromasia, a distinct colour change, can occur when dye molecules bind so closely that they interact with each other.

4 *Trichrome stains:* these were originally introduced to demonstrate selectively collagen, muscle, fibrin. The selectivity is believed to depend on the relative pore size of the fixed tissue components and the molecular size of the various anionic dyes used. The section is first exposed to a dye of small molecular size such as acid fuchsin or ponceau 2 R. This is displaced from the collagen by treatment with phosphomolybdic or phosphotungstic acid and the latter then stained by a dye of large molecular size such as light green or aniline blue. The nuclei are usually stained with an iron haematoxylin.

5 *Reticulin fibres (Type 3 collagen):* these fibres have an affinity for certain metals and the silver impregnation is useful for demonstrating them. They are found in the trabecular meshwork, in basement membranes and the walls of blood vessels. They are also laid down in the stroma of malignant melanomata.

6 *Elastic fibres:* numerous methods have been described for demonstrating elastic fibres. The mechanism of the staining is not known for certain. Of the methods in use, the most popular are:

- Verhoeff's method using haematoxylin with ferric chloride and iodine
- Orcein
- Weigert's resorcin fuchsin (or numerous modifications)
- Alehyde fuchsin

7 *Melanin* has the ability to reduce ammoniacal silver nitrate to metallic silver and melanin granules are blackened and thus rendered more easily visible. This is exploited in the Masson–Fontana method. Some lipofuscins, argentaffin and chromaffin granules are also stained by this method.

8 *Ferric iron* may be detached from protein by dilute hydrochloric acid and precipitated as ferric ferrocyanide (Prussian blue) by treatment with potassium ferrocyanide. This is the basis of Perls' reaction.

9 *Amyloid* has an affinity for certain dyes such as Congo red and the related Sirius red which is believed to depend on the linearity of the dye molecule and the very regular beta-pleated sheet configuration of amyloid. The almost crystalline regularity of the dye precipitation leads to its showing different absorption maxima in different planes in polarised light and hence the characteristic green dichroism.

10 *Bacteria:* the well-known Gram's stain for bacteria can be applied to tissue sections. The method employs crystal violet with neutral red as a counterstain. Some fungi and actinomycetes are also well stained by Gram's method.

Mycobacteria have a lipid capsule which makes them resistant to staining by Gram's method, but they may be stained by hot carbol-fuchsin. Once stained, they resist decolourisation by acid alcohol. This is the basis of the Ziehl–Neelsen reaction. *Mycobacterium leprae* is less resistant to acid alcohol than *M. tuberculosis* and the standard method is modified to take account of this.

Bibliography

Bancroft, J. D. & Stevens, A. eds (1982) *The Theory and Practice of Histological Techniques*. Churchill Livingstone, Edinburgh. New York.

General bibliography

Albert, D. M. & Puliafilo, C. A. (1979) *Foundations of Ophthalmic Pathology*. Appleton-Century-Crofts, New York. (Reprints of classic papers.)

Apple, D. J. & Rabb, M. F. (1985) *Ocular Pathology. Clinical Applications and Self-Assessment*, 3rd edn. C. V. Mosby Co., St Louis.

Boniuk, M., ed. (1964) *Ocular and Adnexal Tumours, New and Controversial Aspects*. C. V. Mosby Co., St Louis.

Fine, B. S. & Yanoff, M. (1979) *Ocular Histology, A Text and Atlas*, 2nd edn. Harper & Row, Hagerstown.

Garner, A. & Klintworth, G. K. (1982) *Pathobiology of Ocular Disease. A Dynamic Approach*, Parts A & B. Dekker, New York.

Jakobiec, F. A., ed. (1978) *Ocular and Adnexal Tumours*. Aesculapius, Birmingham, Ala.

Jensen, O. A. (1986) *Human Ophthalmic Pathology*. Munksgaard, Copenhagen.

Naumann, G. O. H. & Rabb, D. J. (1986) *Pathology of the Eye*. Springer Verlag, New York. (Translation and update of *Pathologie des Auges*, by G. O. H. Naumann, 1980.) Springer Verlag, Berlin.)

Nicholson, D. H., ed. (1980) *Ocular Pathology Update*. Masson, New York.

Rahi, A. H. S. & Garner, A. (1976) *Immunopathology of the Eye*. Blackwell Scientific Publications, Oxford.

Reese, A. B., ed. (1976) *Tumours of the Eye*, 3rd Edn. Harper & Row, Hagerstown.

Silverstein, A. M. & O'Connor, G. R., eds (1979) *Immunology and Immunopathology of the Eye*. Masson, New York.

Spencer, W. H., ed. (1985–6) *Ophthalmic Pathology. An Atlas and Text*, vols 1–3, 3rd Edn. W. B. Saunders Co., Philadelphia.

Yanoff, M. & Fine B. S. (1982) *Ocular Pathology. A Text and Atlas*, 2nd edn. Harper & Row.

Zimmerman, L. E. & Sobin, L. H. (1980) *Histological Typing of Tumours of the Eye and its Adnexa*. International Histological Classification of Tumours No. 24, World Health Organisation, Geneva.

Index

INDEX

Sunlight exposure
  cataracts and 145, 146
  retinal damage and 166

QUEEN ELIZABETH HOSPITAL
KINGS LYNN
KL01355

King's Lynn & Wisbech Hospitals
NHS Trust

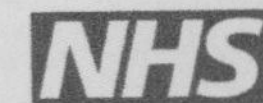

Library/Knowledge Services
The Queen Elizabeth Hospital
King's Lynn
Tel: 01553-613613 – ext. 2827
for renewal

Due for return:

- 6 MAY 2003